Unit Conversion Factors and Useful Constants and Equations

Unit conversion:

Length	1 ft = 12 in. = 30.48 cm = 0.3048 m
	1 cm = 0.394 in. = 0.03280 ft
Volume	1 L = 1000 cm^3 (cc) = 0.001 m^3
	1 ft^3 = 0.028317 m^3
Pressure	1 mmHg = 133.3 N/m^2 = 1333 dyn/cm^2
	1 atm = 14.696 lb/in.^{2} = 760 mmHg
Power	1 hp = 550 ft lb/s = 745.7 W
Density	1 lb_m/ft^3 = 16.018 kg/m^3 = 0.016018 g/cm^3
Viscosity	1 centi Poise (cP) = 10^{-2} Poise (P)
	1 P = 1 dyn s/cm^2 = 1 g/(cm s) = 0.1 N s/m^2 = 0.1 Pa s

Fluid parameters:

Density (ρ): ρ_{water} = 999 $kg/m^3 \approx 1\ g/cm^3$

ρ_{air} = 1.22 kg/m^3 at standard atmospheric temperature and pressure

$\rho_{wholeblood}$ = 1060 kg/m^3 = 1.06 g/cm^3; ρ_{plasm} = 1035 kg/m^3 = 1.035 g/cm^3

Viscosity (μ): μ_{water} = 1.0 cP

μ_{plasma} = 1.2 cP; $\mu_{wholeblood}$ = 3.5 cP at shear rates >100 s^{-1}

Fluid mechanics governing equations:

Fluid constitutive laws:

Newtonian fluid: $\tau = \mu \dfrac{\partial u}{\partial y}$

Casson fluid: $\sqrt{\tau} = \sqrt{\tau_y} + k_c\sqrt{\dot{\gamma}}$

Power law:

$$\tau = K_{pl}\dot{\gamma}^n \quad n \neq 1$$

Equations of motion (incompressible, Newtonian fluid):

Conservation of mass (continuity equation): $\nabla \cdot \vec{V} = 0$

Conservation of momentum: $\frac{\partial \vec{V}}{\partial t} + (\vec{V} \cdot \nabla)\vec{V} = -\frac{1}{\rho}\nabla p + \vec{g} + \frac{\mu}{\rho}\nabla^2 \vec{V}$

Hydrostatics: $\Delta p = \rho g h$

One-dimensional flow:

Conservation of mass: incompressible fluid (ρ = constant): $\bar{V}_1 A_1 = \bar{V}_2 A_2$

Bernoulli equation (conservation of energy)—steady flow—inviscid fluid:

$$p + \frac{\rho V^2}{2} + \rho g h = H(Const.)$$

Poiseuille equation: fully developed steady flow—Newtonian fluid:

$$V_z(r) = \left[\frac{\Delta p R^2}{4\mu L}\right]\left[1 - \left(\frac{r}{R}\right)^2\right] = V_{max}\left[1 - \left(\frac{r}{R}\right)^2\right]$$

$$Q = \frac{\pi \Delta p R^4}{8\mu L} = \frac{\pi \Delta p d^4}{128\mu L}$$

Wall shear stress in cylindrical tube: $\tau_w = -\frac{d}{4}\frac{\Delta p}{L}$

Poiseuille flow wall shear stress: $|\tau_w| = \frac{4\mu Q}{\pi R^3}$

Reynolds number: $Re = \frac{\rho V d}{\mu}$

Entry length: $L_e = 0.06 \cdot d \cdot Re$ for laminar flow

Womersley parameter for pulsatile flow: $\alpha = \frac{d}{2}\sqrt{\frac{\rho\omega}{\mu}}$

SECOND EDITION

Biofluid Mechanics

THE HUMAN CIRCULATION

SECOND EDITION

Biofluid Mechanics

THE HUMAN CIRCULATION

Krishnan B. Chandran
Stanley E. Rittgers
Ajit P. Yoganathan

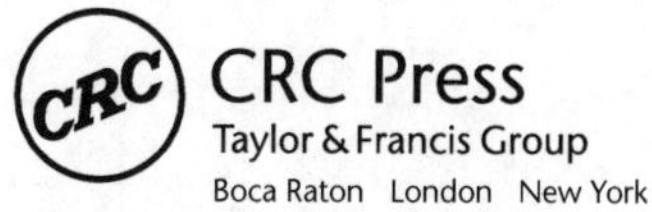

CRC Press is an imprint of the
Taylor & Francis Group, an **informa** business

CRC Press
Taylor & Francis Group
6000 Broken Sound Parkway NW, Suite 300
Boca Raton, FL 33487-2742

Printed in the United States of America on acid-free paper
Version Date: 20111222

International Standard Book Number: 978-1-4398-4516-5 (Hardback)

Library of Congress Cataloging-in-Publication Data

Chandran, K. B.
Biofluid mechanics : the human circulation / Krishnan B. Chandran, Ajit P. Yoganathan, Stanley E. Rittgers. -- 2nd ed.
p. ; cm.
Includes bibliographical references and index.
ISBN 978-1-4398-4516-5 (hardcover : alk. paper)
I. Yoganathan, A. P. (Ajit Prithiviraj), 1951- II. Rittgers, Stanley E., 1947- III. Title.
[DNLM: 1. Blood Circulation--physiology. 2. Cardiovascular Physiological Phenomena. 3. Heart Valves--physiology. WG 103]

612.1'181--dc23 2011051920

Visit the Taylor & Francis Web site at
http://www.taylorandfrancis.com

and the CRC Press Web site at
http://www.crcpress.com

To Vanaja, Aruna and Kelly, and Anjana and Jaime, for their loving support.

Krishnan B. Chandran

To my wife, Eva, and sons, David and Andrew, who have taught me so much.

Stanley E. Rittgers

To my wife, Tripti, and my children, Anila and Anant, for their love, encouragement, and support.

Ajit P. Yoganathan

Contents

PART I Fluid and Solid Mechanics and Cardiovascular Physiology

PART II Biomechanics of the Human Circulation

PART III Cardiovascular Implants, Biomechanical Measurements, and Computational Simulations

Preface

The field of biomedical engineering has seen rapid growth in the last two decades, and numerous new undergraduate and graduate programs have been established in many universities. With the increasing number of students enrolled in these programs, there is also an increase in demand for suitable textbooks. This work is an attempt to provide such a textbook for a course in the application of fluid mechanics to the study of the human circulatory system. This book is intended as a first course on fluid mechanics in the human circulation, which is suitable for senior undergraduate or for first-year graduate students in biomedical engineering. The topics contained in the various chapters have been organized based on the experience that we gained in teaching courses on cardiovascular fluid mechanics in our respective programs.

The book is organized into three parts. Part I consists of introductory review material on fluid and solid mechanics as well as a review of cardiovascular physiology pertinent to the topics covered in the subsequent chapters. Chapters 1 and 2 introduce foundational material on fluid and solid mechanics for those students who have not had prior exposure to these topics. Likewise, Chapter 3 provides a general background on normal cardiovascular physiology as well as basic concepts of one of its primary diseases atherosclerosis. In curricula where students have previously enrolled in courses on fluid mechanics, mechanics of deformable bodies, and human physiology, Part I may serve as a brief review.

Part II deals with fluid mechanics in the human circulation, primarily applied to blood flow at the arterial level. Chapter 4 discusses the viscometry and the rheological behavior of human blood. The solid mechanics of the arterial wall subject to transmural pressure is also discussed briefly in this chapter since the interaction between blood and the arterial wall needs to be considered in unsteady flow simulation. The application of steady flow models to derive some useful diagnostic parameters such as vascular resistance and Gorlin's equations to describe time-averaged flow behavior past heart valves is treated in Chapter 5. Chapter 6 briefly describes the Windkessel model for unsteady flow followed by a detailed treatment of the Moens–Korteweg and Womersley models of pulsatile flow in the human circulation. The relationship between flow-induced stresses and the initiation and growth of atherosclerosis is also discussed with qualitative treatment of flow in curved vessels, branches, and bifurcations, as well as unsteady flow past stenoses and aneurysms. Chapter 7 deals with flow through native heart valves and cardiac chambers.

Part III deals with vascular implants and measurements in the cardiovascular system. Chapter 8 discusses in detail the design and fluid mechanical evaluation of artificial heart valves. Chapter 9 deals with the fluid mechanical alterations related to vascular graft and stent implants. Chapter 10 details the measurement of blood flow, pressure, velocity, and vascular impedance and concludes with discussions on sophisticated fluid mechanical measurements employed *in vitro* and *in vivo* to assess the complex time-dependent three-dimensional flow in the human circulation.

Chapter 11, which has been added since the first edition, describes in detail the various considerations and approaches involved in performing computational modeling of relevant cardiovascular diseases and therapies.

As a first course textbook for exposing students to fluid mechanics in the human circulation, only the heart and major arteries are considered while flow in other organ systems, such as the lungs, the kidneys, and the brain, or flow in the microcirculation is not included. The figures in this book have been selectively included from the publications of numerous eminent researchers in this field, and the captions include the sources from which the figures have been obtained with permission. Citations of these references, however, have not been included in the text so as not to distract the reader from the subject matter. These are, instead, listed as references at the end of each chapter. Students are also referred to leading journals that deal with relevant subject matter (e.g., the *Annals of Biomedical Engineering*; the *Journal of Biomechanical Engineering*; the *Journal of Biomechanics*; *Medical Engineering and Physics*; *Atherosclerosis*; *Circulation*; *Circulation Research*; the *Journal of Thoracic and Cardiovascular Surgery*; the *Journal of Cardiovascular Engineering and Technology*; and the *Annals of Thoracic Surgery*) and numerous other sources for current advances in the field.

We have made several modifications from the first edition to update and enhance the contents in order to reflect changes in the field of biofluid mechanics of the human circulation. We have extensively revised the book with updated material, improved figures, and additional examples in the text as well as in the problems at the end of each chapter (specifically Chapters 1, 2, 4, 5, 6, and 10). We have also added a new chapter (Chapter 11) on computational fluid dynamic (CFD) analysis of the human circulation in order to introduce the students to the rapid development in the application of computational simulations both in research and in the clinical arena.

We are indebted to numerous individuals who have helped in many ways toward the second edition of this book. Professors H. S. Udaykumar and Sarah Vigmostad of the University of Iowa helped in reviewing and providing material for the new chapter on CFD. Many thanks also go to Professor Raghavan of the University of Iowa who provided a number of problems that have been incorporated in the various chapters of the book and who also helped in numerous ways with the enhancement of several figures in the second edition. Vijay Govindarajan and Keshav Venkat Chivikula, graduate students in Professor Chandran's laboratory, were instrumental in the simulation results on Poiseuille flow and flow past stenoses and aneurysms presented in the new chapter on computational simulations.

We also appreciate the support of Michael Slaughter and Marsha Pronin of Taylor & Francis Group in working with us to complete this second edition.

List of Symbols

English

A	Cross-sectional area, amplitude (Chapter 6)
B_0	Main magnetic field strength (Chapter 10)
C	Compliance
C_i	Molar concentration of species i
c	Wave speed
D, d	Diameter
D_i	Diffusion coefficient (Chapter 3); distensibility (Chapter 6)
D_L	Diffusing capacity
E	Elastic modulus (Young's Modulus)
E_{inc}	Incremental elastic modulus
E_p	Pressure elastic modulus
E, F, G	Convective flux vectors (Chapter 11)
E_v, F_v, G_v	Viscous flux vectors (Chapter 11)
G	Shear modulus
g	Gravitational acceleration
H	Total head, total energy per unit volume, head loss
H, Hct	Hematocrit
J	Jacobian (Chapter 11)
J_υ	Bessel function of first kind and υth order
K	Consistency index
K_D	Solubility coefficient
K_s	Spring constant
k	Bulk modulus
ℓ_0	Initial length
ℓ	Instantaneous length
M_t'	Modulus (Chapter 6)
N_D	Dean number
N_i	Molar flux of species i
p	Hydrostatic pressure
p_s	Systolic pressure
p_d	Diastolic pressure
P, F	Axial load, force
Q	Flow rate; vector containing flow variables (Chapter 11)
R	Radius
r, θ, z; r, φ, z	Cylindrical coordinates
r, θ, φ	Spherical coordinates
Re	Reynolds number
R_s	Resistance—Eliminated the same four rows above
SA node	Sino atrial node

T	Torque, truncation error (Chapter 11)
u, v, w	Velocity components
V	Volume
V_0	Initial volume
x, y, z	Cartesian coordinates
Z	Impedance
Z_0	Characteristic impedance
1D (2D, 3D)	One-dimensional

Greek

α	Womersley parameter
γ	Shear strain
$\dot{\gamma}$	Rate of shear strain, velocity gradient
δ	Increment in length
ε	Normal strain (engineering strain)
ε_i	Phase angle (Chapter 6)
ε_t	True strain
$\dot{\varepsilon}$	Normal rate of strain
ξ, η, ζ	Generalized coordinates (Chapter 11)
η, ς, ξ	Tube wall displacements in the r, θ, z directions (Chapter 6)
ρ	Density
μ	Viscosity coefficient
μ_{app}	Apparent viscosity
μ_p	Plasma viscosity
ν	Poisson's ration (solid); kinematic viscosity (μ/ρ) in fluids
σ	Normal stress
σ_{ult}	Ultimate stress
σ_y	Yield stress
Γ	Diagonal matrix (Chapter 11)
τ	Shear stress
ω, Ω	Angular velocity

List of Abbreviations

AAA	Abdominal aortic aneurysm
ALE	Arbitrary Lagrangian-Eulerian (Chapter 11)
AV	Atrioventricular valve (Chapter 3)
AVF	Arteriovenous fistula
bpm	Beats per minute
CDFM	Color Doppler flow mapping
CFD	Computational fluid dynamics
CO	Cardiac output
CT	Computed tomography
CVP	Central venous pressure
CW	Continuous wave
CX	Circumflex coronary artery
DVT	Deep vein thrombosis
EC	Endothelial cell
ECG	Electrocardiogram
EDV	End diastolic volume
EF	Ejection fraction
EMF	Electromagnetic flow meter
e-PTFE	Expanded polytetrafluoroethylene (Teflon)
ESV	End systolic volume
FSI	Fluid–structure interaction
HDL	High-density lipoprotein
HR	Heart rate
IH	Intimal hyperplasia
IMA	Internal mammary artery
LAD	Left anterior descending coronary artery
LDA	Laser Doppler anemometry
LDL	Low-density lipoprotein
LDV	Laser Doppler velocimetry
MAP	Mean arterial pressure
MRI	Magnetic resonance imaging
PET	Polyethylene terephthalate (Dacron)
PIV	Particle image velocimetry
PRF	Pulse repetition frequency
PRU	Peripheral resistance unit
PTA	Percutaneous transluminal angioplasty
PTCA	Percutaneous transluminal coronary angioplasty
PTFE	Polytetrafluoroethylene (Teflon)
RF	Radio frequency
RMS	Root mean square
RV	Regurgitant volume

SG	Specific gravity
SMC	Smooth muscle cell
SV	Stroke volume
SVC, IVC	Superior, inferior vena cava
SVG	Saphenous vein graft
SVHD	Single ventricle heart defect
TEE	Trans-esophageal echocardiography
WSR	Wall shear rate
WSS	Wall shear stress
WSSG	Wall shear stress gradient
ZCC/ZCD	Zero-crossing counter/zero-crossing detector

Part I

Fluid and Solid Mechanics and Cardiovascular Physiology

1 Fundamentals of Fluid Mechanics

1.1 INTRODUCTION

Before considering the mechanics of biological fluids in the circulation, it is necessary to first consider some key definitions and specific properties. Once established, we will use these "pieces" to construct important laws and principles which are the foundation of fluid mechanics. To begin, we will define what we mean by a *fluid*. In general, a material can be characterized as a *fluid* if it deforms continuously under the action of a *shear stress* produced by a force that acts parallel to the line of motion. In other words, a fluid is a material that cannot *resist* the action of a shear stress. Conversely, a fluid at rest cannot *sustain* a shearing stress. For our applications, we will treat a fluid as a continuum (i.e., it is a homogeneous material) even though both liquids and gases are made up of individual molecules. On a macroscopic scale, however, fluid properties such as density, viscosity, and so on are reasonably considered to be continuous.

1.2 INTRINSIC FLUID PROPERTIES

The intrinsic properties of a fluid are considered to be its density, viscosity, compressibility, and surface tension. We will discuss and define each of these individually.

1.2.1 Density

Density, commonly denoted by the symbol, ρ, is defined as the mass of a fluid per unit volume and has units of [M/L^3]. In the meter/kilogram/second (MKS) system, this would be represented by (kg/m^3) or by (g/cm^3) in the centimeter/gram/second (CGS) system where $1\,g/cm^3 = 10^3\ kg/m^3$. Values of density for several common biofluids are

$\rho_{water} = 999\,kg/m^3$ at 15°C ($\approx 1\,g/cm^3$)
$\rho_{air} = 1.22\,kg/m^3$ at standard atmospheric temperature and pressure
$\rho_{whole\ blood} = 1060\,kg/m^3$ at 20°C (6% higher than water)

A related property of a fluid is its *specific gravity*, denoted as SG, which is defined as its density divided by the density of water at 4°C (a reference value that is quite repeatable). Thus, for whole blood at 20°C, $SG = 1.06$. The specific weight of a fluid, denoted as γ (not to be confused with $\dot{\gamma}$, the symbol for rate of shear), is the weight of a fluid per unit volume, or ρg. For blood at 20°C, $\gamma = 1.04 \times 10^4\ N/m^3$.

1.2.2 Viscosity

As we said earlier, a fluid is defined as a material that deforms under the action of a shear force. The *viscosity* of a fluid (or its "stickiness"), denoted by the symbol, μ, is related to the rate of deformation that a fluid experiences when a shear stress is applied to it. Just as with a solid, fluid shear stress is defined as shear force per unit area applied tangentially to a surface and is denoted by τ. To illustrate this, consider two parallel plates each of cross-sectional area A (cm^2) with fluid of viscosity μ between them as shown in Figure 1.1.

If a tangential force F_t is applied to the top plate as shown, it will result in the plate moving with a velocity U (cm/s) relative to the lower plate. The fluid adjacent to the top plate will move with the same velocity as that of the plate since the fluid is assumed to stick to the plate (known as the "no-slip" condition). Similarly, the fluid adjacent to the bottom plate will be at rest since it sticks to a stationary surface. Thus, a velocity gradient, or change in velocity per unit change in height, is produced within the fluid as shown. The shearing force F_t divided by the area, A, over which it acts is defined as the *shearing stress*, τ, having the units [$ML^{-1}T^{-2}$]. The velocity gradient, also referred to as the *rate of shear*, $\dot{\gamma}$, is the ratio U/h where h is the distance between the two parallel plates. Thus, the rate of shear has the dimension of s^{-1}. In general, the rate of shear is defined as $\partial u/\partial y$ where y is the distance perpendicular to the direction of shear as shown in the figure. The viscous properties of all fluids are defined by the relationship between the shear stress and the rate of shear over a range of shear rates.

The relationship between viscous shear stress, τ, viscosity, μ, and shear rate, $\partial u/\partial y$, for flow in the x-direction is given in Equation 1.1 with the derivative taken in the y-direction, perpendicular to the direction of flow:

$$\tau = \mu \frac{\partial u}{\partial y} \tag{1.1}$$

The coefficient in this relationship is known as the *dynamic viscosity* [$ML^{-1}T^{-1}$] and is usually expressed as either Pa·s (kg/m·s) in the MKS system or as Poise (g/cm·s) in the CGS system. In many biological applications, it is convenient to define a centiPoise (cP) where 1 cP = 0.01 P due to the relatively low values of this property. The constitutive relationship expressed in Equation 1.1 can be plotted in a shear stress

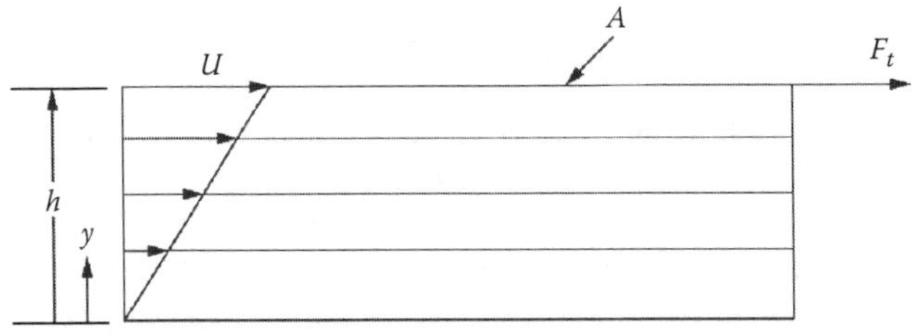

FIGURE 1.1 Fluid subjected to simple shearing stress.

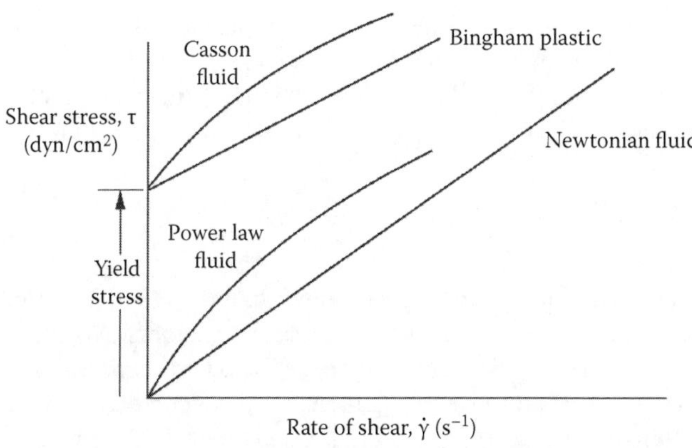

FIGURE 1.2 Shear stress versus rate of shear plots for Newtonian and non-Newtonian fluids.

versus rate of shear plot as shown in Figure 1.2. (*Note*: *Kinematic viscosity*, $\upsilon = \mu/\rho$, is commonly used to condense the density and viscosity into a single variable, especially for liquids where the density is relatively constant.)

A fluid in which the viscosity is *constant* is known as a *Newtonian* fluid and the relationship between viscous shear stress and shear rate is represented in the figure by a straight line passing through the origin with a slope equal to μ. In reality, many fluids do not follow this ideal linear relationship. Those fluids in which the shear stress is *not* directly proportional to the rate of shear are generally classified as *non-Newtonian* fluids. In this case, the ratio of shear stress to the rate of shear at any point of measurement is referred to as the *apparent viscosity*, μ_{app}. The apparent viscosity is not a constant but depends on the rate of shear at which it is measured. There are several classes of non-Newtonian fluids whose constitutive relationships are shown in Figure 1.2. For example, many fluids that exhibit a nonlinear relationship between shear stress and rate of shear and pass through the origin are expressed by the relationship

$$\tau = K_{pl}\dot{\gamma}^n \tag{1.2}$$

where $n \neq 1$. Such fluids are classified as *power law* fluids. Another class of fluids is known as *Bingham plastics* because they will initially resist deformation to an applied shear stress until the shear stress exceeds a *yield stress*, τ_y. Beyond that point, there will be a linear relationship between shear stress and rate of shear. The constitutive relationship for a Bingham plastic is given by

$$\tau = \tau_y + \mu_b\dot{\gamma} \tag{1.3}$$

where

τ_y is the yield stress
μ_b is the plastic viscosity

Fluids that exhibit a yield stress and also a nonlinear relationship between shear stress and rate of shear may be classified as *Casson fluids*. The specific empirical relationship for such fluids that deviate from the ideal Bingham plastic behavior is known as the Casson equation, or

$$\sqrt{\tau} = \sqrt{\tau_y} + k_c\sqrt{\dot{\gamma}} \tag{1.4}$$

As pointed out earlier, it is important in many biomedical applications to know the rheological characteristics of blood. In order to understand the relationship between the shear stress and the rate of shear for blood, experimental measurements are necessary. From those experiments, it has been determined that blood behaves as a Newtonian fluid only in regions of relatively high shear rate (>100 s^{-1}). Thus, for flow in large arteries where the shear rate is well above 100 s^{-1}, a value of 3.5 cP is often used as an estimate for the (assumed) constant viscosity of blood. In the microcirculation (i.e., small arteries and capillaries) and in veins where the shear rate is very low, blood must be treated as a non-Newtonian fluid (see Section 4.1.3).

The viscosity of a fluid is also strongly dependent upon its temperature. Generally, the viscosity of liquids decreases with increasing temperature, while the viscosity of gases increases with increasing temperature.

1.2.3 Compressibility

The *compressibility* of a fluid is quantified by the pressure change required to produce a certain increment in either the fluid's volume or density. This property, known as the *bulk modulus*, *k*, is defined as

$$k = \frac{\Delta p}{dV/V} = \frac{\Delta p}{d\rho/\rho} \tag{1.5}$$

Thus, for an incompressible fluid, $k = \infty$. For water, $k = 2.15 \times 10^9$ N/m^2, indicating that it is practically incompressible. Since the transmission of sound through a fluid such as air or water is simply the movement of pressure waves through the fluid, the speed of sound, *c*, depends on the fluid's bulk modulus and density as

$$c = \sqrt{k/\rho} \tag{1.6}$$

Thus, for water at 15°C,

$$c = (2.15 \times 10^9/999)^{0.5} = 1470 \text{ m/s}$$

The speed of sound in biological tissues and blood is used in various ultrasound modalities to obtain anatomic images and also blood flow velocities (see Section 10.6).

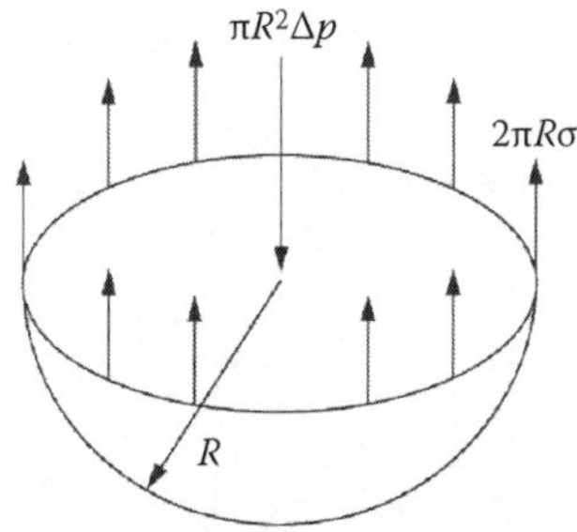

FIGURE 1.3 Pressure-surface tension force balance for a hemispherical drop.

1.2.4 Surface Tension

The surface layer between two different liquids behaves like a stretched membrane due to intermolecular forces. An expression can be found for the surface tension in a fluid, σ, by considering a hemispherical fluid drop of radius, R, as shown as follows (Figure 1.3).

Assuming static equilibrium between the pressure and surface forces and applying a force balance in the vertical direction,

$$2\pi R\sigma = \Delta p\pi R^2$$

and hence,

$$\sigma = \frac{R\Delta p}{2} \tag{1.7}$$

The effect of surface tension is particularly important in the pulmonary airways as it is what maintains the openings in the alveoli (the smallest regions of the lung where gas exchange occurs) and, thus, enables us to breath sufficient air in and out.

1.3 HYDROSTATICS

While most fluids in the body exist in a state of continuous motion, there are important effects on the fluid which are due to static forces. A fluid at rest in a gravitational field, for example, is in hydrostatic equilibrium as shown in Figure 1.4. Under these conditions, the weight of the fluid is exactly offset by the net pressure force supporting the fluid. Here, the pressure at the base of the fluid element is p while that at a distance dz above the base is p plus the gradient of pressure in the z-direction, dp/dz, times the incremental elevation, dz, where p is the gage pressure referenced to the atmospheric pressure, p_a (=1.01 × 10^5 N/m^2). Thus, if we sum the pressure and gravitational forces acting on the element in the vertical direction, we get

$$p\,dA - \left(p + \frac{dp}{dz}dz\right)dA - \rho g\,dA\,dz = 0 \tag{1.8}$$

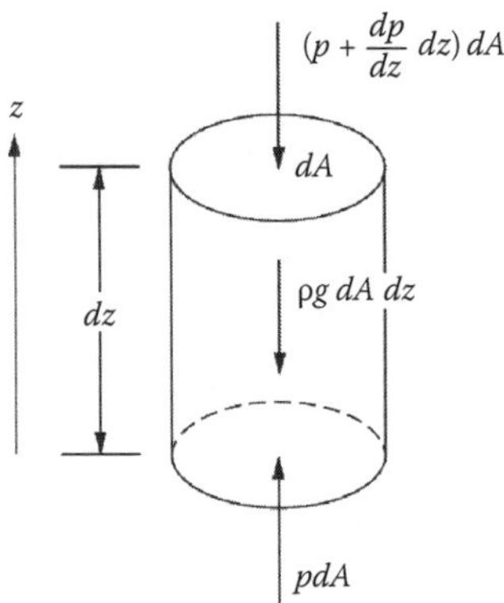

FIGURE 1.4 Hydrostatic equilibrium of a fluid element.

which requires that the pressure gradient be

$$\frac{dp}{dz} = -\rho g \tag{1.9}$$

where g is the gravitational acceleration. The negative sign for the pressure gradient indicates that p decreases as z increases. Integrating the previous equation between the base and the top of the element, z_1 and z_2, respectively, with corresponding pressures, p_1 and p_2, yields

$$\int_{p_1}^{p_2} dp = -\int_{z_1}^{z_2} \rho g\, dz \tag{1.10}$$

or

$$p_2 - p_1 = -\rho g (z_2 - z_1) \tag{1.11}$$

Thus,

$$\Delta p = \rho g h \tag{1.12}$$

for any element of height h. An equivalent expression would be $\Delta p = \gamma h$.

Example 1.1

For the case of a column of mercury where $\rho_{Hg} = 1.35 \times 10^4$ kg/m³, the pressure increase over a height of 1 mm would be

$$\begin{aligned}\Delta p &= 1.35 \times 10^4 (\text{kg/m}^3) \times 9.81 (\text{m/s}^2) \times 10^{-3} (\text{m}) \\ &= 133 \text{ N/m}^2 \\ &= 133 \text{ Pa}\end{aligned}$$

1.4 MACROSCOPIC BALANCES OF MASS AND MOMENTUM

The ultimate goal of fluid mechanics is to identify relationships between variables so that we can determine the value of one or more of these variables in terms of given conditions. In order to do this, we will begin with basic balances of properties or "conservation laws" which, in turn, involve multiple variables of interest. Initially, we will do so on a *macroscopic* basis where we consider the dynamics associated with a relatively large volume of fluid. Later, in Section 1.5, we will reevaluate these laws relative to an infinitesimal, or *microscopic* volume. By doing so, we will be able to determine relatively simple, gross parameters (i.e., flow rate, reaction forces, etc.) with the macroscopic approach but more complex, detailed parameters (i.e., local velocities, pressures, etc.) with the microscopic approach. Classically, the three properties of a fluid that are considered in this analysis are: mass, momentum, and energy. We will establish balances for each based upon the *Reynolds transport theorem*. This theorem relates the time rate of change of each of these properties in a *system* relative to corresponding changes that occur within and across a *control volume* and is given by

$$\frac{dB_{sys}}{dt} = \frac{\partial}{\partial t}\int_{CV} b\rho\, dV + \int_{CS} b\rho V\, dA \tag{1.13}$$

where

B denotes the extensive (i.e., absolute) property

b denotes the intrinsic property (i.e., the amount of that property per unit mass, or, $b = B/m$)

CV denotes the control volume

CS denotes the control surfaces of that volume

1.4.1 Conservation of Mass

The requirement, or "law," of conservation of mass applies to all materials and is thus the logical starting point for an introduction to fluid motion. To begin, we consider a conceptual three dimensional (3D) space or, *control volume*, which is enclosed by a surface across which fluid can move (Figure 1.5). This control volume is constant in size and location over time and does not necessarily coincide with any physical boundaries—that is, it is purely a tool for the analysis of physical systems. If we apply Equation 1.13 for the property mass, then the time rate of change of B_{sys} would be zero since mass of a system is constant by definition. Thus, the law of *conservation of mass* (also known as the "continuity equation") states that any change in mass within this control volume must be equal to the mass of fluid that enters the volume (mass in) minus the mass that exits (mass out). Therefore, for a given period of time, Δt,

$$\boxed{(\text{Rate of mass in}) - (\text{Rate of mass out}) = \text{Rate of change of mass within the tube}}$$

The rate of mass carried across a surface is equal to the density times the flow rate, ρQ, where Q is the volume flow rate, or $\rho V_n A$, and V_n is the component of velocity

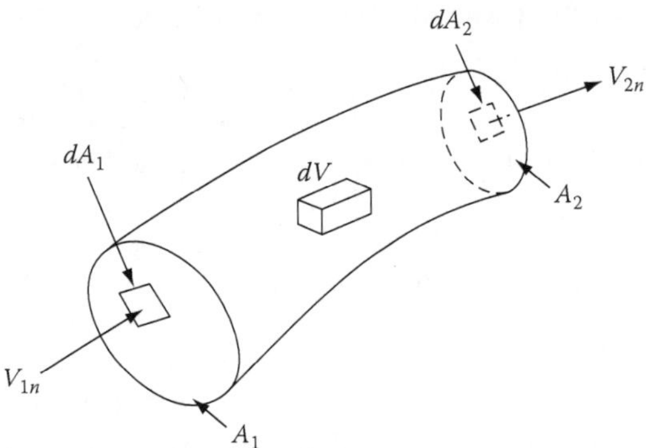

FIGURE 1.5 Mass flux balance for a stream tube.

normal to the cross section. Furthermore, the rate of change of mass within the tube is given by

$$\frac{\partial}{\partial t}\int_{CV} \rho \, dV$$

Thus, for the case shown in Figure 1.5,

$$\text{Rate of mass in} = \int_{A_1} \rho V_{1n} \, dA$$

and

$$\text{Rate of mass out} = \int_{A_2} \rho V_{2n} \, dA$$

where V_{1n} and V_{2n} are the velocities normal to the differential areas at cross sections 1 and 2, respectively.

Inserting these into the law of conservation of mass gives us

$$-\int_{A_2} \rho V_{2n} \, dA + \int_{A_1} \rho V_{1n} \, dA = \frac{\partial}{\partial t}\int_{V} \rho \, dV \tag{1.14}$$

For liquids in general and blood in particular, a very good assumption is that the fluid is incompressible—that is, its density, ρ, is constant. This, together with the fixed size of the control volume, causes the time rate of change of mass within the control volume to be zero. Furthermore, if the flow is steady and there are only two surfaces across which fluid flows (Surfaces 1 and 2), then the mean velocities ($\bar{V}$) and cross-sectional areas (A) can be related as shown in Equation 1.15:

$$A_1\bar{V}_1 = A_2\bar{V}_2 = Q \text{ (constant)} \tag{1.15}$$

If the velocity varies over the cross section as a function of radius, *r*, then the mean velocities must first be obtained by

$$\bar{V}_1 = \frac{1}{A_1}\int_{A_1} V_1(r)\,dA \quad \text{and} \quad \bar{V}_2 = \frac{1}{A_2}\int_{A_2} V_2(r)\,dA$$

Example 1.2

A patient is undergoing a cardiac catheterization procedure in which radiopaque dye is injected into his heart through a 2-m long catheter to obtain x-ray images of his left ventricle (Figure 1.6).

a. If the dye is injected from a syringe outside the body which is 2 cm in diameter, what must be the velocity of the plunger in order to deliver 8.5 cm^3 in 1 s?
b. What would be the average velocity of the dye as it exits the catheter tip if the catheter has a diameter of 2 mm (≈6 Fr)?

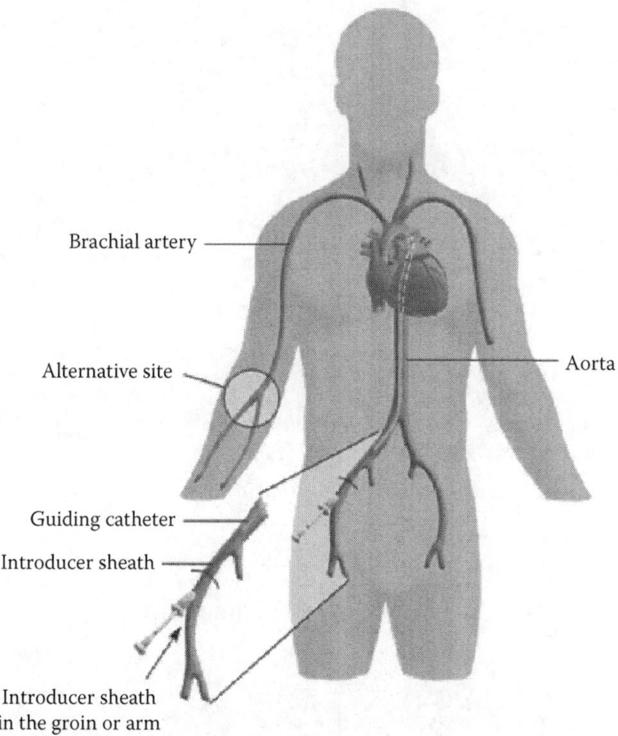

FIGURE 1.6 Cardiac catheter being introduced into the left ventricle via an access site in the iliac artery. (With permission from the Cleveland Clinic Foundation, Cleveland, OH.)

Solution

a. Assuming that the dye has a constant density and that the injection is performed steadily, we can simplify the conservation of mass to Equation 1.15. Then, the volume flow rate, Q, can be calculated as

$$Q = 8.5\,\text{cm}^3/1\,\text{s} = 8.5\,\text{cm}^3/\text{s}$$

Since there is only one outlet at the catheter tip,

$$\begin{aligned} Q &= A_{plunger} \times V_{plunger} \\ &= [\pi(2\,\text{cm})^2/4] \times V_{plunger} \\ &= 3.14 \times V_{plunger} \end{aligned}$$

Thus,

$$\begin{aligned} V_{plunger} &= 8.5\,\text{cm}^3/\text{s}/3.14\,\text{cm}^2 \\ &= 2.71\,\text{cm/s} \end{aligned}$$

b. If we further assume that the velocity exiting the catheter tip is uniform, that is, constant over the cross section, then

$$\begin{aligned} Q &= A_{catheter} \times V_{catheter} \\ &= [\pi(0.2\,\text{cm})^2/4] \times V_{catheter} \\ &= 0.0314 \times V_{catheter} \end{aligned}$$

Thus,

$$\begin{aligned} V_{catheter} &= 8.5\,\text{cm}^3/\text{s}/0.0314\,\text{cm}^2 \\ &= 271\,\text{cm/s}\ (=2.71\,\text{m/s}) \end{aligned}$$

1.4.2 Conservation of Momentum

The principle of *conservation of momentum* was initially formulated from Newton's second law of motion, which states that *the sum of the forces* $\left(\sum \vec{F}\right)$ *acting on an object is equal to its mass (m) times its acceleration* ($\vec{a}$), or

$$\sum \vec{F} = m\vec{a} \tag{1.16}$$

Rewriting $\vec{a}$ as $d\vec{V}/dt$ and bringing m inside the differential (since it is constant for a system) results in

$$\sum \vec{F} = m\left(\frac{d\vec{V}}{dt}\right) = \frac{d(m\vec{V})}{dt} \tag{1.17}$$

where the derivative is now the *time rate of change of momentum.*

Therefore, an alternative way of stating Newton's second law of motion is that for a *system*:

Sum of the external forces acting on the system = Time rate of change of linear momentum of the system

$$\sum \vec{F}_{sys} = \frac{D}{Dt} \int_{sys} \vec{V} \rho \, dV \tag{1.18}$$

When the *system* and the *control volume* are coincident at an instant of time, the forces acting on the system and the forces acting on the control volume are identical, or

$$\sum \vec{F}_{sys} = \sum \vec{F}_{CV} \tag{1.19}$$

Considering the change in linear momentum for such a system and coincident control volume (Equation 1.18 right-hand side [RHS]), the *Reynolds transport theorem* allows us to write

Time rate of change of linear momentum in a system = Time rate of change of linear momentum in control volume + Net rate of change of linear momentum through control volume surfaces

or,

$$\frac{D}{Dt} \int_{sys} \vec{V} \rho \, dV = \frac{\partial}{\partial t} \int_{CV} \vec{V} \rho \, dV + \int_{CS} \vec{V} \rho \vec{V} \cdot \vec{n} \, dA \tag{1.20}$$

Therefore, for a control volume that is fixed (i.e., with respect to an inertial reference) and nondeforming,

$$\sum \vec{F}_{CV} = \frac{\partial}{\partial t} \int_{CV} \vec{V} \rho \, dV + \int_{CS} \vec{V} \rho \vec{V} \cdot \vec{n} \, dA \tag{1.21}$$

The previous equation is called the *linear momentum equation* because we only consider motion acting in an axial direction. The forces in this equation acting on the control volume are both body forces and surface forces and can be expressed as

$$\sum \vec{F}_{CV} = \int_{CV} \rho \vec{g} \, dV + \int_{CS} \vec{t} \, dA \tag{1.22a}$$

where

$\vec{g}$ is the body force per unit mass acting on the control volume contents

$\vec{t}$ is the stress vector acting on the control volume surfaces

When viscous effects are important, the surface area integral of the stress vector is nonzero and must be determined empirically (i.e., from experimental data) and given as *friction factors* or *drag coefficients* (i.e., constants relating drag forces to other variables). However, if viscous effects are *negligible*, then the stress vector is given by

$$\vec{t} = -\hat{n}p \tag{1.22b}$$

where
$\hat{n}$ is the outward directed unit vector normal to the surface
p is the pressure

Example 1.3

In Example 1.2, what is the peak force required to propel the radiopaque dye (ρ = 1.3 g/cm^3, μ = 0.04 P) into the heart if the mean systolic pressure, p_{sys}, is 120 mmHg?

Solution

First, we will consider a control volume, CV, defined by the boundary between the dye and the syringe and catheter surfaces. Then, we can set up a force balance according to Equation 1.21. Furthermore, if the syringe is moved steadily, the time rate of change term becomes negligible, or

$$\frac{\partial}{\partial t}\int_{CV} \vec{V}\rho\, dV = 0$$

Thus, Equation 1.21 reduces to

$$\sum \vec{F}_{CV} = \int_{CS} \vec{V}\rho\vec{V}\cdot\vec{n}\, dA$$

where the sum of the forces, $\sum F_{CV}$, consists of the pressure force produced by the plunger, the pressure force of the blood resisting the motion and the shear, or frictional, force along the dye/catheter interface. Thus,

$$\sum F_{CV} = F_{plunger} - F_{catheter} - F_{friction}$$

The desired unknown force, $F_{plunger}$, acts at the interface of the dye and the syringe plunger, while at the catheter tip, motion is resisted by the blood pressure force

$$\begin{aligned} F_{catheter} &= p_{sys}\cdot A_{catheter} \\ &= (120\,\text{mmHg}\cdot 1333\,\text{dyn/cm}^2/\text{mmHg})[\pi(0.2\,\text{cm})^2/4] \\ &= (1.60\cdot 10^5\,\text{dyn/cm}^2)(0.0314\,\text{cm}^2) \\ &= 5023\,\text{dyn} \end{aligned}$$

The friction force depends upon the fluid viscosity, the fluid/wall shear rate, and the surface area over which it acts (see Section 1.5.3.2 for further details). In this example, this force is given as

$$\begin{aligned} F_{friction} &= 8\pi\mu\ell V \\ &= 8(3.14)(0.04\,\text{dyn s/cm}^2)(200\,\text{cm})(2.71\,\text{cm/s}) \\ &= 545\,\text{dyn} \end{aligned}$$

Again, if we assume uniform velocities at the syringe plunger and at the catheter tip, the momentum integral over those control surfaces can be rewritten as

$$\begin{aligned} \int_{CS} \vec{V}\rho\vec{V}\cdot\vec{n}\,dA &= \sum \vec{V}(\rho\vec{V}\cdot\hat{n})A \\ &= \vec{V}_{plunger}(\rho\vec{V}_{plunger}\cdot\hat{n})A_{plunger} + \vec{V}_{catheter}(\rho\vec{V}_{catheter}\cdot\hat{n})A_{catheter} \end{aligned}$$

Here, the term $(\rho\vec{V}\cdot\hat{n})$ can be thought of as the axial momentum per unit volume, which "carries" the intrinsic property of interest—in this case, momentum/unit mass = $\vec{V}$ (see Equation 1.13).

Thus,

$$\sum \vec{V}(\rho\vec{V}\cdot\hat{n})A = V_{plunger}[\rho(-V_{plunger})A_{plunger}] + V_{catheter}[\rho(+V_{catheter})A_{catheter}]$$

where (+) velocity is along the axis of flow.

If we substitute values into the simplified Equation 1.21, we obtain

$$\begin{aligned} F_{plunger} - 5023 - 545 &= 1.3\,\text{g/cm}^3\,\{[(2.71\,\text{cm/s})\,(-2.71\,\text{cm/s})\,(3.14\,\text{cm}^2)] \\ &\quad + [(271\,\text{cm/s})(271\,\text{cm/s})(0.0314\,\text{cm}^2)]\} \\ &= 1.3\,\text{g/cm}^3\,\{-23.1 + 2306\} \\ &= 2968\,\text{dyn} \end{aligned}$$

Thus,

$$F_{plunger} = 8536\ \text{dyn}$$

The previous two balances of mass and momentum are called *macroscopic* or *integral* balances because they consider the control volume as a large, discrete space and are written in terms of bulk flow variables. In order to derive more general forms of these equations which provide spatial detail throughout the flow field, we need to take a *microscopic* or *differential* approach. Such an approach leads us to what are commonly referred to in the fluid mechanics literature as the *continuity* and the *Navier–Stokes equations*, for conservation of mass and momentum, respectively.

1.5 MICROSCOPIC BALANCES OF MASS AND MOMENTUM

1.5.1 Conservation of Mass

We begin by considering an infinitesimal control volume, CV, of dimension $\Delta x\Delta y\Delta z$ (Figure 1.7a).

A fluid flowing through the control volume will have a velocity denoted by the vector,

$$\vec{V} = u\hat{i} + v\hat{j} + w\hat{k} \tag{1.23}$$

where each of these variables may be a function of time.

The conservation of mass principle states that for a system

The net rate of mass flux *across* the control surface + The rate of change of mass *inside* control volume	$= 0$

Treating each of the aforementioned terms individually, we get

1. The net rate of mass flux *across* the control surfaces (Figure 1.7b) in the x-direction:

$$(\rho u|_x - \rho u|_{x+\Delta x})\Delta y\Delta z$$

y-direction:

$$(\rho v|_y - \rho v|_{y+\Delta y})\Delta x\Delta z$$

z-direction:

$$(\rho w|_z - \rho w|_{z+\Delta z})\Delta x\Delta y$$

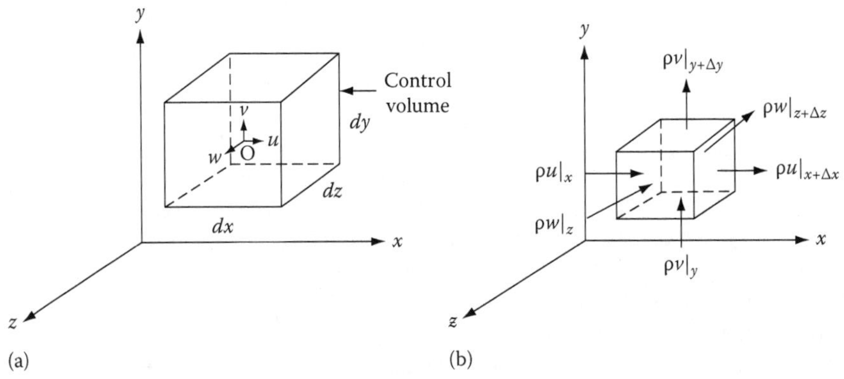

FIGURE 1.7 (a) Differential control volume in rectangular coordinates and (b) mass flux across surfaces of control volume.

2. The rate of change of mass *inside* the control volume

$$\frac{\partial}{\partial t}(\rho\Delta x\Delta y\Delta z)$$

Combining terms and rearranging yields

$$(\rho u|_{x+\Delta x}-\rho u|_x)\Delta y\Delta z+(\rho v|_{y+\Delta y}-\rho v|_y)\Delta x\Delta z+(\rho w|_{z+\Delta z}-\rho w|_z)\Delta x\Delta y$$

$$=-\frac{\partial}{\partial t}(\rho\Delta x\Delta y\Delta z) \tag{1.24}$$

Furthermore, each of the mass flux terms can be equivalently written as the gradient of mass flux in that coordinate direction times the distance moved, or

$$(\rho u|_{x+\Delta x}-\rho u|_x)=\frac{\partial(\rho u)}{\partial x}\cdot\Delta x$$

and so on.

Since the volume within the control element is time *invariant*, we can divide each term by $\Delta x\Delta y\Delta z$. Then, in the limit as $\Delta x\Delta y\Delta z$ approaches zero, we obtain

$$\frac{\partial}{\partial x}(\rho u)+\frac{\partial}{\partial y}(\rho v)+\frac{\partial}{\partial z}(\rho w)+\frac{\partial\rho}{\partial t}=0 \tag{1.25}$$

which is equivalent to

$$\nabla\cdot\rho\vec{V}+\frac{\partial\rho}{\partial t}=0 \tag{1.26}$$

The previous equation is known as the *continuity equation* where the "del" vector operator, ∇, is defined as

$$\nabla=\vec{i}\frac{\partial}{\partial x}+\vec{j}\frac{\partial}{\partial y}+\vec{k}\frac{\partial}{\partial z} \tag{1.27}$$

A fluid such as blood is incompressible, and thus, ρ = constant, so that the continuity equation becomes

$$\rho\nabla\cdot\vec{V}=0P \tag{1.28}$$

or

$$\nabla\cdot\vec{V}=0 \tag{1.29}$$

Note that this equation is valid for both *steady* and *unsteady* (including pulsatile, 3D) flows of an incompressible fluid.

If we return to Equation 1.25 and differentiate each numerator, we obtain

$$\frac{\partial\rho}{\partial t}+u\frac{\partial\rho}{\partial x}+v\frac{\partial\rho}{\partial y}+w\frac{\partial\rho}{\partial z}+\rho\left(\frac{\partial u}{\partial x}+\frac{\partial v}{\partial y}+\frac{\partial w}{\partial z}\right)=\frac{D\rho}{Dt}+\rho\left(\frac{\partial u}{\partial x}+\frac{\partial v}{\partial y}+\frac{\partial w}{\partial z}\right)=0 \quad (1.30)$$

or,

$$\frac{D\rho}{Dt}+\rho\nabla\cdot\vec{V}=0 \quad (1.31)$$

where

$$\frac{D}{Dt}=\frac{\partial}{\partial t}+u\frac{\partial}{\partial x}+v\frac{\partial}{\partial y}+w\frac{\partial}{\partial z}$$

is called *substantive derivative.*

The substantive derivative represents the time derivative of a scalar or vector quantity, which follows the motion of the fluid. For example, for a scalar quantity such as temperature, T, the substantive derivative would be expressed as

$$\frac{DT}{Dt}=\frac{\partial T}{\partial t}+u\frac{\partial T}{\partial x}+v\frac{\partial T}{\partial y}+w\frac{\partial T}{\partial z} \quad (1.32)$$

where

$\partial T/\partial t$ is the local time rate of change of temperature

the terms $u(\partial T/\partial x) + v(\partial T/\partial y) + w(\partial T/\partial z)$ represent the rate of change of temperature due to fluid motion (also known as *convection*)

Finally, for many fluid dynamic situations such as the consideration of liquids or gases at low speeds, it is quite common to assume an incompressible fluid where ρ = constant. In this case, Equation 1.31 can be further reduced to

$$\nabla\cdot\vec{V}=0$$

1.5.2 Conservation of Momentum

In deriving the differential form of this law, we once again consider the dynamics associated with a fluid control volume $-\Delta V = \Delta x\Delta y\Delta z$ shown in Figure 1.7b. We now apply Newton's second law of motion as written in Equation 1.16 in terms of the time rate of change of momentum

Sum of the external *forces* acting on the *control volume* = Net rate of efflux of *linear momentum across control volume* + Time rate of change of *linear momentum within* the *control volume*

In general, linear momentum per unit volume of fluid can be expressed as $\rho\vec{V}$ so that by multiplying this term by the rate of volume change, we can obtain the time rate of change of linear momentum. To determine the flux of a property *across* the control volume surface, the appropriate expression for the rate of volume change is $(\vec{V}\cdot\hat{n})dA$ where $\hat{n}$ is the outward directed normal to a particular surface. For change of a property *within* the control volume, the rate of volume change is simply given by dV/dt. As with the derivation of the continuity equation, the control volume considered is constant and we can express the aforementioned equality as

$$\lim_{\Delta V\to 0}\frac{\Sigma\vec{F}}{\Delta x\Delta y\Delta z}=\lim_{\Delta V\to 0}\iint\frac{\rho\vec{V}(\vec{V}\cdot\vec{n})dA}{\Delta x\Delta y\Delta z}+\lim_{\Delta V\to 0}\frac{\partial}{\partial t}\iiint\frac{\rho\vec{V}\,dV}{\Delta x\Delta y\Delta z}\tag{1.33}$$

if we take the limit of $\Delta V=\Delta x\Delta y\Delta z$ as it approaches zero.

Each of these terms can be evaluated separately as follows:

1. Sum of the external forces

$$\lim_{\Delta V\to 0}\frac{\Sigma\vec{F}}{\Delta x\Delta y\Delta z}=d\vec{F}$$

2. Net rate of momentum efflux across the control volume

$$\lim_{\Delta V\to 0}\iint\frac{\rho\vec{V}(\vec{V}\cdot\vec{n})dA}{\Delta x\Delta y\Delta z}=\frac{\partial}{\partial x}(\rho\vec{V}u)+\frac{\partial}{\partial y}(\rho\vec{V}v)+\frac{\partial}{\partial z}(\rho\vec{V}w)$$

$$=\vec{V}\left[\frac{\partial}{\partial x}(\rho u)+\frac{\partial}{\partial y}(\rho v)+\frac{\partial}{\partial z}(\rho w)\right]+\rho\left[u\frac{\partial\vec{V}}{\partial x}+v\frac{\partial\vec{V}}{\partial z}+w\frac{\partial\vec{V}}{\partial z}\right]$$

At this point, we can also use the continuity equation to substitute terms

$$\frac{\partial}{\partial x}(\rho u)+\frac{\partial}{\partial y}(\rho v)+\frac{\partial}{\partial z}(\rho w)=-\frac{\partial\rho}{\partial t}\tag{1.34}$$

and reduce this limit to

$$\lim_{\Delta V\to 0}\iint\frac{\rho\vec{V}(\vec{V}\cdot\vec{n})dA}{\Delta x\Delta y\Delta z}=-\vec{V}\frac{\partial\rho}{\partial t}+\rho\left[u\frac{\partial\vec{V}}{\partial x}+v\frac{\partial\vec{V}}{\partial y}+w\frac{\partial\vec{V}}{\partial z}\right]$$

3. Time rate of change of momentum within the control volume

$$\lim_{\Delta V\to 0}\iiint\frac{\vec{V}\rho\,dV}{\Delta x\Delta y\Delta z}=\frac{\partial}{\partial t}(\rho\vec{V})=\rho\frac{\partial\vec{V}}{\partial t}+\vec{V}\frac{\partial\rho}{\partial t}$$

Substituting for the limits and combining terms gives

$$d\vec{F} = \rho\left[u\frac{\partial\vec{V}}{\partial x} + v\frac{\partial\vec{V}}{\partial y} + w\frac{\partial\vec{V}}{\partial z}\right] + \rho\frac{d\vec{V}}{dt} \tag{1.35}$$

We have now expressed the change of momentum in terms of its component velocities. Let us now look at the external forces in more detail. The external forces consist of the sum of the *body* forces, $\vec{F}_B$, and the *surface* forces, $\vec{F}_S$. The body forces are typically due to the presence of gravitational, electromagnetic, and electrostatic fields. If the only body force is gravity, then

$$F_{Bx} = \rho g_x \Delta x \Delta y \Delta z \tag{1.36}$$

The surface forces acting on the control volume are those due to the normal, σ, and the shear, τ, stresses. These stresses can be assumed to vary continuously from their nominal value at the center of the control volume in each of the coordinate directions. Figure 1.8 depicts the normal and shear stresses acting on the control volume in the x-direction alone. Similar figures can be constructed for the normal and shear stresses acting in the y- and z-directions. Thus, the net surface force acting in the x-direction is given by

$$F_{Sx} = \left(\frac{\partial\sigma_{xx}}{\partial x}\right)\Delta x\Delta y\Delta z + \left(\frac{\partial\tau_{yx}}{\partial y}\right)\Delta x\Delta y\Delta z + \left(\frac{\partial\tau_{zx}}{\partial z}\right)\Delta x\Delta y\Delta z \tag{1.37}$$

The total force acting on the control volume in the x-direction then becomes

$$F_x = F_{Bx} + F_{Sx} \tag{1.38}$$

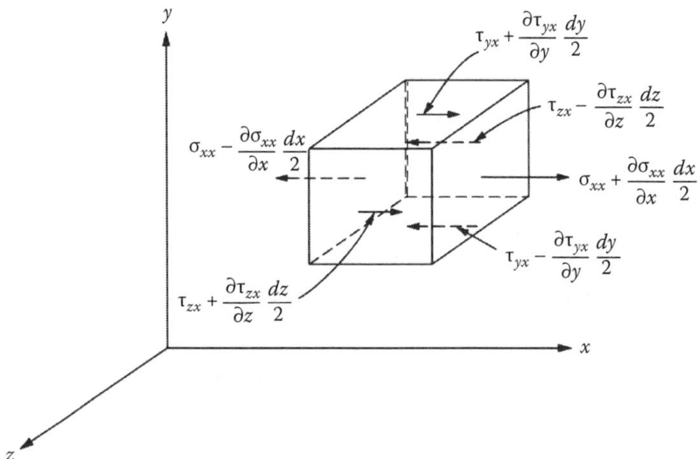

FIGURE 1.8 Normal and shear stresses along the x-coordinate in the control volume.

which, in the limit, can be expressed as

$$dF_x = \rho g_x + \frac{\partial \sigma_{xx}}{\partial x} + \frac{\partial \tau_{yx}}{\partial y} + \frac{\partial \tau_{zx}}{\partial z} \tag{1.39a}$$

Similarly, the differential force components in the *y*- and *z*-directions are

$$dF_y = \rho g_y + \frac{\partial \sigma_{yy}}{\partial y} + \frac{\partial \tau_{xy}}{\partial x} + \frac{\partial \tau_{zy}}{\partial z} \tag{1.39b}$$

$$dF_z = \rho g_z + \frac{\partial \sigma_{zz}}{\partial z} + \frac{\partial \tau_{xz}}{\partial x} + \frac{\partial \tau_{yz}}{\partial y} \tag{1.39c}$$

Substituting the results of the previous expressions (1.39a through 1.39c) back into the expression for Newton's second law (Equation 1.17) yields

$$\rho g_x + \frac{\partial \sigma_{xx}}{\partial x} + \frac{\partial \tau_{yx}}{\partial y} + \frac{\partial \tau_{zx}}{\partial z} = \rho\left(\frac{\partial u}{\partial t} + u\frac{\partial u}{\partial x} + v\frac{\partial u}{\partial y} + w\frac{\partial u}{\partial z}\right) \tag{1.40a}$$

$$\rho g_y + \frac{\partial \tau_{xy}}{\partial x} + \frac{\partial \sigma_{yy}}{\partial y} + \frac{\partial \tau_{zy}}{\partial z} = \rho\left(\frac{\partial v}{\partial t} + u\frac{\partial v}{\partial x} + v\frac{\partial v}{\partial y} + w\frac{\partial v}{\partial z}\right) \tag{1.40b}$$

$$\rho g_z + \frac{\partial \tau_{xz}}{\partial x} + \frac{\partial \tau_{yz}}{\partial y} + \frac{\partial \sigma_{zz}}{\partial z} = \rho\left(\frac{\partial w}{\partial t} + u\frac{\partial w}{\partial x} + v\frac{\partial w}{\partial y} + w\frac{\partial w}{\partial z}\right) \tag{1.40c}$$

In this form, we can see that the RHS of the previous equations actually represents density (mass/volume) × acceleration, or force/volume, where the acceleration terms can be separated into *local acceleration* ($\partial u/\partial t$, etc.) and *convective acceleration* ($u\partial u/\partial x$, etc.) components. The total acceleration can be expressed in terms of the substantive derivative as

$$\frac{Du}{Dt} = \frac{\partial u}{\partial t} + u\frac{\partial u}{\partial x} + v\frac{\partial u}{\partial y} + w\frac{\partial u}{\partial z} \tag{1.41}$$

Equations 1.40a through 1.40c represent the complete form of the differential conservation of momentum balances. These equations cannot be solved, however, because there are more unknowns (i.e., dependent variables) than equations. Thus, it is necessary to derive additional information in order to provide those equations. In practice, we will consider the special, although not uncommon, case of incompressible, Newtonian fluids. Here, the *normal* and *shear* stresses can be expressed as

$$\sigma_{xx} = -p + 2\mu\frac{\partial u}{\partial x} \quad \tau_{xy} = \tau_{yx} = \mu\left(\frac{\partial u}{\partial y} + \frac{\partial v}{\partial x}\right) \tag{1.42a}$$

$$\sigma_{yy} = -p + 2\mu\frac{\partial v}{\partial y} \quad \tau_{yz} = \tau_{zy} = \mu\left(\frac{\partial w}{\partial y} + \frac{\partial v}{\partial z}\right) \tag{1.42b}$$

$$\sigma_{zz} = -p + 2\mu\frac{\partial w}{\partial z} \quad \tau_{zx} = \tau_{xz} = \mu\left(\frac{\partial u}{\partial z} + \frac{\partial w}{\partial x}\right) \tag{1.42c}$$

By substituting these relationships into Equations 1.40a through 1.40c, we obtain the *equations of motion* in *scalar* form along the three coordinate axes as

$$\rho g_x - \frac{\partial p}{\partial x} + \mu\left(\frac{\partial^2 u}{\partial x^2} + \frac{\partial^2 u}{\partial y^2} + \frac{\partial^2 u}{\partial z^2}\right) = \rho\left(\frac{\partial u}{\partial t} + u\frac{\partial u}{\partial x} + v\frac{\partial u}{\partial y} + w\frac{\partial u}{\partial z}\right) \tag{1.43a}$$

$$\rho g_y - \frac{\partial p}{\partial y} + \mu\left(\frac{\partial^2 v}{\partial x^2} + \frac{\partial^2 v}{\partial y^2} + \frac{\partial^2 v}{\partial z^2}\right) = \rho\left(\frac{\partial v}{\partial t} + u\frac{\partial v}{\partial x} + v\frac{\partial v}{\partial y} + w\frac{\partial v}{\partial z}\right) \tag{1.43b}$$

$$\rho g_z - \frac{\partial p}{\partial z} + \mu\left(\frac{\partial^2 w}{\partial x^2} + \frac{\partial^2 w}{\partial y^2} + \frac{\partial^2 w}{\partial z^2}\right) = \rho\left(\frac{\partial w}{\partial t} + u\frac{\partial w}{\partial x} + v\frac{\partial w}{\partial y} + w\frac{\partial w}{\partial z}\right) \tag{1.43c}$$

The equivalent *vector* form of the previous equations is

$$\rho\vec{g} - \nabla p + \mu\nabla^2\vec{V} = \rho\frac{D\vec{V}}{dt} \tag{1.44}$$

which can be alternatively written as

$$\frac{\partial\vec{V}}{\partial t} + (\vec{V}\cdot\nabla)\vec{V} = -\frac{1}{\rho}\nabla p + \vec{g} + \nu(\nabla^2\vec{V}) \tag{1.45}$$

by expanding the material derivative for acceleration and dividing by ρ.

The previous equations (in either scalar or vector form) are commonly called the *Navier–Stokes equations* for Newtonian incompressible fluids in honor of the mathematicians who originally derived these relationships.

The *continuity* and *Navier–Stokes* equations can also be derived in other coordinate systems and, thus, are given in Cartesian, cylindrical, and spherical coordinates in Table 1.1.

TABLE 1.1
Continuity and Momentum Equations in Cartesian, Cylindrical (Polar), and Spherical Coordinate Systems

a. Cartesian coordinate system

$$\frac{\partial u}{\partial x}+\frac{\partial v}{\partial y}+\frac{\partial w}{\partial z}=0$$

$$\rho\left[\frac{\partial u}{\partial t}+u\frac{\partial u}{\partial x}+v\frac{\partial u}{\partial y}+w\frac{\partial u}{\partial z}\right]=\rho B_x-\frac{\partial p}{\partial x}+\mu\left[\frac{\partial^2 u}{\partial x^2}+\frac{\partial^2 u}{\partial y^2}+\frac{\partial^2 u}{\partial z^2}\right]$$

$$\rho\left[\frac{\partial v}{\partial t}+u\frac{\partial v}{\partial x}+v\frac{\partial v}{\partial y}+w\frac{\partial v}{\partial z}\right]=\rho B_y-\frac{\partial p}{\partial y}+\mu\left[\frac{\partial^2 v}{\partial x^2}+\frac{\partial^2 v}{\partial y^2}+\frac{\partial^2 v}{\partial z^2}\right]$$

and

$$\rho\left[\frac{\partial w}{\partial t}+u\frac{\partial w}{\partial x}+v\frac{\partial w}{\partial y}+w\frac{\partial w}{\partial z}\right]=\rho B_z-\frac{\partial p}{\partial z}+\mu\left[\frac{\partial^2 w}{\partial x^2}+\frac{\partial^2 w}{\partial y^2}+\frac{\partial^2 w}{\partial z^2}\right]$$

b. Cylindrical coordinate system

$$\nabla\cdot\vec{V}=\frac{1}{r}\frac{\partial(rV_r)}{\partial r}+\frac{1}{r}\frac{\partial V_\theta}{\partial\theta}+\frac{\partial V_z}{\partial z}=0$$

$$\rho\left[\frac{\partial V_r}{\partial t}+V_r\frac{\partial V_r}{\partial r}+\frac{V_\theta}{r}\frac{\partial V_r}{\partial\theta}-\frac{V_\theta^2}{r}+V_z\frac{\partial V_r}{\partial z}\right]$$

$$=F_r-\frac{\partial p}{\partial r}+\mu\left(\frac{\partial^2 V_r}{\partial r^2}+\frac{1}{r}\frac{\partial V_r}{\partial r}-\frac{V_r}{r^2}+\frac{1}{r^2}\frac{\partial^2 V_r}{\partial\theta^2}-\frac{2}{r^2}\frac{\partial V_\theta}{\partial\theta}+\frac{\partial^2 V_r}{\partial z^2}\right)$$

$$\rho\left[\frac{\partial V_\theta}{\partial t}+V_r\frac{\partial V_\theta}{\partial r}+\frac{V_\theta}{r}\frac{\partial V_\theta}{\partial\theta}+\frac{V_rV_\theta}{r}+V_z\frac{\partial V_\theta}{\partial z}\right]$$

$$=F_\theta-\frac{1}{r}\frac{\partial p}{\partial\theta}+\mu\left(\frac{\partial^2 V_\theta}{\partial r^2}+\frac{1}{r}\frac{\partial V_\theta}{\partial r}-\frac{V_\theta}{r^2}+\frac{1}{r^2}\frac{\partial^2 V_\theta}{\partial\theta^2}+\frac{2}{r^2}\frac{\partial V_r}{\partial\theta}+\frac{\partial^2 V_\theta}{\partial z^2}\right)$$

and

$$\rho\left[\frac{\partial V_z}{\partial t}+V_r\frac{\partial V_z}{\partial r}+\frac{V_\theta}{r}\frac{\partial V_z}{\partial\theta}+V_z\frac{\partial V_z}{\partial z}\right]$$

$$=F_z-\frac{\partial p}{\partial z}+\mu\left(\frac{\partial^2 V_z}{\partial r^2}+\frac{1}{r}\frac{\partial V_z}{\partial r}+\frac{1}{r^2}\frac{\partial^2 V_z}{\partial\theta^2}+\frac{\partial^2 V_z}{\partial z^2}\right)$$

(*continued*)

TABLE 1.1 (continued)
Continuity and Momentum Equations in Cartesian, Cylindrical (Polar), and Spherical Coordinate Systems

c. Spherical coordinate system

$$\frac{\partial V_r}{\partial r}+\frac{2V_r}{r}+\frac{1}{r}\frac{\partial V_\theta}{\partial \theta}+\frac{V_\theta \cot\theta}{r}+\frac{1}{r\sin\theta}\frac{\partial V_\varphi}{\partial \varphi}=0$$

$$\rho\left(\frac{\partial V_r}{\partial t}+V_r\frac{\partial V_r}{\partial r}+\frac{V_\theta}{r}\frac{\partial V_r}{\partial \theta}+\frac{V_\varphi}{r\sin\theta}\frac{\partial V_r}{\partial \varphi}-\frac{V_\theta^2}{r}-\frac{V_\varphi^2}{r}\right)$$

$$=F_r-\frac{\partial p}{\partial r}+\mu\left(\begin{array}{l}\frac{\partial^2 V_r}{\partial r^2}+\frac{2}{r}\frac{\partial V_r}{\partial r}-\frac{2V_r}{r^2}+\frac{1}{r^2}\frac{\partial^2 V_r}{\partial \theta^2}+\frac{\cot\theta}{r^2}\frac{\partial V_r}{\partial \theta}+\frac{1}{r^2\sin^2\theta}\frac{\partial^2 V_r}{\partial \varphi^2}-\frac{2}{r^2}\frac{\partial V_\theta}{\partial \theta}\\ -\frac{2V_\theta\cot\theta}{r^2}-\frac{2}{r^2\sin\theta}\frac{\partial V_\varphi}{\partial \varphi}\end{array}\right)$$

$$\rho\left(\frac{\partial V_\theta}{\partial t}+V_r\frac{\partial V_\theta}{\partial r}+\frac{V_rV_\theta}{r}+\frac{V_\theta}{r}\frac{\partial V_\theta}{\partial \theta}+\frac{V_\varphi}{r\sin\theta}\frac{\partial V_\theta}{\partial \varphi}-\frac{V_\varphi^2\cot\theta}{r}\right)$$

$$=F_\theta-\frac{1}{r}\frac{\partial p}{\partial \theta}+\mu\left(\begin{array}{l}\frac{\partial^2 V_\theta}{\partial r^2}+\frac{2}{r}\frac{\partial V_\theta}{\partial r}-\frac{V_\theta}{r^2\sin^2\theta}+\frac{1}{r^2}\frac{\partial^2 V_\theta}{\partial \theta^2}+\frac{\cot\theta}{r^2}\frac{\partial V_\theta}{\partial \theta}\\ +\frac{1}{r^2\sin^2\theta}\frac{\partial^2 V_\theta}{\partial \varphi^2}+\frac{2}{r^2}\frac{\partial V_r}{\partial \theta}-\frac{2\cot\theta}{r^2\sin\theta}\frac{\partial V_\varphi}{\partial \varphi}\end{array}\right)$$

and

$$\rho\left(\frac{\partial V_\varphi}{\partial t}+V_r\frac{\partial V_\varphi}{\partial r}+\frac{V_rV_\varphi}{r}+\frac{V_\theta}{r}\frac{\partial V_\varphi}{\partial \theta}+\frac{V_\theta V_\varphi\cot\theta}{r}+\frac{V_\varphi}{r\sin\theta}\frac{\partial V_\varphi}{\partial \varphi}\right)$$

$$=F_\varphi-\frac{1}{r\sin\varphi}\frac{\partial p}{\partial \varphi}+\mu\left(\begin{array}{l}\frac{\partial^2 V_\varphi}{\partial r^2}+\frac{2}{r}\frac{\partial V_\varphi}{\partial r}-\frac{V_\varphi}{r^2\sin^2\theta}+\frac{1}{r^2}\frac{\partial^2 V_\varphi}{\partial \theta^2}+\frac{\cot\theta}{r^2}\frac{\partial V_\varphi}{\partial \theta}\\ +\frac{1}{r^2\sin^2\theta}\frac{\partial^2 V_\varphi}{\partial \varphi^2}+\frac{2}{r^2\sin\theta}\frac{\partial V_r}{\partial \varphi}+\frac{2\cot\theta}{r^2\sin\theta}\frac{\partial V_\theta}{\partial \varphi}\end{array}\right)$$

1.5.3 Mathematical Solutions

As mentioned earlier, in order to solve a set of equations, we must have at least as many constraints as we have dependent variables. Examination of Equations 1.43a through 1.43c shows that there are *four* dependent variables—pressure (p) and the three velocity components (u, v, and w) defined in terms of *four* independent variables—time (t) and the three position coordinates (x, y, and z) but only *three* equations. (*Note*: Similar results would be found with the cylindrical and spherical coordinate systems as well.) However, by including the continuity equation, we obtain a fourth constraint which will allow us to uniquely define each dependent variable. Mathematically, Equations 1.31 (*continuity*) and 1.44 (*Navier–Stokes*) are first and second order partial differential equations, respectively. Furthermore, Equations 1.43a through 1.43c is nonlinear because of the presence of product terms such as $u\partial u/\partial x$, $v\partial u/\partial y$, and so on. Unfortunately, no exact analytical solution has been defined for equations of this form. Therefore, in practice, two approaches have been taken. One is to first simplify the equations until they have a mathematical form for which there is a solution while the other is to solve them numerically.

1.5.3.1 Couette Flow

One example of obtaining a solution to the continuity and Navier–Stokes equations by simplifying the number of spatial and temporal variables used is that of flow between two parallel plates as shown in Figure 1.9. We will assume that the upper plate is moving at a steady velocity U while the lower plate is fixed. Furthermore, there is no variation into or out of the plane (z-axis), so we can consider this as a two-dimensional (2D) problem with flow along only one axis. These two assumptions, then, allow us to eliminate all terms involving $\partial/\partial t$ due to steady flow and two of the velocity components (v and w) due to uniaxial flow. Since the flow is in the x-direction only, Equation 1.31 reduces to

$$\frac{\partial u}{\partial x} = 0$$

or,

$$u = f(y) + C$$

where C is the integration constant.

Furthermore, Equation 1.43a reduces to

$$\frac{\partial p}{\partial x} = \mu\left(\frac{\partial^2 u}{\partial y^2}\right)$$

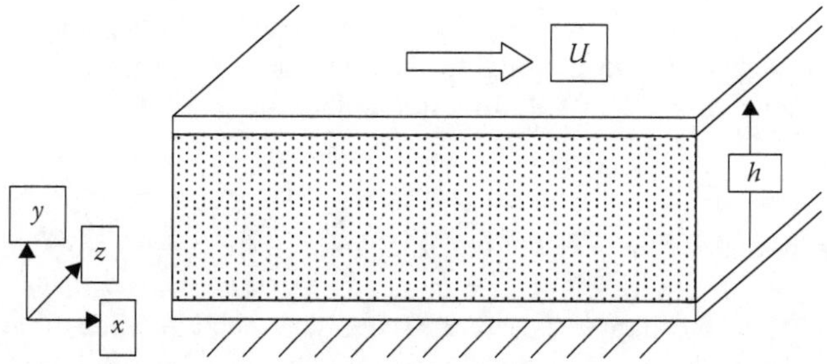

FIGURE 1.9 Flow between two infinite, flat plates.

where it is now possible to solve for $u(y)$ as an explicit function of p. Integrating twice, we obtain

$$\frac{\partial u}{\partial y} = \left[\frac{1}{\mu}\frac{\partial p}{\partial x}\right] y + C_1$$

and

$$u(y) = \left[\frac{1}{2\mu}\frac{\partial p}{\partial x}\right] y^2 + C_1 y + C_2$$

where C_1 and C_2 are constants of integration which can be evaluated by applying specific boundary conditions for the problem. In this case, for example, we know that the near-wall velocity is the same as that of the walls due to the "no-slip" criteria. Thus, $u(y = 0) = 0$ and $u(y = h) = U$. Furthermore, there is no pressure gradient in the x-direction. Applying these boundary and driving force conditions, $C_2 = 0$ and $C_1 = U/h$, yielding a velocity solution or "profile" of

$$u(y) = \left(\frac{U}{h}\right) y$$

as shown.

An alternate configuration is that the flow is driven by a pressure gradient in the x-direction between two stationary plates. In that case, $dp/dx \neq 0$ but $u(y = 0) = u(y = h) = 0$. Applying these constraints, we find that $C_2 = 0$ but now, $C_1 = [(1/2\mu)\,\partial p/\partial x]h$. The resulting velocity profile becomes

$$u(y) = \left[\frac{1}{2\mu}\frac{\partial p}{\partial x}\right](y^2 - hy)$$

This is the classical *Couette relationship* for steady flow between stationary boundaries.

1.5.3.2 Hagen–Poiseuille Flow

If we now apply the Navier–Stokes equations in cylindrical coordinates (Table 1.1) to the case of steady flow in a straight, circular, horizontal tube (Figure 1.10), the momentum balance in the z-(axial) direction reduces to

$$-\frac{\partial p}{\partial z} + \mu\left[\frac{1}{r}\frac{\partial}{\partial r}\left(r\frac{\partial V_z}{\partial r}\right)\right] = 0 \tag{1.46}$$

since the time rate of change (i.e., $\partial/\partial t$), secondary velocity (i.e., V_r and V_θ), and circumferential velocity gradient (i.e., $\partial V_z/\partial\theta$) terms are zero. As a consequence, the conservation of mass balance results in $\partial V_z/\partial z$ also being zero.

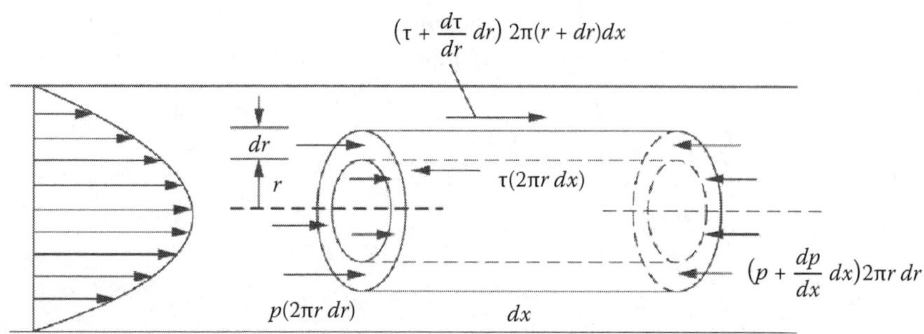

FIGURE 1.10 Force balances for steady flow through a straight, horizontal, circular tube.

Rearranging terms then yields

$$\frac{\partial p}{\partial z} = \mu\left[\frac{1}{r}\frac{\partial}{\partial r}\left(r\frac{\partial V_z}{\partial r}\right)\right] \tag{1.47}$$

Since pressure is *only* a function of length and axial velocity is *only* a function of radius, this equation can equivalently be written in terms of ordinary derivatives, or

$$\frac{dp}{dz} = \mu\left[\frac{1}{r}\frac{d}{dr}\left(r\frac{dV_z}{dr}\right)\right] \tag{1.48}$$

We can further observe that, for the two terms of the equation (i.e., left-hand side [LHS] and RHS) to be equal for *all* values of the independent variables r and z (each of which is only present in one of the terms), each term must be constant. Equation 1.48 can then be integrated twice to yield

$$\frac{dV_z}{dr} = \frac{1}{2\mu}\left(\frac{dp}{dz}\right)r + \frac{c_1}{r}$$

$$V_z = \frac{1}{4\mu}\left(\frac{dp}{dz}\right)r^2 + c_1 \ln r + c_2 \tag{1.49}$$

The constant terms, c_1 and c_2, can be evaluated by applying known values of axial velocity at specific boundary locations. For example, $V_z = 0$ at $r = R$ due to the "no-slip" condition at the tube wall. The value of V_z, however, is not known at the tube center, $r = 0$, although we can assume that it is a maximum at that point due to overall symmetry of the tube. Thus, the appropriate boundary condition here is that $dV_z/dr = 0$, which requires that $c_1 = 0$ and which also constrains all velocities to be finite.

Evaluating c_2 and substituting it into Equation 1.49 results in

$$V_z = \frac{1}{4\mu}\left(\frac{dp}{dz}\right)[r^2 - R^2] \tag{1.50}$$

If we replace the differential pressure gradient term by the pressure gradient along the *entire* tube, $\Delta p/L$, then the velocity variation or "profile" in a tube is given by

$$V_z(r) = \left[\frac{\Delta p R^2}{4\mu L}\right]\left[1-\left(\frac{r}{R}\right)^2\right]$$

or,

$$V_z(r) = V_{max}\left[1-\left(\frac{r}{R}\right)^2\right] \tag{1.51}$$

where

V (m/s) is the velocity of the fluid at a distance r (m) from the center of the tube
V_{max} (m/s) is the maximum (centerline) velocity
R (m) is the radius of the tube
Δp (Pa) is the pressure drop along a length L (m) of the tube

By integrating this velocity profile over the tube's cross section and dividing by the area, we can obtain the average velocity

$$V_{ave} = \frac{V_{max}}{2} \tag{1.52}$$

Since flow rate in the tube, Q (m^3/s), is equal to the average velocity, V_{ave}, times the cross-sectional area, we can write

$$Q = V_{ave}(\pi R^2) = \frac{V_{max}}{2}(\pi R^2)$$

$$= \left(\frac{\Delta p R^2}{8\mu L}\right)(\pi R^2) = \frac{\Delta p \pi R^4}{8\mu L} \tag{1.53}$$

In terms of tube diameter, this becomes

$$Q = \frac{\Delta p \pi d^4}{128\mu L} \tag{1.54}$$

Solving for the pressure difference, we obtain

$$\Delta p = 128\frac{\mu L Q}{\pi d^4} \tag{1.55}$$

which is commonly known as the *Hagen–Poiseuille equation.*

Finally, the shear rate along the inner tube wall can be obtained by differentiating Equation 1.51 and evaluating it at $r = R$, or

$$\left.\frac{\partial V_z(r)}{\partial r}\right|_{r=R} = V_{max}\left.\left(\frac{-2r}{R^2}\right)\right|_{r=R} = \frac{-2V_{max}}{R}$$

Recalling Equation 1.1, we can now solve for wall shear stress as

$$\tau = \mu\left.\frac{\partial V_z(r)}{\partial r}\right|_{r=R} = \frac{-2\mu V_{max}}{R}$$

where the negative sign indicates that the shear stress acts in the direction opposite to the flow.

1.5.3.3 Numerical Solutions

This approach is more complex but provides the ability to solve problems without making unrealistic simplifying assumptions. The basic technique is to first subdivide the flow into many small regions, or *elements*, over which the governing equations are applied. Rather than use the differential form of the equations, however, they are rewritten in algebraic form in terms of changes that occur in variables due to incremental changes in position and time. Solutions are then obtained locally at specific locations, or *nodes*, on the finite elements across a *mesh* of elements (Figure 1.11). This set of

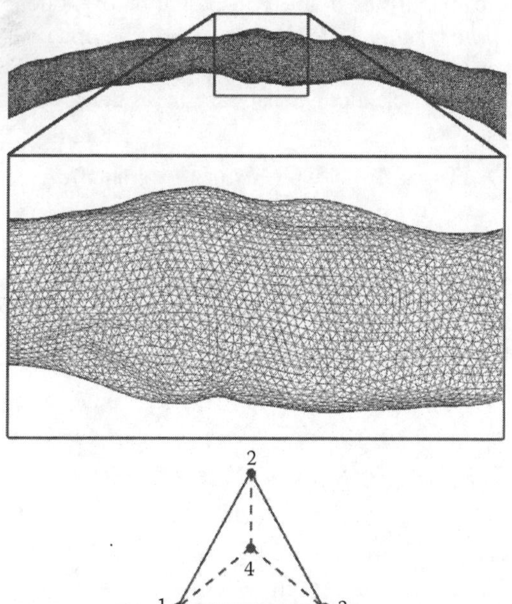

FIGURE 1.11 CFD mesh for a reconstructed human coronary artery with a stenosis segment. It can be observed that a finer mesh is employed in the area of stenosis in order to obtain more accurate results in this region of interest.

solutions is then updated at subsequent time intervals over the entire mesh until some acceptable level of accuracy, or *tolerance*, is achieved based upon convergence between successive values of certain output variables. Obviously, this can be a very detailed and time-consuming process depending upon the complexity of the geometry being analyzed and the initial and boundary conditions imposed. Furthermore, additional features are sometimes included in the equations, for example, to allow for simulation of non-Newtonian fluids and turbulent flow conditions. While it is always important to validate such results, these *computational fluid dynamic* (CFD) software programs are increasingly being used to solve challenging biomedical flow problems unapproachable by any other means. A thorough discussion of this topic is given in Chapter 11.

1.6 BERNOULLI EQUATION

One particularly useful tool known as the *Bernoulli equation* can be obtained by simplification of the *Navier–Stokes* equations (Equations 1.43a through 1.43c). Specifically, flow is assumed to be inviscid (i.e., the viscous forces are negligible), which then allows the Navier–Stokes equations to be simplified to what is known as *Euler's equation of motion* (Equation 1.46):

$$\frac{\partial \vec{V}}{\partial t} + (\vec{V} \cdot \nabla)\vec{V} = -\frac{1}{\rho}\nabla p + \vec{g} \tag{1.56}$$

As can be seen, the shear stress terms have been set equal to zero since there is no friction in the system. To further simplify the equation of motion, we will focus on flow along a *streamline* (Figure 1.12). A streamline is an imaginary line in the flow field drawn so that it is always tangential to the velocity vectors. The sum of the forces acting on a fluid particle along the streamline is given by

$$\sum F_S = p\,dA - \left(p + \frac{\partial p}{\partial s}ds\right)dA - \rho g(\sin\theta)\,dA\,ds \tag{1.57}$$

where $\sin\theta = dz/ds$.

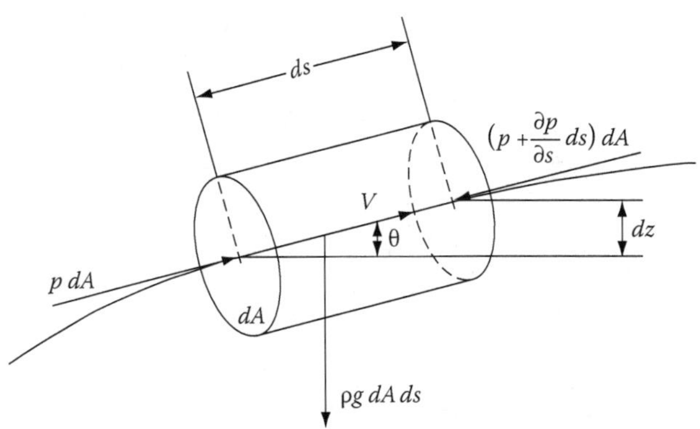

FIGURE 1.12 Force balance for a fluid particle along a streamline.

Substituting this and simplifying Equation 1.57 results in

$$\sum F_S = \left(-\frac{\partial p}{\partial s} ds - \rho g\, dz \right) dA \tag{1.58}$$

Furthermore, fluid acceleration along the streamline curve consists of temporal and spatial components given by

$$\left. \frac{d\vec{V}}{dt} \right|_{tan} = \frac{\partial \vec{V}}{\partial t} + \vec{V} \frac{\partial \vec{V}}{\partial s} \tag{1.59}$$

where $\vec{V}$ has been substituted for $\partial s/\partial t$.

Taking the mass of the particle as $\rho\, dA\, ds$ and inputting Equations 1.58 and 1.59 into Newton's second law of motion gives us

$$\rho\, dA\, ds \left(\frac{\partial \vec{V}}{\partial t} + \vec{V} \frac{\partial \vec{V}}{\partial s} \right) = \left(-\frac{\partial p}{\partial s} ds - \rho g\, dz \right) dA \tag{1.60}$$

Since an equivalent mathematical expression for the term $\vec{V}\partial \vec{V}/\partial s$ is $\partial/\partial s(\vec{V}^2/2)$, we will now substitute this into Equation 1.59 and integrate between any two arbitrary points 1 and 2 to obtain

$$\rho \int_1^2 \frac{\partial \vec{V}}{\partial t} ds + \rho \frac{\left(V_2^2 - V_1^2 \right)}{2} + (p_2 - p_1) + \rho g (z_2 - z_1) = 0 \tag{1.61}$$

Equation 1.61 is known as the *unsteady* form of the *Bernoulli equation* where p_1, V_1, and z_1 are the pressure, velocity, and height at the upstream location, and p_2, V_2, and z_2 are the pressure, velocity, and height at the downstream location. The integral term accounts for the flow acceleration or deceleration between the two locations and for *steady* flow conditions (where $\partial/\partial t = 0$), it becomes zero. Furthermore, since the points 1 and 2 are arbitrary, we can write a general expression of the steady flow Bernoulli equation as

$$p + \rho \frac{V^2}{2} + \rho g z = H \tag{1.62}$$

where p, V, and z are evaluated at any point along the streamline. Here, H is a constant and is referred to as the "total head" or total energy per unit volume of fluid. This terminology is used because even though we derived this equation based on conservation of momentum principles, the terms in Equation 1.62 all have the units of F/L^2 which can equivalently be written as FL/L^3, or energy/volume.

In the absence of frictional losses, then, the Bernoulli equation states that the total mechanical energy per unit volume at any point remains constant. The mechanical energy of a system consists of a pressure energy component (due to static pressure), a kinetic energy component (due to motion), and a potential energy component (due to height) assuming there are no thermal energy changes. Thus, between any two points, the form of the mechanical energy may change from kinetic to potential and vice versa, for example, but the total mechanical energy does not change.

Example 1.4

A syringe is filled with water and held vertically as shown in Figure 1.13. A pressure of 100 mmHg is applied to the fluid by pushing on the plunger. What is the velocity of the fluid leaving the syringe tip and how high will the stream go?

Using Bernoulli equation (1.62), we can solve for the total head, H, by assuming that the elevation in the barrel is zero and that its velocity is negligible (this is reasonable since the cross-sectional areas of the barrel and tip are in a ratio of 100:1). Thus,

$$H = p_1 = 100 \text{ mmHg} \times 1{,}330 \text{ dyn/cm}^2/\text{mmHg}$$

$$= 133{,}000 \text{ dyn/cm}^2$$

The water velocity leaving the syringe tip, V_2, can be calculated knowing that the local (gauge) pressure, p_2, is zero since it is the same as atmospheric. Thus,

$$0 + \frac{1}{2}\rho V_2^2 + \rho g h_2 = 133{,}000 \text{ dyn/cm}^2$$

and

$$V_2 = 514 \text{ cm/s } (=5.14 \text{ m/s})$$

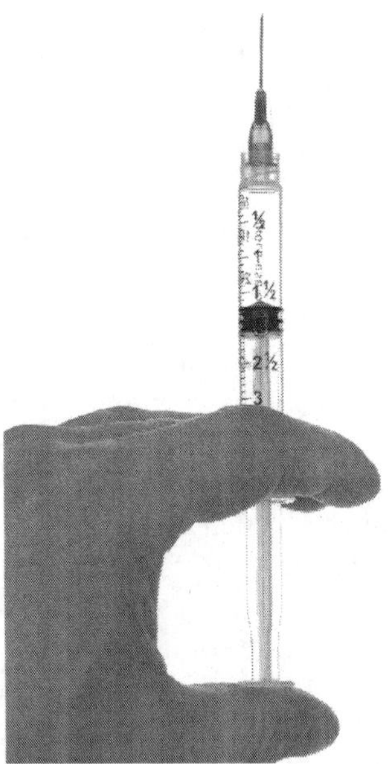

FIGURE 1.13 A jet of flow from a pressurized syringe. (Image purchased from 123rf.com)

Finally, the elevation of the stream, h_3, can be calculated by knowing that it occurs when the local velocity, V_3, becomes zero. Thus,

$$0 + 0 + \rho g h_2 = 133{,}000 \text{ dyn/cm}^2$$

and

$$h_3 = 137 \text{ cm } (=1.37 \text{ m})$$

(*Note*: By conservation of mass, the velocity in the syringe barrel, V_1, would actually be $V_2/100 = 5.14$ cm/s and lead to an error of $\ll$1%.)

The Bernoulli equation also states that the pressure drop between two points located along a streamline at similar heights is only a function of the velocities at these points. Thus, for $z_1 = z_2$, Bernoulli equation simplifies to

$$p_1 - p_2 = \frac{1}{2}\rho(V_2^2 - V_1^2) \tag{1.63}$$

Finally, when the downstream velocity is much higher than the upstream velocity (i.e., $V_2 \gg V_1$), ρV_1^2 can be neglected, and Equation 1.63 can then be further simplified to

$$p_1 - p_2 = \frac{1}{2}\rho V_2^2 \tag{1.64}$$

In the specific case of *blood flow* where we can assume a density of 1.06 g/cm³, Equation 1.64 becomes

$$p_1 - p_2 = 4V_2^2 \tag{1.65}$$

where

p_i is in mmHg
V_2 is in m/s
the constant term, 4, has units of (mmHg/(m/s)²)

Equation 1.65 is referred to as the *simplified Bernoulli equation*, and has found wide application clinically in determining pressure drops across *stenoses*, or vascular obstructions, using velocity measurements made from noninvasive instruments such as Doppler ultrasound and magnetic resonance phase velocity mapping (see Sections 10.6 and 10.8).

It is important to keep in mind that the Bernoulli equation is *not* valid in cases where viscous forces are significant, such as in long constrictions with a small lumen diameter, or in flow separation regions. In addition, it does *not* account for turbulent energy losses in cases of severe stenosis since they are time varying. Such losses should be taken into account in any calculation because they may substantially reduce the energy content of the fluid.

Example 1.5

A patient has a stenotic aortic valve producing a pressure drop between the left ventricle and the aorta. The mean velocity in the left ventricle proximal (upstream) to the valve is 1 m/s while the mean velocity in the aorta distal (downstream) of the valve is 4 m/s. Applying Equation 1.65, the pressure drop across the valve is

$$\begin{aligned} p_1 - p_2 &= 4V_2^2 \\ &= 4(4\,\text{m/s})^2 \\ &= 64\,\text{mmHg} \end{aligned}$$

By comparison, if we include the proximal velocity in the calculation, then the pressure drop reduces to

$$\begin{aligned} p_1 - p_2 &= 4\left(V_2^2 - V_1^2\right) \\ &= 4[(4\,\text{m/s})^2 - (1\,\text{m/s})^2] \\ &= 60\,\text{mmHg} \end{aligned}$$

This example demonstrates an important clinical use of the Bernoulli equation, since the degree of pressure drop is a good indicator of the severity of the stenosis, and thus, of the need for treatment. Unfortunately, it is a somewhat risky and complicated procedure to obtain pressure data directly since it requires inserting a catheter manometer (pressure meter) into the aorta. A much simpler and noninvasive technique (see Section 10.6) is capable of measuring the flow velocity in the valve, thus enabling an estimate of the pressure drop by means of the simplified Bernoulli equation. Several cautions should be observed in using this approach, however, due to the basic assumptions made in deriving the original Bernoulli equation and those made in further simplifying it which may either over- or underestimate its true value.

1.7 DIMENSIONAL ANALYSIS

If we return to the general form of the conservation of momentum or the Navier–Stokes equations, we can write

$$\rho\frac{\partial\vec{V}}{\partial t} + \rho\vec{V}\cdot\nabla\vec{V} = -\nabla p + \rho\vec{g} + \mu\nabla^2\vec{V} \tag{1.66}$$

where

$\rho\partial\vec{V}/\partial t$ is the local acceleration

$\rho\vec{V}\cdot\nabla\vec{V}$ is the convective acceleration

$-\nabla p$ is the pressure force per unit volume

$\rho\vec{g}$ is the body force per unit volume

$\mu\nabla^2\vec{V}$ are the viscous forces per unit volume

If we represent

$$\vec{g} = -\nabla\varphi \tag{1.67}$$

where

$$\varphi = -(g_x x + g_y y + g_z z) \tag{1.68}$$

then

$$-\nabla p + \rho\vec{g} = -\nabla p - \rho\nabla\varphi = -\nabla(p + \rho\varphi) = -\nabla p \tag{1.69}$$

or

$$\rho\frac{\partial\vec{V}}{\partial t} + \rho\vec{V}\cdot\nabla\vec{V} = -\nabla p + \mu\nabla^2\vec{V} \tag{1.70}$$

Based on the principles of *dimensional analysis*, the dependent variables, $\vec{V}$ and p, are functions of the independent variables, x, y, z, and t, as well as the constants, ρ, μ, and $\vec{g}$, along with any other parameters that appear in the boundary conditions. Furthermore, examination of the previous equation shows that each term has units of force per unit volume, or F/L^3. Multiplying numerator and denominator by L results in an equivalent expression $(F \cdot L)/(L^3 \cdot L)$, or energy/(volume $\cdot L$). Now, if we divide each term by a constant having those same units, we would obtain a *dimensionless* equation. For the moment, let us designate a characteristic (i.e., reference or representative) length and a characteristic velocity as L_o and V_o, respectively. Now, the ratio of $\rho V_o^2/L_o$ also has the dimension of $(F \cdot L)/(L^3 \cdot L)$, so multiplying every term by $L_o/\rho V_o^2$ would result in

$$\frac{\partial(\vec{V}/V_o)}{\partial(tV_o/L_o)} + \left(\frac{\vec{V}}{V_o}\right)\cdot(L_o\nabla)\left(\frac{\vec{V}}{V_o}\right) = (L_o\nabla)\left(\frac{p}{\rho V_o^2}\right) + \left(\frac{\mu}{\rho V_o L_o}\right)(L_o^2\nabla^2)\left(\frac{\vec{V}}{V_o}\right) \tag{1.71}$$

where individual terms have been grouped into dimensionless variables defined as

$\Psi = \left(\dfrac{\vec{V}}{V_o}\right)$ dimensionless velocity

$\tilde{\nabla} = L_o\nabla$ dimensionless vector gradient operators

$\mathbf{P} = \left(\dfrac{p}{\rho V_o^2}\right)$ dimensionless pressure

$T = t\left(\dfrac{V_o}{L_o}\right)$ dimensionless time

$Re = \left(\dfrac{\rho V_o L_o}{\mu}\right)$ dimensionless parameter called the Reynolds number

Writing the equation in terms of these dimensionless variables, we get the *dimensionless form* of the *Navier–Stokes equation*:

$$\frac{\partial \Psi}{\partial T} + \Psi \cdot \tilde{\nabla}\Psi = -\tilde{\nabla}p + \frac{1}{Re}\tilde{\nabla}^2\Psi \tag{1.72}$$

For *incompressible* flows, the *dimensionless continuity equation* becomes

$$\tilde{\nabla} \cdot \Psi = 0 \tag{1.73}$$

Examination of Equations 1.72 and 1.73 shows that, for a given value of Re, there is only *one solution* to these equations for each driving function, $\tilde{\nabla}p$. One consequence of this is that by matching values of Re for various systems that are similar but of different scales, it is possible to achieve *dynamic similarity* and obtain predictive information about prototypes from scaled model measurements.

Example 1.6

It is desired to study the fluid dynamics in a coronary artery (diameter = 3 mm) using a laser Doppler velocimetry (see Section 10.7). However, the resolution of the LDV system is 300 μm, resulting in a maximum of 10 velocity points across the artery diameter and low accuracy for obtaining wall shear stresses from the fitted velocity profile. In order to improve the resolution by ×10, an *in vitro* model is constructed with a diameter of 3 cm. What flow rate should be used to ensure dynamic similarity between the model and the prototype? (Assume the working fluid has the same kinematic viscosity as blood: $\nu = 0.035\ \text{cm}^2/\text{s}$.)

Since $D_p = 3$ mm, $D_m = 30$ mm, dynamic similarity can only be achieved if

$$Re_m = Re_p$$

or

$$\frac{V_m D_m}{\nu_m} = \frac{V_p D_p}{\nu_p}$$

For $\nu_m = \nu_p$,

$$V_m = \frac{D_p}{D_m} V_p = 0.1 V_p$$

Therefore, flow in the model must be

$$Q_m = V_m\left(\frac{\pi D_m^2}{4}\right) = 0.1 V_p\left(\frac{\pi (10 D_p)^2}{4}\right) = 10 Q_p$$

1.8 FLUID MECHANICS IN A STRAIGHT TUBE

Much of the blood flow in the human circulation occurs within tubular structures—arteries, capillaries, veins, and so on. It is for that reason that the study of fluid mechanics in a straight tube is of particular interest in biofluid mechanics.

While the human vasculature is not strictly a series of straight tubes of constant diameter, results from this analysis do provide good estimates or starting points for further evaluation. Before we look at this topic in detail, however, we need to make several definitions of terms that are relevant to common flow conditions.

Blood flow in the circulatory system is invariably unsteady and, in most regions (e.g., the systemic arteries and the microcirculation), it is pulsatile. The term "unsteady" is very general and refers to any type of flow, which is simply not constant. If the flow has a periodic behavior *and* a net directional motion over the cycle (i.e., the average flow is >0), then it is called *pulsatile*. On the other hand, if the flow has a periodic behavior but oscillates back and forth *without* a net forward or reverse output (i.e., the average flow = 0), it is called *oscillatory flow*. Despite the fact that blood flow is unsteady, it is helpful to first describe the principles of fluid flow under more simplified conditions, before moving to complex physiological situations. The simplest case to consider, therefore, is that of steady flow of a Newtonian fluid through a straight, rigid, circular tube aligned in a horizontal position (see Section 1.5.3.2).

1.8.1 Flow Stability and Related Characteristics

The nature of flow of a Newtonian fluid in a straight, rigid, circular tube is controlled by the inertial (accelerating) and the viscous (decelerating) forces applied to the fluid elements. When *viscous* forces dominate, the flow is called *laminar*, and is characterized by a smooth motion of the fluid. Laminar flow can be thought of as if the fluid is divided into a number of layers flowing parallel to each other without any disturbances or mixing between the layers. On the other hand, when *inertial* forces strongly dominate, the flow is called *turbulent*. Here, the fluid exhibits a disturbed, random motion in all directions, which is superimposed on its repeatable, main motion.

1.8.1.1 Steady Laminar Flow

The key characteristic of laminar flow is that it is very orderly and very energy efficient, whereas turbulent flow is chaotic and accompanied by high energy losses. Therefore, turbulent flow is undesirable in the blood circulation because of the excessive workload it would put on the heart and also because of potential damage to blood cells. A useful index used to determine whether the flow in a tube is laminar or turbulent is the ratio of its inertial properties to its viscous properties. This ratio is classically known as the *Reynolds number* (*Re*), which is dimensionless since both terms have the same units $[F \cdot T/L^2]$. It is defined as

$$Re = \frac{\text{Inertial forces}}{\text{Viscous forces}} = \frac{\rho V d}{\mu} \tag{1.74}$$

where

ρ (kg/m^3) is the density of the fluid
V (m/s) is the average velocity of the fluid over the cross section of the tube
d (m) is the tube diameter
μ (kg/m · s) is the dynamic viscosity of the fluid

Although inertial forces obviously begin to dominate for $Re > 1$, it has been determined experimentally that in a smooth-surfaced tube, flow is laminar for all conditions where $Re < 2100$. Within this range, the viscous or "retarding" forces are sufficient to suppress any tendency for the flow to gain so much inertia as to become "chaotic." Due to our assumption in Section 1.5.3.2 that the flow was steady, Equation 1.55 will *only* be valid for laminar flow conditions—that is, $Re < 2100$. Furthermore, if the tube is long enough to have stabilized any entrance effects that are present (see Section 1.8.1.3), then the velocity profile takes on a parabolic shape and the flow is called *fully developed* laminar flow.

1.8.1.2 Turbulent Flow

For $Re > 2100$, the flow starts to become turbulent in parts of the fluid and particle motions begin to vary with time. Such flow is called *transitional flow*, and the range of Re for which this type of flow exists varies considerably, depending upon the application (i.e., system configuration and stability) and the roughness of the tube surface. Usually, flows in a smooth-surfaced tube with $2100 < Re < 4000$ are characterized as transitional. Fully developed *turbulent flow* is observed starting at $Re = 10^4$ for a rough-surfaced tube and starting at $Re = 10^8$ for a smooth-surfaced tube. The velocity profile of fully developed turbulent flow is flatter than that for laminar flow, although it is not considered uniform or "plug" flow (Figure 1.14).

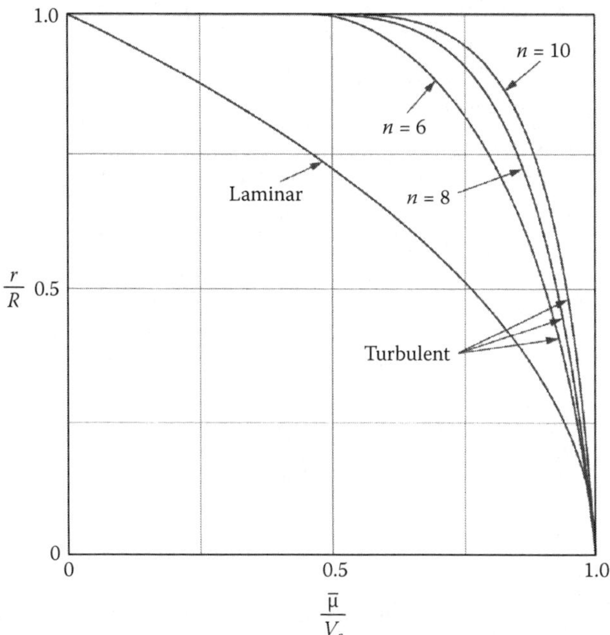

FIGURE 1.14 Plots of laminar (Poiseuille) and turbulent velocity profiles for $n = 6$, 8, and 10.

In order to quantitatively describe turbulent flow, we think of the instantaneous velocity, $V(t)$, at a given radial location as the sum of a time-averaged mean velocity, $\overline{V}$(m/s), and a randomly fluctuating velocity component, V'(m/s), or

$$V(t) = \overline{V} + V' \tag{1.75}$$

Expressing turbulent flow in this way allows us to separate out one component of a given variable which can be quantified and expressed as an analytic function while also allowing us to modify each variable by superimposing a random, disorderly motion on top of it. In the case of velocity, the mean velocity profile (i.e., the quantifiable component) of a fully developed turbulent flow at $Re < 10^5$ is described by

$$\overline{V} = \overline{V}_{max}\left(1 - \frac{r}{R}\right)^{1/n} \tag{1.76}$$

where
$\overline{V}$ (m/s) is the time-averaged velocity at a distance r from the center of the tube
$\overline{V}_{max}$ (m/s) is the maximum (centerline) time-averaged velocity

The exponent, $1/n$ (where $6 < n < 10$), is not constant but decreases as Re increases. When $n = 7$, for example, the average cross-sectional velocity is equal to 4/5 of the maximum centerline velocity. This illustrates the flatter nature of the velocity profile compared with that for the laminar flow case. The reason for this is that axial momentum under turbulent conditions is rapidly transported across the tube diameter due to nonzero radial velocity components, reaching a plateau level closer to the tube wall. Under laminar flow, this can only occur as a result of relatively slow viscous interactions between layers since radial velocity is zero. The amount of turbulence present in a flow field is quantified by the *turbulence intensity*, I, and can be determined by

$$I = \frac{V_{rms}}{\overline{V}_{ave}} 100\% \tag{1.77}$$

where $V_{rms} = \sqrt{\overline{V'^2}}$ is the root mean square of the fluctuating velocity (m/s).

It should be emphasized that blood flow in the circulatory system is normally laminar, although in the ascending aorta it can destabilize briefly during the deceleration phase of late systole; however, this time period is generally too short for flow to become fully turbulent. Certain disease conditions, though, can alter this condition and produce turbulent blood flow, particularly downstream of an arterial stenosis (a vessel narrowing, usually due to atherosclerosis), distal to defective (i.e., stenotic or regurgitant) heart valves or distal to prosthetic heart valves.

1.8.1.3 Flow Development

We should further point out that the aforementioned velocity profiles, both laminar and turbulent, are only valid in a *fully developed flow region*—that is, at a distance in a straight, smooth-surfaced tube that is far enough from the entrance for any upstream disturbances to have dissipated. These disturbances can be caused by a number of geometric changes or discontinuities such as vessel curvature or taper, or presence of a bifurcation, an anastomosis, an aneurysm, or an occlusion, and so on. The effects of these flow disturbances are significant only in the immediate region downstream of the discontinuity. It is in this region that "flow development" or stabilization occurs and, downstream of this region, the flow profile is called "fully developed." Even though these changes are occurring in the flow, it is important to remember that, in both the flow development and the fully developed flow regions, the no-slip condition at the wall remains valid and that the average velocity across the tube will remain the same for a constant cross-sectional area because of the *principle of mass conservation.*

An illustration of a flow development region can be seen in Figure 1.15, which shows the flow field in a small diameter tube downstream of a gradual outlet from a large tank.

Immediately after entering the tube, the flow profile is essentially flat since the flow is dominated by higher velocity particles near the tube center. Just downstream of the entrance, the layer of fluid closest to the wall decelerates as some particles adhere to the wall (dashed lines in Figure 1.15). It then slows adjacent inner fluid layers through viscous (shear) forces. At the same time, the fluid layers near the center of the tube accelerate since the axial pressure drop is not opposed by large frictional forces in this region. This acceleration is also necessary in order to satisfy the mass conservation principle. The region of flow near the tube inner surface where viscosity effects alter the velocity profile is called the *boundary layer.*

For *laminar* flow, the thickness of this boundary layer, δ, increases with distance downstream because of the continued action of significant drag or retarding forces acting on the fluid through its viscosity by the tube wall. When the boundary layer finally grows enough to fill the entire tube cross section (i.e., $\delta = D/2$), the flow is said to have become *fully developed*—that is, there is no room left for further adjustment to take place. From this position on, all flow conditions (velocity profile, pressure gradient, etc.) remain constant. For *turbulent* flow, the viscous forces are insignificant compared with inertial forces (as seen by the extremely high *Re* values

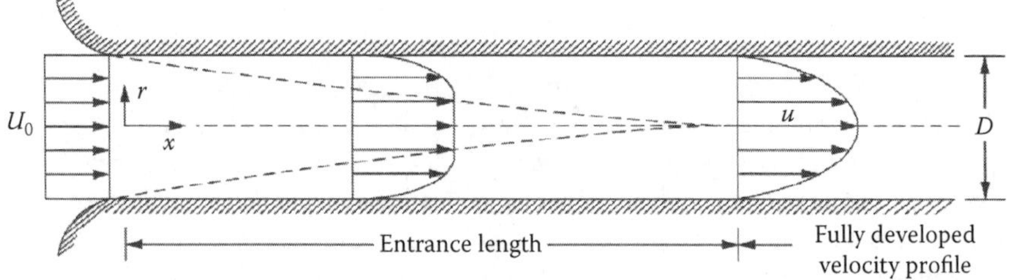

FIGURE 1.15 Flow development from a uniform to a parabolic velocity profile in the entrance region of a pipe (dashed lines indicate the viscous boundary layer).

required for turbulence) everywhere except in a small region very close to the wall. Here, there is a laminar (since the local Re is relatively low) boundary layer that is very thin. For both laminar and turbulent cases, the axial length required for this flow development to occur, known as the *entrance length*, L_e, can be estimated as

$$L_e = 0.06 \cdot d \cdot Re \quad \text{for } laminar \text{ flow} \tag{1.78}$$

$$L_e = 0.693 \cdot d \cdot Re^{1/4} \quad \text{for } turbulent \text{ flow} \tag{1.79}$$

Example 1.7

For flow in the proximal aorta with a diameter of ~2.5 cm (0.025 m) and an average velocity of ~0.25 m/s, the Reynolds number would be

$$Re = \frac{\rho VD}{\mu} = (1.07\,\text{g/cm}^3 \times 25\,\text{cm/s} \times 2.5\,\text{cm})/(0.035\,\text{P}) \quad \text{(in CGS system)}$$
$$\approx 1900$$

This would result in an entrance length on the order of 2.5–3 m. Since an adult human aorta is <1 m in length, this means that flow would be within an entrance length in the *entire* aorta, implying that it never becomes fully developed.

Example 1.8

Flow in the intercostal arteries derives from the thoracic aorta (diameter of ~2.0 cm) as they branch off to perfuse the musculature of the chest wall. These vessels have a diameter of ~2 mm with an average velocity of ~10 cm/s. Therefore, the Reynolds number would be

$$Re = \frac{\rho VD}{\mu} = (1.07\,\text{g/cm}^3 \times 10\,\text{cm/s} \times 0.2\,\text{cm})/(0.035\,\text{P})$$
$$\approx 60$$

In this case, the entrance length would be on the order of 0.7 cm. As a result, flow development occurs in a relatively short distance and the majority of the intercostal artery (several centimeters long) experiences Poiseuille-type flow (in the mean).

1.8.1.4 Viscous and Turbulent Shear Stress

In the study of hemodynamics and, in particular, of vascular disease, one of the most important variables is the shear stress, τ (N/m^2), at the vessel wall (τ_w). Wall shear stress has considerable clinical relevance because it provides information about both the magnitude of the force that the blood exerts on the vessel wall as well as the force exerted by one fluid layer on another. In healthy blood vessels, the shear stress is generally low (~15–20 dyn/cm^2) and is not harmful either to the blood cells or to the cells that line the inner surface of the vessel, called *endothelial cells*. Shear stress varies with flow conditions (cardiac output [CO], heart rate [HR], etc.) as well as with the local geometry of the vessel (curves, branches, etc.) as will be discussed in later sections. Excessively high levels of shear stress caused, for example, by atherosclerotic lesions or artificial heart valves, may damage the red blood cells (a condition called "hemolysis") or the endothelium of the vessel wall. Other abnormal shear stresses, such as very low or strongly oscillatory shear stresses, may also change the biological behavior of some cells such as platelets in the blood stream in which they become activated, leading to thrombus formation. These stresses may also act on endothelial cells lining the vessel wall which then secrete vasoactive compounds, leading to vessel constriction or wall hypertrophy. (*Note*: Each of the above topics will be discussed in greater detail in Sections 6.4 and 6.5.)

Based on our earlier discussions, we can readily determine the shear stress for laminar flow of a Newtonian fluid as being linearly related to the shear rate (du/dr) according to Equation 1.1 expressed in terms of cylindrical coordinates:

$$\tau = \mu \frac{\partial u}{\partial y} \tag{1.1}$$

where

u is the velocity (m/s) at radial position r (m)

μ is the dynamic viscosity (N s/m^2) of the fluid

For turbulent flow, we said that the boundary layer is very thin and the velocity profile is flatter than for laminar flow. The combination of a flatter profile with the no-slip condition at the wall results in much higher shear rates and, thus, wall shear stresses for turbulent flow are large as compared with laminar flow. For either case (laminar or turbulent), the wall shear stress can be determined from a force balance within a control volume if the pressure drop, Δp, is known along a length L of the tube (refer again to Figure 1.10):

$$\tau_w = -\frac{d}{4}\frac{\Delta p}{L}$$

or,

$$\tau_w = \frac{4\mu Q}{\pi R^3} \tag{1.80}$$

after substituting the expression for Δp in Hagen–Poiseuille flow from Equation 1.55.

As mentioned earlier, both viscous and turbulent shear stresses, if large enough, can potentially activate or lyse (i.e., rupture) blood cells. However, the origin, and consequently, the scale of viscous and turbulent shear stresses are different. Viscous shear stresses act on a molecular scale—that is, they arise from the tendency of one molecule to remain in close proximity to its neighbors. This is quantified in fluids through the measure of their "viscosity." Since viscous stresses act on a scale much smaller than the diameter of a blood cell (which is on the order of a few microns), blood cells will always experience a viscous shear stress if one is present. In contrast, turbulent shear stresses arise from the inertia contained within the fluctuations of turbulent flow and are defined as the product of the instantaneous velocity fluctuations times the fluid density, or

$$\tau = -\rho(\overline{U'V'}) \tag{1.81}$$

for turbulence along two axes (x and y). These stresses act on a scale comparable with the length of the smallest turbulent fluctuations which are often much larger than the diameter of a blood cell. Thus, if such a turbulent shear stress is present, a blood cell may not experience it, particularly if it resides within a turbulent eddy.

1.8.2 Effect of Flow Pulsatility

The previous section outlined the characteristics of *steady* flow in a tube when the driving pressure gradient is constant. However, we said earlier that blood flow in the heart and arteries is quite pulsatile, meaning that the pressure and velocity profiles vary periodically (here, the period denotes the duration of a cardiac cycle[s]) with time. When the heart contracts during systole, a pressure originates from the left ventricle which then travels out as a *wave* due to the elasticity of the arteries. The most immediate consequence of this is that the pressure in the left ventricle (upstream) exceeds that in the aorta (downstream) resulting in opening of the aortic valve and the blood being ejected from the heart. Due to the compliant nature of the arteries and their finite thickness, the pressure travels like a sound wave at a speed which is much faster than the flow velocity (~500:1). The pulsatile nature of the flow also affects the pressure distribution out into the vessels and the velocity profiles within them as well as the point of transition from a laminar to a turbulent regime. This later effect is due to the fact that flow accelerates rapidly in early systole, when, based on the instantaneous Reynolds number in the ascending aorta, flow would be expected to be turbulent during a major part of systole. Despite this, however, it has been observed that aortic blood flow remains laminar and well streamlined under these conditions. The reason for this is partly due to the stabilizing effect that systolic acceleration has on the flow. One might anticipate, then, that the onset of turbulence would occur during the later part of systole when flow decelerates. This has, in fact, been shown by the presence of erratic fluctuations in velocity recordings (Figure 1.16).

The flow destabilization that occurs in late systole is mainly due to the development of an adverse (i.e., against the flow) pressure gradient during the flow deceleration, but that is not the entire reason. Additionally, flow in the aorta does not become turbulent as soon or to the degree expected based on the instantaneous *Re* values because there is not sufficient time available for flow to become turbulent. To understand this, think of turbulence as a *process* that requires both a minimum amount of energy to be present *and* a triggering or seeding mechanism to initiate it. In this case, the triggering is provided by some "disturbance" to the flow (e.g., a surface roughness or an external vibration) at some site. For "fully developed" turbulence

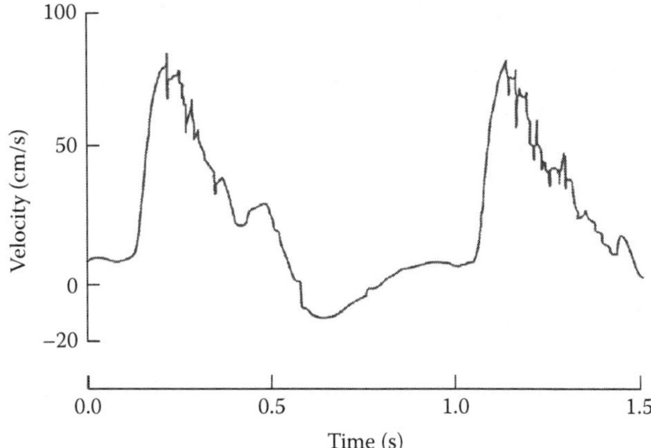

FIGURE 1.16 Disturbances during flow deceleration phase in a pulsatile (periodic unsteady) flow velocity patterns in the aorta. (Redrawn from *Cardiovasc. Res.*, 5, Seed, W.A. and Wood, N.B., 319–330, Copyright (1971), with permission from Elsevier.)

to occur, however, this disturbance must propagate throughout the entire flow field. With steady flow, these conditions are always present but with pulsatile flow, they only exist for a limited time (up to the cycle period) and then they reverse. Therefore, in a healthy artery, turbulence is generally absent because the flow destabilization time interval (mid-to-end systole) is short (~150 ms) and is immediately followed by diastole when the velocity and instantaneous *Re* are low. When the subsequent systolic phase begins, a new acceleration phase restabilizes the flow. It should be pointed out here that, although complex vortex-containing flows are present in regions like bifurcations or branches, such flow is not necessarily turbulent in the sense that it is either random or unpredictable. Many of these flows contain very laminar flow behavior, just not simply in linear directions.

Based on the earlier discussion, *Re* alone is clearly not enough to completely characterize pulsatile flow. Another dimensionless parameter, the *Womersley number* (denoted as α), is also used to characterize the periodic nature of blood flow. The definition of α is

$$\alpha = \frac{d}{2}\sqrt{\frac{\rho\omega}{\mu}} \tag{1.82}$$

where ω (radians/s) is the HR. The Womersley number in unsteady flow has a physical significance similar to that of *Re* in steady flow in that it provides a comparison between *unsteady* inertial forces and viscous forces. In the human circulatory system, α ranges from 10^{-3} in capillaries to nearly 20 in the ascending aorta at rest. When α < 1.0, viscous forces dominate in every region in the tube and the conditions are known as *quasi-steady* flow. As α increases, the inertial forces become more important and start to dominate, initiating at the center of the tube. As a result, a delay (with respect to the driving pressure gradient) can be observed in the bulk flow, and the velocity profile becomes flat in the central region of the tube.

Example 1.9

The ascending aorta has a diameter $d = 2.5$ cm, and the HR is 70 bpm. The density, ρ, and the viscosity of blood, μ, are 1.06 g/cm^3 and 0.035 P, respectively. Based on these data, the Womersley parameter would be

$$\alpha = \frac{d}{2}\sqrt{\frac{\rho\omega}{\mu}}$$

$$= \frac{2.5}{2}\sqrt{\frac{1.06 \cdot 2\pi(70/60)}{0.035}}$$

$$= 18.6$$

What this example illustrates is that flow in the major arteries is characterized by both large mean flow and large oscillatory flow components due to the intermittent nature of the heart pump. As we will see later in Chapter 6, the Womersley parameter is an important index of the net amount of forward flow and the shape of the local velocity profile.

1.9 BOUNDARY LAYER SEPARATION

As we described earlier for flow development in a circular tube, when a moving fluid contacts a solid boundary, the fluid immediately adjacent to the boundary takes on the same velocity as the boundary. Since this velocity is usually different from that of the free stream, a transition must occur between the two locations, and, thus, a *boundary layer* is formed (Figure 1.10). The boundary layer is the region in which flow velocity changes from zero (relative to the wall) to the value of the free stream. Although boundary layers may actually be extremely thin, they are very important because it is *only* in this region of the flow that viscous effects are significant. This may seem paradoxical since the fluid has the same viscosity everywhere. However, for a force to be exerted between fluid layers (i.e., presence of a shear stress), there must be both a nonzero viscosity *and* a nonzero shear rate. These requirements are satisfied in the boundary layer where velocity varies with distance but they are not satisfied in the main flow where velocity is nearly uniform. As the fluid proceeds downstream, viscous diffusion occurs further into the free stream as slower near-wall layers interact with faster free stream layers and viscous effects are felt at a greater depth from the wall—thus, it is said that the boundary layer "grows."

When a fluid encounters a solid object and flows over it, it is forced to deviate from an axial direction and, thus, changes direction in order to pass around the body (Figure 1.17). For this redirection to occur, a pressure gradient must exist. The presence of an *adverse pressure gradient* (i.e., a pressure gradient acting *against* the flow direction and tending to decrease the fluid velocity) may have a magnitude that is large enough to cause the fluid within the boundary layer to stop and deflect away from the surface. When this happens, *boundary layer separation* is said to have occurred. Boundary layer separation begins at a *separation point* on the boundary, which is defined as a location where not only is the flow velocity, u, equal to zero, but the rate of change of u along a direction normal to the surface, n, is also zero,

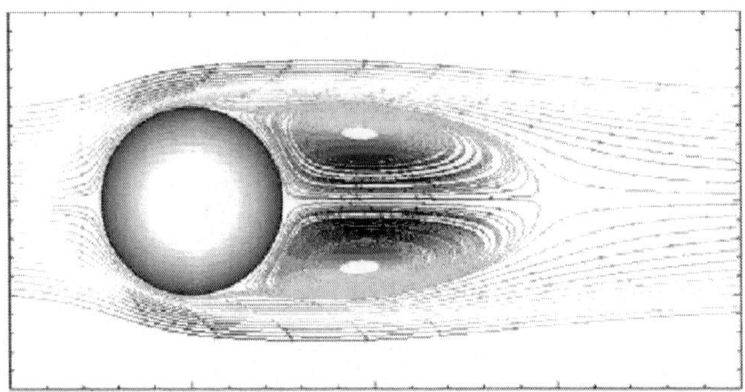

FIGURE 1.17 Laminar flow past a sphere (Re = 250), streamlines: symmetrical plane. (With permission from Computer Systems Support, College of Engineering, The University of Iowa, Iowa City, IA.)

or $\partial u/\partial n = 0$. Beyond the separation point, there may exist a region of reversed, turbulent, or disturbed flow where recirculating or vortical flows are commonly seen. These characteristics are important biologically since they can lead to reverse and/or oscillatory shear stresses and to long particle residence times, both of which can have a wide variety of clinical implications, including the initiation of atherosclerosis (see Sections 6.5 and 6.7).

In pulsatile flows, flow separation can be generated by a geometric adverse pressure gradient or by time-varying changes in the driving pressure. Geometric adverse pressure gradients, for example, are present behind all prosthetic heart valves because of their small orifice areas. As the area downstream of a prosthetic heart valve increases, the mean flow velocity must decrease in accordance with the continuity equation. This decrease in velocity is also accompanied by an adverse pressure gradient due to the energy balance. Similar effects are seen as a result of the contractile nature of the heart in which blood flow experiences both acceleration and deceleration during a cardiac cycle. An adverse pressure gradient exists during the deceleration phase of a particular flow and may lead to boundary layer separation. Consequently, flow separation is even more likely in regions where *both* geometric and temporal adverse pressure gradients exist (e.g., arterial stenoses, stenotic heart valves, prosthetic heart valves, and aneurysms).

PROBLEMS

1.1 For *Hagen–Poiseuille* flow, show that the shear stress at the tube wall ($\tau_w = \tau_{r=R}$) can be written as

$$|\tau_w| = \frac{4\mu Q}{\pi R^3}$$

1.2 For a laminar flow of a Newtonian fluid in a tube of circular cross section,

a. Show that the mean velocity over the cross section is ½ of the peak velocity in the tube.

b. Show that the ratio of mean shear to the wall shear rate is 2/3.

1.3 What *pressure* will be required to force 1 cm^3/s of blood serum through an intravenous tube of radius 0.50 mm and length 3 cm and into an artery with a mean pressure of 100 mmHg?
(*Assume*: Blood serum viscosity, $\mu = 7 \times 10^{-3}$ P)

1.4 A patient has atherosclerosis that produces a stenosis of his aorta of 16% diameter reduction.

a. What is the resultant *reduction in flow rate*?
b. Assuming laminar flow, how much *pressure increase* is necessary to compensate for this reduction?

REFERENCE

Seed, W. A. and Wood, N. B. (1971) Velocity patterns in the aorta. *Cardiovasc. Res.* 5: 319–330.

2 Introduction to Solid Mechanics

As blood flows throughout the arterial system in the human circulation, there is a constant interaction between the flowing blood and the wall of the arteries. In order to study the unsteady blood flow dynamics in the arteries, it becomes necessary to consider the material behavior of the arterial wall. In this chapter, the basic stress–strain relationship for an elastic material is reviewed and basic relationships for stresses in thin-walled and thick-walled cylindrical tubes are derived that will be useful in modeling unsteady blood flow in the arteries. A brief discussion on viscoelastic behavior of materials is also included as this has significance in the force-deformation behavior of the arterial wall.

2.1 INTRODUCTION TO MECHANICS OF MATERIALS

2.1.1 Elastic Behavior

A material is defined to be *elastic* if it deforms when a force is applied to it, but returns to its original configuration without energy dissipation when the applied force is removed. Consider the uniform thin cylindrical wire shown in Figure 2.1a with an undeformed length ℓ_0 subjected to a normal tensile load P. The wire will elongate by a magnitude δ due to the axial load. The average normal stress that the wire is subjected to can be computed as $\sigma = P/A$, where A is the cross-sectional area of the wire in the *undeformed* configuration. The normal stress has the units of force per unit area. In the SI system, stress has the dimensions of N/m^2 and is referred to as pascal (Pa). The magnitudes for stress occurring in engineering practice are relatively large and hence prefixes such as kPa (kilopascal = 10^3 Pa), MPa (megapascal = 10^6 Pa), or GPa (gigapascal = 10^9 Pa) are usually employed. When the wire is stretched in the axial direction, there will be a reduction in the cross-sectional area. This fact can be demonstrated easily by stretching an elastic band and it can be observed that the cross-sectional area decreases with increase in axial stretch. The decrease in dimensions is not large enough to be observed by visual inspection in most engineering materials. In usual engineering practice, the stress is defined based on the cross-sectional area of the undeformed configuration rather than the instantaneous value and the error introduced will be negligible.

The ratio of the increment in length over the initial length is defined as the normal strain. This relationship is given by

$$\varepsilon = \frac{\ell - \ell_0}{\ell_0} = \frac{\delta}{\ell_0} \tag{2.1}$$

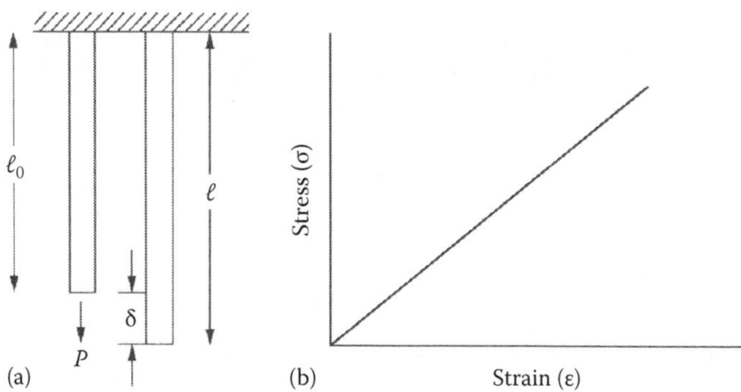

FIGURE 2.1 Stress–strain behavior of Hookean elastic material: (a) a specimen with an initial length ℓ_0 is shown to deform to the final length ℓ with an axial load P; (b) the resulting linear stress–strain plot for a material that follows the Hooke's law.

In this equation, ℓ is the instantaneous length. By varying the load, the applied stress can be varied and by measuring the increase in length, the corresponding strain can be obtained. The normal strain, ε, defined earlier is the ratio of length units and hence is dimensionless. However, it is a common practice to specify normal strain as m/m or mm/mm. In engineering applications, the strain will be very small and will be in the range of 10^{-6} m/m or μm/m.

The stress–strain relationship for an ideal linear elastic material is shown in Figure 2.1b. The slope of the stress–strain plot is a constant, E referred to as the *elastic modulus* or *Young's modulus*. A material exhibiting a linear stress–strain relationship is known as a *Hookean* elastic material named after Robert Hooke who demonstrated such a behavior in 1678. The Hookean relationship can be expressed as

$$\sigma = E\varepsilon \tag{2.2}$$

It is apparent that the elastic modulus will have the same units as of stress. A material is said to be *homogeneous* if the elastic modulus, E, is same at every point of the bar. This will result in the elongation being uniformly distributed along the length of the bar. A material is defined as *isotropic* if the stress–strain behavior does not change if the direction of loading is changed. The stress–strain diagram will be linear until the proportionality limit is reached and then the relationship will become nonlinear. Engineering materials can be divided into two broad categories based on the stress–strain relationship. Figure 2.2 shows the typical stress–strain relationship for a *ductile* and for a *brittle* material. For a ductile material, the stress initially increases linearly with strain until a critical value of the yield stress, σ_y, is reached. If the applied stress exceeds the yield stress for the material, the material will be subject to a large deformation with a small increase in load exhibiting plastic deformation. After the maximum value of stress, or the ultimate stress, σ_{ult} has been reached, the diameter of a region of the specimen decreases significantly—this phenomenon is referred to as *necking*. After necking occurs, a lower load is sufficient to induce further deformation of the specimen until rupture takes place. The load to induce rupture is known as the breaking strength, σ_b, of the material. In the case of a brittle material, there is no noticeable change in the rate of elongation before rupture

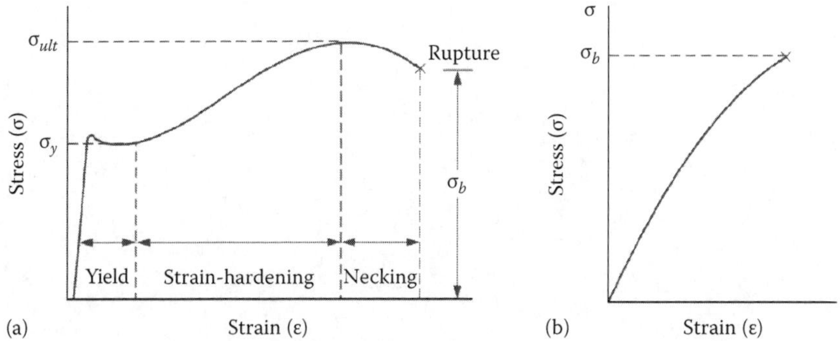

FIGURE 2.2 Stress–strain diagrams for typical ductile (a) and brittle (b) material.

takes place. In such a material, the ultimate strength and the breaking strength are the same. Any material for which the stress–strain curve does *not* follow the linear relationship is classified as being nonlinear. We will observe later that most biological materials generally do not exhibit a linear stress–strain relationship.

2.1.2 Engineering and True Strain

In Equation 2.1, we defined strain as

$$\varepsilon = \frac{\ell - \ell_0}{\ell_0} = \frac{\delta}{\ell_0}$$

This relationship is defined as the engineering strain where the ratio of the elongation δ and the initial length of the specimen ℓ_0 are used. However, strain can also be computed by using the successive values of the instantaneous length as they are recorded. Taking the value of the instantaneous length and the corresponding increment in length, the true strain, ε_t, can be defined as

$$\varepsilon_t = \sum \Delta\varepsilon = \sum \frac{\Delta\ell}{\ell}$$

Replacing the summation by integrals, the true strain can be expressed as

$$\varepsilon_t = \int_{\ell_0}^{\ell} \frac{d\ell}{\ell} = \ln\frac{\ell}{\ell_0} \tag{2.3}$$

The relationship between the true strain and the engineering strain can be obtained as

$$\varepsilon_t = \ln(1+\varepsilon) \tag{2.4}$$

In most of the engineering materials undergoing small deformations and strains, the magnitude of engineering strain will be very close to that of the true strain.

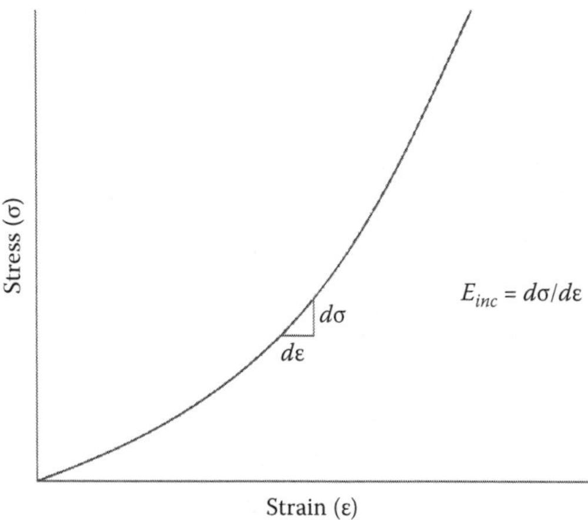

FIGURE 2.3 Schematic of a nonlinear stress versus strain relationship for biological soft tissue.

2.1.3 Incremental Elastic Modulus

As shown in Figure 2.1, any material that follows Hooke's law will exhibit a linear stress–strain relationship. However, when the material does not follow Hooke's law, it will have a nonlinear stress–strain relationship as shown in Figure 2.3. In such cases, an elastic modulus can be defined as the slope of the curve at any value of the stress and the corresponding strain. This value is called the *incremental modulus* and is given by the relationship

$$E_{inc} = \frac{d\sigma}{d\varepsilon} \tag{2.5}$$

The incremental elastic modulus (and the material stiffness) increases with the increase in slope of the nonlinear stress–strain curve schematically shown.

2.1.4 Poisson's Ratio

As discussed earlier, when a slender bar is loaded axially (Figure 2.4), an axial elongation takes place and a linear stress–strain relationship is observed within the elastic limit. In this case, the normal strain can be given by the relationship (from Equation 2.2)

$$\varepsilon_x = \frac{\sigma_x}{E} \tag{2.6}$$

In this equation, subscript x denotes the coordinate along the axial direction. It was also pointed out earlier that when the bar elongates axially there would be a corresponding contraction in the transverse directions. In other words, even if there is

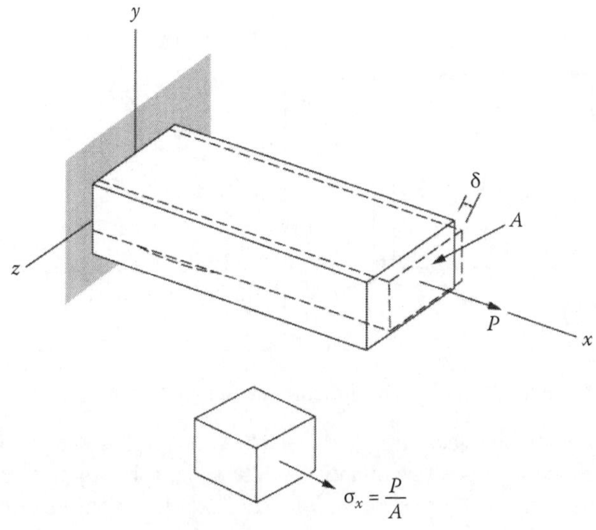

FIGURE 2.4 An axially loaded slender bar.

no applied stress in the transverse directions, there will be strains present in those directions. The *Poisson's ratio* is defined as

$$\nu = \left| \frac{\text{lateral strain}}{\text{axial strain}} \right|$$

or

$$\nu = -\frac{\varepsilon_y}{\varepsilon_x} = -\frac{\varepsilon_z}{\varepsilon_x} \tag{2.7}$$

In this relationship, the material is assumed to be isotropic so that the transverse strain in the *y*- and *z*-directions is the same. The negative sign in Equation 2.7 is introduced to make the Poisson's ratio a positive quantity since ε_y will be negative for a positive ε_x and *vice versa*. From Equations 2.6 and 2.7, we can derive

$$\varepsilon_x = \frac{\sigma_x}{E} \quad \text{and} \quad \varepsilon_y = \varepsilon_z = -\nu \frac{\sigma_x}{E} \tag{2.8}$$

2.1.5 Shearing Stresses and Strains

In Figure 2.5, a planar element is shown which is subjected to *shearing stresses* τ_{xy} and τ_{yx}. The first subscript of each variable denotes that the shearing stress acts on a plane perpendicular to the axis denoted by that subscript and the second subscript denotes the direction of the shear stress. The effect of such stresses will be to deform the element such that two of the angles are reduced from $\pi/2$ to $(\pi/2) - \gamma_{xy}$ while the other two angles are increased from $\pi/2$ to $(\pi/2) + \gamma_{xy}$. The small angle γ_{xy}, expressed in radians, is defined as the *shearing strain*. When the deformation results in a reduction

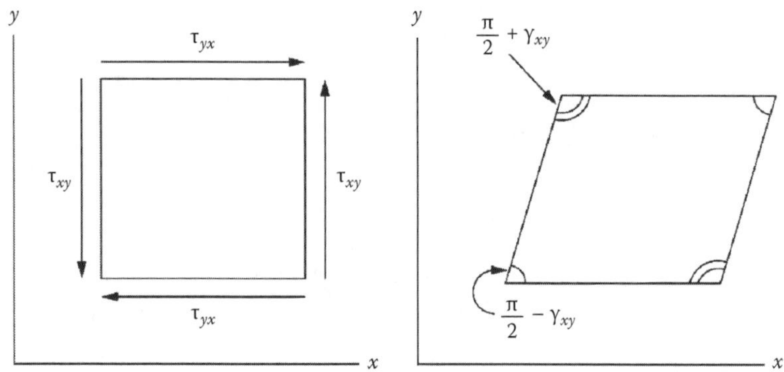

FIGURE 2.5 An element subjected to shearing stresses.

of an angle formed by two faces oriented toward the positive x- and y-axes, the shearing strain is defined as a *positive* quantity—otherwise, it is negative. By measuring the values of the shearing strains for various values of the shearing stresses, a shear stress–strain diagram can be plotted for each material. The plots will be similar to those obtained for the axial stress–strain relationship. For shearing stress values that do not exceed the elastic limit, a Hooke's law for shear can be written as

$$\tau_{xy} = G\gamma_{xy} \tag{2.9}$$

In this relationship, G is the *modulus of rigidity* or the *shear modulus*. In a similar manner for a homogeneous isotropic material, two additional relationships can be written as

$$\tau_{yz} = G\gamma_{yz} \quad \text{and} \quad \tau_{zx} = G\gamma_{zx} \tag{2.10}$$

2.1.6 Generalized Hooke's Law

Consider the general stress condition represented in Figure 2.6. As long as none of the stresses represented here exceed the proportional or elastic limit, the *principle of superposition* can be applied and we can write the generalized Hooke's law as given as follows:

$$\begin{aligned}
\varepsilon_x &= \frac{\sigma_x}{E} - \frac{\nu\sigma_y}{E} - \frac{\nu\sigma_z}{E} \\
\varepsilon_y &= \frac{\sigma_y}{E} - \frac{\nu\sigma_x}{E} - \frac{\nu\sigma_z}{E} \\
\varepsilon_z &= \frac{\sigma_z}{E} - \frac{\nu\sigma_x}{E} - \frac{\nu\sigma_y}{E} \\
\gamma_{xy} &= \frac{\tau_{xy}}{G}; \quad \gamma_{yz} = \frac{\tau_{yz}}{G}; \quad \gamma_{zx} = \frac{\tau_{zx}}{G}
\end{aligned} \tag{2.11}$$

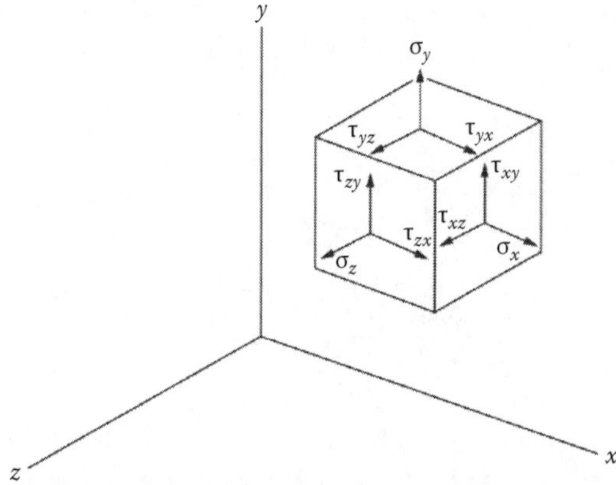

FIGURE 2.6 General stress conditions on a cubic element.

Here, σ_x, σ_y, and σ_z are the normal stresses in the respective coordinate directions and ε_x, ε_y, and ε_z, the corresponding normal strains. The normal strain, ε, is a measure of the elongation or contraction of a line segment in the body. Hence, normal strains cause a change in the volume of a rectangular element shown in Figure 2.6. τ_{xy}, τ_{yz}, and τ_{zx} are the shear stresses and γ_{xy}, γ_{yz}, and γ_{zx} are the corresponding shear strains. In these terms, the first subscript indicates the plane normal to the coordinate direction on which the stress acts and the second subscript indicates the direction of the stress. The shear strain is a measure of the change in angle between two small line segments that are originally perpendicular to each other and, thus, represents a change in the shape of the rectangular element.

The previous equation can be rewritten to express stress in terms of strain as follows:

$$\begin{aligned}
\sigma_x &= \frac{E}{(1+\nu)(1-2\nu)}[(1-\nu)\varepsilon_x + \nu(\varepsilon_y + \varepsilon_z)] \\
\sigma_y &= \frac{E}{(1+\nu)(1-2\nu)}[(1-\nu)\varepsilon_y + \nu(\varepsilon_z + \varepsilon_x)] \\
\sigma_z &= \frac{E}{(1+\nu)(1-2\nu)}[(1-\nu)\varepsilon_z + \nu(\varepsilon_x + \varepsilon_y)] \\
\tau_{xy} &= G\gamma_{xy} \\
\tau_{yz} &= G\gamma_{yz} \\
\tau_{zx} &= G\gamma_{zx}
\end{aligned} \tag{2.12}$$

In Equation 2.11, if $\sigma_z = 0$, stresses exist only in the *x-y* plane. Such problems are considered as *plane stress analysis*. In such cases, the stresses can be expressed in terms of strain as

$$\begin{aligned} \sigma_x &= \frac{E}{(1-\nu^2)}(\varepsilon_x + \nu\varepsilon_y) \\ \sigma_y &= \frac{E}{(1-\nu^2)}(\varepsilon_y + \nu\varepsilon_x) \end{aligned} \tag{2.13}$$

In the case of blood vessels, a subject of interest in this textbook, the vessel geometry can be approximated as a tube and hence the use of polar (r, θ, z) coordinates will be appropriate. The Hooke's law in polar coordinates can be written as

$$\begin{aligned} \varepsilon_r &= \frac{\sigma_r}{E} - \frac{\nu\sigma_\theta}{E} - \frac{\nu\sigma_z}{E} \\ \varepsilon_\theta &= \frac{\sigma_\theta}{E} - \frac{\nu\sigma_z}{E} - \frac{\nu\sigma_r}{E} \\ \varepsilon_z &= \frac{\sigma_z}{E} - \frac{\nu\sigma_r}{E} - \frac{\nu\sigma_\theta}{E} \end{aligned} \tag{2.14a}$$

The previous equation can be rewritten to express stress in terms of strain as follows:

$$\begin{aligned} \sigma_r &= \frac{E}{(1+\nu)(1-2\nu)}[(1-\nu)\varepsilon_r + \nu(\varepsilon_\theta + \varepsilon_z)] \\ \sigma_\theta &= \frac{E}{(1+\nu)(1-2\nu)}[(1-\nu)\varepsilon_\theta + \nu(\varepsilon_z + \varepsilon_r)] \\ \sigma_z &= \frac{E}{(1+\nu)(1-2\nu)}[(1-\nu)\varepsilon_z + \nu(\varepsilon_r + \varepsilon_\theta)] \end{aligned} \tag{2.14b}$$

and the corresponding expressions for shear stresses are

$$\begin{aligned} \tau_{r\theta} &= G\gamma_{r\theta} \\ \tau_{\theta z} &= G\gamma_{\theta z} \\ \tau_{zr} &= G\gamma_{zr} \end{aligned} \tag{2.14c}$$

In the case of plane stress analysis (where $\sigma_z = 0$), the stresses can be written in terms of strains as

$$\sigma_r = \frac{E}{(1-\nu^2)}(\varepsilon_r + \nu\varepsilon_\theta)$$
$$\sigma_\theta = \frac{E}{(1-\nu^2)}(\varepsilon_\theta + \nu\varepsilon_r) \tag{2.15}$$

2.1.7 Bulk Modulus

Consider a cubic element (Figure 2.6) where each side of the cube has a unit length. If only normal stresses σ_x, σ_y, and σ_z are present, the cube will deform to the shape of a rectangular parallelepiped. The volume of the deformed element is

$$V = (1+\varepsilon_x)(1+\varepsilon_y)(1+\varepsilon_z) \tag{2.16}$$

Since the strains are much smaller than unity, their products will even be smaller and can be neglected and, thus, V can be written as

$$V = 1+\varepsilon_x+\varepsilon_y+\varepsilon_z \tag{2.17}$$

Since the original volume $V_0 = 1$, the change in volume is given by

$$V - V_0 = \Delta V = \varepsilon_x+\varepsilon_y+\varepsilon_z$$

The change in volume per unit volume, also referred to as the *volumetric strain* or *cubical dilatation*, is given by

$$\frac{\Delta V}{V_0} = \varepsilon_x+\varepsilon_y+\varepsilon_z \tag{2.18}$$

By rewriting the expressions for the strains in terms of stresses from Equation 2.12, we have

$$\frac{\Delta V}{V_0} = \frac{(1-2\nu)}{E}(\sigma_x+\sigma_y+\sigma_z) \tag{2.19}$$

This expression shows that when the Poisson's ratio is 0.5, the volumetric strain will be equal to zero. A special case to be considered is when the body is subjected to a uniform hydrostatic pressure p. Then, each of the stress components is equal to $-p$ and the aforementioned relationship can be rewritten as

$$\frac{\Delta V}{V_0} = \frac{-3(1-2\nu)}{E}p \tag{2.20}$$

Introducing the constant $k = E/3(1 - 2\nu)$, we have

$$\frac{\Delta V}{V_0} = -\frac{p}{k} \tag{2.21}$$

The constant k is defined as the *bulk modulus* or the *modulus of compression*. A body subjected to a uniform compressive force will decrease in volume and, hence, the volumetric strain will be negative, yielding a positive value for the bulk modulus. A material with an infinite bulk modulus is known as an *incompressible* material. Water has a relatively high bulk modulus (300,000 psi) and, hence, can be considered as incompressible for most applications. In general, blood is also considered as an incompressible fluid in the analysis of flow in the human circulation.

For a *homogeneous isotropic material*, an expression relating E, G, and ν can be derived as

$$G = \frac{E}{2(1+\nu)} \tag{2.22}$$

Therefore, the complete material description of an isotropic, linear elastic material can be specified by two independent constants where the third is derived using the aforementioned relationship.

2.2 ANALYSIS OF THIN-WALLED CYLINDRICAL TUBES

As a first approximation, the geometry of major blood vessels can be considered as thin-walled elastic tubes of circular cross section. Therefore, in order to model the dynamics of vascular tissues, we will develop a relationship for the stresses present in the walls of tubes of cylindrical geometry. A cylindrical thin-walled vessel of internal radius R and a thickness t is shown in Figure 2.7. Since the vessel walls offer little resistance to bending, it can be assumed that the forces developed in the wall are *tangential* to the surface of the vessel as shown in the figure. Due to the axisymmetric geometry, no shear forces are generated and only the normal stresses along the axial and circumferential directions exist. The normal stress in the circumferential direction is the *hoop stress* and in the axial direction, it is the *longitudinal stress*. In order to derive an expression for the hoop stress, σ_θ, we will consider a segment of the tube as shown in Figure 2.8a. The forces acting on the segment are also shown in the figure. The pressure p in the figure denotes the *transmural pressure*, which is the difference between the inside and outside pressures. In employing this analysis for blood vessels,

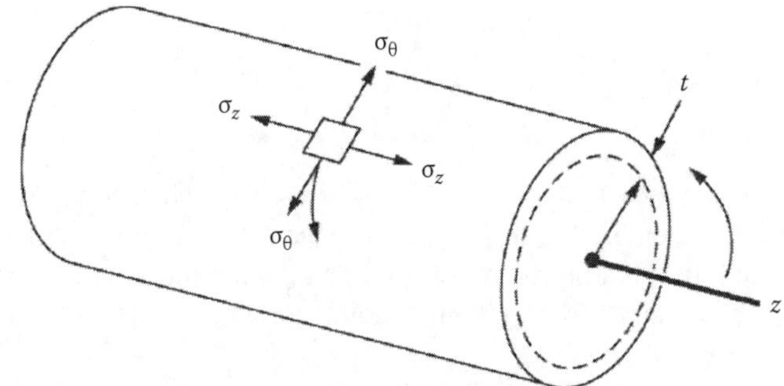

FIGURE 2.7 Stresses on a thin-walled cylindrical vessel.

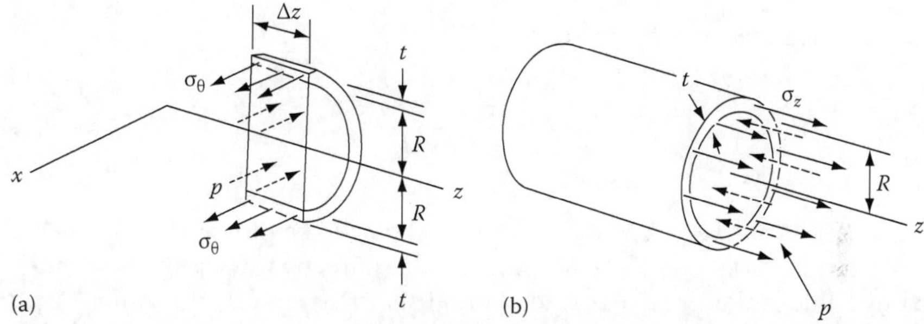

FIGURE 2.8 Forces on segments of the thin-walled cylindrical pressure vessel: (a) schematic of the forces in the diametrical plane for hoop stress, σ_θ; (b) forces in the axial direction for axial stress, σ_z.

the pressure acting on the outer surface of the vessel is usually neglected and the blood pressure is the transmural pressure load resulting in the deformation of the vessel.

Static force equilibrium in the θ direction can be written as

$$2\sigma_\theta t\Delta z - p(2R\Delta z) = 0 \tag{2.23}$$

and solving this equation, we obtain

$$\sigma_\theta = \frac{pR}{t} \tag{2.24}$$

Similarly, assuming a close-ended vessel as in Figure 2.8b, force equilibrium along the z-direction will yield the relationship

$$\sigma_z(2\pi Rt) - p(\pi R^2) = 0 \tag{2.25}$$

An expression for the longitudinal stress is derived from this as

$$\sigma_z = \frac{pR}{2t} \tag{2.26}$$

From Equations 2.24 and 2.26, we note that

$$\sigma_\theta = 2\sigma_z \tag{2.27}$$

In open-ended tubes, $\sigma_z = 0$ and only the hoop stress will exist. Note that the radius R used in this derivation is the *internal* radius of the tube. The initial circumferential length is $2\pi R$ and, if the radius increases by a small amount, ΔR, due to the applied internal pressure, then the circumferential strain can be computed as

$$\varepsilon_\theta = \frac{[2\pi(R+\Delta R) - 2\pi R]}{2\pi R} = \frac{\Delta R}{R} \tag{2.28}$$

and the Young's modulus expressed as

$$E = \frac{\sigma_\theta}{\varepsilon_\theta} = \frac{pR^2}{t\Delta R} \tag{2.29}$$

In this derivation, we assumed the cylindrical tube to be thin-walled and, hence, neglected the variation of stresses in the radial direction. Usually, the assumption of a thin-walled vessel is made only if the ratio is <0.1. When this condition is *not* satisfied, the stresses developed in a *thick-walled vessel* need to be considered.

2.3 ANALYSIS OF THICK-WALLED CYLINDRICAL TUBES

If $t/R \geq 0.1$, then the thick-walled cylinder formulation needs to be employed in the analysis of deformation under internal pressure loading. For many cardiovascular applications of interest, the wall thickness-to-radius ratio of arteries generally requires us to use the thick-walled cylindrical formulation. The arterial wall is also tethered and hence a plane strain formulation (displacement in the axial direction is neglected) is commonly used.

2.3.1 EQUILIBRIUM EQUATION

Consider an open-ended thick cylinder with an internal radius, R_1, and external radius, R_2, with an internal pressure, p_1, and external pressure, p_2, as shown in Figure 2.9. A differential element of thickness, dz, together with the radial and circumferential stresses acting on the element, is also shown in the figure. Due to the axisymmetric geometry and loading, there are no shear stresses generated at either the inner or the outer surfaces of the cylinder. An equilibrium equation obtained by summation of forces in the radial direction yields

$$(\sigma_r + d\sigma_r)(r + dr)d\theta\, dz - \sigma_r r\, d\theta\, dz - 2\sigma_\theta dr\, dz \sin\frac{d\theta}{2} = 0 \tag{2.30}$$

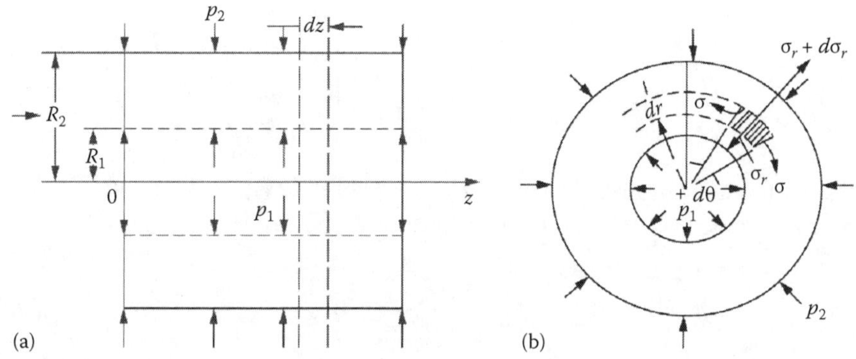

FIGURE 2.9 Stresses on a thick-walled open-ended vessel: (a) schematic of the thick-walled cylindrical vessel subjected to internal and external pressure; (b) forces acting on a small element of the thick-walled vessel.

Since $\sin(d\theta/2) \cong d\theta/2$ for small angles, after gathering terms, discarding higher order terms, and dividing by $rdrd\theta dz$, we obtain

$$\frac{d\sigma_r}{dr} + \frac{(\sigma_r - \sigma_\theta)}{r} = 0 \tag{2.31}$$

The previous equation is the equilibrium equation for axisymmetric cylinders.

2.3.2 Compatibility Condition

The strain displacement and stress–strain relations are developed as follows. Displacements are functions of r only. All points deform radially, although points at different radii deform by different amounts. From the definition of strain, the radial and circumferential strains are written as

$$\varepsilon_r = \frac{du}{dr} \tag{2.32}$$

and

$$\varepsilon_\theta = \frac{2\pi(r+u) - 2\pi r}{2\pi r} = \frac{u}{r} \tag{2.33}$$

where u is the radial displacement. Substituting the aforementioned compatibility conditions into the stress–strain relationship, we have

$$\sigma_r = \frac{E}{1-\nu^2}(\varepsilon_r + \nu\varepsilon_\theta) = \frac{E}{1-\nu^2}\left(\frac{du}{dr} + \nu\frac{u}{r}\right) \tag{2.34}$$

and

$$\sigma_\theta = \frac{E}{1-\nu^2}(\varepsilon_\theta + \nu\varepsilon_r) = \frac{E}{1-\nu^2}\left(\frac{u}{r} + \nu\frac{du}{dr}\right) \tag{2.35}$$

Substituting the above relationship into the equilibrium equation (Equation 2.31), we obtain the second-order differential equation:

$$\frac{d^2u}{dr^2} + \frac{1}{r}\frac{du}{dr} - \frac{u}{r^2} = 0 \tag{2.36}$$

The previous equation incorporates equilibrium, stress–strain, and compatibility conditions. The equation can be written in the form

$$\frac{d}{dr}\left[\frac{1}{r}\frac{d}{dr}(ur)\right] = 0 \tag{2.37}$$

Following two integrations, a function $u(r)$ satisfying the previous equation is given as

$$u = c_1 r + \frac{c_2}{r} \tag{2.38}$$

where c_1 and c_2 are constants of integration. Substitution of Equation 2.38 into Equations 2.34 and 2.35 yields

$$\sigma_r = \frac{E}{1-\nu^2}\left[(1-\nu)c_1 - \frac{1-\nu}{r^2}c_2\right] \tag{2.39}$$

and

$$\sigma_\theta = \frac{E}{1-\nu^2}\left[(1-\nu)c_1 + \frac{1-\nu}{r^2}c_2\right] \tag{2.40}$$

The constants c_1 and c_2 in Equations 2.39 and 2.40 are evaluated by applying the boundary conditions. From Figure 2.9, the boundary conditions can be specified as $\sigma_r = -p_1$ at $r = R_1$ (inner surface) and $\sigma_r = -p_2$ at $r = R_2$ (outer surface). The negative signs in the previous equations indicate that the pressures act into the surface as shown in Figure 2.9. Substituting for c_1 and c_2 in the previous equations, the radial and circumferential stresses are derived as

$$\sigma_r = p_1\left[\frac{R_1^2}{R_2^2 - R_1^2}\right]\left[1 - \frac{R_2^2}{r^2}\right] - p_2\left[\frac{R_2^2}{R_2^2 - R_1^2}\right]\left[1 - \frac{R_1^2}{r^2}\right] \tag{2.41}$$

and

$$\sigma_\theta = p_1\left[\frac{R_1^2}{R_2^2 - R_1^2}\right]\left[1 - \frac{R_2^2}{r^2}\right] - p_2\left[\frac{R_2^2}{R_2^2 - R_1^2}\right]\left[1 - \frac{R_1^2}{r^2}\right] \tag{2.42}$$

The stress equations (2.41) and (2.42) were first published in 1833 and are known as the *Lame relationships.*

In the stress analysis of blood vessels, the external pressure p_2 is generally assumed to be zero and the force acting on the vessel wall is the transmural blood pressure. The expression for the radial displacement in an artery considered as a thick-walled tube is given by the expression

$$u = \left\{\frac{p_1R_1^2(1+\nu)(1-2\nu)}{(R_1^2 - R_2^2)}\frac{r}{E}\right\} + \left\{\frac{p_1R_1^2R_2^2(1+\nu)}{(R_1^2 - R_2^2)r^2}\frac{r}{E}\right\} \tag{2.43}$$

While the previous equation can be used to determine the deformation of thick-walled cylinder with known internal pressure and material properties, in practice it is used to determine the material property employing the deformation measured experimentally. Rearranging the previous equation in terms of the elastic modulus, we obtain

$$E = \left\{\frac{p_1R_1^2(1+\nu)(1-2\nu)}{(R_1^2 - R_2^2)}\frac{r}{u}\right\} + \left\{\frac{p_1R_1^2R_2^2(1+\nu)}{(R_1^2 - R_2^2)r^2}\frac{r}{u}\right\} \tag{2.44}$$

Bergel (1961a, b) obtained an expression for the *incremental modulus* corresponding to an increase in outer radial dimension ΔR_2 due to an increase in internal pressure Δp. By replacing p_1 with Δp, r with R_2, and u with ΔR_2 in the previous equation, the incremental modulus can be shown to be

$$E_{inc} = \frac{2(1-\nu^2)R_1^2R_2\Delta p}{(R_2^2 - R_1^2)\Delta R_2} \tag{2.45}$$

In this expression, $(R_2^2 - R_1^2)$ is a constant since the wall is assumed to be incompressible and the vessel wall is tethered. This expression requires measurement of the internal pressure, the radius, and the wall thickness of the blood vessels *in situ*. The magnitude of the incremental modulus will depend upon the mean pressure at which it was computed.

In several cases (including blood vessels *in vivo*), the internal pressure and the external radius can be measured. In such cases, a *pressure-strain modulus*, E_p, is given by

$$E_p = \Delta p\frac{R_2}{\Delta R_2} \tag{2.46}$$

This relationship ignores the tube wall thickness and, thus, E_p represents a structural modulus rather than the elastic property of the tube material.

2.4 VISCOELASTICITY

The relationships for material properties derived earlier are applicable for *purely elastic material* in which a load applied to the material produces an instantaneous response in the form of deformation. Upon removal of the external load, the specimen will instantaneously return to the undeformed state (assuming inertial effects are small). In the presence of *viscous behavior*, however, recovery of deformation will not occur instantly. This is because the applied shear stress in viscous material is a function of *rate of shear*, as is discussed in Section 1.2. Material behaviors that incorporate both elastic and viscous characteristics are referred to as *viscoelastic*. The elastic component for such materials, in a one-dimensional (1D) form, can be represented by a linear elastic spring with a spring constant K_s (Figure 2.10a) and is given by the relationship

$$\sigma = K_s \varepsilon \tag{2.47}$$

The viscous behavior can be represented by a dashpot as shown in Figure 2.10b with the relationship between the stress, σ, and the rate of strain, $\dot{\varepsilon} = d\varepsilon/dt$, being given by

$$\sigma = \mu\dot{\varepsilon} \tag{2.48}$$

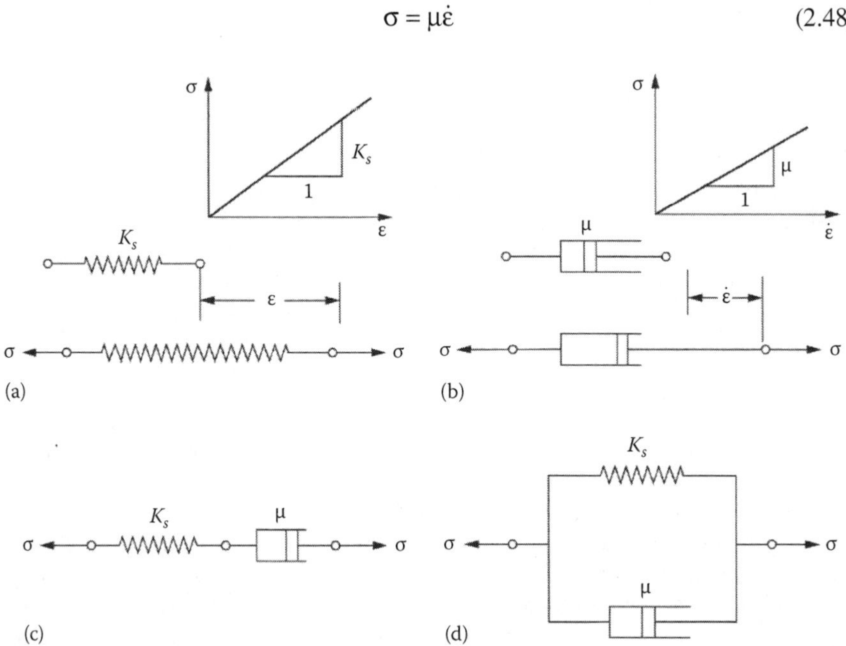

FIGURE 2.10 A typical viscoelastic material schematically represented by (a) a linear spring representing the elastic component with the corresponding stress–strain relationship and (b) the viscous component represented by a dashpot with the corresponding stress–strain rate relationship. The combined viscoelastic behavior of a solid represented by (c) a Maxwell model with the spring and dashpot in series and (d) a Kelvin model with spring and dashpot in parallel.

where μ is the viscosity coefficient. The combined viscoelastic behavior of a solid is represented by the spring and dashpot in series (the *Maxwell model*) or in parallel (the *Kelvin* or *Voigt model*). In the case of the Maxwell model (Figure 2.10c), the constitutive relationship is given by

$$\frac{\dot{\sigma}}{K_s} + \frac{\sigma}{\mu} = \dot{\varepsilon} \tag{2.49}$$

In the case of the Kelvin model (Figure 2.10d), the constitutive relationship can be expressed as

$$\sigma = K_s\varepsilon + \mu\dot{\varepsilon} \tag{2.50}$$

These two-element models are not generally adequate to represent the viscoelastic behavior of real materials and, thus, models with three or more elements are employed which can incorporate the flexibility needed to describe the response of actual materials. *Creep* and *stress relaxation* experiments are generally performed to describe the viscoelastic properties of materials. In the case of creep tests (Figure 2.11), the viscoelastic specimen is subjected to an instantaneous *constant stress* σ_0 and the strain (creep response) is measured as a function of time. For the stress relaxation experiment (Figure 2.12), the specimen is subjected to an instantaneous *constant strain* and the stress (relaxation) is measured as a function of time. Thus, in

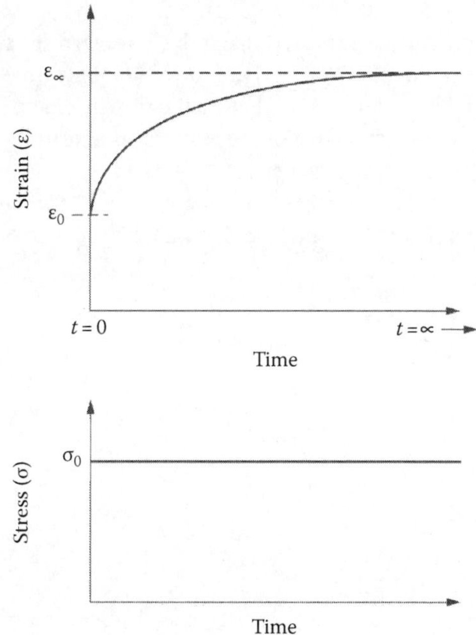

FIGURE 2.11 Creep test for a viscoelastic material.

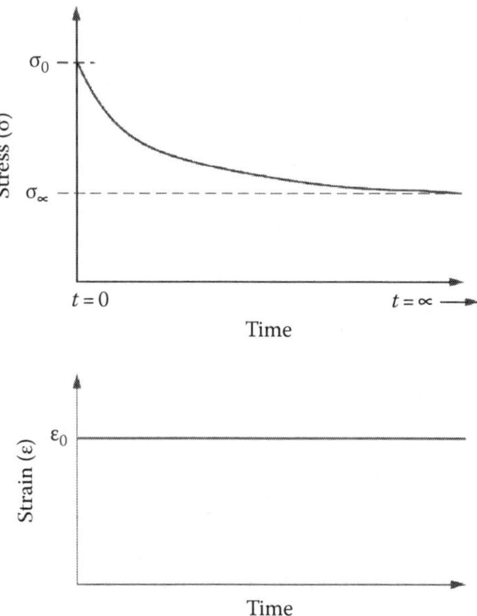

FIGURE 2.12 Stress relaxation experiment for a viscoelastic material.

viscoelastic material including blood vessels, a finite time is required after the application of the load before the complete deformation is attained with a static load. With such a material, the radius of the tube for a step increase in pressure will take a finite time to increase to its steady state value (Figure 2.13). The same phenomenon will also occur when the pressure is removed instantly. To determine the elastic modulus under *static conditions* of applied internal pressure, adequate time should be allowed for the vessel to expand to its final radius before the measurement is made. With such experiments, only the elastic response of the material is determined and no information is obtained about the viscous properties.

To determine the viscoelastic behavior of the material, *dynamic experiments* are performed with the application of sinusoidally varying pressure. A typical response

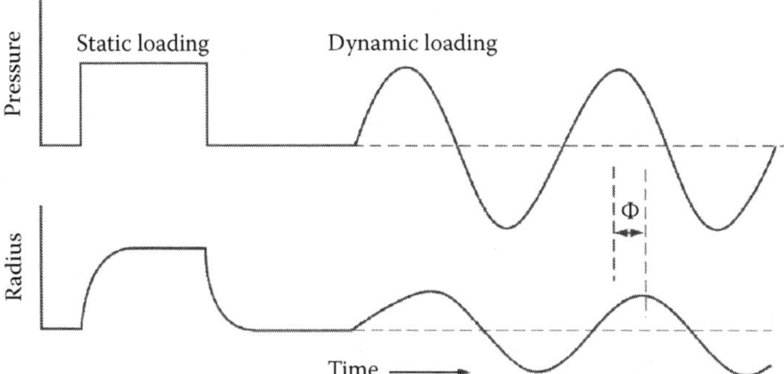

FIGURE 2.13 Response to time-dependent pressure loading of a viscoelastic structure.

to such loading is shown in Figure 2.13. Even though the oscillations of the radius have the same frequency as that of the applied pressure, the effect of viscosity is to delay the response by a phase angle, ϕ. Moreover, it is also observed that the value of peak distension under sinusoidal loading is smaller than that for static deflection. This is due to the fact that before the delayed response can attain its peak, the load has already reached its down slope and thus reversing the process so that the amplitude of the distension is smaller.

Due to the phase difference between the applied pressure and the radial changes, the ratio of stress to resultant strain will be a complex quantity, which can be expressed by the relationship

$$E_c = |E_c| e^{i\phi} = |E_c| \cos\phi + i\,|E_c| \sin\phi \tag{2.51}$$

The modulus, E_c, is a function of the applied oscillatory frequency and its values can be determined by applying sinusoidal loading at varying frequencies. For the case of dynamic loading in viscoelastic material, the incremental elastic modulus expression given in Equation 2.45 can be modified as

$$E_{inc} = \frac{2(1-\nu^2)R_1^2 R_2}{(R_2^2 - R_1^2)} \frac{\Delta p}{\Delta R_2} e^{i\phi} \tag{2.52}$$

As pointed out earlier, the measured strains obtained in dynamic testing of viscoelastic materials will be smaller than those measured under static conditions, and, hence, the dynamic elastic modulus will be higher than the corresponding static value.

PROBLEMS

2.1 Derive the relationship between the Young's modulus E, shear modulus G, and the Poisson's ratio given in Equation 2.22.

2.2 Following a uniaxial extension test, to calculate the stress–strain data from load-extension data, engineering stress and strain are given as stress, $\sigma = F/A_0$, where F is force and A_0 is the original cross-sectional area, and strain, $\varepsilon = (l - l_0)/l_0$, where l_0 is the original length and l is the current length. However, the cross-sectional area actually diminishes with extension (or strain). Therefore, it is only appropriate that the true stress be defined as true stress, $\sigma_{true} = F/A$, where A is the "true" diminished cross-sectional area which would be dependent on extension (and therefore strain) and the compressibility of the tissue. Assuming that the arterial tissue is perfectly incompressible (i.e., the volume of the specimen is a constant throughout the test) and that the specimen shape is always rectangular, derive a relationship for "A" as a function of A_0 and ε, and consequently show that $\sigma_{true} = (F/A_0)(1 + \varepsilon)$.

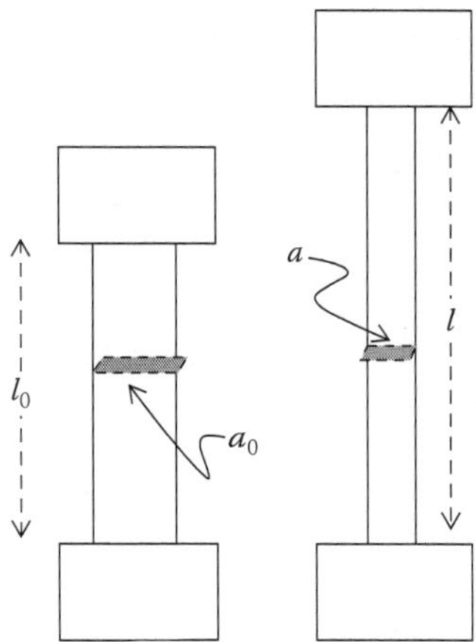

2.3 A circular aluminum tube 40 cm in length is subjected to a tensile load of 2 kN. The outside and inside diameters of the tube are 4.2 and 4.0 cm, respectively. What is the amount of tensile stress on the bar? Aluminum has an elastic modulus of 73.1 GPa. Determine the axial strain and the increase in length of the bar for the given load. Assuming a typical elastic modulus of about 0.1 MPa for a typical artery, what would be the corresponding tensile load on an arterial specimen of the same dimension that would result in the same axial strain?

2.4 A high strength steel rod (E = 200 GPa and ν = 0.32) with a diameter of 5 cm is being subjected to a compressive load of 10 KN. Determine the increase in diameter of the tube after the load is applied.

2.5 A brass specimen 10 mm in diameter and a length of 50 mm is loaded with a 20 kN force in tension. If the length increases by 0.12 mm, determine the elastic modulus of the brass. If the diameter of the bar decreases by 0.0083 mm, calculate the Poisson's ratio of the material.

2.6 An aluminum soda can (E = 73.1 GPa) has a radius to thickness ratio of 200:1 and holds soda under pressure. When the lid is opened to release the pressure, the strain in the longitudinal direction is measured as 170 μm/m. What was the internal pressure in the can? Express your answer in the units of mmHg. Compare this pressure magnitude with the typical mean blood pressure in an artery.

REFERENCES

Bergel, D. H. (1961a) The static elastic properties of the arterial wall. *J. Physiol.* 156: 445–457.

Bergel, D. H. (1961b) The dynamic elastic properties of the arterial wall. *J. Physiol.* 156: 458–469.

3 Cardiovascular Physiology

3.1 INTRODUCTION

This chapter contains a brief review of the cardiovascular physiology relevant to fluid mechanics in the human circulation. For a detailed study, the reader is referred to any textbook on physiology (e.g., Guyton and Hall (2000) or Silverthorn (2001) or their most recent editions). The cardiovascular system includes the heart and blood vessels of the systemic and pulmonary circulation. Fundamental requirements of the circulatory system are to provide adequate blood flow without interruption and to regulate blood flow according to the various demands of the body (Rushmer, 1976). The contracting heart supplies the energy required to maintain the blood flow through the vessels. The pressure gradient developed between the arterial and the venous end of the circulation is the driving force causing blood flow through the blood vessels. The energy is dissipated in the form of heat due to the frictional resistance. Blood picks up oxygen in the lungs and nutrients in the intestine and delivers them to the cells in all parts of the body. The circulating blood also removes cellular wastes and carbon dioxide from the cells for excretion through the kidneys and the lung, respectively. The circulating blood also maintains the visceral organs such as the heart, the kidney, the liver, and the brain at a constant temperature by convecting the heat generated in the core body region and dissipating the same through transfer across the skin. In the following brief review of the cardiovascular system, we will concentrate on the mechanical aspects of circulation.

3.2 HEART

3.2.1 Overview

The human heart consists of four chambers whose function is to pump blood throughout the body. The four chambers of the heart are schematically illustrated in Figure 3.1. The arrows indicate the direction of blood flow through the heart which is ensured by the presence of the heart valves. The heart consists of two pumps in series circulating blood through the pulmonary and systemic circulations, respectively. The right ventricle, a low-pressure pump, supplies the pulmonary circulation, whereas the left ventricle, a high-pressure pump, supplies the systemic circulation.

The fundamental skeleton of the heart is formed by the four rings of interconnected dense tissue which secure the valves (Figure 3.2). The atrial chambers are attached to the superior surface of the annulus of the atrioventricular (AV) valves while the trunks of the aorta and the pulmonary artery are attached to the annulus of the semilunar valves. The right and left ventricles are attached below and around the

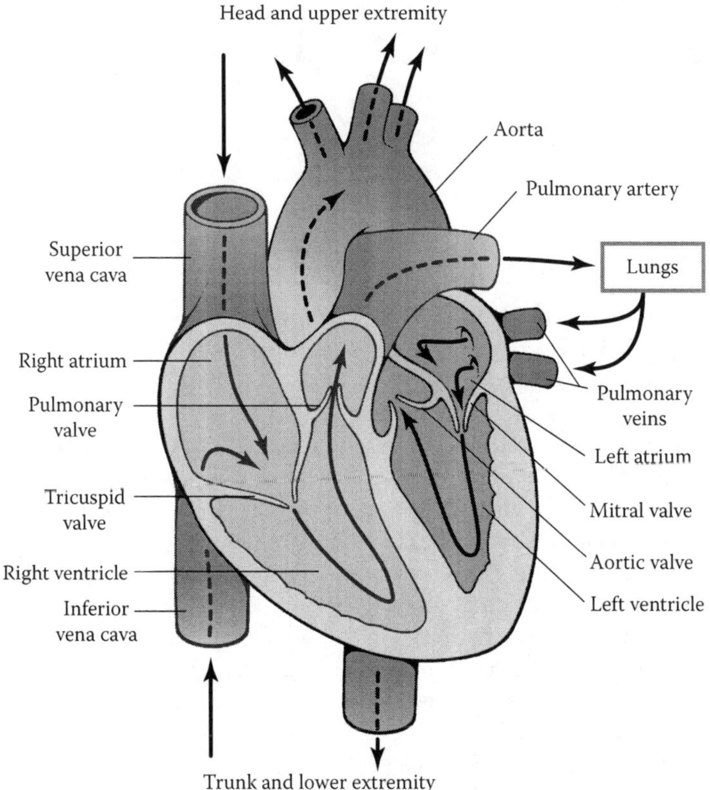

FIGURE 3.1 Schematic diagram of the four chambers of the heart and the heart valves. The arrows indicate the direction of blood flow. (Redrawn from Guyton, A.C. and Hall, J.E., *A Textbook of Medical Physiology*, 10th edn., W.B. Saunders Company, Philadelphia, PA, 2000. With permission.)

circumference of the fibrous skeleton and the interventricular septum is attached to the line of fusion between the mitral and tricuspid valve rings (Rushmer, 1976). The right atrium receives venous blood from the superior and inferior venae cavae (SVC and IVC, respectively). During ventricular relaxation, blood flows through the tricuspid valve into the right ventricle. During ventricular contraction, blood is pumped through the pulmonary arteries into the capillaries of the lung where carbon dioxide is excreted and oxygen absorbed from the air in the alveolar sac. The oxygenated blood returns to the heart via the pulmonary veins and is collected by the left atrium. Blood then fills the left ventricle through the open mitral (bicuspid) valve during ventricular relaxation. Upon subsequent ventricular contraction, blood is pumped through the aortic valve into the systemic circulation via the aorta.

The heart muscle, or *myocardium*, consists of three major types—atrial, ventricular, and specialized excitatory or conducting muscle. The atrial and ventricular muscles contract due to electrical excitation causing an increase in the blood pressure that induces pumping of the blood. The excitatory and conducting fibers conduct the electrical activity to all parts of the heart. These specialized conducting fibers contain

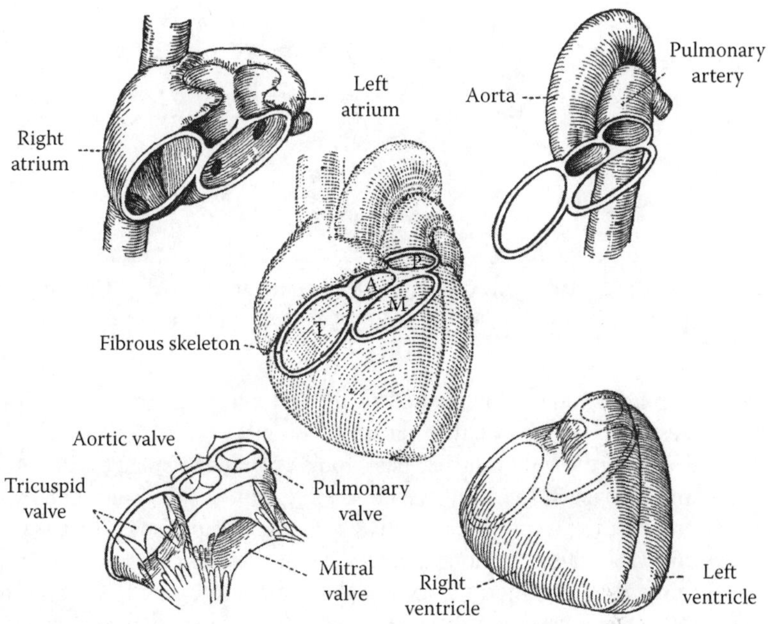

FIGURE 3.2 The fibrous skeleton and the four chambers of the heart. (Redrawn from Rushmer, R.F., *Cardiovascular Dynamics*, W.B. Saunders Company, Philadelphia, PA, 1976. With permission.)

few contractile fibrils and thus contract very feebly. The cardiac (atrial and ventricular) muscle consists of myofibrils containing actin and myosin filaments. The actin and myosin filaments slide across each other during the excitation-contraction function of the cardiac muscles producing contraction. Individual cardiac muscle cells are separated by intercalated discs giving the cardiac muscle a striated appearance. Even though these intercalated discs separate myocardial cells anatomically, the electrical resistance through the discs is low. Thus, the cardiac muscle cells can functionally be considered to be a continuum and referred to as a functional *syncytium*.

3.2.2 Cardiac Structure

Figure 3.3 schematically illustrates the geometry of the left and right ventricles. The left ventricle has a more circular cross section, whereas the right ventricle assumes a semilunar shape which wraps around part of the left ventricle. The anatomical features of the ventricles are adapted to the type of work done by the respective chambers. For example, the left ventricle is the high-pressure pump and has a cavity surface area, which is small relative to the blood volume because of its cylindrical shape. The contraction of the left ventricle involves both a reduction in the diameter of the cylindrical portion and a shortening along the longitudinal direction. The contraction of the circumferential fibers in the relatively thick-walled left ventricle induces a very high internal pressure. This high pressure supplies energy for flow of blood through the high-resistance systemic circulation.

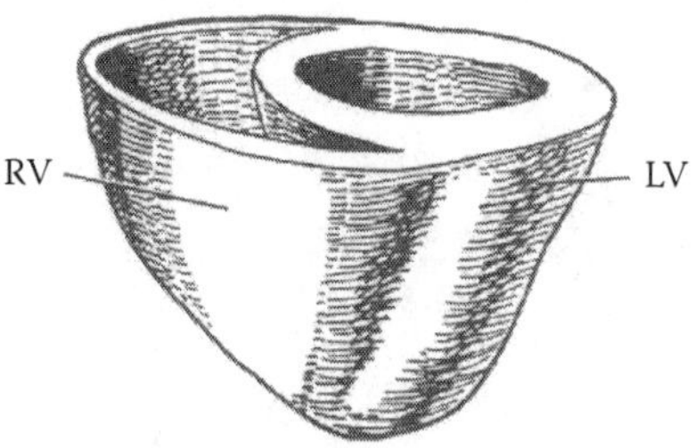

FIGURE 3.3 A schematic drawing depicting the left and right ventricles. The left ventricle has a more rounded shape whereas the right ventricle has a semilunar shape and wraps around the left ventricle.

If a large pumping volume is demanded of the left ventricle, the left ventricular chamber dilates to accommodate the increased volume.

On the other hand, the right ventricle has a roughly triangular shape with a convex septal wall, and a concave free wall, yielding a crescent-shaped ventricular cavity. The surface area of the cavity wall is relatively high in comparison with the volume of blood within the chamber. Blood pumped from the right ventricle is affected by (1) shortening of the longitudinal axis of the chamber, (2) the free wall moving toward the interventricular septum, and (3) contraction of the circumferential fibers of the right ventricle resulting in a greater curvature of the septal wall. Thus, pumping of blood from the right ventricle resembles the action of a bellows, where a large volume of fluid is displaced at a relatively low pressure. This pumping action is suitable for the pulmonary circulation where the resistance to flow is relatively small and high pressures are not needed. However, if the pulmonary resistance increases due to disease, the right ventricular myocardium cannot produce the sustained high pressures needed and, hence, failure of the right ventricle (clinically known as congestive heart failure [CHF]) will result.

3.2.3 Cardiac Conduction

Figure 3.4 illustrates the anatomical details of the cardiac conduction system. The sinoatrial (SA) node is a specialized group of autorhythmic cells located in the posterior wall of the right atrium in the vicinity of the SVC. The SA node has intrinsic rhythmicity that produces approximately 70–80 action potentials per minute in the normal adult human heart. These action potentials spread through the atrial muscle at a speed of about 0.3 m/s.

As the cardiac impulse spreads through the atria, the muscles contract and pump the blood through the AV valves into the ventricles. A few specialized conducting fibers in the atrial muscle conduct the impulse rapidly to the AV node and the impulse reaches the AV node approximately 40 ms after the start of the impulse in the SA node. The AV node complex consists of junctional fibers, the node, transitional fibers, and the AV bundle. The atrial muscles are electrically separated from the ventricular muscles with the exception of the AV bundle, which is the only pathway through which the electrical activity is conducted from the atrial to the ventricular chambers. A delay of ~110 ms occurs as the impulse is conducted through

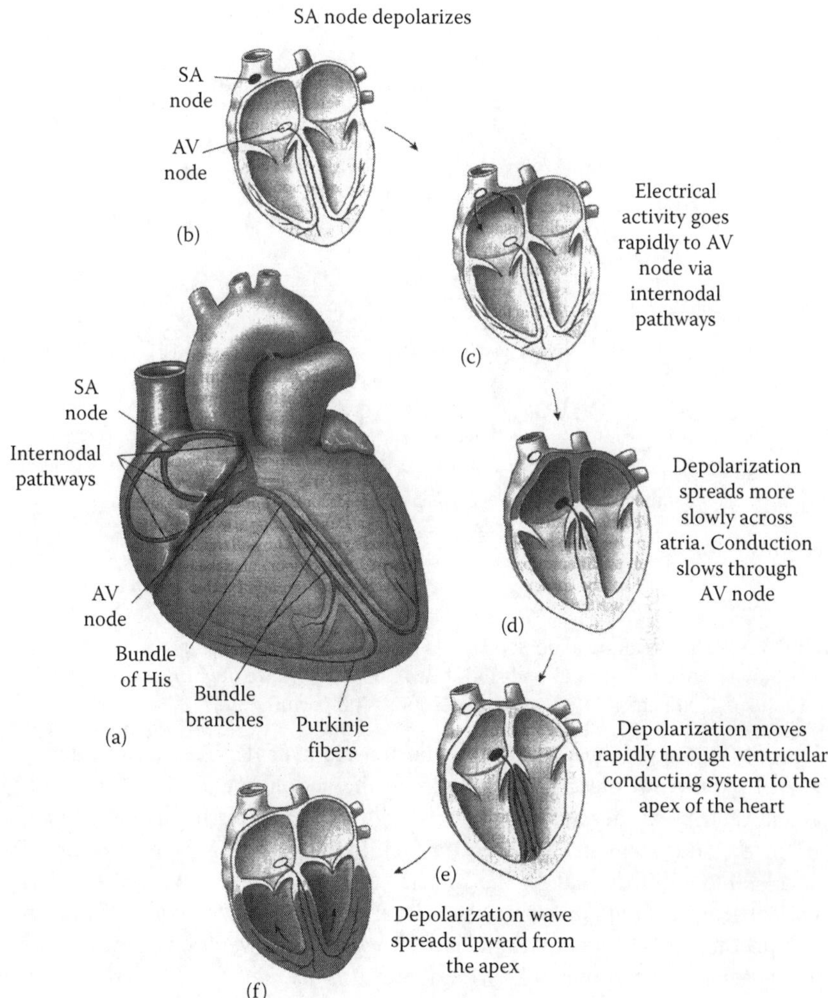
SA node depolarizes
SA node
AV node
(b)
Electrical activity goes rapidly to AV node via internodal pathways
(c)
SA node
Internodal pathways
AV node
Bundle of His
Bundle branches
Purkinje fibers
(a)
Depolarization spreads more slowly across atria. Conduction slows through AV node
(d)
Depolarization moves rapidly through ventricular conducting system to the apex of the heart
(e)
Depolarization wave spreads upward from the apex
(f)

FIGURE 3.4 The electrical conduction of the heart: (a) schematic of the conducting system of the heart including the SA node, the internal pathways, the AV node, and the conducting fibers in the ventricular chambers; (b) depolarization of the SA node; (c) electrical activity travels to the AV node; (d) depolarization spreads in the atria and the conduction is slowed through the AV node; (e) depolarization moves rapidly to the apex; and (f) depolarization spreads upwards from the apex. (Redrawn from Silverthorn, D.U., *Human Physiology: An Integrated Approach*, 2nd edn., Prentice Hall, Upper Saddle River, NJ, 2001. With permission.)

this complex. This electromechanical delay allows sufficient time for blood from the atrial contraction to be pumped into the ventricles prior to ventricular contraction.

The *Purkinje fibers* are specialized conducting fibers in the ventricles. The *bundle of His* starts from the AV complex and is large in diameter. It conducts the electrical impulses into the ventricular muscles at a velocity of 1.5–2.5 m/s. The AV bundle divides into left and right bundle branches below the valves at the interventricular septum and spreads toward the apex of the respective ventricle before turning toward

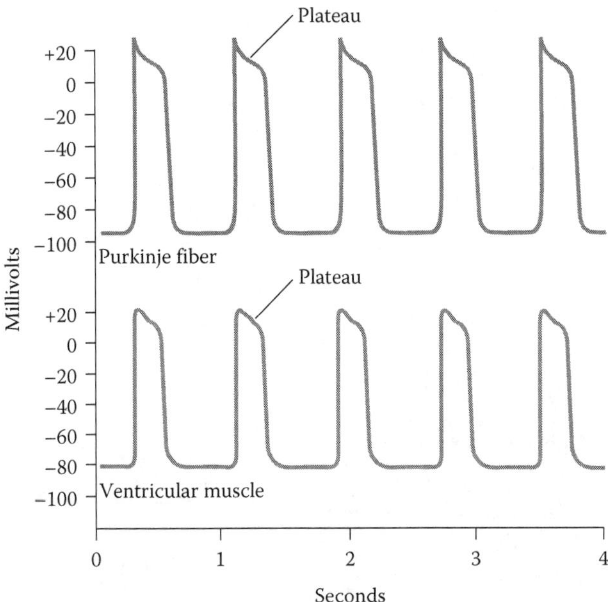

FIGURE 3.5 The rhythmic action potentials of the Purkinje fiber, and the ventricular muscle. (Redrawn from Guyton, A.C. and Hall, J.E., *A Textbook of Medical Physiology*, 10th edn., W.B. Saunders Company, Philadelphia, PA, 2000. With permission.)

the base of the heart. Thus, the ventricular muscle near the apex is activated first, followed by the basal muscle. The details of the action potentials of the Purkinje fibers and ventricular muscle are shown in Figure 3.5. The resting membrane potential of the SA node is about −55 to −60 mV while the potential for the Purkinje fiber is about −90 to −100 mV and for the ventricular muscles it is about −80 to −85 mV. Upon electrical excitation, however, the cells are depolarized to about +20 mV inside with respect to the outside environment. The phases of a ventricular muscle action potential include a sharp upstroke from the resting membrane potential (0), a brief overshoot (1), a plateau region (2), rapid recovery or repolarization (3), and electrical diastole (4) as depicted in Figure 3.5. In the action potential of the SA node, each time the resting membrane potential is reestablished; the potential gradually decays until it reaches the threshold for self-excitation. At this point, depolarization takes place and the action potential is established. The action potential of the SA node repolarizes within about 15 ms after depolarization, whereas 15–30 ms time delay is required for the other cardiac muscles. During this plateau region, or the *refractory period*, only extremely high electrical stimulation can initiate a new spike and the normal cardiac impulses cannot initiate a new spike in these muscles.

The intrinsic discharge or depolarization rate of the SA node is 70–80 times a minute. For the Purkinje fibers, it is 40–60 times a minute and for the ventricular muscles it is 15–40 times a minute. In the absence of excitation from the SA node, the AV node or the Purkinje fibers can provide rhythmic excitation of the heart. Since the SA node excitation is relatively fast, its action potential normally controls the rhythmicity of the heart. The period between the beginnings of the rhythmic excitation

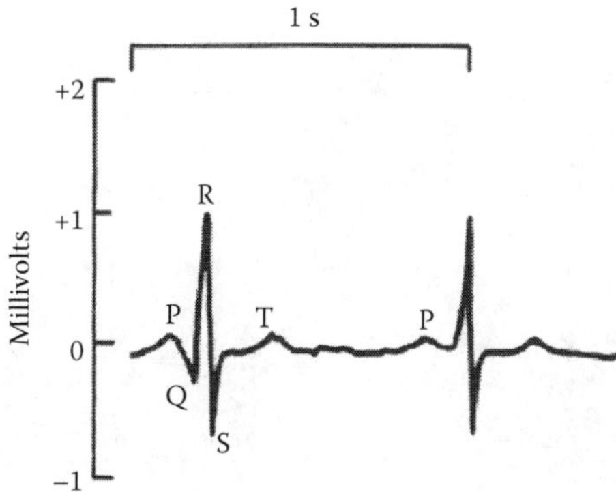

FIGURE 3.6 A typical normal electrocardiogram.

of the SA node to the next excitation is defined as a *cardiac cycle*. The contractile motion of the ventricular muscle also follows the order in which the action potential reaches the particular region. Hence, the interventricular septum starts contracting first followed by the endocardial surface of the apical region and the contraction spreads toward the base (Figure 3.4). From a mechanical point of view, this sequence of contraction enables an efficient ejection of blood from the ventricles to the respective blood vessels through an effective "squeezing" of the heart.

Electrical potentials generated by the heart also spread to the surrounding tissues and this electrical activity can be recorded by placing electrodes on the surface of the skin. Such a recording is known as the electrocardiogram (ECG) and a typical ECG signal is shown in Figure 3.6. The *P wave* and the *QRS complex* shown in the figure are depolarization waves. The electrical currents cause the P wave as the atrial muscles depolarize followed by the contraction of the atrial muscles. The QRS complex represents the depolarization of the ventricular muscles that is followed by the ventricular muscular contraction. The *T wave* is generated as the ventricular muscles repolarize and, hence, it is known as the repolarization wave. In Figure 3.6, the time between consecutive R waves is 0.8 s or, in other words, the heart rate (HR) is 75 cycles or beats per minute (bpm). For a normal adult, the HR is between 70 and 75 bpm under resting conditions.

3.2.4 Cardiac Function

The cardiac cycle has two phases—*diastole* and *systole*. Diastole is that portion of the cardiac cycle in which the cardiac muscles are relaxing while systole is the time during which the cardiac muscles are contracting (Figure 3.7). At the beginning of diastole, both the atrial and ventricular muscles are relaxing and blood from the venae cavae and the pulmonary veins is filling into the right and left atrium, respectively. The AV (i.e., the mitral and tricuspid) valves between the atria and the ventricles open and blood flows into the ventricles, increasing the ventricular volume. Atrial systole follows with the depolarization of the SA node resulting in contraction of the atrial muscles, which pumps blood into the ventricles. After the depolarization wave moves through the AV node and the Purkinje fibers in the ventricles, the

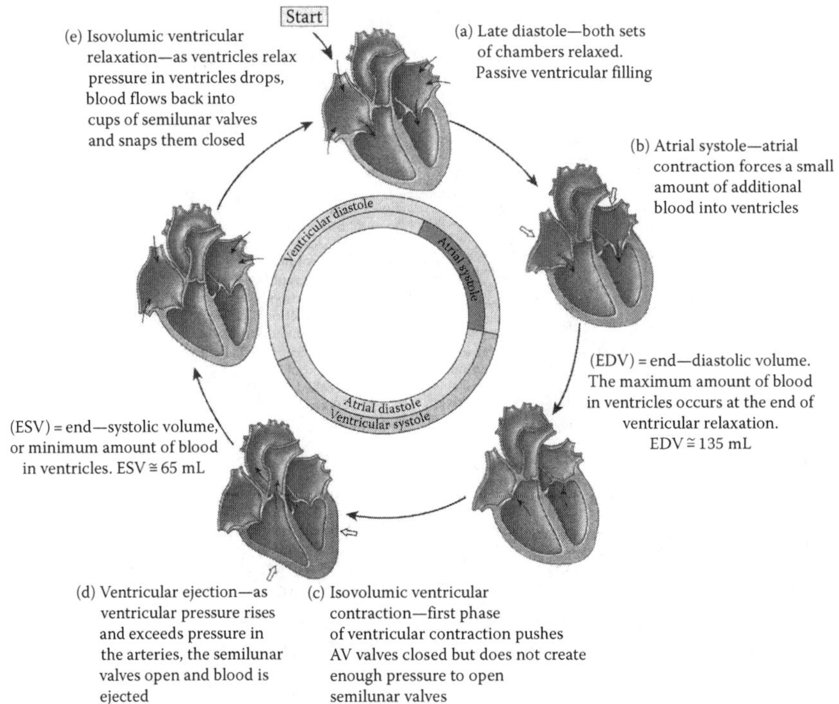

FIGURE 3.7 Schematic of the cardiac cycle with the atrial and ventricular systolic and diastolic phases: (a) late diastole; (b) atrial systole; (c) isovolumic contraction; (d) ventricular ejection; and (e) isovolumic relaxation. (Redrawn from Silverthorn, D.U., *Human Physiology: An Integrated Approach*, 2nd edn., Prentice Hall, Upper Saddle River, NJ, 2001. With permission.)

ventricular muscles start contracting from the apex toward the base of the ventricle. Ventricular pressure increases with the ventricular contraction and the AV valves close to prevent blood from flowing back to the atria. Ventricular muscles continue to contract while both the AV and the semilunar (i.e., the aortic and pulmonary) valves remain closed. Ventricular chamber pressures rise rapidly during the isovolumic contraction and, once they exceed those of the pulmonary or aortic arteries, the semilunar valves open and blood is forced out into the pulmonary and systemic circulations. At the end of systole, the ventricular muscles begin to relax and the chamber pressures fall rapidly. As soon as the arterial pressures exceed that of the ventricular chambers, the semilunar valves close and the ventricles continue to relax isovolumically. When the ventricular pressures fall below those of the atria, the AV valves open and the next cardiac cycle begins.

The relationship between the ventricular chamber pressure and volume can be represented by the pressure-volume curve shown in Figure 3.8 for the left ventricle. Panel A in the figure depicts the ventricular filling phase when the blood volume increases from about 80 to 160 mL and represents the *end diastolic volume* (EDV) and is the maximum ventricular volume during a cardiac cycle. With the beginning of ventricular contraction, the chamber pressure rises resulting in the closure of the mitral valve (and the aortic valve remains closed) and the isovolumic contraction

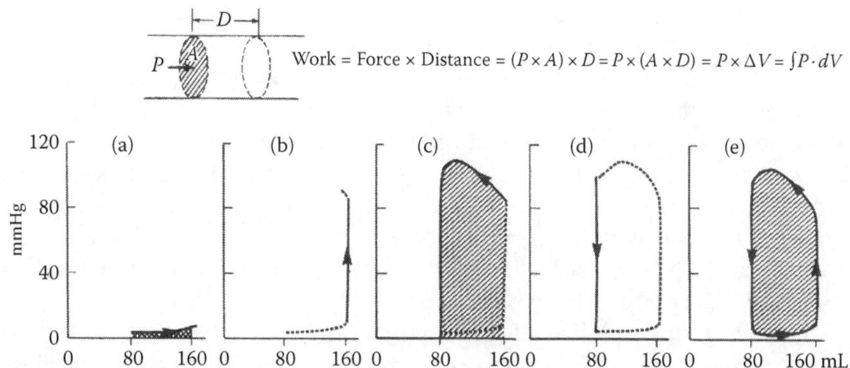

FIGURE 3.8 A ventricular pressure-volume curve: (a) filling phase; (b) isovolumic contraction; (c) ventricular ejection; (d) isovolumic relaxation; and (e) the complete cardiac cycle. (From Burton, A.C., *Physiology and Biophysics of the Circulation*, Year Book Medical Publishers, Chicago, IL, 1971.)

phase shown in Panel B. During this phase, the ventricular volume remains the same with a rapid increase in blood pressure. As the ventricular pressure exceeds that of the aorta and the aortic valve opens, and the blood is being rapidly ejected into the aorta (Panel C). The ventricular muscles continue to contract increasing the chamber pressure (along with the pressure in the aorta) while ejecting the blood into the aorta; hence, the ventricular volume decreases. The amount of blood left in the ventricle at the end of contraction (about 80 cc in the figure) is the *end systolic volume* (ESV) and represents the minimum ventricular volume in a cardiac cycle. The difference between the EDV and the ESV is called the *stroke volume* (SV):

$$\text{SV(mL/beat)} = \text{EDV} - \text{ESV} \tag{3.1}$$

SV represents the volume of blood pumped out by the left ventricle into the systemic circulation in a cardiac cycle (mL/beat). At the end of contraction, the ventricular muscles start to relax, the ventricular pressure falls below that of the aorta and the aortic valve closes. The ventricular muscles continue through the isovolumic relaxation (Panel D) and the cardiac cycle starts again. The amount of blood that is pumped out of the ventricles in 1 min is referred to as the cardiac output (CO) and is the product of the SV and the HR:

$$\text{CO(mL/min)} = \text{SV(mL/beat)} \cdot \text{HR(beats/min)} \tag{3.2}$$

A similar pressure-volume curve can also be constructed for the right ventricle with the pressures generated in the right ventricles being smaller. From elementary thermodynamics, we know that the total work done in a heat cycle is the area under the pressure-volume curve. This follows from the fact that mechanical work is the product of force and distance and, since force is the product of pressure and area, the work done can be written as (pressure × area) × distance or pressure × volume. Thus, the mechanical work done by the ventricles can be computed from the pressure-volume curve for a cardiac cycle. Panel A in Figure 3.8 represents the *filling phase* of the cardiac cycle where work is being done by the blood on the left ventricle to increase the ventricular volume. During the *isovolumic contraction phase*, no work is done and the energy is stored as elastic energy in the muscles. During the *ejection phase*, work is done by the cardiac muscles on blood and no work is done during the isovolumic relaxation phase. The area within the pressure-volume curve represents the net work done by the ventricle on blood as shown in Panel E. The heart muscles receive the energy to perform this work from the oxygen in the blood. Computing the input and output energies, efficiency of the heart can be computed. Typically, the work done by the heart amounts to only 10%–15% of the total input energy and the remainder of the energy is dissipated as heat.

A combined representation of the electrical activity of the heart (ECG), the pressure pulses in the cardiac chambers and the aorta, and the ventricular blood volume is illustrated in the Wiggers diagram (Figure 3.9). The heart sounds generated during the cardiac cycle are also illustrated as phonocardiography recording. Ventricular systole begins at the apex of the heart and the blood is squeezed toward the base of the heart during the ventricular contraction. The increase in pressure in the ventricular chambers and the blood pushing upward on the ventricular side of the atrioventricular (mitral and tricuspid) valves keeps the leaflets closed so that blood does not flow back into the atria. Vibration induced following the closure of the valves generates the first heart sound (1st in Figure 3.9) that can be heard through

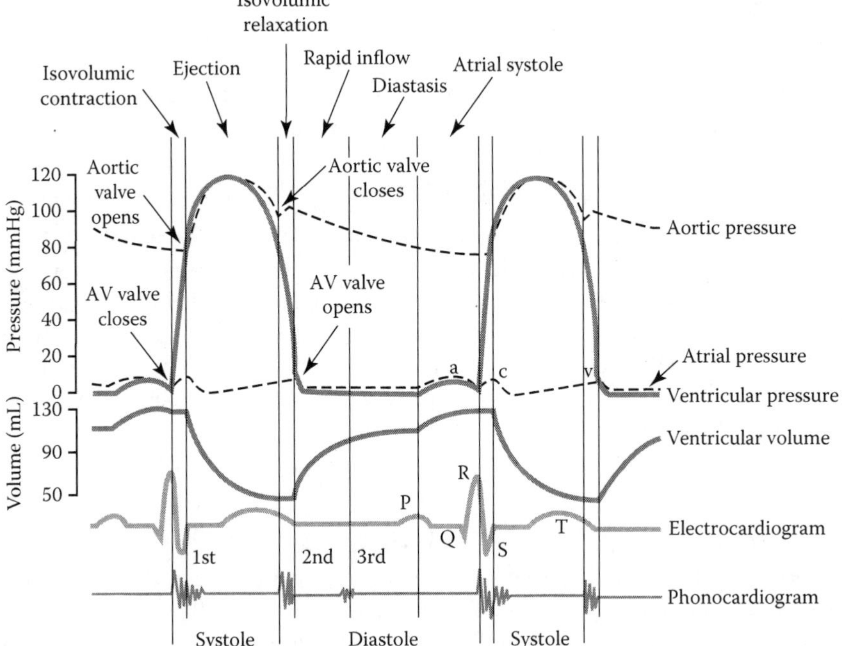

FIGURE 3.9 The Wiggers diagram depicting the relationship between the electrocardiogram, the ventricular and the atrial pressures, the heart sounds, and the volume changes in the ventricular chamber. (Redrawn from Guyton, A.C. and Hall, J.E., *A Textbook of Medical Physiology*, 10th edn., W.B. Saunders Company, Philadelphia, PA, 2000. With permission.)

a stethoscope. Similarly, at the end of contraction, the ventricles relax with a rapid pressure reduction in the chambers. Once the ventricular pressure falls below that of the arteries, blood starts to flow back toward the ventricles and the semilunar (i.e., aortic and pulmonary) valves close. The second heart sound (2nd) is generated due to the induced vibrations with the closure of the semilunar valves. The third heart sound (3rd) is generated due to turbulent or agitated flow of blood into the ventricles during the filling phase. The fourth heart sound has also been reported in the literature (not illustrated in the figure) and is associated with turbulence created by the atrial contraction. Diseased states such as stenosed (i.e., stiffer) or incompetent (i.e., leaking) valve leaflets will result in changes in characteristics of the heart sounds such as frequency and amplitude. Hence, heart sounds can also be used in diagnosis of valvular diseases.

3.3 CARDIAC VALVES

As is evident from the earlier description, the function of the heart valves is to prevent back flow of blood from the ventricles into the atria or from the great arteries (i.e., the aorta and pulmonary a.) into the ventricles. The valves open and close passively. They open and close relatively rapidly and, when closed, completely seal their respective orifices. The thin leaflets of the valves withstand very high repetitive loads for billions of cycles during the human lifetime. Cross-sectional and frontal views of the heart with the four valves are shown in Figure 3.10. The AV valves consist of the tricuspid valve between the right atrium and the right ventricle and the bicuspid (mitral) valve between the left atrium and the left ventricle. The pulmonary valve between the right ventricle and the pulmonary artery and the aortic valve between the left ventricle and the aorta have three symmetrical valve cusps in the shape of a half moon and, hence, are called the semilunar valves. The systolic phase of the cardiac cycle with the AV valves closed and the semilunar valves open is shown in the top panels and the diastolic phase is illustrated in the bottom panel.

Behind the aortic valve cusps, there are three aortic sinuses called the *sinuses of Valsalva*. Two of these sinuses have openings for the origin of the coronary arteries where presence of the sinuses prevents the obstruction of the coronary arteries by the valve cusps in the fully open position. During systole, the three cusps open to the full dimensions of the valve ring resulting in axial flow of blood into the aorta. The AV valves have two large opposing cusps and small intermediary cusps at each end. For the mitral valve, *chordae tendineae* originating from the edge of the two larger leaflets are connected to two *papillary muscle* groups. The chordae tendineae from the tricuspid valves are attached to three groups of papillary muscles. The mitral valve consists of a large anteromedial cusp that hangs like a curtain at the fully open position and a shorter posterolateral cusp. The combined surface area of the two leaflets is almost twice the valve ring area. In the open position, the upper portion of the mitral valve resembles that of a funnel. During contraction of the ventricle, the papillary muscles also contract and pull the valve leaflets toward the ventricle for efficient closure of the valves at the beginning of systole. The anatomy and function of the tricuspid valve is similar to that of the mitral valve. The detailed analysis of fluid mechanics of the heart valves is included in Chapter 7.

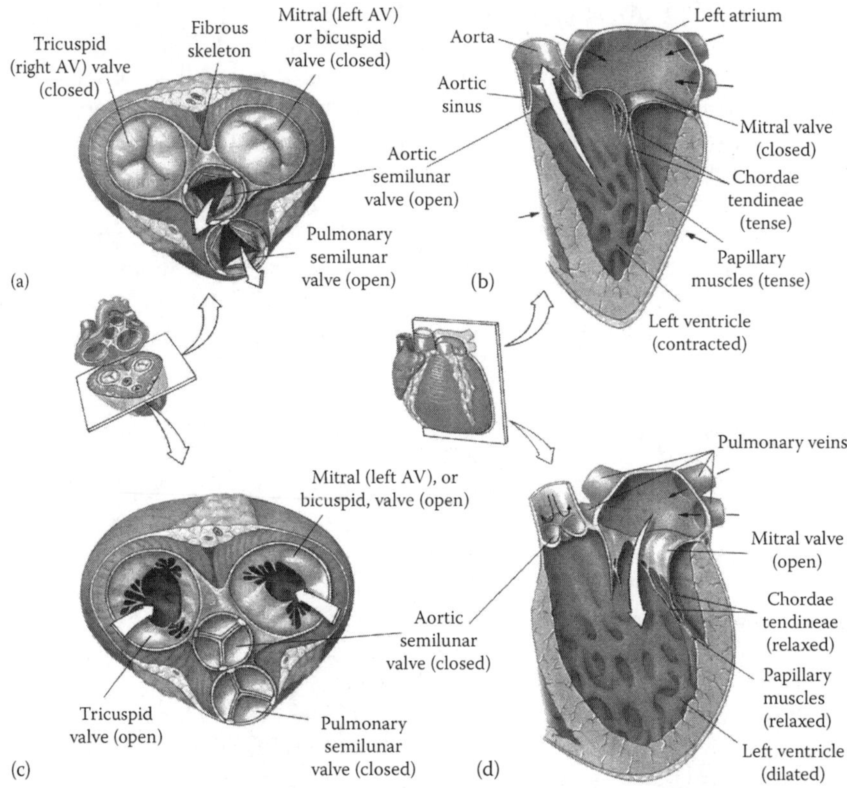

FIGURE 3.10 Illustration of the four heart valves during the systolic and diastolic phases of a cardiac cycle: (a) transverse section view and (b) frontal section view depicting the ventricular contractile phase with the atrioventricular valves in the closed position and the semilunar valves in the open position; (c) transverse section view and (d) frontal section view depicting the ventricular filling phase with the atrioventricular valves in the open position and the semilunar valves in the closed position. (Redrawn from Silverthorn, D.U., *Human Physiology: An Integrated Approach*, 2nd edn., Prentice Hall, Upper Saddle River, NJ, 2001. With permission.)

3.4 SYSTEMIC CIRCULATION

A schematic of the human circulatory system is shown in Figure 3.11. The flow of blood from the left ventricle into the aorta to the peripheral regions of the body and back to the right atrium is defined as the systemic circulation. The arteries and the arterioles carry the blood to the capillaries in the tissues and the blood returns to the right atrium through the venules and the veins. Blood flow from the right ventricle into the lungs and back to the left atrium is defined as the pulmonary circulation. The pulmonary artery distributes blood from the right ventricle into the lungs and the blood returns to the left atrium via the pulmonary vein. Blood is pumped through the pulmonary and systemic circulations at a rate of about 5–6L/min

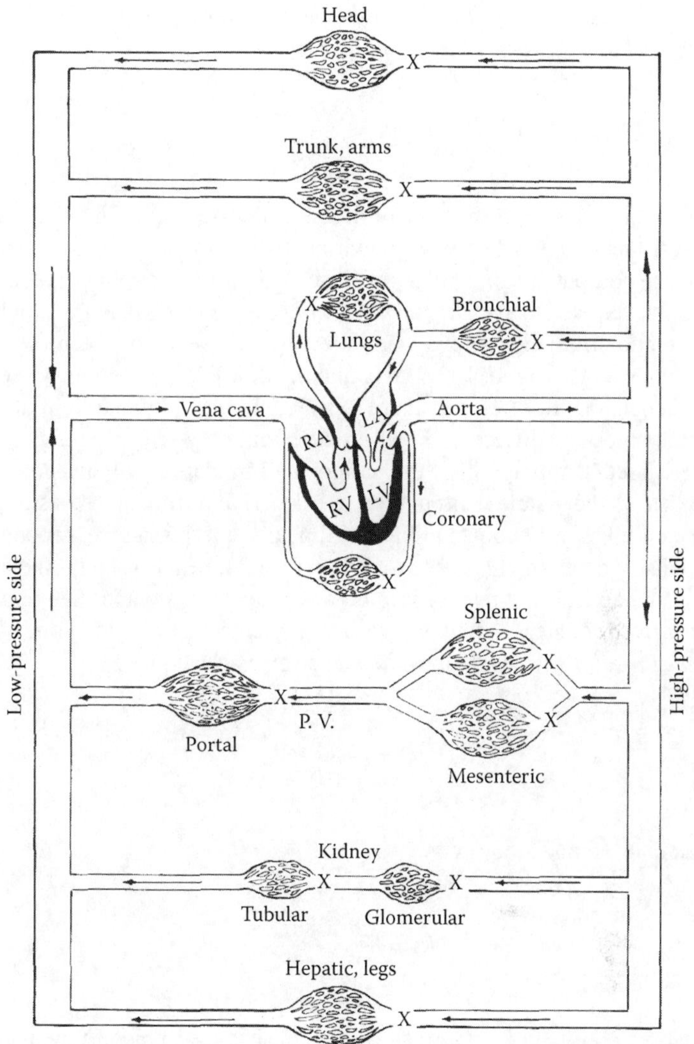

FIGURE 3.11 Schematic of blood flow to the visceral organs of systemic and pulmonary circulation. (From Burton, A.C., *Physiology and Biophysics of the Circulation*, Year Book Medical Publishers, Chicago, IL, 1971.)

under normal conditions. The driving force for propelling blood through any segment of the circulatory system is the pressure gradient across the segment. Even though the blood flow through the arterial segments is highly pulsatile, and thus, not amenable to the steady flow *Hagen–Poiseuille* model (Section 1.8), a basic relationship between the pressure difference and the flow rate can be determined if we consider the time-averaged values. If Δp is the time-averaged pressure difference across an arterial segment (i.e., difference between mean arterial pressure [MAP] at the aortic root and the venous pressure in the right atrium in the case of systemic circulation) and Q is the time-averaged flow rate (i.e., CO), then from basic fluid mechanics, we have the relationship

$$R_S = \frac{\Delta p}{Q} \tag{3.3}$$

where R is the resistance to the flow of blood in that segment. Under these conditions, the resistance to blood flow is predominantly due to the viscous shear stresses. The resistance computed using units of pressure in mmHg and flow rate in mL/s in Equation 3.3 is referred to as *peripheral resistance units* (PRUs). For example, in the normal systemic circulation, if the mean pressure difference between the systemic arteries and the veins is about 100 mmHg and the flow rate through the systemic circulation is about 100 mL/s, the resistance is 1 PRU. In the pulmonary circulation, the time-averaged pressure difference between the pulmonary artery and the left atrium is normally about 10 mmHg. Since the pulmonary circulation will also maintain the same flow ratc as the systemic circulation over a period of time, the resistance in the pulmonary circulation is about 0.1 PRU. Clinically, the resistance is computed in "Woods Units" where mmHg is used for pressure and L/min is used for the flow rate.

Again, in Chapter 1, the relationship between the flow rate and the pressure gradient was derived for steady flow of a viscous fluid through a rigid cylindrical pipe. The *Hagen–Poiseuille* flow relationship was given by the equation

$$Q = \frac{\Delta p \pi R^4}{8\mu L} \tag{1.53}$$

From Equations 3.3 and 1.53, we get

$$R_S = \frac{\Delta p}{Q} = \frac{8\mu L}{\pi R^4} \tag{3.4}$$

From Equation 3.4, it can be observed that the resistance to blood flow is inversely proportional to the fourth power of tube radius. Thus, small changes in the radius of arteries and arterioles will significantly alter the vascular resistance. This is important since one of the characteristics of blood vessel walls is that they are very responsive to stimulation. With sympathetic stimulation, the tone of the vessel walls increases, causing a decrease in diameter and, thereby, a significant increase in resistance to flow of blood. On the other hand, with sympathetic inhibition, the tone of the vessels decreases resulting in an increase in the vessel diameter and a corresponding decrease in flow resistance. Thus, sympathetic stimulation or inhibition is effectively used in controlling the flow rate of blood through any region of the body and this control is affected at the arteriolar level. For example, an increase in vessel diameter of just 5% would produce a reduction in resistance of over 21%.

The ratio of change in volume to a change in pressure gives a measure of the distensibility of the blood vessel. In practice, the increase in volume normalized to the initial volume is used to define the volumetric strain of the vessel. The definition for *vascular compliance*, *C*, is given by

$$C = \frac{\Delta V/V}{\Delta p} = \frac{\Delta V}{V\Delta p} \tag{3.5}$$

where

ΔV is the change in volume
V is the initial volume

A pressure-volume curve can be used to describe the relationship between the pressure and volume for a vessel. Figure 3.12 shows such a relationship for the arterial and venous system in man. The effect of sympathetic stimulation is to reduce the distensibility of the vessel, whereas sympathetic inhibition has the opposite effect. In the venous system, a large increase in blood volume results in a relatively *small* increase in pressure when compared with the arterial system. In other words, the venous system has a greater distensibility or capacitance. As a result, the veins act as the primary volume reservoir for blood in the circulatory system.

The aorta and other major arteries are high-pressure conduits transporting blood to the various regions and visceral organs in the body. The normal arterial wall is made up of three layers—the *intima*, *media*, and *adventitia*. The intimal layer of the artery consists of a layer of *endothelial cells* attached to a *basement membrane*. The medial layer consists of vascular smooth muscle cells, collagen, and elastin fibers in an extracellular matrix. The adventitial layer consists of connective tissue that

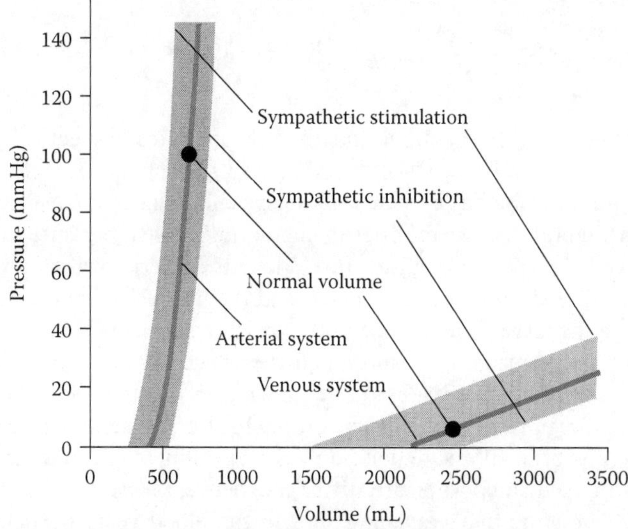

FIGURE 3.12 Pressure-volume curves for the arterial and venous system. (Redrawn from Guyton, A.C. and Hall, J.E., *A Textbook of Medical Physiology*, 10th edn., W.B. Saunders Company, Philadelphia, PA, 2000. With permission.)

is attached, or tethered, to the surrounding organs in the body. Since blood flows under high pressures through the arteries, these vessels have strong walls. The arterial walls are also less compliant compared with the venous vessels as shown in Figure 3.12. In the systemic arteries, relatively small increases in arterial volume will result in large increases in pressure. Therefore, the systemic arteries serve as a pressure reservoir (Rushmer, 1976). The small arteries further branch into arterioles that also have strong muscular walls where the vascular tone is controlled by regulatory mechanisms. Thus, the blood flow distribution to various regions of the body is controlled by changes in resistance offered by various arterioles. The blood from the arterioles then enters into capillaries where the exchange of nutrients between the blood and the interstitial space takes place. The capillary walls are very thin and permeable to small molecular substances to allow for an efficient exchange of nutrients. Blood from the capillaries is collected into venules that coalesce into larger veins which eventually return it to the right atrium. Table 3.1 shows the total cross-sectional area, the time-averaged velocity of blood, and the percentage of blood at any given time in the various vessels in the systemic circulation (Milnor, 1989).

At the root of the aorta, the systolic pressure of a normal adult is about 120 mmHg and the diastolic pressure is about 80 mmHg. The difference between the systolic and diastolic pressures is referred to as the *pulse pressure.* A typical pressure pulse in the aorta as a function of time is shown in Figure 3.13. The pressure pulse in systole starts with a steep rise which gradually decreases to a plateau at peak pressure. This is followed by a sharp incisura, or *dicrotic notch*, due to the closing of the aortic valve. During diastole, there is essentially an exponential decay of the pressure pulse. Systole lasts for about one-third of the cardiac cycle followed by diastole for about two-thirds of the cardiac cycle. The MAP over a cardiac cycle can be computed as

$$MAP = \frac{(p_s + 2p_d)}{3} \tag{3.6}$$

where p_s and p_d represent the systolic and diastolic pressures, respectively. The mean aortic pressure for the waveform shown in Figure 3.13 is about 93 mmHg.

The magnitudes of blood pressures in the systemic and pulmonary circulations are shown in Figure 3.14. At the root of the aorta, a pulse pressure of 40 mmHg can be observed. The pressure pulses travel along the arterial wall at a speed much greater than the blood velocity in the vessels and, as the pressure pulse travels downstream through the larger arteries, the pulse pressure increases. The velocity of the pressure pulse in the aorta is ~3–5 m/s and increases to ~7–10 m/s in the large arteries and ~35 m/s in small arteries. It will be shown later that the velocity of transmission of the pressure pulses is directly proportional to the stiffness of the arterial wall. The augmentation of the pressure pulse downstream is due to several factors: (1) the blood vessels in the distal portion are stiffer and, hence, the velocity of transmission increases; (2) curvature and branching sites in the blood vessels reflect the pulse wave and the reflected wave interacts with the waves in the forward direction; and (3) the high-pressure portion of the pressure pulse travels faster than the other parts of the pulse and results in nonlinear interactions.

TABLE 3.1
Cross-Sectional Area of Various Blood Vessels in the Systemic and Pulmonary Circulation Along with the Percentage Volume of Blood for a 20 kg Dog

Vessels	Mean Diameter (mm)	Number of Vessels	Mean Length (mm)	Total Cross Section (cm^2)	Total Volume (mL)	Percentage of Total Blood Volume
Systemic circulation						
Aorta	(19–45)	1		(2.0–16.0)	60	
Arteries	4.000	40	150.0	5.0	75	
Arteries	1.300	500	45.0	6.6	30	
Arteries	0.450	6,000	13.5	9.5	13	11
Arteries	0.150	110,000	4.0	19.4	8	
Arterioles	0.050	2.8×10^6	1.2	55.0	7	
Capillaries	0.008	2.7×10^9	0.65	1357.0	88	5
Venules	0.100	1.0×10^7	1.6	785.4	126	
Veins	0.280	660,000	4.8	406.4	196	
Veins	0.700	40,000	13.5	154.0	208	
Veins	1.800	2.100	45.0	53.4	240	67
Veins	4.500	110	150.0	17.5	263	
Venae cavae	(5–14)	2		(0.2–1.5)	92	
					1,406	
Pulmonary circulation						
Main artery	1.600	1	28.0	2.0	6	
Arteries	4000	20	10.0	2.5	25	3
Arteries	1000	1,550	14.0	12.2	17	
Arterioles	0.100	1.5×10^8	0.7	120.0	8	
Capillaries	0.008	2.7×10^9	0.5	1357.0	68	4
Venules	0.110	2.0×10^6	0.7	190.0	13	
Veins	1.100	1,650	14.0	15.7	22	
Veins	4.200	25	100.0		35	5
Main veins	8.000	4	30.0		6	
					200	
Heart						
Atria		2			30	
Ventricles		2			54	5
					84	
					1,690	100

Source: From Milnor, W.R., *Hemodynamics*, 2nd edn., Williams & Wilkins, Baltimore, MD, 1989.

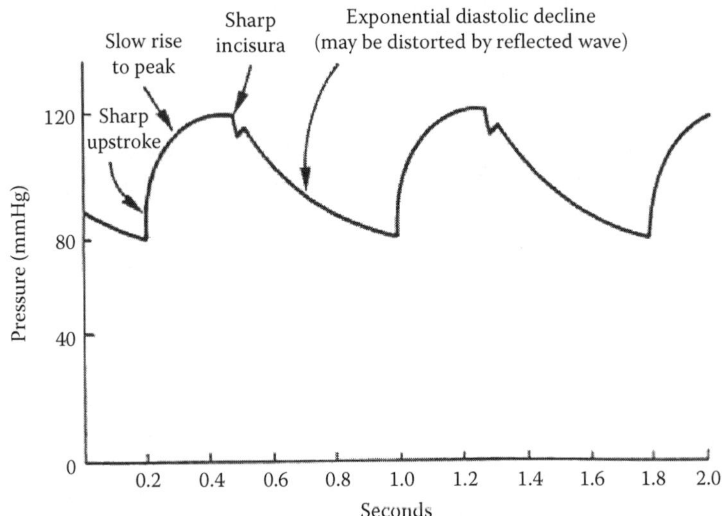

FIGURE 3.13 Schematic of a normal pressure pulse in the aorta depicting the sharp pressure rise in the beginning of systole and the exponential pressure decay during diastole. The incisura during the pressure decay represents the closing of the aortic valve.

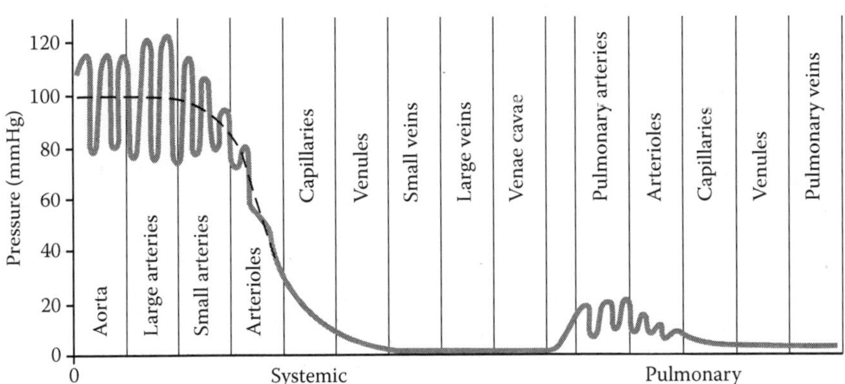

FIGURE 3.14 Pressure pulses in the systemic and pulmonary circulation. (Redrawn from Guyton, A.C. and Hall, J.E., *A Textbook of Medical Physiology*, 10th edn., W.B. Saunders Company, Philadelphia, PA, 2000. With permission.)

Blood traveling downstream has to overcome the resistance to flow in the smaller vessels and, hence, the blood pressure decreases in the distal arteries. As pointed out earlier, the major resistance to flow is provided by the arteriolar segments and, thus, a sharp decrease in blood pressure is observed at the origin of the capillaries where the pressure pulse is minimal. This continues through the veins so that at the end of the venae cavae, as the blood enters the right atrium, the blood pressure is close to 0 mmHg (<5 mmHg). Since all the blood from the venous system empties into the right atrium, measurement of the right atrial pressure is also referred to as the *central venous pressure* (CVP). The CVP is modulated by the ability of the heart to pump blood forward and by the amount of blood that flows back from the peripheral circulation (called the *venous return*). If the heart is not pumping efficiently, the CVP will tend to rise and vice versa.

Venous valves and the "venous pump" also play a major role in the transport of blood back to the heart. If a person is standing, the pressure in the veins in the legs could be as high as 90 mmHg relative to that of the right atrium due to hydrostatic forces. With the contraction of muscles surrounding the veins in the legs due to normal activity, however, the veins are compressed and the blood is "pumped" toward the heart. Venous valves prevent flow back to the legs which would normally occur due to gravity. A defect in the venous valves which allows blood to leak back toward the legs will result in venous distention and stasis that may progress to the development of *varicose veins* and *deep venous thrombosis* (DVT).

3.5 CORONARY CIRCULATION

Nutrients are supplied to the heart muscles by the coronary arteries. The distribution of the main coronary arteries around the heart is illustrated in Figure 3.15. The top panel shows the origin of the left and right coronary arteries from the left and right coronary sinuses. The bottom panel illustrates the principal branches of the left and right coronary arteries. The openings for the coronary arteries, the coronary ostia, are situated in the right and left sinuses of Valsalva. The left coronary artery originates from the left aortic sinus and divides immediately into the left anterior descending and the left circumflex branches. The left coronary artery supplies most of the left ventricle, the anterior two-thirds of the interventricular septum, the anterior left margin of the free wall of the right ventricle, the apex, the left atrium, and the lower half of the interatrial septum. The right coronary artery, originating from the right coronary sinus, supplies the anterior and posterior walls of the right ventricle, the right atrium and the sinus node, the posterior one-third of the interventricular septum, the atrioventricular node, the upper half of the interatrial septum, and the posterior base of the left ventricle. In approximately one-half of humans, more blood flows through the right coronary artery while the left coronary flow is predominant in about 20% of humans. The coronary flow from the large conduit arteries, which are on the *epicardium* (i.e., surface of the heart), branch into arterioles and then capillaries that supply the heart muscle. The blood from the capillaries circulates through the venules and the large conduit veins back to the heart. Eighty-five percent of the returning venous blood drains through the coronary sinus. The remaining 15% flows through the anterior superficial veins and the thebesian veins and directly empties into the cardiac chambers (Marcus, 1983).

The coronary artery circulation has been extensively studied because of the importance of the coronary blood supply in maintaining the proper function of the heart. The resting coronary blood flow is about 225 mL/min, or about 0.8 mL/min/g of the heart muscle. When the heart muscles work harder, for example, during exercise conditions, the coronary blood supply can increase by 4–10 times the resting blood flow rate. The rate of blood flow through the coronary arteries during a cardiac cycle is illustrated in Figure 3.16. During systole, when the heart muscles are contracted, very little flow occurs in the coronary arteries due to the constriction

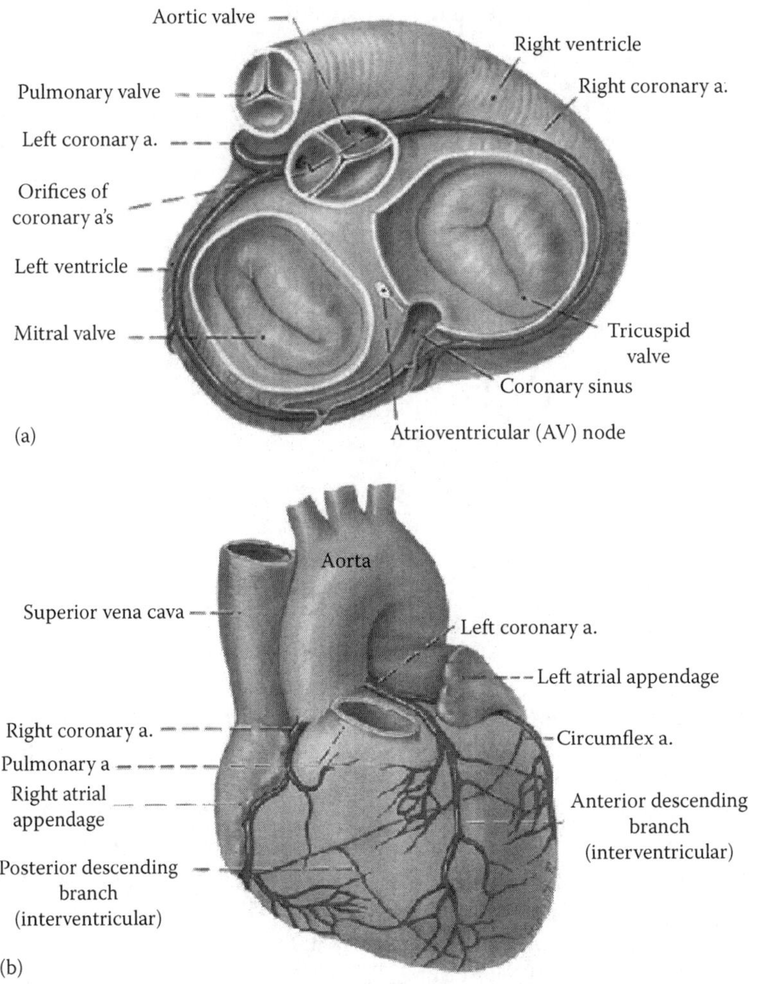

FIGURE 3.15 The anatomical details of the left and right coronary arteries: (a) top view showing the left and right coronary ostia and the origin of the coronary arteries and (b) main branches of the coronary vessels and its perfusion field. (Redrawn from Jacob, S.W. and Francone, C.A., *Structure and Function in Man*, 3rd edn., W.B. Saunders, Philadelphia, PA, 1974. With permission.)

of the intramuscular branch vessels of the coronary arteries. During diastole, the heart muscles are relaxed, the lumen of the intramuscular arteries open fully, and the major portion of the coronary flow occurs. Measurements of coronary blood flow with electromagnetic flow meters have indicated that the flow through the arteries in systole constitutes from 7% to 45% of the total coronary flow during a cardiac cycle (Rushmer, 1976).

During resting conditions, 65% of the oxygen is extracted from the coronary arterial blood as it passes through the heart. The rate of blood flow through the coronary arteries is regulated by the myocardial oxygen demand. Under severe exercise

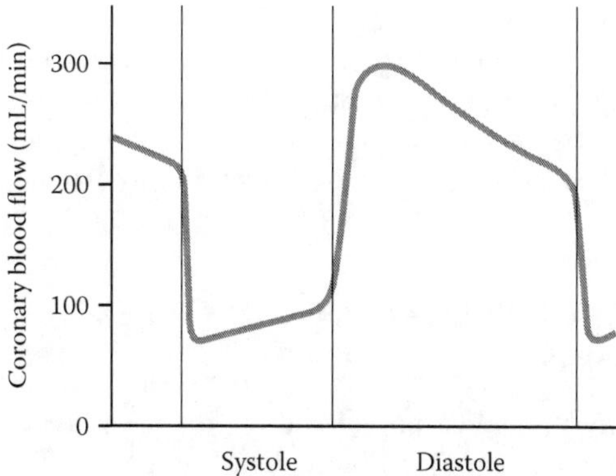

FIGURE 3.16 The blood flow rate in the human left coronary vessels in systole and diastole extrapolated from dog data. (Redrawn from Guyton, A.C. and Hall, J.E., *A Textbook of Medical Physiology*, 10th edn., W.B. Saunders Company, Philadelphia, PA, 2000. With permission.)

conditions, the CO can increase three to six times the resting value. To meet the increased oxygen demand as the cardiac muscles are working harder to increase the CO, the coronary blood flow also increases by several folds. The fact that coronary blood flow is regulated in response to the myocardial oxygen demand can be illustrated by occluding the coronary arteries for a few seconds and then releasing the occlusion. The myocardium distal to the occlusion has a reduction in blood supply and oxygen during the occlusion. Hence, immediately after the occlusion is released, the blood flow through the vessel increases significantly and stays high for a length of time depending upon the length of occlusion. This phenomenon, referred to as *reactive hyperemia*, is illustrated in Figure 3.17.

Chest pain, or *angina pectoris*, results if the myocardium receives inadequate oxygen supply. Angina pectoris can be initiated by physical exertion or emotional stress and is usually relieved by rest or administration of nitrites (drugs that dilate the arteries). *Myocardial infarction* (MI) is the result of acute occlusion of coronary vessels.

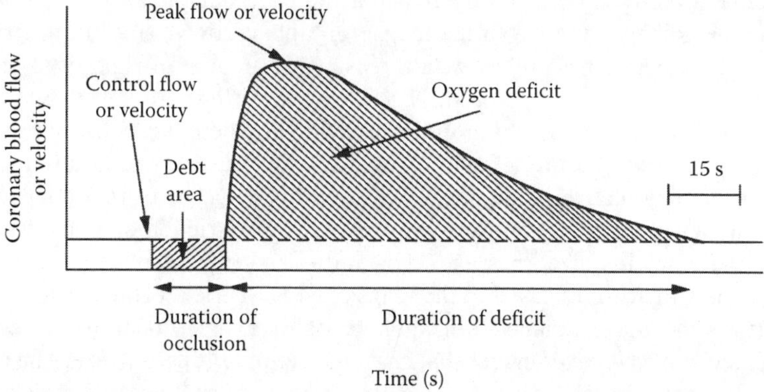

FIGURE 3.17 Schematic of reactive hyperemia caused by occlusion of the coronary vessels.

Coronary artery occlusion is due to the presence of vascular lesions called *atherosclerosis* and will result in lack of blood supply to the portion of the myocardium perfused by the artery together with injury or death to the affected segment. A description of this disease, its predilection, and attempts to relate abnormal flow–induced stresses to the etiology of these lesions are discussed later in this chapter and in subsequent chapters in this book.

3.6 PULMONARY CIRCULATION AND GAS EXCHANGE IN THE LUNGS

The exchange of oxygen and carbon dioxide in the lung takes place between the air in the alveolar sac and the blood in the lung capillaries. The lungs contract or expand due to the upward or downward movement of the diaphragm and by the depression or elevation of the ribs to increase the anterior-posterior diameter of the chest cavity, although normal, quiet breathing is principally accomplished by movement of the diaphragm alone. The diaphragm motion is downward, pulling the lower surfaces of the lung along with it during inspiration. The diaphragm then relaxes and the elastic lung tissue recoils during expiration. In heavy breathing, such as during exercise, additional forces due to the contraction of abdominal muscles assist in the motion of the diaphragm. The lung is surrounded by a thin layer of pleural fluid that lubricates the movement of the lung within the thoracic cavity. The pressure within the pleural space between the lungs and the thoracic cavity is slightly negative (approximately −5 cm of water) at the beginning of inspiration and as the expansion of the thoracic cavity pulls the lungs outward and the pleural pressure becomes more negative (approximately −7.5 cm water). Obviously, when no air is moving in and out of the lungs, the pressure in all parts of the respiratory track, including the alveoli, is equal to atmospheric pressure. During inspiration, the pressure in the alveoli falls to about −1 cm water with respect to atmospheric pressure and about 0.5 L of air fills the lung. During expiration, the alveolar pressure increases to +1 cm water to expire an equal amount of air. The breathed air passes through the trachea, several generations of bronchi, and the bronchioles before reaching the alveolar sacs. Under normal respiratory conditions, a pressure gradient between the atmosphere and alveoli of 1 cm of water is sufficient to maintain airflow into and out of the lungs. Multiple cartilage rings in the trachea and bronchi provide these tubes with a reasonable amount of rigidity to prevent collapse and to allow passage of air. These cartilage rings are not present in the later generations of the bronchi or in the bronchioles where the walls in these segments are composed mainly of smooth muscles. Obstructive diseases in the lung (e.g., chronic obstructive pulmonary disease [COPD]) occur from the narrowing of the smaller bronchi and bronchioles due to the constriction of smooth muscle cells in these smaller sized passages. Histamine and slow reactive substances of anaphylaxis which are released in the lungs due to allergic reactions (caused, e.g., by pollen in the air) can induce bronchiolar constriction. The respiratory passages are kept moist by a layer of mucus that coats the entire luminal surface. The mucus also traps small particles from the inspired air and keeps most of the particles from reaching the alveoli. The respiratory passages are also lined with epithelial

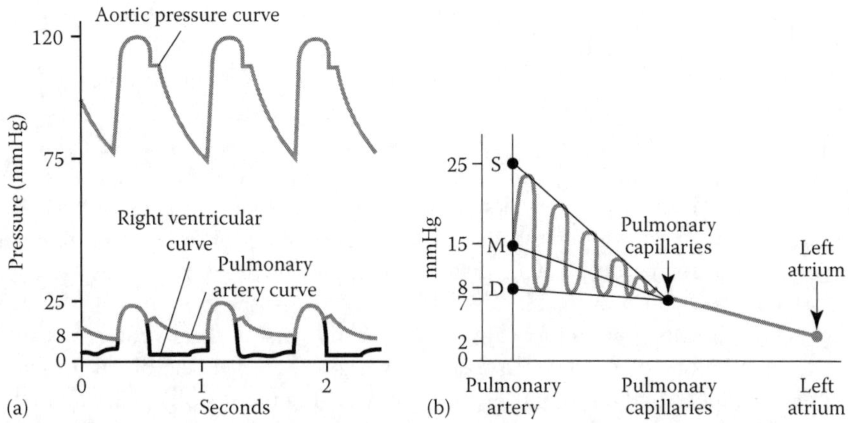

FIGURE 3.18 (a) Typical pressure pulses in the right ventricle, pulmonary artery, and the aorta; and (b) distribution of pressures in the blood vessels in the lung. (Redrawn from Guyton, A.C. and Hall, J.E., *A Textbook of Medical Physiology*, 10th edn., W.B. Saunders Company, Philadelphia, PA, 2000. With permission.)

cells containing about 200 *celia*, or flagella, in each cell. These celia beat continually at a rate of 10–20 times per second, inducing motion of the mucus toward the pharynx which, together with the entrapped particles, is either swallowed or coughed out to the exterior.

Blood flow to the lungs is provided by the contraction of the right ventricle into the pulmonary artery that extends about 4 cm beyond the pulmonary valve before branching into the right and left pulmonary arteries that feed the two lungs. The pressure pulse curve for the right ventricle is compared with that of the aorta in Figure 3.18a and the pressures in the blood vessels of the lung are shown in Figure 3.18b. The systolic and diastolic right ventricular pressures are about 22 and 0 mmHg, respectively. In the pulmonary artery, the corresponding pressures are 22 and 8 mmHg with a pulse pressure of 14 mmHg. By conservation of mass, the rate of blood flow from the right ventricle into the lungs averaged over time must be the same as the rate at which blood is pumped by the left ventricle into the systemic circulation. Thus, the flow rate through the lungs is very high compared with that of other organs because the entire CO must flow through the lungs to become oxygenated. This is possible fluid dynamically because the distance traversed by the blood in the pulmonary circulation is relatively short compared with that in the systemic circulation and because the pulmonary arterioles are larger in size and more distensible than their systemic counterparts, causing the resistance in the pulmonary circulation to be low. Therefore, the lower pressures generated by the right ventricle are still sufficient to maintain the same CO through the pulmonary circulation and back into the left atrium (see Equation 1.54). The lungs themselves are supplied with oxygenated blood for nutrition through the bronchial arteries that originate from the systemic circulation. The flow in this circuit amounts to only 1%–2% of the CO. The bronchial circulation supplies oxygen to supporting tissues of the lungs, including connective tissue as well as the bronchi. The blood from the bronchial circulation empties into the pulmonary veins and returns to the left atrium, thus bypassing the lung capillaries (i.e., alveoli).

Due to the low pulmonary pressures, distribution of blood flow in the lung capillaries is noticeably affected by gravity. More specifically, when a person is in the standing position, pressure in the base (inferior) region is higher than in the apical (superior) region of the lung. Another important phenomenon is that the capillaries in the alveolar walls are distended by blood pressure but are also compressed by air pressure in the alveoli. Hence, in the regions where the alveolar air pressure becomes larger than that of the capillary blood pressure, the capillaries collapse and prevent blood flow. Therefore, in the basal regions of the lungs where the blood pressure is always higher than that of the alveolar pressure, there is continuous blood flow. In the apical zones, however, the blood pressure becomes higher than the alveolar pressure only during the systolic phase and thus results in an intermittent flow through the capillaries. During exercise when there is an increase in CO, the flow through the lungs may increase by fourfold up to sevenfold. This additional flow is accomplished by increasing the number of open capillaries, distension of the capillaries, and by an increase in the pulmonary arterial pressure.

The exchange of oxygen from the fresh inspired air in the alveolar sac to blood in the pulmonary capillaries and carbon dioxide in the opposite direction takes place through the process of *diffusion* from a region of high to low species concentration. One dimensional transport of nonelectrolytes across a membrane is governed by *Fick's law* that is expressed as

$$N_i = -D_i \frac{dC_i}{dz} = -D_i \frac{\Delta C_i}{\delta} \tag{3.7}$$

where

N_i is the molar flux of the species i
D_i is the diffusion coefficient
C_i is the molar concentration
δ is the thickness of the membrane across which the mass transport occurs

The diffusion flux can also be expressed in terms of the partial pressure of the species dissolved in air or in blood. The partial pressure of the dissolved gas is given by Henry's law $\Delta C_i = K_D \Delta p_i$ where K_D is the solubility coefficient and Δp is the partial pressure difference. The transport of gases in the lung is induced by the difference in partial pressures between the alveolar air and the pulmonary capillary blood across the respiratory membrane. The respiratory membrane consists of a layer of fluid lining the alveolus containing a *surfactant* (to reduce the surface tension of the alveolar air), the *alveolar epithelium*, an *epithelial basement membrane*, a thin interstitial space, a capillary basement membrane, and the *capillary endothelial cell layer.* The thickness of the respiratory membrane averages about 6 μm and the total surface area of the respiratory membrane in normal adults is about 70 m^2 for efficient exchange of gases. The total amount of gas transported across the respiratory membrane can be obtained as the product of the mass flux and the area of the respiratory membrane available for the transport and is given by

$$w = -\frac{D_i K_{Di} A}{\delta} \Delta p_i = -D_{Li} \Delta p_i \tag{3.8}$$

In this equation, w is the total amount of gas transported across the respiratory membrane cross-sectional area, A. Since A and δ are very difficult to determine accurately, all the parameters in the equation are lumped together as the diffusing capacity D_L. Under resting conditions, the diffusing capacity of O_2 is 21 mL/min · mmHg and that of CO_2 is 400–450 mL/min · mmHg. The time-averaged partial pressure difference across the respiratory membrane under resting conditions is about 11 mmHg and the total amount of oxygen transferred across the respiratory membrane is about 252 mL/min. The total amount of CO_2 transferred is about 200 mL/min. Since the solubility of oxygen in aqueous solution is rather poor, oxygen diffuses across the red blood cell membrane in the capillary and then reacts with hemoglobin in the intracellular fluid volume so that it is transported principally as *oxyhemoglobin*.

3.7 CEREBRAL AND RENAL CIRCULATIONS

3.7.1 Cerebral Circulation

Blood circulation to the brain is supplied by the carotid arteries and the vertebral arteries. The brachiocephalic, left common carotid, and left subclavian arterial branches originate from the aortic arch. The brachiocephalic artery further divides into the right subclavian and the right common carotid arteries. In the neck region, the carotid arteries bifurcate into the internal and external carotid arteries. The external carotid arteries supply blood to the face and the skull, while the internal carotids feed the cranial cavity. In addition, vertebral arteries branch out from the two subclavian arteries and ascend to the cranial cavity protected by the bony arches of the cervical vertebrae. The vertebral arteries join to form the basilar artery in the hind (back) brain which is connected to the internal carotid arteries through the *Circle of Willis* as shown in Figure 3.19.

The Circle of Willis is a protective mechanism in that blood flow can be shunted to different parts of the brain around the circle if one of the feeding arteries is occluded. The normal blood flow to the brain is about 750 or 50–55 mL/min per 100 g of brain matter. The control of blood supply to the brain is such that it is maintained at this level even under severe conditions.

3.7.2 Renal Circulation

The right and left renal arteries originate from the descending aorta and supply blood to the two kidneys. In addition to removing the body waste material that is either ingested or produced by metabolism, the kidneys also regulate water and electrolyte balances, body fluid osmolality and electrolyte concentration, acid-base balance, and blood pressure and volume. The two kidneys lie on the posterior wall of the abdomen, outside the peritoneal cavity. The renal circulation is unique in that it

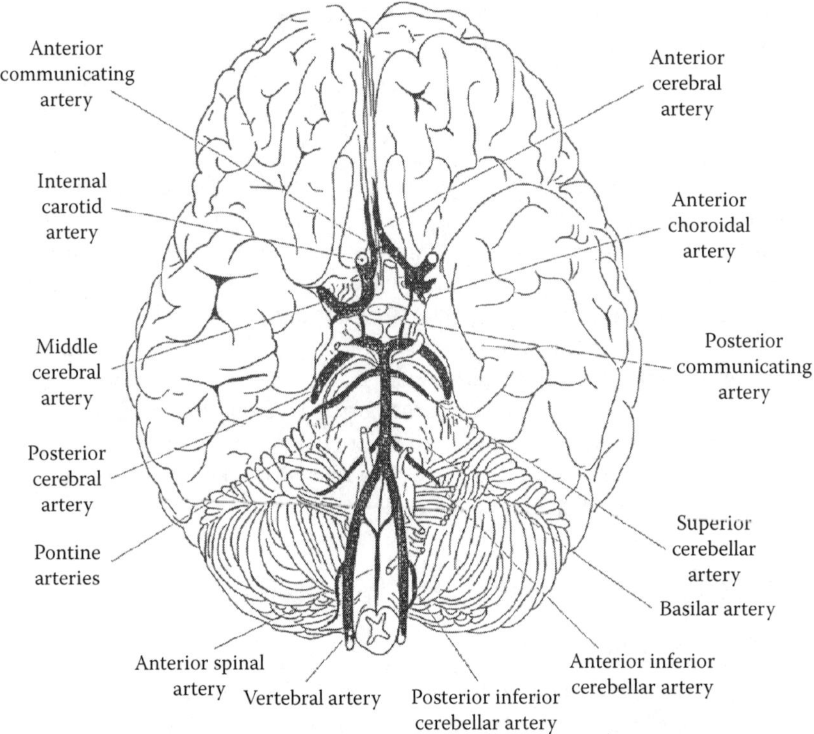

FIGURE 3.19 Schematic of blood flow in the human brain showing the Circle of Willis connecting flow from the vertebral and carotid arteries. (Redrawn from DeArmond, S.J., Fusco, M.M., and Dewey, M.M, *Structure of the Human Brain*, 1974, by permission of Oxford University Press.)

has two capillary beds, the glomerular and peritubular capillaries. The blood flow rate to the kidneys is about 1100 to 1200 mL/min or about 25% of the CO. The renal artery branches progressively to form the interlobar arteries, arcuate arteries, and interlobular (also called radial arteries) arteries that lead into the afferent arterioles. The glomerular capillaries that lie at the end of the afferent arterioles filter large amounts of fluid and solutes, except for the plasma proteins, to begin the process for urine formation. High hydrostatic pressures in the glomerular capillaries cause rapid filtration across these capillaries into the Bowman's capsule (Figure 3.20). Distally, these capillaries coalesce to form the efferent arterioles leading to the peritubular capillaries. Lower hydrostatic pressures in these capillaries enable fluid to be rapidly absorbed from the filtrate transported from the Bowman's capsule via the tubules traversing adjacent to the capillary bed. By adjusting the resistances of the afferent and efferent arterioles, the kidneys can alter the amount of glomerular filtrate as well as the amount of fluid reabsorbed based on the body's demand. The peritubular capillaries empty into the interlobular veins that progressively coalesce into the arcuate veins, interlobar veins, and into the renal veins. These vessels join the venous circulation (IVC) that returns the blood to the right atrium.

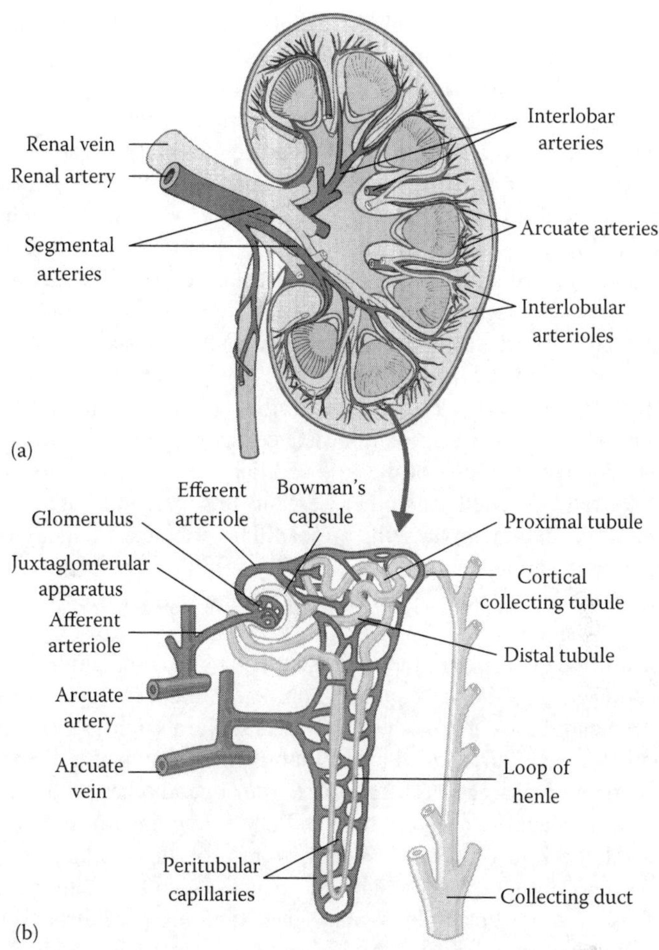

FIGURE 3.20 Schematic of the blood supply to the kidneys: (a) renal artery and vein and (b) details of the afferent and efferent arterioles along with the Bowman's capsule used in the filtration of blood of waste products. (Redrawn from Guyton, A.C. and Hall, J.E., *A Textbook of Medical Physiology*, 10th edn., W.B. Saunders Company, Philadelphia, PA, 2000. With permission.)

3.8 MICROCIRCULATION

In the previous sections, we reviewed blood flow in both the systemic and pulmonary circulations. We started with the contractile function of the heart in generating a sufficient pressure gradient in order to induce flow along the circulatory system. We also discussed the arterial system that acts as the main conduits transporting blood to the various visceral organs and the peripheries of the human body. In large blood vessels, the typical size (i.e., diameter) of the blood vessel is several magnitudes larger than the formed elements of blood, such as the red blood cells and the white blood cells, so that blood may be treated as a homogeneous fluid. These large vessels mainly function as conduits for supplying blood to the capillary network.

The exchange of nutrients and cellular excreta between the tissues and the flowing blood occurs at the level of capillaries. The fluid mechanics within the arterioles and capillaries are characteristically different from those in large arteries. Hence, flow of blood in the system of blood vessels consisting of arterioles, capillaries, and venules is termed the *microcirculation*. The arteries divide into arterioles and the diameters of arterioles can range up to 100 μm. The walls of the arterioles are highly muscular and have the ability to alter the vessel diameter several fold and hence vary the resistance to flow across the microvascular bed. The arterioles divide into metarterioles with diameters of about 20 μm. The musculature in the metarterioles is not continuous as smooth muscle fibers are found intermittently surrounding the wall. The branching pattern of the capillary network varies from tissue to tissue as well as within any one bed. Some of the capillary vessels (referred to as "true capillaries") that branch from the metarterioles have pre-capillary sphincters at their origin. The sphincters consist of one or two smooth muscle cells wrapped around the arteriolar-capillary junction. The diameter of the true capillary ranges from 5 to 8 μm barely large enough for red blood cells and other elements to squeeze through. Some of the capillaries are large and do not have the pre-capillary sphincters and are referred to as the "preferential channels." If the pre-capillary sphincters constrict, the blood is shunted through the low-resistance preferential channels and hence the microvascular bed unit is bypassed.

The concentration of oxygen in the tissue supplied by the unit regulates the degree of opening and closing of the pre-capillary sphincters and amount of blood flowing through the true capillaries. The wall of the true capillaries consists of a unicellular layer of endothelial cells surrounded by a thin basement membrane of about 0.5 μm in thickness. Pores or passageways, far apart from one another with a fraction of the lumen surface area, are present in the capillary membrane through which water and water-soluble substances pass between the lumen of the capillary and the interstitial fluid. Several of these water-soluble substances, such as sodium and chloride ions and glucose, are not lipid-soluble and hence can only pass through the pores. Transport of fluid between the capillary lumen and the interstitial fluid depends on the hydrostatic and colloid osmotic pressure difference between the capillary blood and the interstitial fluid. The rate at which water-soluble substances transport across the pores depends upon the permeability of the capillary pores. The diameter of the pores is about 80–90 Å. Water molecules are much smaller than the pore diameter and hence have a larger permeability compared with that of the plasma protein molecules. Lipid-soluble substances such as oxygen and carbon dioxide are transported by means of diffusion across the cell membrane into the capillary. The amount of diffusion is directly proportional to the concentration difference across the two sides of the membrane. At the distal end, the capillaries merge into post capillaries and then into *venules*. In the systemic circulation, venules merge into larger veins terminating in the SVC and IVC which drain the blood into the right atrium. The lymphatic circulation drains the excess fluid from the interstitial locations. Lymphatic capillaries are blind-ended sacs present in the interstitial space around the collecting venules and which merge into collecting lymphatics. These become lymphatic vessels that run parallel to the veins and that drain via the thoracic duct into the subclavian vein in the neck.

Even the largest arterioles in the microvascular bed have a diameter that is only about 15 times larger than that of the red blood cells. The true capillary diameter is about the same size or smaller than that of the red blood cell and, thus, the cells must squeeze through the capillaries. In such flow situations, the blood cannot be considered as a continuum and the interaction between particulates (i.e., cells) and the plasma must be taken into account. Due to the small diameters and low velocities in the microcirculation, viscous effects dominate over inertial effects and the magnitude of the Reynolds number ranges between 0.005 and 0.5. However, the velocity gradient at the wall or the wall shear rates in the microcirculation is of the order of $1000\,s^{-1}$ and are relatively large compared with that of those in the arteries as we will observe in subsequent chapters. The study of microcirculatory dynamics is beyond the scope of this textbook but can be found in treatises such as Caro et al. (1978) and Fung (1984).

3.9 REGULATION OF THE CIRCULATION

The human body has mechanisms for regulation of the heart function and the circulation based on the needs of the various regions and the visceral organs of the body. Regulation of the circulation consists of systemic control as well as the ability for each tissue to control its own blood flow based on its metabolic needs. The metabolic needs include the delivery of oxygen and nutrients such as glucose, amino acids, and fatty acids, removal of carbon dioxide and hydrogen ions from the tissues, transport of hormones, and maintenance of a concentration balance of other ions. Acute control of local blood flow is achieved by altering the resistance to blood flow into the region by rapid changes in the tone of the arterioles, metarterioles, and pre-capillary sphincters within a few seconds to several minutes. The widely accepted mechanism through which the local vascular tone is altered is that with higher metabolism of a tissue, the availability of oxygen and other metabolites decreases. In response, the tissue releases vasodilators such as adenosine and carbon dioxide, among others, in order to reduce the vascular resistance and increase blood flow to the tissue. Another possible mechanism is that, due to lack of sufficient oxygen, the blood vessels naturally relax and dilate to allow more blood flow. A typical example of the local regulation of blood flow is the *reactive hyperemia* in the coronary circulation described earlier (Figure 3.17). The local mechanism for increasing blood flow into the tissues is dilation of the microvessels in the tissue. Rapid flow of blood in the arterioles and small arteries also causes an increase in the wall shear stress acting on the endothelial cells. The endothelial cells respond to this stimulus by releasing *endothelial-derived relaxing factor* (EDRF), or, nitric oxide. Nitric oxide acts to relax the local arterial wall and, hence, the vessels dilate locally. Both the kidneys and the brain have special mechanisms for control of blood flow. In the case of kidneys, the composition of the fluid in the early distal tubule is monitored by a tubular epithelial structure called the *macula densa*. When too much fluid is filtered through the glomerular capillaries into the tubular system, feedback signals from the macula densa constrict the afferent and efferent arterioles in the kidneys to reduce the renal blood flow and the glomerular filtrate. In the brain, the concentration of carbon dioxide and hydrogen ions also influences the blood flow rate to the organ in addition to the effect of changes in tissue oxygen concentration.

Long-term control of local blood flow (i.e., effecting changes over a period of weeks or months) in proportion to the needs of the tissue is the result of increase or decrease of the physical size and number of blood vessels supplying the tissue. If the metabolic rate in a given tissue is increased over a prolonged period, the vascularity is also increased. Growth of new blood vessels to increase vascularity results from the presence of various peptides such as *vascular endothelial growth factor* (VEGF), *fibroblast growth factor*, and *angiogenin* among others. Another mechanism for increasing the vascularity is by development of a collateral circulation. When a blood vessel is blocked, collateral vessels develop in the region around the blocked vessel over a period of time in order to compensate for the decrease in blood supply. For example, collateral blood supply is an important mechanism for keeping the cardiac muscles viable and, possibly preventing a heart attack, after thrombosis of a coronary vessel.

The global nervous control of circulation and cardiac function is performed by the autonomic *sympathetic* and *parasympathetic* nervous systems. The control of both these nervous systems is affected by the vasomotor center in the brain. The sympathetic vasomotor nerve fibers pass through the spinal cord and innervate the visceral organs and the heart, as well as the vasculature in the peripheral region. Parasympathetic nerve fibers do not play a major role in the control of circulation, but control the heart by the nerve fibers contained in the vagus nerve. The sympathetic nerve fibers carry a large number of vasoconstrictor fibers that secrete norepinephrinc. Constriction of the blood vessels by norepinephrine increases the resistance to blood flow (due to a reduction in the radius of the vessels), resulting in an increase in the blood pressure. The large veins are also constricted and, hence, blood from these highly distensible vessels is displaced toward the heart. Thus, the volume of ventricular filling increases, resulting in increased CO through the *Frank-Starling* mechanism. With increase in the filling volume, the heart muscles contract with increased force and, hence, the SV (and the CO) increases together with an increase in blood pressure. The sympathetic nervous system also directly acts on the heart by *increasing* both the HR and the force of contraction. Parasympathetic nerve fibers, on the other hand, *decrease* the HR and cause a slight decrease in heart contractility resulting in a reduction in CO and blood pressure.

Baroreceptors or pressoreceptors are stretch receptors in the nervous control system that helps to control the arterial blood pressure. These receptors are located particularly in the wall of the aortic arch and in the walls of the internal carotid artery slightly above the bifurcation in the carotid sinus. The baroreceptors respond rapidly to *changes* in blood pressure (rather than to the MAP). Should the blood pressure rapidly rise, the signals from the baroreceptors inhibit the vasoconstrictor nerves and excite the vagal parasympathetic nerves. The net result is the dilation of the peripheral blood vessels while the HR and force of contraction of the cardiac muscles are reduced. Should the blood pressure rapidly decrease, the opposite effects will take place resulting in an increase in blood pressure. The nervous control system can act to rapidly control the blood pressure for a short time on the order of minutes.

The kidneys play an important role in the long-term control of blood pressure and in the development of hypertension (i.e., high blood pressure). When the body contains too much extracellular fluid, the blood volume and mean arterial pressure rise. The kidneys react to the increased blood pressure by excreting excess body fluid and return the blood pressure to its normal value. This phenomenon of increasing urinary output to control the blood pressure is known as *pressure diuresis*. Aside from using changes in the extracellular fluid in the kidneys to control blood pressure, the renin-angiotensin system in the kidneys also plays an important role in blood pressure control. With a decrease in the blood pressure, renin is released in the kidneys. This enzyme reacts chemically with plasma proteins to release angiotensins I and II. Intense vasoconstriction caused by the effect of *angiotensin II* in the artery results in an increase in blood pressure. Mild constriction of the veins displaces additional blood to the heart, resulting in increase in ventricular filling and CO and an increase in blood pressure as well. When the MAP rises to magnitudes above 110 mmHg (along with corresponding increases in systolic and diastolic blood pressures), this condition is referred to as *hypertension*. Hypertension can be a result of release of large quantities of renin in the kidneys due to malfunction of the renin-secreting juxtaglomerular cells. Chronic high blood pressure will result in excess workload and eventual failure of the heart, rupture of blood vessels, particularly in the brain, renal hemorrhage, and renal failure.

3.10 ATHEROSCLEROSIS

Diseases in the blood vessels and in the heart, such as heart attack and stroke, are responsible for nearly half of the deaths in the United States. The underlying cause for these events is the formation of lesions, known as *atherosclerotic plaques*, in the large and medium-sized arteries in the human circulation. These plaques can grow and occlude the artery and hence prevent blood supply to its distal bed. Plaques with calcium in them can also rupture and initiate the formation of blood clots (*thrombus*). The clots can form *emboli* that are carried in the bloodstream and occlude smaller vessels, resulting in interruption of blood supply to the distal bed. Plaques formed in coronary arteries can lead to heart attacks while those formed in the cerebral circulation can result in stroke. There are a number of risk factors for the presence of atherosclerotic lesions. Those for which we have no control include gender, age, and familial history of early cardiovascular disease. *Risk factors* that can be controlled to minimize the occurrence of atherosclerosis include smoking, obesity, sedentary life style, elevated serum cholesterol and triglycerides, untreated high blood pressure, and diabetes mellitus.

3.10.1 Morphology of Atherosclerosis

Atherosclerosis is associated with lipid deposition in the subendothelial space, intimal thickening, SMC proliferation, and plaque formation. It is an inflammatory response of the arterial wall to injury resulting from fluid dynamics, local oxidation of lipoproteins, or toxins (carbon monoxide). Increased accumulation of lipid and lipoprotein particles underneath the endothelium is made possible by locally enhanced permeability. Oxidation of lipoproteins within the intima leads to activation of endothelial cells and expression of receptors for monocytes and lymphocytes (immune response).

In the presence of elevated plasma cholesterol and high levels of *low-density lipoproteins* (LDL), oxidation within the intima, formation of foam cells from monocytes and mast cells, and their continued accumulation in the intima lead to an atherosclerotic lesion or *fatty streak*. With the continuing effect of hypercholesterolemia, endothelial cell injury, and abnormal hemodynamics, the fatty streak will grow into a fibro-fatty lesion containing multiple layers of SMC, connective tissue, macrophages, and T lymphocytes (Figure 3.21). With further growth, a fibrous cap will form to create an *advanced lesion*.

The role of elevated blood cholesterol levels in the development of atherosclerosis is well-established. Cholesterol is a lipid that is absorbed in the digestive tract and is not soluble in aqueous solutions. Cholesterol combines with a lipoprotein molecule so that it can dissolve in the plasma. Cholesterol that combines with *high-density lipoproteins* (HDL) is associated with lower risk of heart attacks, whereas elevated levels of LDL-cholesterol is associated with arterial disease. The LDL carrier is necessary for cholesterol uptake into all of the body cells. The LDL portion of the complex combines with an LDL receptor in the cell membrane and the receptor-LDL-cholesterol complex enters into the cell by *endocytosis*. However, if LDL-cholesterol is not absorbed into the cells and remains in the blood, the excess LDL-cholesterol will move into the walls of the arteries.

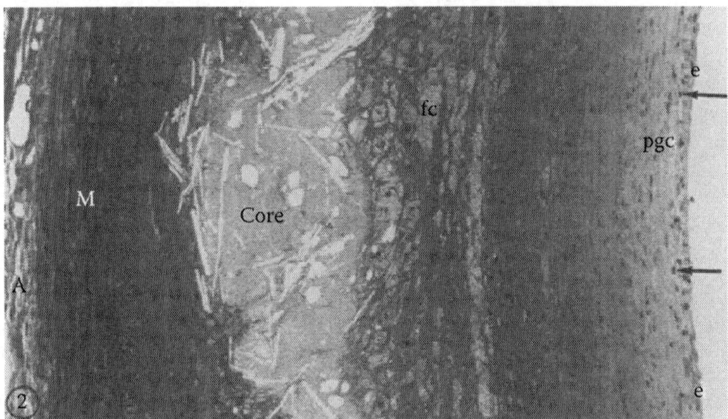

FIGURE 3.21 Photomicrograph of thick part of an advanced atherosclerotic lesion in a coronary artery. Core of extracellular lipid includes cholesterol crystals. Macrophage foam cells (fc) overlie core on aspect toward lumen. Macrophages that are not foam cells (arrows) occupy proteoglycan layer (pgc) adjacent to the endothelium (e) at lesion surface. A indicates adventitia; M, media. Fixation by pressure perfusion with glutaraldehyde. Maraglas embedding. One micron thick section. Magnification 220×. (Reprinted from Stary, H.C. et al., AHA Medical/Scientific Statements, American Heart Association, Dallas, TX, 1995. With permission.)

3.10.2 Sequence of Growth of the Lesion

The initiation and development of atherosclerotic plaques is schematically depicted in Figure 3.22. In the early stages of the lesion formation, the excess LDL-cholesterol accumulates in the acellular layer between the endothelium and the connective tissue. There it is oxidized and absorbed by the macrophages

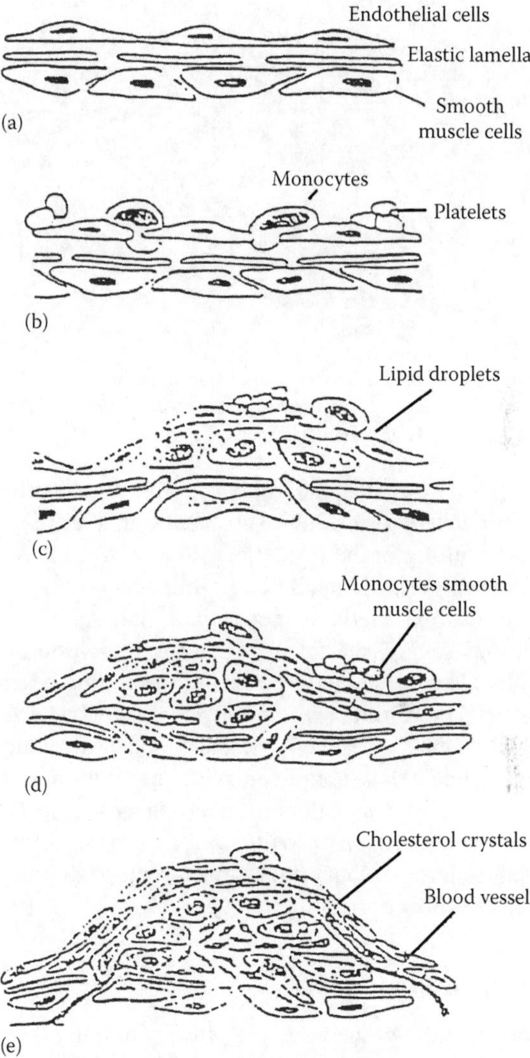

FIGURE 3.22 Postulated sequence of events in the pathogenesis of atherosclerosis: (a) normal vessel wall; (b) endothelial injury leading to attachment of monocytes and platelets; (c) infiltration of monocytes into the intima and accumulation of lipids; (d) smooth muscle cells migrating into the subendothelial space; and (e) foam cell population consisting of lipid-containing macrophages and smooth muscle cells continuously building up. (From White, R.A. and Cavaye, D.M., *A Text and Atlas of Arterial Imaging—Modern and Developing Technology*, Cavaye, D.M. and White, R.A., eds., 1993.)

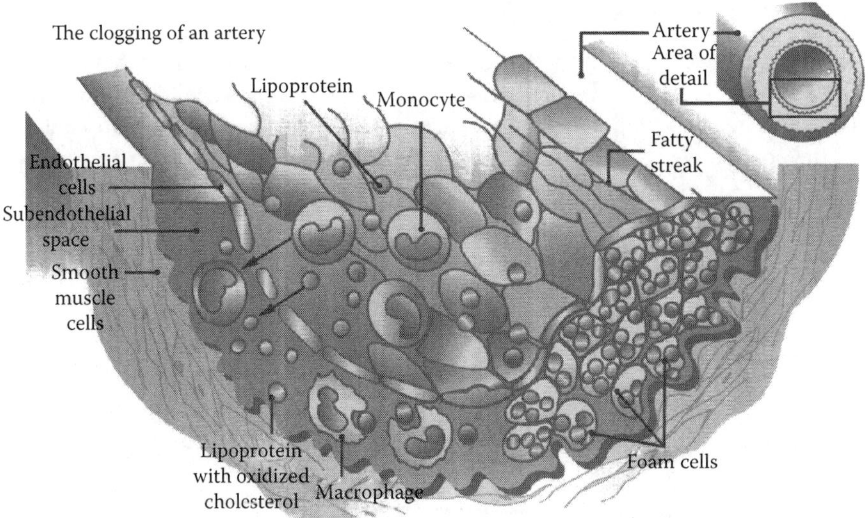

FIGURE 3.23 Schematic of the components involved in the development of atherosclerosis. (From Kleinstreuer et al., Chapter 1 in *Cardiovascular Techniques*, C. Leondes, ed., CRC Press, Boca Raton, FL, 2001. With permission.)

through *phagocytosis*. When the macrophages are filled with oxidized LDL-cholesterol, they produce *paracrines*—substances that attract smooth muscle cells to the region, resulting in the formation of *fatty streaks*. When these events occur, newly formed cells in the media begin migrating into the intima and lay down additional fibrous extracellular matrix material. As cholesterol continues to accumulate, fibrous scar tissue forms around the cholesterol. The migrating smooth muscle cells also divide, and as a result, the intima begins to thicken, or become hyperplastic. The resultant *intimal hyperplasia* (IH) is a serious chronic response of arterial tissue to changes in local blood flow, which may result in arterial occlusion. When IH is combined with the abnormal accumulation of excess fatty material, as well as calcium, macrophages from the blood stream, and necrotic tissue, then an *atherosclerotic plaque* is said to form (Figure 3.23). The enlarging atherosclerotic plaque then starts to protrude into the lumen until it eventually becomes a flow obstruction.

3.10.3 Physiological Implications

To compensate for expanding atheroma, the arteries initially remodel by distending and becoming thinner to maintain the arterial lumen cross section for normal blood flow. Once the remodeling limit is reached, however, the lesion protrudes into the lumen forming a *stenosis*. In the advanced stages of the lesion, the cells in the plaque may die and form calcified scar tissue. The deposits of calcium create the hardening of the arteries which reduces the distensibility in the region of the atherosclerotic plaques. If the plaques have a rough surface or if they rupture, platelets will stick to the damaged area and with each other to form a thrombus on

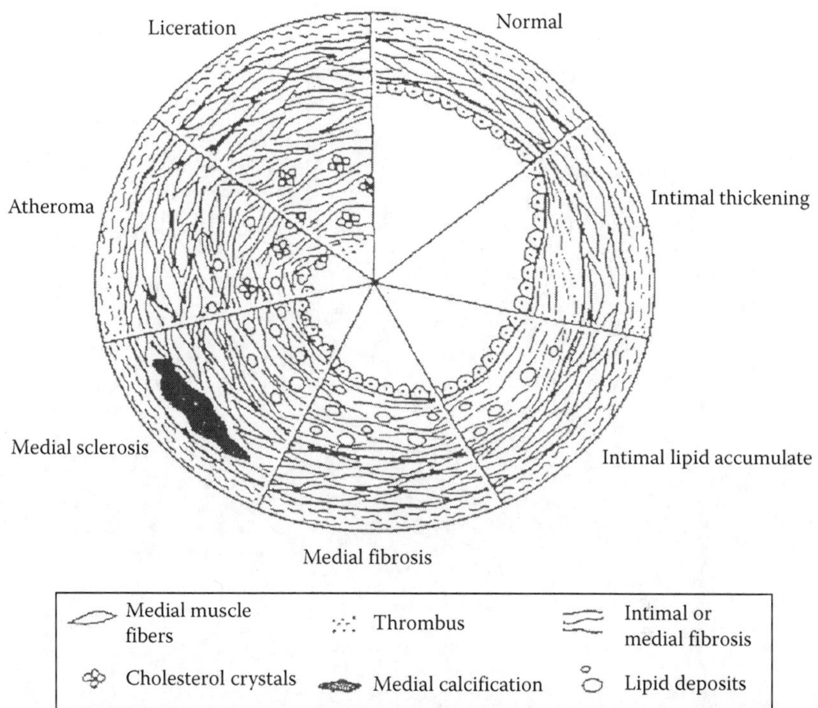

FIGURE 3.24 Schematic of the cross section of a blood vessel illustrating the growth of atherosclerotic lesions progressively reducing the lumen area available for blood flow to the distal beds supplied by the vessel. (Redrawn from Engeler et al., *Am. J. Roentgenol.*, 156, 1087, 1991.)

the arterial wall. Figure 3.24 shows the progression of initial fatty lesions to calcified plaques in the intimal layer of a blood vessel and the gradual decrease in the lumen cross section available for blood flow.

The common sites of predilection of atherosclerosis in the human circulation are shown in Figure 3.25. These include the coronary arteries, the branching of the subclavian and common carotids in the aortic arch, the bifurcation of the common carotid to the internal and external carotids, especially in the carotid sinus region distal to the bifurcation, the renal arterial branching in the descending aorta and in the ileofemoral bifurcations of the descending aorta. The common feature for the development of the lesion is the presence of curvature, branching, and bifurcation present in these sites. Besides the geometry, the fluid dynamics at these sites can be anticipated to be considerably different from that at other segments of arteries that are relatively straight and devoid of any branching segments. Hence, a number of investigators have attempted to link fluid dynamically induced stresses with the formation of atherosclerotic lesions in the human circulation. Hemodynamic theories for the genesis of atheromatous plaques and detailed descriptions of the fluid dynamics at corresponding sites will be the topic of discussion in subsequent chapters where steady and unsteady flow models in the human circulation will be considered.

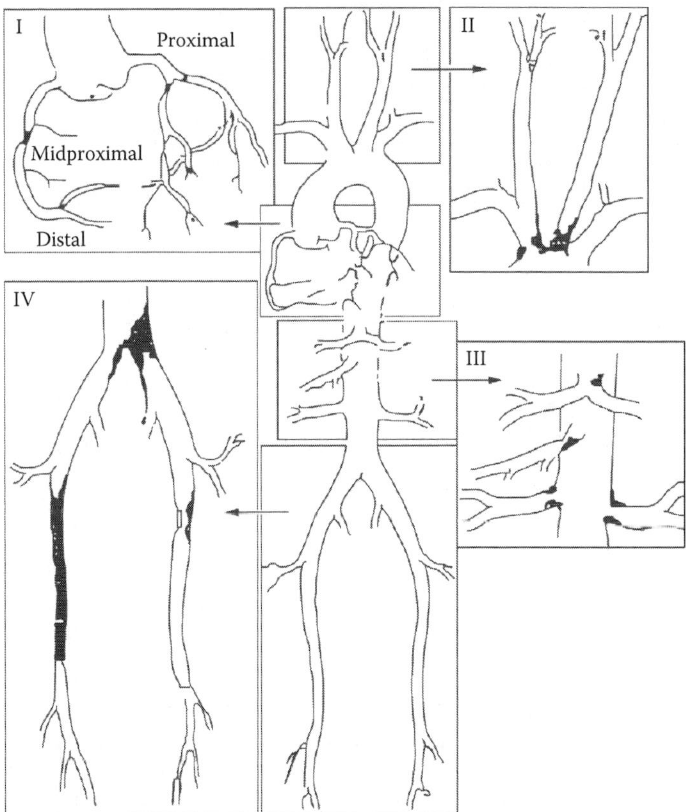

FIGURE 3.25 Common sites for the presence of atherosclerotic plaques in the human circulation. (Redrawn from DeBakey et al., *Ann. Surg.*, 201, 115, 1985.)

PROBLEMS

3.1 Under normal conditions, the mean systemic arterial pressure at the aortic root is 95 mmHg and the corresponding CVP is 0 mmHg. The corresponding pressures in the pulmonary artery and the left atrium are 13 and 4 mmHg, respectively. If the CO is 5.2 L/min, compute the peripheral resistance in the systemic and pulmonary circulation. Express your answers in PRUs as well as in SI units. In the case of moderate exercise, the mean aortic pressure rose to 150 mmHg and the CO increased by three times the normal value. Compute the percentage change in the systemic peripheral resistance. (Conversion factor: 1 mmHg = 133.3 Pa.)

3.2 In a clinical situation, the SV for a patient was measured at 45 mL/stroke and the HR was recorded to be 85 bpm. Compute the CO for the patient. Cardiac index is expressed as the ratio of CO over the body surface area. Assuming that the human body can be approximated to be a cylinder, compute the cardiac index (lpm/m^2) for the patient if the height and average diameter for the patient were measured to be 5.6 and 0.95 ft, respectively.

3.3 The resting coronary blood flow in a normal human is 225 mL/min assuming that 19.4 mL of oxygen is transported by the blood for every 100 mL of blood and 65% of oxygen is absorbed by the myocardium as the blood passes through the coronary arteries, compute the amount of oxygen consumed by the heart muscles each minute.

3.4 In a typical human aortic segment of 10 cm length and an average diameter of 2.5 cm, a 8% increase in diameter is measured for a pulse pressure of 40 mmHg. Compute the compliance of the aortic vessel.

3.5 Estimate the work done by the left ventricle of the heart in 1 day, in lbf · ft using the pressure-volume diagram for the cardiac cycle shown in Figure 3.8. This estimate is smaller than the actual work done by the heart. Why? How far could one raise a 100 lb weight with this amount of work?

3.6 The amount of work done per cycle computed in Problem 3.5 is the left ventricular work output. For a HR of 70 bpm, the left ventricular output per minute can be computed. The amount of oxygen consumed by the myocardial muscle per minute computed in Problem 3.3 can be converted as work input to the heart (1 mL of O_2 consumed = 20 J = 14.75 lbf · ft). Compute the efficiency of the heart as the ratio of work output to the work input.

REFERENCES

Burton, A. C. (1971) *Physiology and Biophysics of the Circulation*, Year Book Medical Publishers, Chicago, IL.

Caro, C. G., Pedley, T. J., Schroter, R. C., and Seed, W. A. (1978) *The Mechanics of the Circulation*, Oxford Medical Publications, Oxford, U.K.

DeArmond, S. J., Fusco, M. M., and Dewey, M. M. (1974) *Structure of the Human Brain*, Oxford University Press, London, U.K.

DeBakey, M. E., Lawrey, G. M., and Glaeser, G. H. (1985) Patterns of arteriosclerosis and their surgical significance. *Ann. Surg*. 201: 115–131.

Engeler, C. E., Edlicky, J., Letourneau, J. W., Castaneda-Auniga, J. G., Hunger, W. R., and Amplat, D. W. (1991) Intravascular sonography in the detection of arteriosclerosis and evaluation of vascular interventional procedures. *AJR* 156: 1087–1090.

Fung, Y. C. (1984) *Biodynamics: Circulation*, Springer-Verlag, New York.

Guyton, A. C. and Hall, J. E. (2000) *A Textbook of Medical Physiology*, 10th edn., W.B. Saunders Company, Philadelphia, PA.

Jacob, S. W. and Francone, C. A. (1974) *Structure and Function in Man*, 3rd edn., W.B. Saunders, Co., Philadelphia, PA.

Kleinstreuer, C., Buchanan Jr., J. R., Lei, M., and Truskey, G. A. (2001) Computational analysis of particle hemodynamics and prediction of the onset of arterial diseases. In *Cardiovascular Techniques*, Leondes, C. ed., CRC Press, Boca Raton, FL, pp. I-1–I-69.

Marcus, M. L. (1983) *The Coronary Circulation in Health and Disease*, McGraw-Hill, New York.

Milnor, W. R. (1989) *Hemodynamics*, 2nd edn., Williams & Wilkins, Baltimore, MD.

Rushmer, R. F. (1976) *Cardiovascular Dynamics*, W.B. Saunders Company, Philadelphia, PA.

Silverthorn, D. U. (2001) *Human Physiology: An Integrated Approach*, 2nd edn., Prentice Hall, Upper Saddle River, NJ.

Stary, H. C., Chandler, A. B., Dinsmore, R. E., Fuster, V., Glagov, S., Insull, W., Jr., Rosenfeld, M. E., Schwartz, C. J., Wagner, W. D., and Wissler, R. W. (1995) A definition of advanced types of atherosclerotic lesions and a histological classification of atherosclerosis. A report from the Committee on Vascular Lesions of the Council of Arteriosclerosis, American Heart Association. *Circulation* 92: 1355–1374.

White, R. A. and Cavaye, D. M. (1993) In *A Text and Atlas of Arterial Imaging—Modern and Developing Technology*, Cavaye, D. M. and White, R. A., eds., W. W. Lippincott, Philadelphia, PA.

Part II

Biomechanics of the Human Circulation

4 Rheology of Blood and Vascular Mechanics

4.1 RHEOLOGY OF BLOOD

Rheology is the study of deformation and flow of material. An object or body is said to have deformed if its shape or size is altered due to the action of appropriate forces on the same. If the degree of deformation changes continuously with respect to time, the body is considered to be flowing. This chapter will deal with the behavior of blood as it flows in the blood vessels. A basic understanding of the rheological or flow characteristics of blood *in vivo* under normal conditions will help us delineate the effect of abnormal flow conditions such as stenosed valves and obstructed arteries on the formed elements of blood. The understanding of the fluid dynamics past prosthetic devices such as heart valves, vascular grafts, and artificial hearts and the effect of such flow conditions on blood will also help us in improving the designs of the implants. Several extracorporeal flow devices such as blood oxygenators, dialyzers, and ventricular assist devices are commonly used in modern medicine. A thorough knowledge of blood flow behavior through such devices will also aid in design improvement so as to minimize trauma to blood and optimize the functioning of the devices.

4.1.1 Viscometry and Theory for Capillary, Coaxial Cylindrical, and Cone and Plate Viscometers

The viscosity coefficient as an intrinsic property of any fluid was defined and the basic constitutive relationship between the shear stress and rate of shear for a Newtonian fluid as well as various classes of non-Newtonian fluid were discussed in Chapter 1.

Before discussing the viscous properties of blood, we will briefly look into various methods for measurement of viscosity. Detailed treatment of viscometry can be found in several textbooks including that of Dinsdale and Moore (1962). Since rates of shear and shear stresses are quantities that are difficult to measure directly, relationships are derived with them and other quantities that can be measured relatively easily and accurately. Three basic types of devices for measurement of fluid viscosity are (1) capillary viscometer, (2) coaxial cylinder viscometer, and (3) cone and plate viscometer. The principles behind each type of viscometer are outlined in the following.

4.1.1.1 Capillary Viscometer

Capillary viscometry is based on the *Poiseuille flow* relationship for steady flow in a long, circular, cylindrical tube that was derived from the equations of motion, or the

Navier–Stokes equations, in Chapter 1 (Equations 1.43a through 1.43c). There, the relationship between the flow rate and the pressure gradient was found to be

$$Q = \frac{\Delta p \pi R^4}{8\mu L} \tag{1.53}$$

Keep in mind that one of the fundamental assumptions behind this equation is that the flow is *fully developed* or $L \gg 2R$. The nature of flow developing in the entrance region of a tube is discussed in Section 1.8 where an approximate relationship for the entry length prior to fully developed flow is derived. One way to achieve this condition is to use a very narrow or "capillary" tube.

Thus, in a capillary viscometer of radius R and length L, if the flow rate and pressure drop of a fluid can be accurately measured, the viscosity coefficient can be determined as

$$\mu = \frac{\Delta p \pi R^4}{8QL} \tag{4.1}$$

Referring to Figure 4.1, the net force pushing the fluid to the right is

$$F_p = p_1 \pi r^2 - p_2 \pi r^2 = (p_1 - p_2)\pi r^2$$

while the shear force that retards the motion acts on the circumferential surface of the fluid element and is given by

$$F_\tau = \tau 2\pi r L$$

In fully developed, steady flow, these two forces balance each other and we obtain

$$(p_1 - p_2)\pi r^2 = \tau(2\pi r L)$$

which can be rearranged to give

$$\tau = (p_1 - p_2) r / 2L$$

From this expression for the shear stress, the magnitude of the shear stress at the wall will be

$$|\tau_w| = \left.\frac{(\Delta p) r}{2L}\right|_{r=R} = \frac{\Delta p R}{2L} \tag{4.2}$$

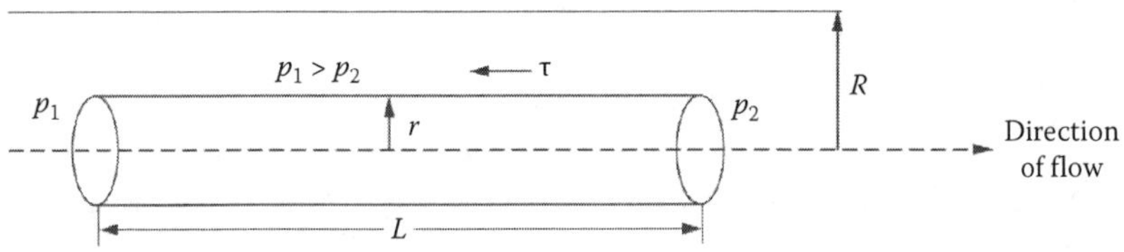

FIGURE 4.1 Steady flow of Newtonian fluid through a straight tube of circular cross section.

Furthermore, the constitutive law for a Newtonian fluid (Section 1.2) is given in cylindrical coordinates by

$$\tau = -\mu \frac{du}{dr}$$

where u is the velocity of the fluid. Hence, the shear rate at the wall is given by

$$|\dot{\gamma}_w| = \frac{\Delta p R}{2\mu L}$$

Using the relationship for Δp from Equation 1.53, wall shear rate becomes

$$|\dot{\gamma}_w| = \frac{4Q}{\pi R^3} \tag{4.3}$$

Thus, having obtained values for wall shear stress and wall shear rate in terms of measured Δp and Q (Equations 4.2 and 4.3), respectively, one can calculate fluid viscosity from their ratio.

Capillary viscometers include devices that measure the absolute viscosity coefficient as well as the viscosity relative to fluids of known viscosity. The flow through the capillary may be induced by an externally applied pressure gradient or by gravitational forces. There are several precautions that need to be observed in using these instruments. The derivation of the relationship given in Equation 4.3 included several assumptions such as laminar (streamlined), steady, fully developed flow and that the fluid is Newtonian. To avoid the effects of turbulent flow in deviating from the derived relationship, experiments must be performed at lower Reynolds numbers where streamlined flow will be assured. The assumptions of steady and fully developed flow imply that the velocity profile within the capillary is parabolic and no acceleration of the fluid is occurring within the viscometer. In most types of capillary viscometers, part of the applied pressure is used to induce kinetic energy to the fluid. Moreover, a small amount of energy is also expended in overcoming the viscous forces at the converging and diverging streamlines at the entrance and exit to the capillary. Kinetic energy and Couette corrections, respectively, need to be taken into account to correct for the errors due to these two effects and are detailed in Dinsdale and Moore (1962). In viscometers with externally applied pressure, the effective pressure gradient includes the externally applied pressure gradient as well as the hydrostatic head of the fluid in the viscometer. Hydrostatic corrections are also needed to account for the constantly decreasing hydrostatic head (Dinsdale and Moore, 1962). The use of this device on Newtonian fluids is not only *required* for the Poiseuille relation to hold, but it is also essential due to the variable shear rate within the tube. Differentiation of the parabolic velocity profile shows that the rate of shear is not constant but is a function of radial position, r. Thus, a fluid particle near the wall would be exposed to a high shear rate while one at the tube center would experience zero shear rate. If the fluid viscosity were shear rate–dependent, that is, $\mu(\dot{\gamma})$, then a range of viscosities would be seen and no meaningful value would be obtained. The relationships between pressure gradient and flow rate for non-Newtonian fluids in straight circular tubes are discussed later in this chapter.

4.1.1.2 Coaxial Cylinder Viscometer

Rotational viscometers are particularly useful in analyzing the rheological characteristics of *non-Newtonian* fluids because one sample of fluid can be used to study the viscous behavior at different rates of shear or when continuous measurements are required to study the effect of time-varying conditions on the flow properties. A simple coaxial cylinder rotational viscometer is shown schematically in Figure 4.2.

In the case of the coaxial cylinder viscometer, the inner cylinder, also referred to as the "bob," with a radius R_1 and height h remains stationary. The outer cylinder, also referred to as the "cup," with a radius R_2 which contains the test fluid is rotated at a constant speed, Ω (rad/s), and the resultant torque, T (dyn · cm), is measured by the angular deflection of the inner cylinder which is suspended by fine wire. It is assumed that the flow of the fluid between the cylinders is steady and laminar and that the end effects are negligible.

Fluid viscosity measurements are derived from the following analysis. Consider a volume of fluid between the stationary inner cylinder and an arbitrary radius r. If ω is the angular velocity of the fluid at radius r, then the torque exerted on the fluid at this radius is

$$T = F_t r$$

or

$$T = \tau_r(2\pi rh)r$$

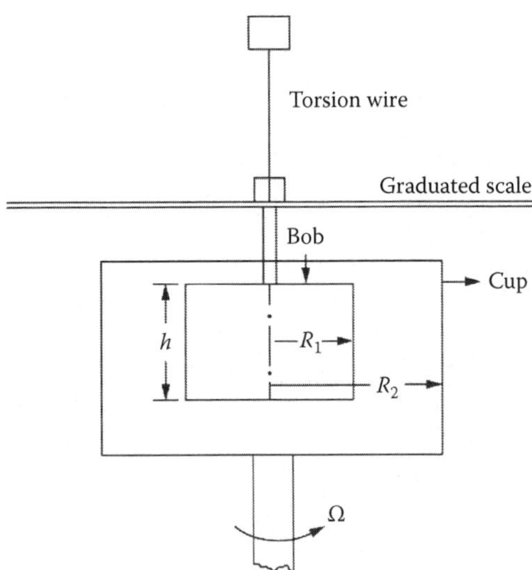

FIGURE 4.2 Schematic of a coaxial (Couette) cylinder viscometer.

The torque, T, measured at the surface of the inner cylinder must be the same as the torque at any arbitrary radius r since the motion is steady. Rewriting in terms of the shear stress, we get

$$\tau_r = \frac{T}{2\pi r^2 h}$$

It can be observed from the aforementioned relationship that the shearing stress is inversely proportional to the square of the distance from the axis of rotation. It is interesting to note, however, that by using an annular gap that is small compared with the cylinder radii (i.e., $dr \ll R_1, R_2$), the shearing stress on the fluid will be almost constant throughout the volume of the testing fluid and, thus, approaches the case of *Couette* flow. (Couette flow is a classic configuration of flow between two infinitely large flat plates where either one plate is in motion [as in this device] or a pressure gradient is present or both [see Section 1.5.3.1].)

The velocity of the fluid at the radius r is

$$V = r\omega$$

and thus, the gradient of velocity, or, rate of shear, will be given by

$$\frac{dV}{dr} = r\frac{d\omega}{dr} + \omega$$

In this expression, the first term on the right-hand side represents the radial velocity gradient and the second term is the angular velocity due to rigid body rotation. Since we are interested in the tangential velocity gradient in the fluid, the second term with the constant angular velocity can be neglected. For a Newtonian fluid, $\tau_r = \mu\dot{\gamma}$, or

$$\tau_r = \mu\dot{\gamma} = \mu\frac{dV}{dr} = \mu r\frac{d\omega}{dr}$$

or

$$\frac{T}{2\pi r^2 h} = \mu r\frac{d\omega}{dr}$$

Consequently,

$$\frac{d\omega}{dr} = \frac{T}{2\pi\mu h r^3}$$

Integrating the previous equation with appropriate boundary conditions results in the expression

$$T = \left[\frac{4\pi h R_1^2 R_2^2}{\left(R_2^2 - R_1^2\right)}\right]\mu\Omega \tag{4.4}$$

or $T = C\mu\Omega$ where C is the instrumentation geometric constant. The same expression will be applicable if the inner cylinder is rotated while the outer cylinder is held stationary. It is also applicable if the torque is applied externally and the resulting rotation of the cylinder is measured. It is to be noted that the relationship derived in Equation 4.4 ignores the effects due to forces on the top and bottom free surfaces of the space between the cylinders. Correction due to the "end effects" must be taken into account especially in fluids with a viscosity lower than 1 P. Various attempts to minimize the errors due to end effects are discussed in Dinsdale and Moore (1962).

4.1.1.3 Cone and Plate Viscometer

In the case of the cone and plate viscometer (Figure 4.3), the fluid sample is contained between a cone of large apical angle and a flat surface (plate) normal to its axis. If the angle between the cone and the plate, ψ, is small, the rate of shear is essentially constant as shown as follows.

Let Ω be the angular velocity at which the cone is rotated. The velocity of the fluid at any radial distance r is then

$$V = \Omega r$$

The rate of shear will be given by the ratio of the linear velocity and the gap between the cone and plate h at that radius. From the figure, it can be observed that $h = r \tan \psi$.

Thus, the shear rate $\dot{\gamma} = \Omega r / r \tan \psi = \Omega / \psi$ provided that the cone angle ψ is small. Furthermore, the shearing stress is also independent of the radius in this configuration and the entire fluid sample is being subjected to a constant rate of shear.

The total torque, T, can be obtained by the expression

$$T = \int_A r\tau_r \, dA$$

where $dA = 2\pi r dS$. However, from the figure, it can be observed that $r = s \cos \psi$. Therefore, $ds = dr/\cos \psi$ or $ds = dr$ if ψ is small.

Hence,

$$T = \tau_r \int_0^R 2\pi r^2 dr$$

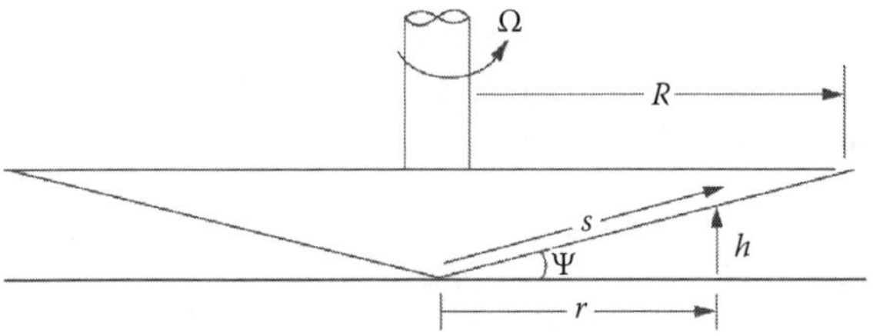

FIGURE 4.3 Schematic of a cone and plate viscometer.

and thus,

$$\tau_r = \frac{3T}{2\pi R^3}$$

For a Newtonian fluid,

$$\mu = \frac{\tau_r}{\dot{\gamma}} = \frac{3T\psi}{2\pi R^3 \Omega} \tag{4.5}$$

In summary, the capillary tube viscometers require only a small volume of fluid, are easy to use, and the results are reproducible. However, for non-Newtonian fluids, measurements must be made over a wide range of rates of shear which are uniformly applied to the entire fluid. Coaxial cylinder or, Couette, viscometers are thus more appropriate because they subject the fluid sample to a relatively constant rate of shear and multiple measurements at various rates of shear can be made with a given blood sample. However, the end effects of these devices discussed earlier will introduce large errors particularly with non-Newtonian fluids and the instruments are expensive. The experiments are also more complicated to perform compared with the tube viscometers. The cone and plate viscometers have the same advantages as those of the Couette viscometers and need a smaller sample of blood for measurements. Although tube viscometers have been used extensively in the past to study the rheology of blood, Couette and cone and plate viscometers are widely used because of their greater accuracy and flexibility.

4.1.2 Physical Properties of Blood

Whole blood consists of formed elements that are suspended in *plasma*. The plasma is a dilute electrolyte solution (0.15 N) containing about 8% by weight of three major types of proteins: fibrinogen, globulin, and albumin in water. When blood clots in the absence of an anticoagulant, the fibrinogen polymerizes into fibrin. If the clot of fibrin and blood cells are left alone, the clot will contract. The portion of the blood without the fibrin is called the serum. Globulin, which may be subdivided into groups, is a carrier of lipids and other water-soluble substances. Globulin also contains antibodies that resist infection from bacteria and viruses. Albumin, with the lowest molecular weight of the three proteins, is the main contributor to the total colloid osmotic pressure of the plasma proteins and is important in the balance of the water metabolism. Plasma is identical to the interstitial fluid in composition except for the presence of plasma proteins. The higher osmotic pressure due to the presence of proteins in the plasma results in the absorption of water from the interstitial fluid into the capillary. When the whole blood is centrifuged with suitable anticoagulants added to prevent clotting, the formed elements will settle to the bottom of the tube. About 45% by volume will consist of formed elements and about 55% will consist of *plasma* in the normal human blood. The formed elements in blood consist of 95% red blood cells, 0.13% white blood cells, and about 4.9% platelets. The white blood cells, also known as leukocytes, consist of monocytes, lymphocytes, neutrophils, eosinophils, and basophils. Monocytes that leave the circulation and enter the tissues develop into macrophages. Neutrophils, monocytes, and macrophages are collectively known as phagocytes because they can engulf and ingest bacteria and other foreign particles. Platelets, which are smaller than red or white blood cells, are anucleated cell fragments produced in the bone marrow from huge cells known as megakaryocytes. The average life of a platelet is about 10 days and the inactivated platelets are discoid in shape. The cytoplasm of platelets contains organelles (a cytoskeleton consisting of microtubules and microfilaments) and granules. The surface membrane expresses various glycoprotein molecules. The platelets can be activated by prolonged exposure to high shear stress or by rapid increases in shear stress. Platelets can also stick to exposed collagen (as a result of vascular injury) and become activated. Upon activation, changes occur in the internal cytoskeleton, which causes the platelets to become spheroid in shape and to release the contents of their internal granules such as serotonin, ADP, and platelet-activating factors (PAF). The release of PAF can cause additional platelets to become activated which promote platelet aggregation and collagen-induced thrombus formation. The initiation of the coagulation cascade results in fibrinogen being converted to fibrin and in fibrin stabilizing the adhered platelets to form a blood clot.

The majority of the formed elements are red blood cells and the measure of the volume percent of formed elements in blood is referred to as the *hematocrit*. The typical shape of a red blood cell is shown in Figure 4.4a and an actual human red blood cell as viewed through an electron microscope is shown in Figure 4.4b. The biconcave-shaped red blood cell consists of hemoglobin surrounded by a flexible red cell membrane. The primary function of hemoglobin in the red blood cell is to transport oxygen from the lungs to the living tissues of the body. The diameter of the red blood cell is about 8.5 μm with transverse dimensions of 2.5 μm at the thickest portion and about 1 μm at the thinnest portion. The volume of the intracellular fluid is about 87 μm^3 and the surface area of the cell is about 163 μm^2. It can be easily shown that a spherical shaped red cell with the same intracellular fluid volume will have about 40% smaller surface area compared with the

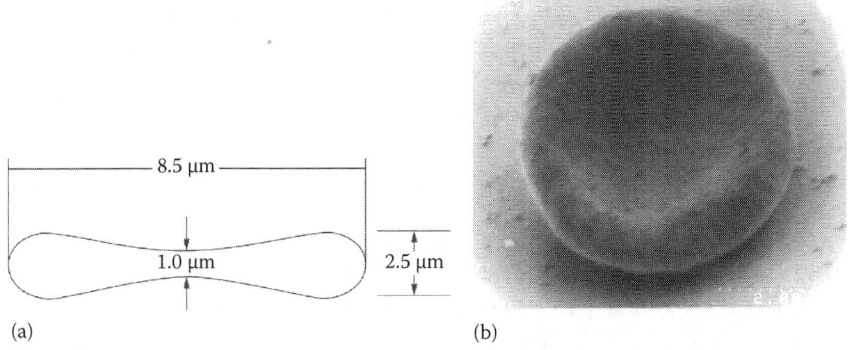

FIGURE 4.4 (a) Schematic of the biconcave shape of the red blood cell with typical dimensions and (b) a scanning electron microscope picture of the human red blood cell magnified 13,000 times.

biconcave shape. Thus, the advantage of the biconcave shape with a larger surface area for efficient gas exchange in the capillaries can be noted. The membrane is flexible and the cell can pass through capillaries of diameter as small as 5 μm by assuming a bent shape.

4.1.3 Viscous Behavior of Blood

4.1.3.1 Plasma

The viscosity of plasma can be measured by obtaining a sample of blood and separating out the formed elements by centrifuging. However, as soon as blood is removed from the body, clotting mechanism is initiated and an anticoagulant must be added to prevent clotting. Typical anticoagulants added are heparin, sequestrate, oxalate, or citrate in isotonic concentration. The addition of the anticoagulant is generally assumed to reduce the actual blood or plasma viscosity even though the specific effect of the various compounds is not clearly established.

Human plasma has a density of about 1.035 g/cc and its viscosity coefficient ranges between 0.011 and 0.016 P compared with 1.0 g/cc and 0.01 P, respectively, for water. The presence of plasma proteins results in the higher viscosity compared with that for water. Experiments using capillary as well as rotating viscometers have suggested that mammalian plasma behaves like a non-Newtonian fluid while other published works have suggested that plasma is a Newtonian liquid. Variability in the protein concentrations in the samples within the species, across species, and also in the experimental techniques may be contributing factors for such contradictory results. The rheological characteristics of plasma in the presence of pathological conditions may also contribute to non-Newtonian behavior. Temperature also has a significant influence on the plasma viscosity causing it to decrease with an increase in temperature. A fall of 2%–3% in the viscosity coefficient per degree Celsius rise in temperature has been reported in the range of 25°C–37°C. For our purposes, we will assume that the plasma behaves as a Newtonian fluid with a constant viscosity at 37°C, which is the human body temperature. We will, for modeling the flows in the arterial system, assume that the plasma viscosity is 1.2 cP.

4.1.3.2 Whole Blood

Samples of whole blood, with the addition of suitable anticoagulants, have been tested in capillary, coaxial cylinder or cone and plate viscometer over a wide range of rates of shear. A description of the instruments used, test samples taken, and experimental conditions for measuring the viscosity of blood from some of the published works are included in Table 4.1. In order to identify the constitutive relationship for whole blood, a plot of shear stress versus rate of shear can be obtained from the data. However, as pointed out before, the viscosity of blood and plasma also differs from sample to sample due to the variations in species and constituents such as protein content. To avoid difficulties in interpreting the data due to the variability in the blood samples, the shear stress is normalized with respect to the plasma viscosity of the sample. A plot of shear stress/plasma viscosity and rate of shear data is shown in Figure 4.5. As can be seen, the data suggest a nonlinear behavior, particularly at low shear rates. It can also be noted that the best-fit curve does not pass through the

TABLE 4.1
Summary of Selected Studies on Blood Viscosity Measurement Reported in the Literature in the 1960s

Viscometer	Blood	Anticoagulant	Hematocrit	Temperature (°C)	Comments
Coaxial cylinder	Human	ACD	0%–40%	20–40	6–200 s^{-1}
Capillary	Human	Heparin	12.5%–70%	25–32	12.8–335 s^{-1} power law
Cone and plate	Dog	Heparin		37	11.45–230 s^{-1}
Cone and plate	Human	ACD	Normal	37	2–100,000 s^{-1}
Coaxial cylinder	Human	Heparin	0%–95%	37	0.052–52 s^{-1}
Coaxial cylinder	Human	Heparin	43%–48%	37	23–230 s^{-1}
Cone and plate	Human	None/heparin oxalate	33%–57%	37	10–250 s^{-1}
Coaxial cylinder	Human	ACD	42.5%	25–37	0.1–20 s^{-1}
Cone and plate	Human	Heparin	0.80%	22–37	2–12 s^{-1}

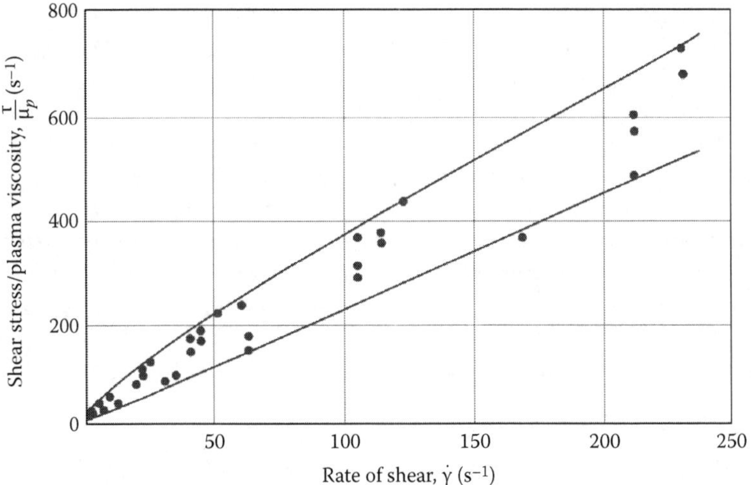

FIGURE 4.5 Shear stress normalized to the plasma viscosity versus rate of shear plot from experimental data. (Redrawn from Whitmore, R.L., *Rheology of Circulation*, Pergamon Press, New York, 1968. With permission.)

origin and exhibits a positive y-intercept indicating that the induced shear stress must exceed a minimum yield stress before blood will flow.

If the constitutive relationship for whole blood follows the power law ($\tau = K_{pl}\dot{\gamma}^n : n \neq 1$), then the data can be represented as a straight line in the logarithmic shear stress versus rate of shear plot (Figure 4.6). Even though the data points exhibit a linear behavior over small ranges of shear rates, a curvilinear relationship is observed over the entire range of shear rates for which data have been obtained.

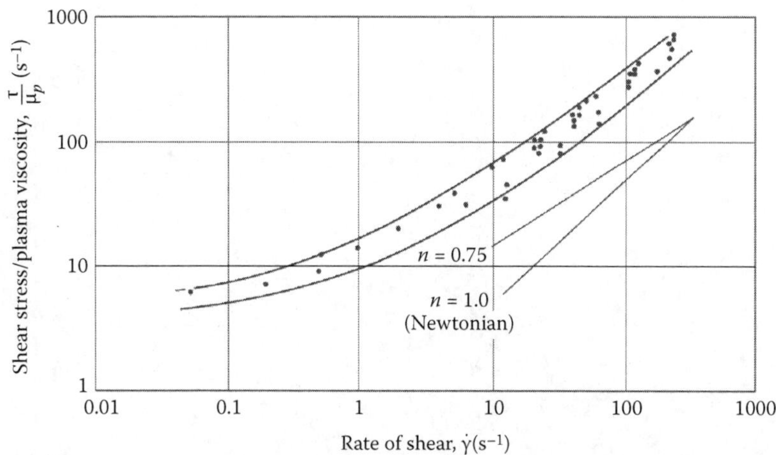

FIGURE 4.6 Shear stress versus rate of shear plot in logarithmic scale. (Redrawn from Whitmore, R.L., *Rheology of Circulation*, Pergamon Press, New York, 1968. With permission.)

Tests conducted with rotational viscometers for shear rates ranging from 5 to 200 s^{-1} follow the power law reasonably well for values of the exponent n between 0.68 and 0.8. Values of n exceeding 0.9 have been reported from results obtained with capillary viscometers.

Inspection of Figure 4.5 once again reveals that even though blood exhibits a yield stress (y-intercept on the plot), the data do not suggest a linear relationship between shear stress and rate of shear particularly at low shear rates, a relationship indicative of an ideal Bingham plastic ($\tau = \tau_y + K_b\dot{\gamma}$). As an alternative, we could consider the constitutive relationship for the Casson fluid $\left(\sqrt{\tau} = \sqrt{\tau_y} + K_c\sqrt{\dot{\gamma}}\right)$ where there is a linear relationship of the square root of shear stress versus the square root of rate of shear. A plot of such a curve together with the data obtained for whole blood is shown in Figure 4.7.

A least square fit of the data yields the relationship

$$\sqrt{\frac{\tau}{\mu_p}} = 1.53\sqrt{\dot{\gamma}} + 2.0 \tag{4.6}$$

The apparent viscosity coefficient for whole blood at any rate of shear can thus be computed from the aforementioned relationship. For example, at a rate of shear of 230 s^{-1}, the apparent viscosity of whole blood is about 3.3 cP using a value of 1.2 cP for plasma viscosity. This value compares favorably with the experimentally determined values ranging from 3.01 to 5.53 cP. Apparent viscosity data from experiments by various investigators for a range of shear rates are shown in Figure 4.8. A plot of the constitutive relationship in Equation 4.6 is also included in the figure. As can be observed, the apparent viscosity increases to relatively large magnitudes at low rates of shear. This is because the red blood cells tend to aggregate into Rouleaux formations and thus exhibit an increase in viscosity at low rates of shear. Aggregates of red blood cells are shown in Figure 4.9. As the rate of shear increases, the aggregates

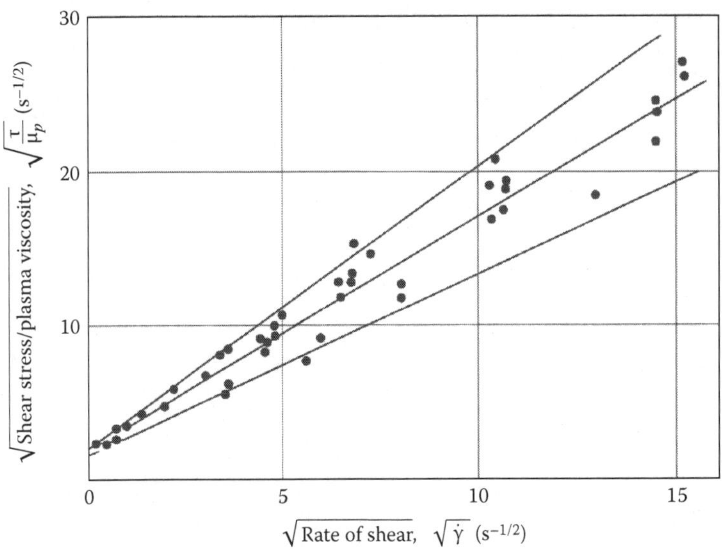

FIGURE 4.7 Square root of shear stress adjusted to plasma viscosity versus square root of shear rate from viscometry data. (Redrawn from Whitmore, R.L., *Rheology of Circulation*, Pergamon Press, New York, 1968. With permission.)

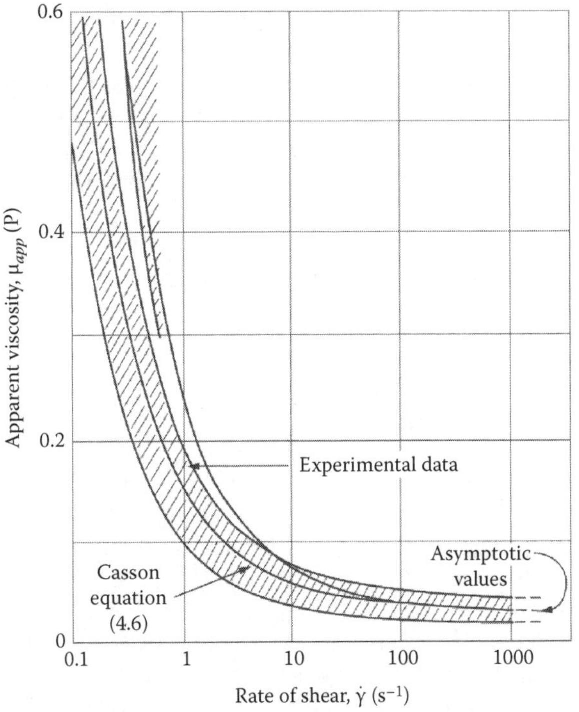

FIGURE 4.8 A plot of apparent viscosity as a function of rate of shear. (Redrawn from Whitmore, R.L., *Rheology of Circulation*, Pergamon Press, New York, 1968. With permission.)

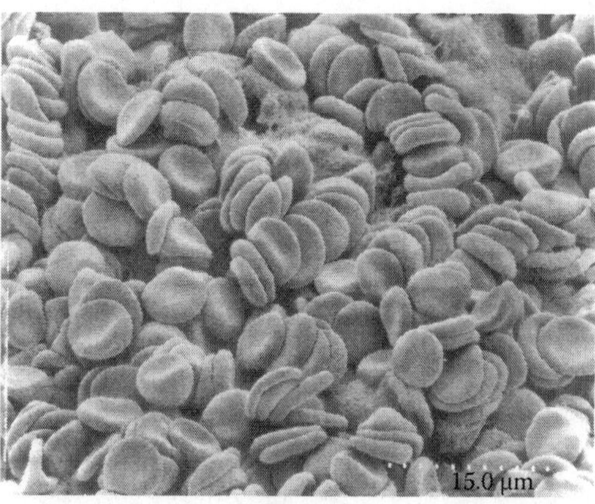

FIGURE 4.9 A scanning electron microscope view of aggregation of red blood cells magnified 2000 times.

gradually break up above a rate of shear of about 50 s^{-1}, and the viscosity coefficient approaches an asymptotic value of about 3.5 cP. Thus, when specifying the viscosity coefficient of blood, it is important to specify the rate of shear at which the measurements were obtained.

As discussed earlier, apart from the fact that the rate of shear has a profound effect on the measured apparent viscosity of whole blood, the variability of samples, the effect of the addition of anticoagulants, and the experimental conditions must also be taken into account. Let us now look into the effect of other variables on the viscosity coefficient of blood.

4.1.3.3 Effect of Hematocrit

The hematocrit for normal human blood varies between 40% and 45%. To study the effect of hematocrit on blood viscosity, the red blood cells are separated out by centrifuging and reconstituted in appropriate proportions with serum, saline, or Ringer's solution before viscometry experiments. A plot of the relative viscosity of blood (with respect to plasma) as a function of hematocrit is shown in Figure 4.10a. (Note that the relative viscosity is plotted in logarithmic scale in this figure.) The viscosity increases with increasing hematocrit and also decreases with increasing rates of shear as observed earlier. The viscosity of rigid spheres suspended in a solution is seen to rise faster than that of blood, thus indicating the effect red blood cell flexibility has in minimizing the viscosity. Figure 4.10b compares the viscosity as a function of hematocrit for normal cells, rigid spheres, and red cells which have been hardened by treating in an aldehyde solution. Once again, the effect of red cell flexibility on reducing the viscosity is clearly demonstrated.

4.1.3.4 Effect of Temperature

As pointed out earlier for the case of plasma, the effect of temperature on the viscosity of blood is still not clearly established so it is the usual practice to keep the temperature at a constant value (preferably at body temperature of 37°C) when measurements are obtained.

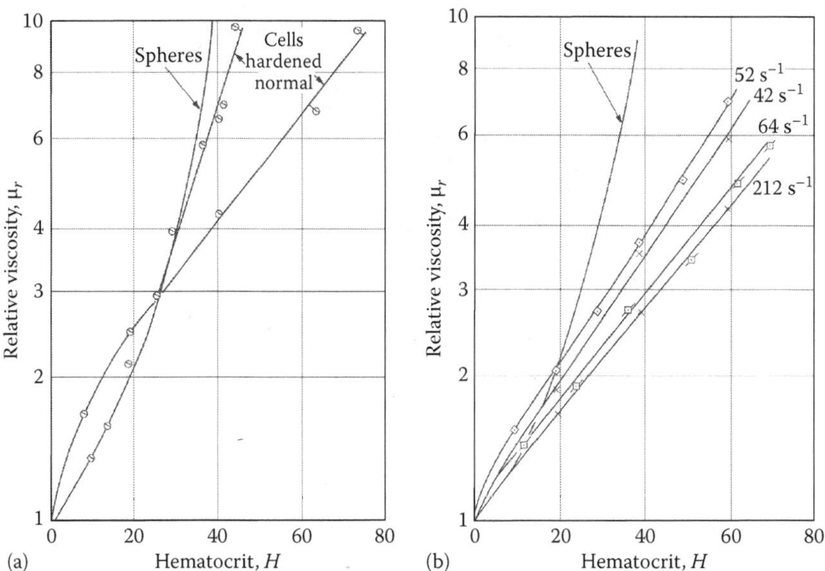

FIGURE 4.10 (a) Effect of hematocrit on the relative viscosity of blood and (b) effect of hardening of the red blood cell on the relative viscosity. (Redrawn from Whitmore, R.L., *Rheology of Circulation*, Pergamon Press, New York, 1968. With permission.)

4.1.3.5 Effect of Protein Content in Plasma

Figure 4.11 shows the plot of viscosity versus rate of shear (at lower shear rates) for whole blood as well as for red blood cells suspended in isotonic solution with one protein of physiological concentration included. The results are presented for 37°C and a hematocrit of 49%. It can be observed that globulin appears to have the dominant effect on increasing the viscosity of blood, whereas albumin moderates the rise in viscosity. Since the concentration level of fibrinogen is very low, its effect on viscosity is minimal.

4.1.3.6 Yield Stress for Blood

A review of the Casson relationship (Figure 4.7) shows that the curve exhibits a *y*-intercept which is the square root of the yield stress. Studies have shown that the yield stress depends strongly on fibrinogen concentration and is also dependent on the hematocrit (Figure 4.12a and b).

Several empirical formulae relating the yield stress to hematocrit and fibrinogen concentration in blood have been reported in the literature (Cooney, 1976). An empirical relationship for the yield stress as a function of hematocrit can be given by

$$\tau_y^{1/3} = \frac{A(H - H_m)}{100} \tag{4.7}$$

where

A is a constant $\{(0.008 \pm 0.002\,\text{dyn/cm}^2)^{1/3}\}$
H is the hematocrit
H_m is the hematocrit below which yield stress vanishes (5%–8%)

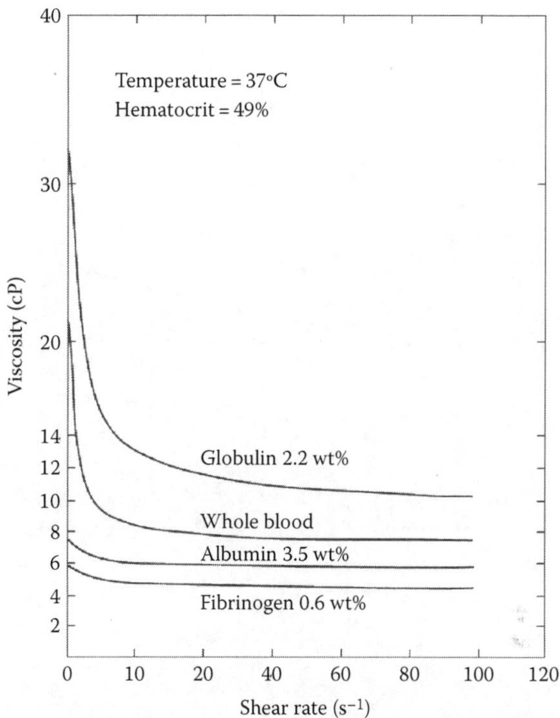

FIGURE 4.11 Effect of plasma proteins on the viscosity of whole blood. (Redrawn from Copley, A.L. and Stainsby, G., eds., *Flow Properties of Blood*, 1960, by permission of Oxford University Press.)

Assuming $H = 45\%$ and $H_m = 5\%$, the yield stress values for normal human blood should be between 0.01 and 0.06 dyn/cm^2. Another empirical formula for the yield stress as a function of hematocrit and fibrinogen concentration is

$$\sqrt{\tau_y} = (H - 0.1)(C_F + 0.5) \tag{4.8}$$

where

C_F is the fibrinogen content in g/100 mL
H is the hematocrit expressed as a fraction

This correlation fits the experimental data satisfactorily and is valid for $0.21 < C_F < 0.46$ and $H > 0.1$. As pointed out earlier, the yield stress appears to vanish below a hematocrit fraction of 0.1.

An estimate can be obtained on the effect of yield stress on blood flow in capillaries by considering the pressure gradient required to maintain steady flow of blood in cylindrical tubes. Assuming Poiseuille flow for this situation, the shear stress will vary linearly with the radius having a magnitude of zero at the center and

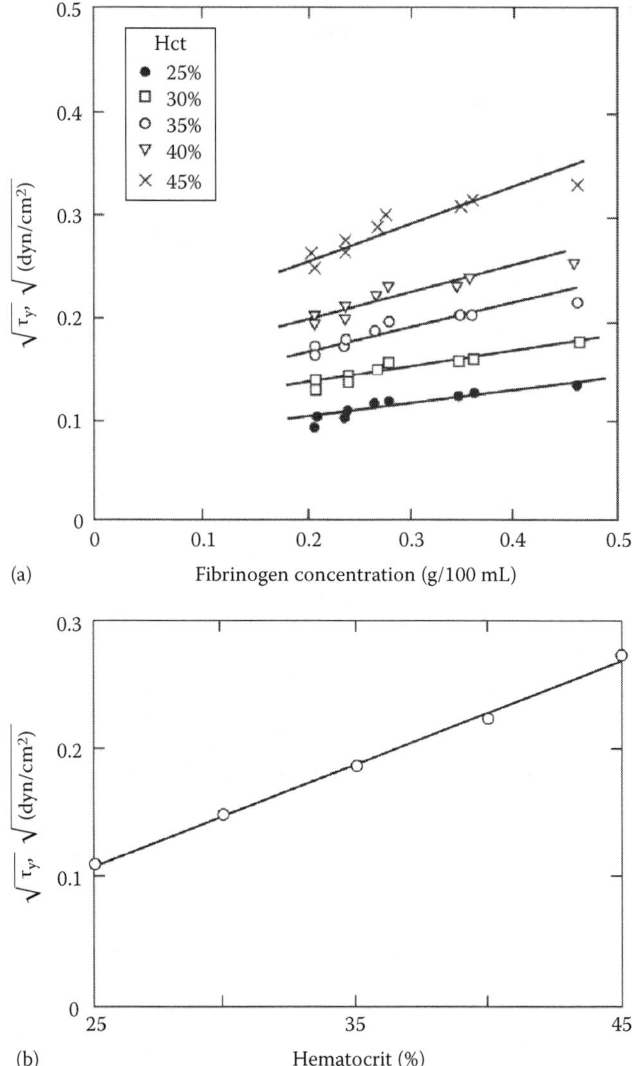

FIGURE 4.12 Effect of (a) fibrinogen concentration and (b) hematocrit on the yield stress for blood. (Redrawn from Merrill, E.W. et al., in *Proceedings of the Fourth International Congress on Rheology*, Providence, RI, Copley, A.L., ed., 1965. With permission.)

a maximum at the wall. To initiate flow, the imposed pressure drop must be large enough so that the wall shear stress

$$\tau_w = \frac{R\Delta p}{2L}$$

will exceed the yield stress for blood. Equating the wall shear stress to the value for the yield stress for blood (0.07 dyn/cm^2), the pressure gradient required to initiate flow can be computed. Assuming a length of 20 cm for a typical capillary viscometer and a radius of 0.1 cm, the required pressure drop can be computed as 0.021 mmHg. Similarly, for a typical systemic capillary with a length of 1 mm and a radius of 5 μm, the pressure drop required is computed to be the same value. In the normal circulation, the magnitude of pressure drop across the systemic capillaries is about 16 mmHg and, hence, the effect of yield stress for blood appears to be negligible under normal flow conditions.

4.1.3.7 Effect of Tube Diameter

A plot of the apparent viscosity of blood as a function of tube radius at a hematocrit of 40% is shown in Figure 4.13. As can be observed, the apparent viscosity for blood has a very low value in very small diameter tubes. The viscosity increases with the increase in tube diameter and approaches an asymptotic value at tube diameters larger than about 0.5 mm. This phenomenon of a decrease in the apparent viscosity in small diameter tubes is referred to as the *Fahraeus-Lindqvist effect*. This effect can be explained on a physical basis as detailed in the following. As the blood flows through a tube, the blood cells tend to rotate as shown in Figure 4.14. Due to the

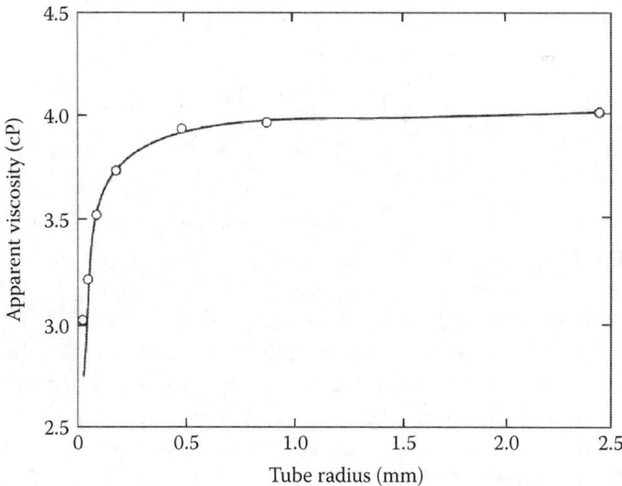

FIGURE 4.13 Plot of apparent viscosity as a function of tube radius.

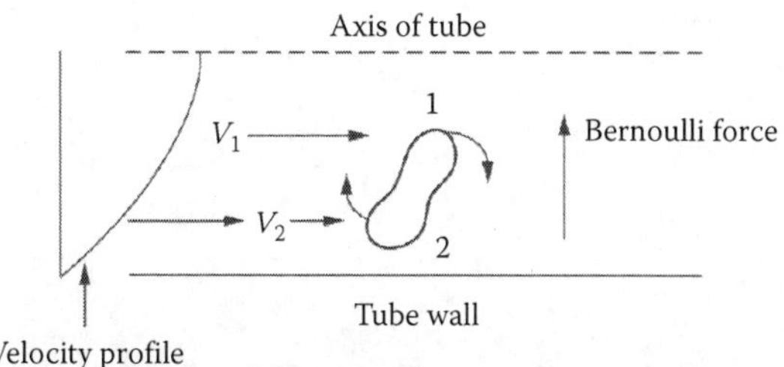

FIGURE 4.14 Schematic describing the rotation of red blood cells under the influence of a velocity gradient.

spinning of the red blood cells, they tend to move toward the center of the tube, and, hence, a cell-free layer, referred to as the plasma-skimming layer, exists near the wall. In tubes with small diameters, the cross-sectional area of the cell-free zone is comparable with the central core. Hence, the net effect of the cell-free zone with a lower viscosity (that of plasma alone) is to reduce the apparent viscosity of flow through the tube. As the tube diameter increases, the effect of the cell-free zone reduces, and, hence, the viscosity coefficient approaches an asymptotic value.

Two mathematical models have been developed to describe the Fahraeus-Lindqvist effect and will be considered in the following.

4.1.3.7.1 Cell-Free Marginal Layer Model

Consider steady flow of blood through a circular tube of radius a as shown in Figure 4.15.

The tube cross section can be divided into a core region and a cell-free plasma region near the wall. The governing equations for both regions can be given by the following equations:

$$-\frac{\Delta p}{L} = \frac{1}{r}\frac{d}{dr}\left[\mu_c r \frac{du_c}{dr}\right] \quad 0 \le r \le R - \delta \tag{4.9}$$

$$-\frac{\Delta p}{L} = \frac{1}{r}\frac{d}{dr}\left[\mu_p r \frac{du_p}{dr}\right] \quad R - \delta \le r \le R \tag{4.10}$$

where

μ_c and μ_p represent the viscosities of the core and periphery, respectively
u_c and u_p represent the velocities of the core and periphery, respectively

The boundary conditions used to obtain a solution for the two differential equations are as follows: (1) the velocity gradient is zero at the center of the tube, (2) no slip occurs at the tube wall, and (3) the velocity and the shear stress is continuous at the interface between the two zones. The equations can be integrated with the previous boundary conditions to solve for the velocity components and to obtain an expression for the flow rate as given as follows:

$$Q = \frac{\pi R^4 \Delta p}{8\mu_p L}\left[1 - \left(1 - \frac{\delta}{R}\right)^4\left(1 - \frac{\mu_p}{\mu_c}\right)\right] \tag{4.11}$$

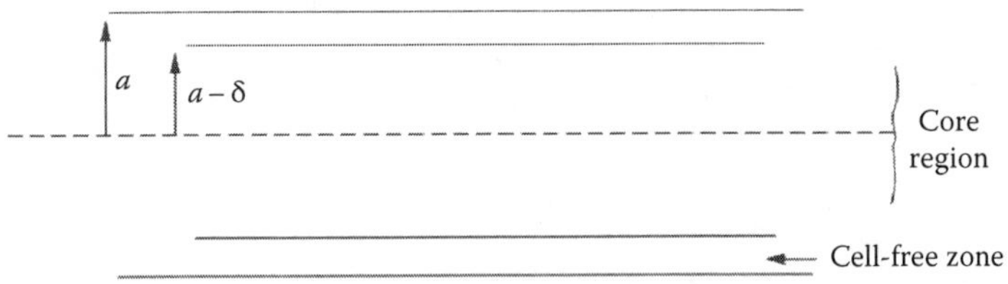

FIGURE 4.15 Schematic of a cell-free zone layer model.

By comparison, the expression for the flow rate for a homogeneous fluid (Poiseuille's equation) was derived earlier as

$$Q = \frac{\pi R^4 \Delta p}{8\mu L}$$

Comparing these two equations, if Poiseuille's law was applied to calculate the viscosity of blood, the apparent viscosity could be written as

$$\mu_{app} = \frac{\mu_p}{[1-(1-(\delta/R))^4(1-(\mu_p/\mu_c))]} \quad (4.12)$$

In the limit as $\delta/R \rightarrow 0$, $\mu_{app} \rightarrow \mu_c$ as would be expected. When the ratio δ/R is small, the higher order terms containing the ratio can be neglected and the relationship for the apparent viscosity reduces to

$$\mu_{app} = \frac{\mu_c}{1+4(\delta/R)((\mu_c/\mu_p)-1)} \quad (4.13)$$

4.1.3.7.2 Sigma Effect

In deriving the Poiseuille formula, the homogeneous fluid was assumed to be a continuum, allowing integration to be performed to obtain the flow rate from the expression for the velocity. The sigma effect theory, however, states that when blood flows through a small diameter tube, the assumption of a continuum is not valid. For example, assume that the tube diameter is so small that there is only room for five red blood cells to move abreast. Then the ensuing velocity profile would not be continuous and would consist of concentric laminae moving axially as demonstrated in Figure 4.16.

An apparent viscosity can be derived for this case by the following analysis. The expression for flow rate from the Poiseuille solution

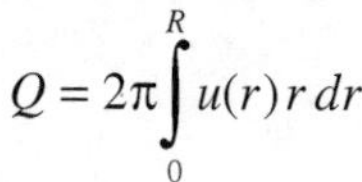

$$Q = 2\pi \int_0^R u(r)\, r\, dr$$

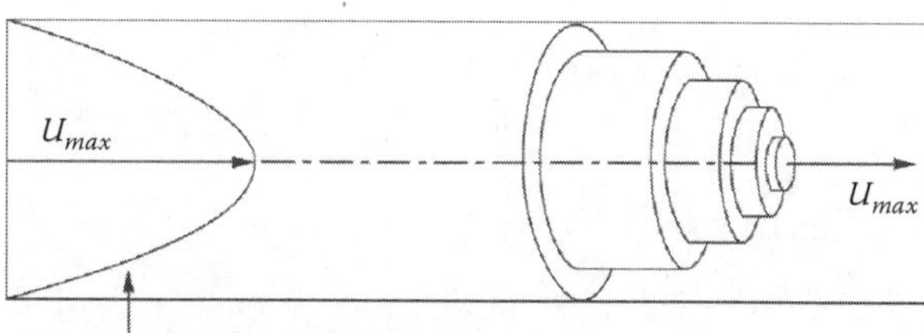

FIGURE 4.16 Concentric layer model for flow in small tubes.

can be rewritten as

$$Q = \pi \int_0^R d[u(r)r^2] - \pi \int_0^R r^2 \frac{du}{dr} dr$$

Applying the "no-slip" condition at the wall, the first integral on the right side will be identically equal to zero. From the parabolic velocity profile characteristic of Poiseuille flow, the expression for the velocity gradient will be given by

$$\frac{du}{dr} = -\frac{\Delta pr}{2\mu L}$$

Substituting this velocity gradient into the flow integral, we obtain

$$Q = \frac{\pi \Delta p}{2\mu L} \int_0^R r^3 dr \tag{4.14}$$

Now, if we assume that flow occurs in N concentric laminae, each of thickness ε, then the radius R of the tube will be equal to $N\varepsilon$ and any general radius r can be replaced by $n\varepsilon$ where $n = 1, 2, \ldots, N$. If $r = n\varepsilon$, then $dr = \varepsilon \Delta n = \varepsilon$ since Δn is equal to unity.

Hence, the integration in Equation 4.14 can be replaced by a summation as

$$Q = \frac{\pi \Delta p}{2\mu L} \sum_{n=1}^{N} (n\varepsilon)^3 \varepsilon \tag{4.15}$$

Employing the mathematical identity,

$$\sum_{n=1}^{N} n^3 = \frac{N^2 (N+1)^2}{4}$$

one can show that

$$\sum_{n=1}^{N} (n\varepsilon)^3 \varepsilon = \varepsilon^4 \sum_{n=1}^{N} n^3 = \varepsilon^4 \frac{N^2 (N+1)^2}{4}$$

Thus, the flow rate can be written as

$$Q = \frac{\pi \Delta p R^4}{8\mu L} \left(1 + \frac{\varepsilon}{R}\right)^2 \tag{4.16}$$

and the apparent viscosity can be given by the formula

$$\mu_{app} = \frac{\mu}{(1+(\varepsilon/R))^2} \tag{4.17}$$

In this relationship, as $\varepsilon/R \rightarrow 0$, the expression reduces to that for Poiseuille flow. It can also be seen that the sigma effect theory and the cell-free zone theory are equivalent if

$$\delta = \frac{\varepsilon\mu_p}{2(\mu_c - \mu_p)} \tag{4.18}$$

Even though the Fahraeus-Lindqvist effect is not important in large arteries from the viscosity coefficient point of view, the cell-free zone is still present. If blood samples are obtained from large arteries at the wall, the measured hematocrit will be lower than the actual value due to the presence of the plasma-skimming layer.

4.1.4 Pressure–Flow Relationship for Non-Newtonian Fluids

For any fluid flowing through a circular tube, the force balance between the pressure gradient and the viscous drag forces yields the relationship

$$\tau = -\frac{r\Delta p}{2L} \tag{4.19}$$

The expression for the velocity profile and the flow rate for steady flow of a Newtonian fluid through a tube were derived earlier in Section 1.8, Equations 1.51 and 1.53, respectively, as well as in the description of the capillary viscometer in Section 4.1.1.1. We will now derive the corresponding relationships for fluids that follow the power law, Bingham plastic, and Casson constitutive relationships.

4.1.4.1 Power Law Fluid

The constitutive relationship for a power law fluid is given by

$$\tau = K_{pl}\dot{\gamma}^n = K_{pl}\left(\frac{du}{dr}\right)^n \tag{4.20}$$

Substituting this term for shear stress yields

$$K_{pl}\left(\frac{du}{dr}\right)^n = -\frac{r\Delta p}{2L}$$

Rewriting,

$$\int du = -\left(\frac{\Delta p}{2K_{pl}L}\right)^{1/n} \int r^{1/n} dr$$

and integrating we get

$$u = -\left(\frac{\Delta p}{2K_{pl}L}\right)^{1/n} \frac{n}{n+1} r^{(n+1)/n} + C$$

Employing the boundary condition that $u = 0$ at $r = R$, we have

$$C = \left(\frac{\Delta p}{2K_{pl}L}\right)^{1/n} \frac{n}{n+1} R^{(n+1)/n}$$

Substituting this value for C, the expression for the velocity profile becomes

$$u = \frac{n}{n+1}\left(\frac{\Delta p}{2K_{pl}L}\right)^{1/n} \left[R^{(n+1)/n} - r^{(n+1)/n}\right] \tag{4.21}$$

Finally, the flow rate, Q, through the tube is given by

$$Q = \int_0^R 2\pi r u \, dr$$

$$= 2\pi \frac{n}{n+1}\left(\frac{\Delta p}{2K_{pl}L}\right)^{1/n} \left[\int_0^R R^{(n+1)/n} r \, dr - \int_0^R r^{(n+1)/n} r \, dr\right]$$

$$= 2\pi \frac{n}{n+1}\left(\frac{\Delta p}{2K_{pl}L}\right)^{1/n} \left[\int_0^R R^{(n+1)/n} r \, dr - \int_0^a r^{(2n+1)/n} dr\right]$$

$$= 2\pi \frac{n}{n+1}\left(\frac{\Delta p}{2K_{pl}L}\right)^{1/n} \left[R^{(n+1)/n} \frac{r^2}{2}\Big|_0^R - \frac{r^{(3n+1)/n}}{(3n+1)/n}\Big|_0^R\right]$$

$$= 2\pi \frac{n}{n+1}\left(\frac{\Delta p}{2K_{pl}L}\right)^{1/n} \left[\frac{R^{(3n+1)/n}}{2} - \frac{R^{(3n+1)/n}}{(3n+1)/n}\right]$$

$$= 2\pi \frac{n}{n+1}\left(\frac{\Delta p}{2K_{pl}L}\right)^{1/n} \left[\frac{((n+1)/n)R^{(3n+1)/n}}{2((3n+1)/n)}\right]$$

which can be reduced to an expression for the flow rate as

$$Q = \frac{n\pi R^3}{3n+1}\left(\frac{R\Delta p}{2K_{pl}L}\right)^{1/n} \tag{4.22}$$

The flow distribution in the tube given by Equation 4.22 depends upon the value for n. The value for n for human whole blood can be approximated to ~0.75 over the range of rates of shear from 10 to 1000 s^{-1}.

4.1.4.2 Bingham Plastic

For the Bingham plastic, the constitutive relationship will be given by

$$\tau = \tau_y + K_b\dot{\gamma} = \tau_y - K_b\left(\frac{du}{dr}\right) \tag{4.23}$$

where

τ_y is the yield stress
K_b is the viscosity coefficient for the Bingham plastic

Again, substituting τ into Equation 4.19, we get

$$\frac{du}{dr} = -\frac{r\Delta p}{2K_bL} + \frac{\tau_y}{K_b} \tag{4.24}$$

or

$$du = -\frac{\Delta p}{2K_bL} r\,dr + \frac{\tau_y}{K_b} dr$$

Integrating, we obtain

$$u = -\frac{\Delta p}{2K_bL}\frac{r^2}{2} + \frac{\tau_y}{K_b} r + C$$

By applying the boundary condition that $u = 0$ at $r = R$, we can evaluate the constant

$$C = \frac{\Delta p}{2K_bL}\frac{R^2}{2} - \frac{\tau_y}{K_b} R$$

The velocity profile is then given by

$$u = -\frac{\Delta p}{2K_bL}\frac{r^2}{2} + \frac{\tau_y r}{K_b} + \frac{\Delta pR^2}{4K_bL} - \frac{\tau_y R}{\mu_b}$$

Rearranging terms,

$$u = \frac{\Delta p}{4K_bL}(R^2 - r^2) - \frac{\tau_y}{K_b}(R - r) \tag{4.25}$$

From the expression for the wall shear stress at the inner surface of the tube ($r = R$) given by

$$|\tau_w| = \frac{R\Delta p}{2L}$$

until the shear stress at the wall, τ_w, exceeds the Bingham plastic yield stress, there is no flow possible through the tube. However, once the wall shear stress exceeds the yield stress, flow is induced through the tube. We can also determine a radius R_c at which the shear stress equals the yield stress:

$$R_c = \frac{2L\tau_y}{\Delta p}$$

The fluid will have a constant velocity u_c between the center of the tube and R_c and the velocity profile will follow Equation 4.25 from R_c to R. Using Equation 4.25, the core velocity can be written as

$$u_c = \frac{\Delta p}{4K_bL}\left(R^2 - R_c^2\right) - \frac{\tau_y}{K_b}(R - R_c)$$

Substituting $\tau_y = R_c\Delta p/2L$, the core velocity is

$$u_c = \frac{\Delta p}{4K_bL}\left(R^2 - R_c^2\right) - \frac{R_c\Delta p}{2L}\frac{1}{K_b}(R - R_c) \tag{4.26}$$

The flow rate through the tube is equal to the sum of the flow through the core and the peripheral regions:

$$Q = Q_{core} + Q_{per}$$

where

$$Q_{core} = u_c\pi R_c^2$$

Thus,

$$Q_{core} = \frac{\Delta p\pi}{K_bL}\left[\frac{\left(R^2 - R_c^2\right)R_c^2}{4} - \frac{R_c^3}{2}(R - R_c)\right] \tag{4.27}$$

Flow in the peripheral region is given by

$$Q_{per} = \int_{R_c}^{R} 2\pi ru\,dr$$

Substituting for τ_y in terms of Δp, the velocity in the periphery will be expressed as

$$u_{per} = \frac{\Delta p}{K_b L}\left[\frac{(R^2 - r^2)}{4} - \frac{R_c}{2}(R - r)\right]$$

and the peripheral flow rate can be expanded as

$$Q_{per} = \frac{\Delta p}{K_b L}\int_{R_c}^{R}\left[\frac{(R^2 - r^2)}{4} - \frac{R_c}{2}(R - r)\right]2\pi r\,dr$$

Integrating,

$$Q_{per} = \frac{\pi \Delta p}{K_b L}\left[\frac{R^4}{8} - \frac{R^2 R_c^2}{4} - \frac{5}{24}R_c^4 - \frac{R_c R^3}{6} + \frac{R R_c^3}{2}\right] \tag{4.28}$$

Adding Equations 4.27 and 4.28,

$$Q = \frac{\pi \Delta p}{K_b L}\left[\frac{R^4}{8} + \frac{R_c^4}{24} - \frac{R_c R^3}{6}\right] \tag{4.29}$$

and substituting for R_c as

$$R_c = \frac{2\tau_y}{\Delta p/L}$$

The relationship for the flow is then given by

$$Q = \frac{\pi R^4 \Delta p}{8 K_b L}\left[1 - \frac{4}{3}\left(\frac{2\tau_y}{R(\Delta p/L)}\right) + \frac{1}{3}\left(\frac{2\tau_y}{R(\Delta p/L)}\right)^4\right] \tag{4.30}$$

If the yield stress becomes zero, the flow relationship will reduce to that of Poiseuille flow for a Newtonian fluid. Equation 4.30 is known as the Buckingham's equation for an idealized Bingham plastic.

4.1.4.3 Casson Fluid

The constitutive relationship for a Casson fluid is given by the relationship

$$\sqrt{\tau} = \sqrt{\tau_y} + K_c\sqrt{\dot{\gamma}} \tag{4.31}$$

Replacing $\dot{\gamma}$ by $-du/dr$ and the expression for the yield stress, we obtain

$$\sqrt{-\frac{du}{dr}} = \frac{1}{K_c}\sqrt{\frac{r\Delta p}{2L}} - \frac{\sqrt{\tau_y}}{K_c}$$

Squaring the previous equation, we get

$$-\frac{du}{dr}=\frac{1}{K_c^2}\frac{r\Delta p}{2L}+\frac{\tau_y}{K_c^2}-\frac{2}{K_c^2}\sqrt{\frac{r\tau_y\Delta p}{2L}}$$

or

$$du=-\frac{1}{K_c^2}\frac{\Delta p}{2L}r\,dr-\frac{\tau_y}{K_c^2}dr+\frac{2}{K_c^2}\sqrt{\frac{\tau_y\Delta p}{2L}}\sqrt{r}dr$$

Integrating,

$$u=-\frac{1}{K_c^2}\frac{\Delta p}{2L}\frac{r^2}{2}-\frac{\tau_y}{K_c^2}r+\frac{2}{K_c^2}\sqrt{\frac{\tau_y\Delta p}{2L}}\frac{r^{3/2}}{3/2}+C$$

applying the boundary condition that $u = 0$ at $r = R$,

$$C=\frac{1}{K_c^2}\frac{\Delta p}{2L}\frac{a^2}{2}+\frac{\tau_y}{K_c^2}R+\frac{2}{K_c^2}\sqrt{\frac{\tau_y\Delta p}{2L}}\frac{R^{3/2}}{3/2}$$

and substituting for C and rearranging terms, we obtain the relationship for the velocity profile as

$$u=\frac{1}{K_c^2}\frac{\Delta p}{4L}(R^2-r^2)+\frac{\tau_y}{K_c^2}(R-r)-\frac{4}{3K_c^2}\sqrt{\frac{\tau_y\Delta p}{2L}}(R^{3/2}-r^{3/2}) \tag{4.32}$$

As we discussed with a Bingham plastic, there will be no flow if $\Delta p/L < 2\tau_y/R$, while if $\Delta p/L > 2\tau_y/R$, flow will exist. Similarly, the velocity profile will be flat in the core region with a Casson velocity profile in the peripheral region.

The radius of the core region is given by

$$R_c=\frac{2L\tau_y}{\Delta p}$$

Substituting for the yield stress mentioned earlier in Equation 4.32, we get the core velocity as

$$u_c=\frac{1}{K_c^2}\frac{\Delta p}{4L}\left(R^2-R_c^2\right)+\frac{1}{K_c^2}\frac{R_c\Delta p}{2L}(R-r)-\frac{4}{3K_c^2}\sqrt{\frac{R_c\Delta p}{2L}}\sqrt{\frac{\Delta p}{2L}}\left(R^{3/2}-R_c^{3/2}\right)$$

Rewriting the equation, we get

$$u_c=\frac{\Delta p/L}{4K_c^2}\left[R^2-\frac{8}{3}\sqrt{R_c}R^{3/2}+2R_cR-\frac{R_c^2}{3}\right] \tag{4.33}$$

For $r > R_c$, the expression for the velocity profile will be

$$u_{per} = \frac{\Delta p/L}{4K_c^2}\left[R^2 - r^2 + 2R_cR - 2R_cR - \frac{8}{3}\sqrt{R_c}R^{3/2} + \frac{8}{3}\sqrt{R_c}R^{3/2}\right] \quad (4.34)$$

The flow rate through the tube is

$$Q = Q_{core} + Q_{per}$$

$$Q_{core} = u_c\pi R_c^2 = \pi R_c^2\frac{\Delta p/L}{4K_c^2}\left[R^2 - \frac{8}{3}\sqrt{R_c}R^{3/2} + 2R_cR - \frac{R_c^2}{3}\right]$$

and the expression for the flow in the core region can be simplified as

$$Q_{core} = \pi\frac{\Delta p/L}{4K_c^2}\left[R^2R_c^2 - \frac{8}{3}R_c^{5/2}R^{3/2} + 2R_c^3R - \frac{R_c^4}{3}\right] \quad (4.35)$$

The flow through the peripheral region can be obtained as

$$Q_{per} = \int_{R_c}^{R} u_{per}2\pi r\,dr$$

$$= 2\pi\frac{\Delta p/L}{4K_c^2}\int_{R_c}^{R}\left[R^2 - r^2 + 2R_cR - 2R_cr - \frac{8}{3}\sqrt{R_c}R^{3/2} + \frac{8}{3}\sqrt{R_c}r^{3/2}\right]r\,dr$$

Integrating the previous expression and simplifying, we get

$$Q_{per} = \pi\frac{\Delta p/L}{4K_c^2}\left[\frac{R^4}{2} - R^2R_c^2 + \frac{13}{42}R_c^4 + \frac{2}{3}R_cR^3 - 2RR_c^3 - \frac{8}{7}\sqrt{R_c}R^{7/2} + \frac{8}{3}R^{3/2}R_c^{5/2}\right] \quad (4.36)$$

Adding Equations 4.35 and 4.36, we get the expression for the flow through the tube as

$$Q = \frac{\Delta p/L\pi}{4K_c^2}\left[\frac{R^4}{2} - \frac{R_c^4}{42} + \frac{2}{3}R_cR^3 - \frac{8}{7}\sqrt{R_c}R^{7/2}\right]$$

Substituting for R_c in terms of the yield stress, the flow rate is given by

$$Q = \frac{\pi R^4\Delta p}{8K_c^2L}\left[1 - \frac{1}{21}\left(\frac{2\tau_y}{(\Delta p/L)R}\right)^4 + \frac{4}{3}\left(\frac{2\tau_y}{(\Delta p/L)}\right) - \frac{16}{7}\left(\frac{2\tau_y}{(\Delta p/L)R}\right)^{1/2}\right] \quad (4.37)$$

Assuming steady flow, one can compute the flow dynamics through a typical artery using the relationships derived earlier for Newtonian and non-Newtonian fluids. For a typical human peripheral vessel, the pressure gradient $\Delta p/L$ can be computed as 6 dyn/cm^3 from the Poiseuille relationship assuming a flow rate of 140 mL/min and a radius of 0.43 cm. Using the Poiseuille relationship, we are assuming a Newtonian behavior for human whole blood with a viscosity coefficient of 3.5 cP. The wall shear stress and the corresponding wall shear rate can be computed as follows:

For $R = 0.43$ cm, $Q = 140$ mL/min and $\mu = 3.5$ cP; $\Delta p/\ell = 8\mu Q/\pi a^4 = 6.0$ dyn/mL Additionally,

$$|\tau_w| = R\Delta p/2\ell = 1.29 \text{ dyn/cm}^2 \quad \text{and} \quad \dot{\gamma} = \tau_w/\mu = 36.9/\text{s}$$

Applying the same wall shear stress and the shear rate in the constitutive relationships for the other fluids, the consistency indices and the corresponding flow rate through the artery can be computed with the magnitudes shown in Table 4.2. The computed velocity profiles for the four fluids described earlier are included in Figure 4.17.

Conversely, by assuming a constant flow rate and the consistency index values computed earlier, one can also compute the pressure drop required for the various fluids and the corresponding wall shear rates. Assuming a yield stress for whole blood of 0.07 dyn/cm^2, the core radius where plug flow exists is very small (0.02 cm). Hence, the core region with a constant velocity is confined to a very small region near the center of the tube in the aforementioned plots. Using the assumed blood flow rate and the radius for the vessel as done early and the consistency indices computed for the various fluids, the computed pressure gradients and the corresponding wall shear stresses for each of the fluids are shown in Table 4.3 when the flow rate through the vessel is assumed to be the same for each case. The corresponding velocity profiles are plotted in Figure 4.18.

TABLE 4.2
Computed Consistency Index Values and the Flow Rates through an Artery Assuming a Constant Pressure Drop for the Various Fluids

	Consistency Index	Flow Rate Q (mL/s)
Newtonian fluid	$\mu = 3.5$ cP	140
Power law fluid ($n = 0.75$)	$k_{pl} = \tau_w/\dot{\gamma}_w^{0.75} = 0.0862$	127
Bingham plastic $\tau_y = 0.07$ dyn/cm^2	$\mu_b = \dfrac{(\tau_w - \tau_y)}{\dot{\gamma}} = 0.0331$	136
Casson fluid $\tau_y = 0.07$ dyn/cm^2	$k_c = \dfrac{\sqrt{\tau_w} - \sqrt{\tau_y}}{\sqrt{\dot{\gamma}}} = 0.1435$	117

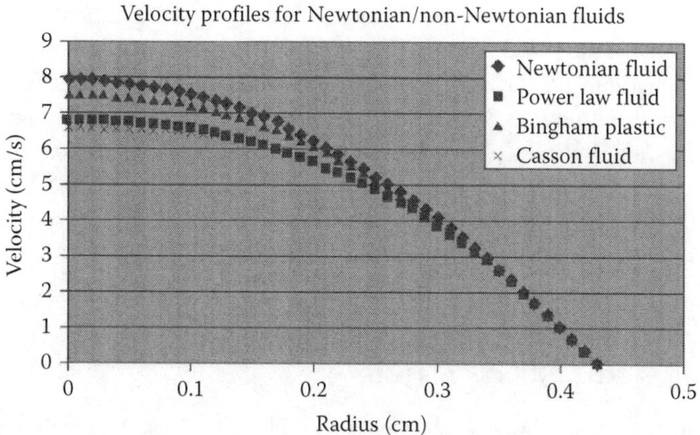

FIGURE 4.17 Velocity profiles computed with the flow rate and consistency index values shown in Table 4.2 for the various fluids. A constant pressure drop was assumed for each case.

TABLE 4.3
The Pressure Gradient and the Wall Shear Stress Computed for the Various Fluids with the Assumption of a Constant Flow Rate

	Newtonian	Power Law	Bingham Plastic	Casson Fluid
Consistency index	0.035	0.0862	0.0331	0.1435
$\Delta p/\ell$ (dyn/cm^3)	6.0	6.37	6.099	6.708
τ_w (dyn/cm^2)	1.29	1.37	1.31	1.44

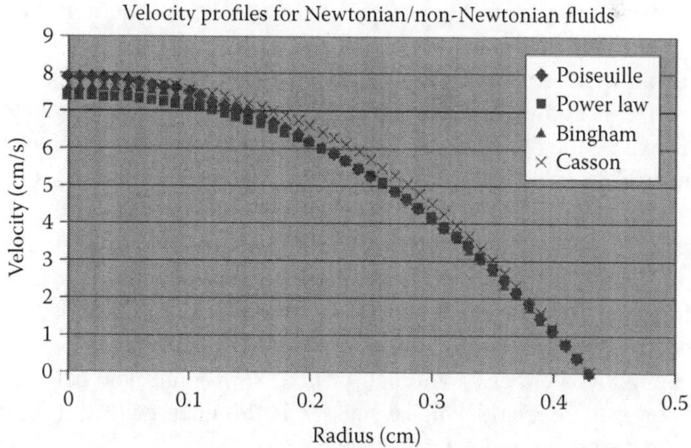

FIGURE 4.18 Velocity profiles for the various fluids assuming a constant flow rate and the computed pressure drops (and wall shear stress) shown in Table 4.3.

It can be observed that there is an increase in pressure gradient of about 12% between the Newtonian fluid and the Casson fluid with the flow rate and tube radius maintained constant and the wall shear stress increased by about 10%. In simulation studies on blood flow in an artery, it is a common practice to assume that blood is Newtonian since the shear rates are expected to be larger than $50\,s^{-1}$ for most of the cardiac cycle. The aforementioned computations demonstrate that the wall shear stress magnitudes can be expected to differ by about 10% if the Casson relationship rather than the Newtonian law is employed in the simulations.

4.1.5 Hemolysis and Platelet Activation with Fluid Dynamically Induced Stresses

We discussed earlier the rheological behavior of blood and the experimental methods to determine the viscous behavior of whole human blood. Whole blood follows a nonlinear constitutive relationship between the shear stress and strain in the form of Casson equation. Furthermore, whole human blood exhibits a yield stress, although its magnitude is too small to be of physiological importance. The apparent viscosity for blood is relatively high at low rates of shear because the red blood cells tend to aggregate, resulting in increased viscosity. As the rate of shear increases, the apparent viscosity reduces to an asymptotic value and, hence, whole blood exhibits a shear-thinning behavior. At relatively large rates of shear, we can approximate the whole blood constitutive relationship by that of a Newtonian fluid. A thorough knowledge of the rheological properties of blood is important for many applications. In order to analyze the blood flow dynamics in the human circulation from the large arteries to the capillary level, and then to the venous circulation, it will be necessary to apply the constitutive equations. In addition, blood analog fluids with rheological behavior similar to that of whole blood are necessary for employing *in vitro* experimental analysis of flow behavior in the various regions of the human circulation. In Chapters 5 and 6, steady and unsteady flow models of blood in large arteries and their applications to the understanding of physiological flow behavior will be discussed.

Comprehensive analysis of blood flow characteristics in the normal circulation will also help in delineating changes in flow behavior under various circulatory diseases. For example, atherosclerosis, or the formation and development of plaques in the large arteries, is known to develop at specific sites within the human circulation (Figure 3.25) where the arteries exhibit curvatures, bifurcations, or branches. Since these geometrical features induce complex flow dynamics and fluid stresses compared with those in arteries with a relatively straight geometry, various theories for the initiation and development of atherosclerotic plaques due to hemodynamic factors have been suggested. Numerous theoretical and experimental studies elucidating flow behavior in curved, bifurcating, or branching geometries have been reported in the literature to support the hemodynamic theories of atheroma development. These studies have employed either Newtonian or non-Newtonian flow behavior with the appropriate constitutive relationships discussed in this chapter. Results of these studies will also be discussed in detail in Chapter 6.

In employing the constitutive relationships for Newtonian or non-Newtonian fluid behavior in blood flow models, blood is treated as a homogeneous fluid, thus ignoring the significant fraction of formed elements (red and white blood cells and platelets) in it. The flow-induced stresses, predominantly shear stresses, can activate or even destroy the blood cells and platelets. Many studies have been performed on the effect of high shear stresses on blood cells. The magnitudes of the shear stresses and the time of exposure of the cells to stresses are important determinants of the destruction or activation of the blood cells. A shear stress versus time of exposure plot for red blood cells hemolysis threshold and for activation or destruction of platelets is shown in Figure 4.19. The data included in the plot are a compilation of experimental data in which the blood was subjected to a range of shear stresses and exposure times collected by various investigators. As illustrated in the figure, hemolysis and platelet activation can result even with relatively lower magnitudes of shear stresses if the formed elements are exposed to foreign surfaces during flow.

Hemolysis of red blood cells will result in the release of hemoglobin into the plasma. Hemoglobin within the red blood cells is the principal material for transport of oxygen from the lungs to the body tissues. Therefore, hemolysis at an elevated rate will result in anemia so that the blood cannot transport sufficient oxygen to the tissues. Platelet activation, on the other hand, can trigger the formation of thrombus within the vessel. Thrombus formation is initiated by the adherence of activated platelets to the subendothelial structures (such as the extracellular matrix, collagen, and the vascular smooth muscle cells) which have been exposed due to local vascular injury or to foreign surfaces in the presence of implantable devices

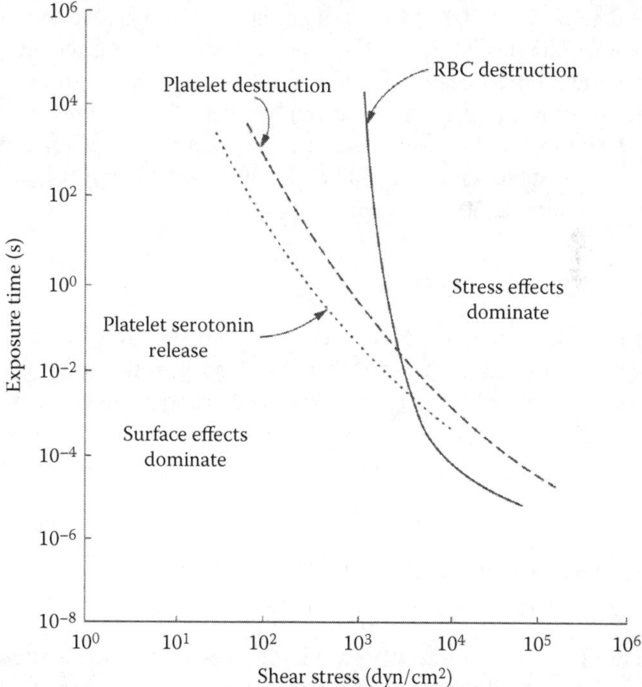

FIGURE 4.19 Shear stress-exposure time plot for threshold hemolysis of red blood cells and destruction of platelets.

such as mechanical heart valves or vascular stents. The thrombus then grows with additional platelet activation and aggregation. With the coagulation of blood, the adhered platelets combine with fibrin to form thrombus or blood clots. If the thrombus breaks apart and forms *emboli* that are transported downstream, they may lodge in smaller vessels and prevent blood supply to the region downstream of those sites. Should emboli lodge in the smaller vessels in the brain, neurological deficits will occur. Heart failure can occur if the emboli affect the smaller vessels in the coronary circulation.

From Figure 4.19, it can be observed that with relatively high shear rates, hemolysis or platelet activation can occur at very short time periods, whereas with lower magnitudes of shear stress, the cells must be under the influence of shear for a longer time before activation can be anticipated. By integrating the area under the shear stress-time plots, a single parameter with units of stress × time has also been proposed as an activation parameter in experimental and computational studies for the prediction of platelet activation and thrombus initiation in flow past devices such as mechanical heart valves. It should also be pointed out that the experiments from which the data for these plots were generated for the activation of platelets were performed with platelet-rich plasma (without the red blood cells) in the sample fluid subjected to prespecified shear stresses for known amount of time. In reality, under normal physiological concentration, there will be four platelets and one white blood cell present for 60 red blood cells. The effect of the red blood cells in the fluid sample on the behavior of platelets is essentially ignored in these experiments in order to relate the flow-induced stresses on platelet activation, aggregation, and thrombus development. The mechanics of thrombus initiation with circulatory implants continues to be an active area of research even today in order to provide design improvements to minimize or prevent thrombus deposition. Thrombus formation and ensuing embolic complications continues to remain as a major problem with circulatory implants such as mechanical heart valves, vascular grafts and stents, and artificial heart and circulatory assist devices.

4.2 VASCULAR MECHANICS

Pulsatile blood flow in the human arterial circulation is the result of constant interaction between the flowing blood and the arterial wall. In the analysis of the fluid mechanics of blood flow in human arteries, we need to understand the behavior of the arterial wall in addition to knowledge about the flow behavior of blood. Therefore, we will briefly review the structural components and the mechanics of the walls of blood vessels.

4.2.1 Structural Components of the Blood Vessel Wall and Their Contribution to Material Behavior

The arterial wall is a composite of three layers, each of which contains varying amounts of elastin, collagen, vascular smooth muscle cells, and extracellular matrices (Figure 4.20). The inner most layer of the artery, called the *intima*, consists of a single layer of endothelial cells and a very thin lamina of elastin. The role of the

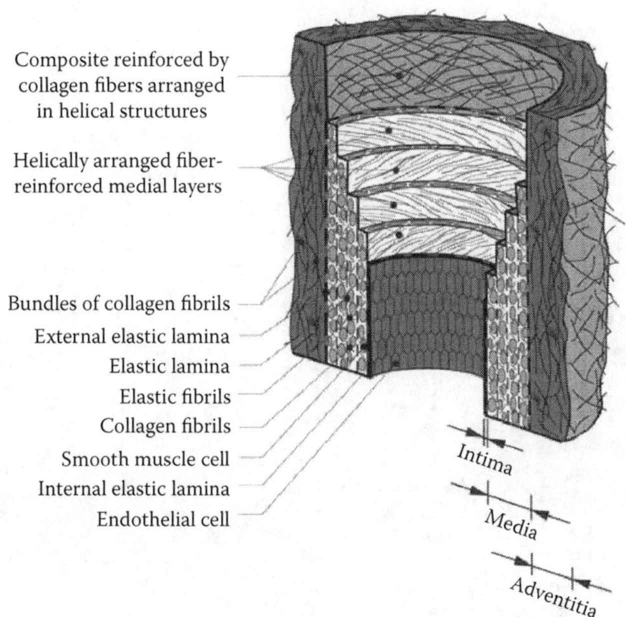

FIGURE 4.20 Schematic of the components of a healthy artery. (From Holzapfel et al., *J. Elast.*, 61, 1, 2000. With permission from Kluwer Academic Publishers.)

endothelial cells lining the inner surface of the artery is to provide a smooth wall and selective permeability to water, electrolytes, sugars, and other substances between the bloodstream and the tissues. The outer layer, the *adventitia*, consists of connective tissue that merges with the surrounding structures. The middle layer, known as the *media*, consists of elastin, collagen, and vascular smooth muscles embedded in an extracellular matrix. Wall diameters, thicknesses, and compositions of various blood vessels are shown in Figure 4.21. Elastin fibers are present in all the vessels except the capillaries and the venules and are very easily stretched. Collagen fibers, which form a network in both the media and the adventitia, are much stiffer than the elastin fibers. However, the collagen fibers are normally found with a degree of slackness, and, thus, their full stiffness is not apparent until after the vessels are stretched to the extent where the slackness is removed. Even though the individual components behave like linear elastic materials, the combination of taut elastin and relaxed collagen fibers results in a nonlinear behavior as illustrated in Figure 4.22. A schematic illustration of the taut elastin and unstretched collagen fibers is shown in Figure 4.22a. A schematic of the force-deformation test for a single elastin fiber is shown in Figure 4.22b whose elastic modulus is about 10^6 dyn/cm^2. A similar schematic for the collagen fiber behavior with an elastic modulus of about 10^9 dyn/cm^2 is shown in Figure 4.22c. For a combination of elastin and collagen fibers, the effect of increasing distension where the collagen fiber becomes taut and reacts to the load will result in a bilinear curve as shown in Figure 4.22d. The continuous recruitment of more collagen fibers with increased load results in a nonlinear force-deformation behavior as illustrated in Figure 4.22e. The function of the elastin and collagen fibers

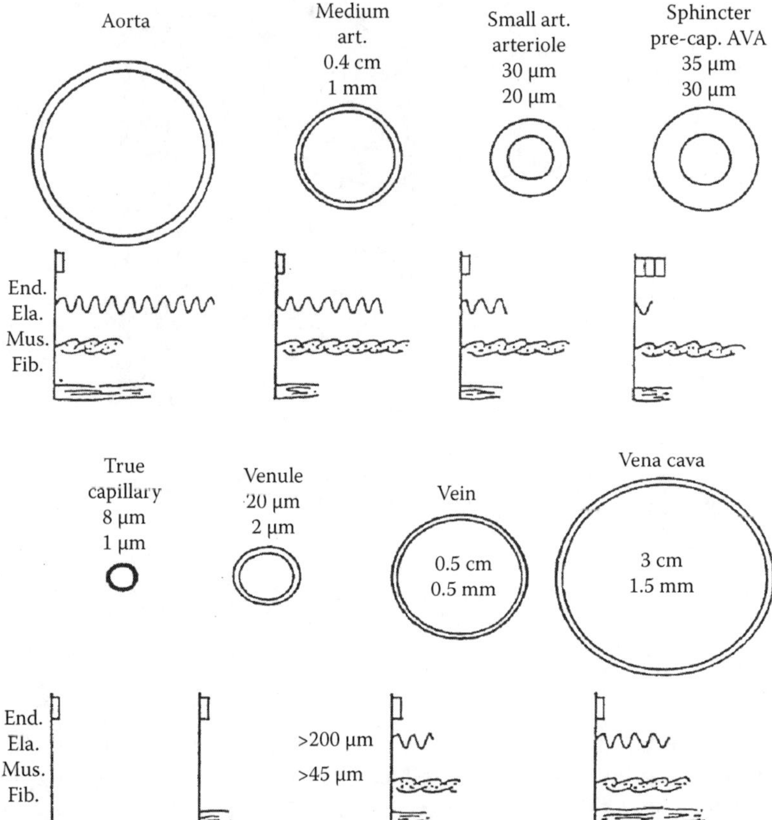

FIGURE 4.21 The diameter, wall thickness, and components of the wall of the various blood vessels in the circulatory system. (Redrawn from Burton, A.C., *Physiology and Biophysics of the Circulation*, Year Book Medical Publishers, Chicago, IL, Copyright 1971, Elsevier.)

is to maintain a steady tension within the vessels to act against the transmural pressure exerted on them. On the other hand, the function of the vascular smooth muscle is to provide an active tension by means of contraction under physiological control. Thus, more smooth muscle content is observed in the smaller arteries and arterioles where vascular resistance can be controlled by the change in the radius of the vessel produced by the tension of the smooth muscles. The elastic modulus for smooth muscles depends upon the relaxed or contracted state of the muscle. The endothelial cells act more as sensors and mediators of physiological changes and offer negligible resistance to mechanical load.

4.2.2 Material Behavior of Blood Vessels

Uniaxial extension tests can be performed *in vitro* on strips of arteries cut in various orientations from the artery (such as circumferential or longitudinal strips) to determine the force-deformation behavior. When biological tissues are subjected to

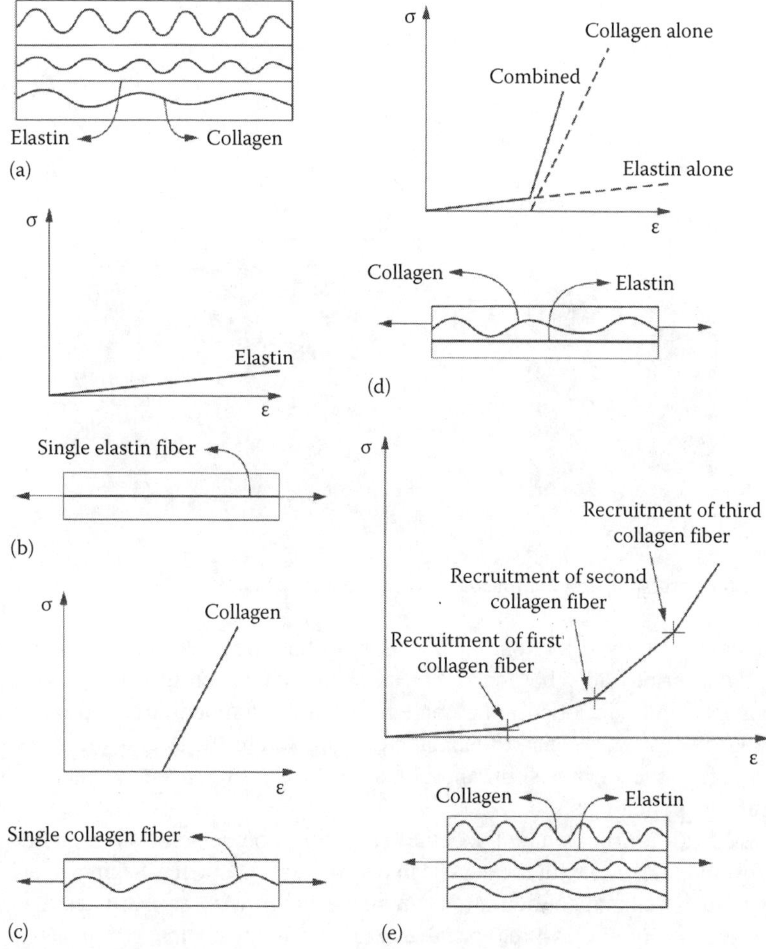

FIGURE 4.22 (a) Schematic of the elastin-collagen complex in an unstretched arterial wall, (b) stress–strain relationship for an elastin and (c) for a collagen fiber, (d) stress–strain behavior of an elastin and collagen fiber combination, and (e) behavior with additional collagen fiber recruitment with increasing load.

load-deformation tests cyclically, the tests will result in a hysteresis loop. In other words, the load-deformation curve during loading will take a different path from the unloading curve, indicating an energy loss during the loading and unloading process. With repeated loading and unloading, the area under the loop will decrease rapidly at first and reach a steady state after a number of cycles. For this reason, data on the load-deformation behavior for biological tissue are obtained only after preconditioning the tissue by loading and unloading for several cycles. Figure 4.23 shows a photograph of a strip of an aorta of a pig gripped between clamps and attached to a testing apparatus. The corresponding measured stress–strain behavior for the specimen is also shown in the figure. Such tests performed with specimens with various orientations (e.g., longitudinal or circumferential) will yield

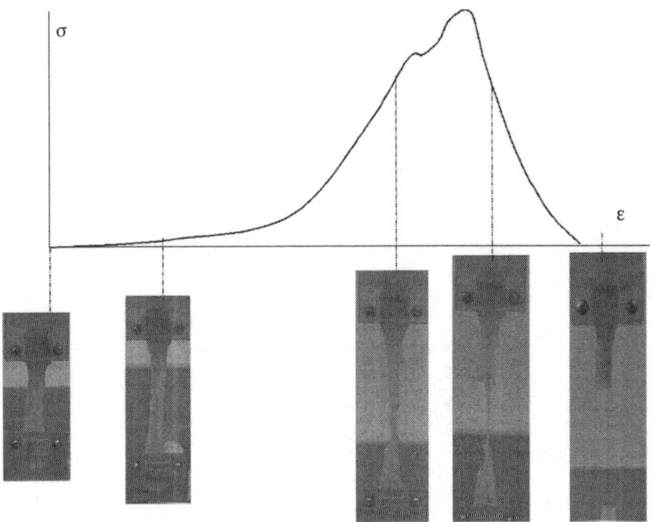

FIGURE 4.23 Images of a pig's thoracic aorta being subjected to a uniaxial test (bottom row); and the corresponding nonlinear stress–strain relationship.

information about the directional dependence of the force-deformation behavior, if any, of the arterial wall. These *in vitro* tests should be performed in a physiological environment with controlled ionic content, moisture, temperature, and other variables. Figure 4.24 represents a schematic comparison of the stress–strain relationship for soft tissue such as skin, and blood vessel with dry bone and steel used in engineering applications.

More useful information on the actual behavior of blood vessels can be obtained by performing the tests with the vessels in their natural geometry. Segments of blood vessels in their original configuration can be used in *in vitro* or *in situ* testing under an applied transmural pressure. For *in vitro* testing, relatively long segments need to

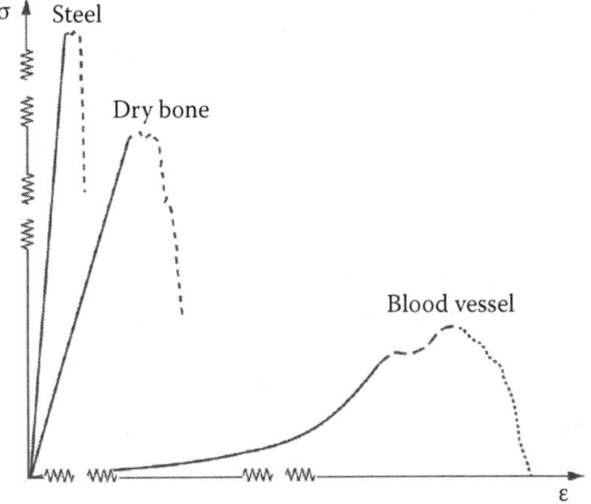

FIGURE 4.24 A comparison of stress–strain relationship for steel, bone, blood vessel, and skin.

be obtained so that making the measurements sufficiently away from the supports can eliminate "end effects." Once again, the physiological environment needs to be maintained during the testing to obtain any meaningful data. Consideration must be given to the changing state of the smooth muscle with *in vitro* specimens. In the absence of stimuli, the smooth muscles tend to relax while they also stiffen after death ("rigor mortis"). When a segment of artery is cut, the length can decrease by as much as 40% of the initial length. Hence, the usual practice with *in vitro* testing is to mark the length of the artery before dissecting it and then stretching the segment back to its original length before performing the tests so that the mechanical tethering will be similar to that *in vivo*.

Either a static pressure or a dynamic pressure pulse is applied to the arterial segment in both the *in vitro* and *in situ* tests and the changes in the radius and the wall thickness are measured to determine the load-deformation behavior. The applied pressure can be measured relatively easily with sensitive pressure transducers. However, measurement of change in radius and, especially, the wall thickness is more complicated. Several techniques using strain gages, differential transformers, or electro-optical methods have been used to measure the change in the outer radius. Measurement of the change in the internal diameter and thereby the change in the wall thickness requires data from angiographic, ultrasonic, or other imaging modalities. In static tests, a change in radius for a corresponding change in a step pressure increase can be measured to determine the incremental modulus as described earlier. Sufficient time must be allowed before the measurement of the diameter change after the application of pressure to allow for creep effects. In dynamic tests, a sinusoidal pressure pulse is applied and the resulting change in diameter is continuously recorded so that viscoelastic properties of the arterial segments can be determined.

In vivo tests can also be performed either by surgically exposing the vessel under study and making direct measurements or by applying noninvasive imaging techniques and inserting a pressure transducer by catheterization to record changes in diameter and the pulse pressure, respectively. A pressure-strain modulus can be computed using the relationship given in Equation 2.46. If the wall thickness change can also be measured, a static elastic modulus can be computed from the measured data using the relationship given in Equation 2.45. On the other hand, if a continuous recording of the diameter changes can be obtained along with the physiological pressure pulse, the signals can be separated into harmonics by the use of the Fourier series analysis. From this, the dynamic elastic modulus values over a range of frequencies can be obtained.

4.2.2.1 Assumptions in the Analysis

The data on changes in pressure, radii, and wall thickness, obtained from *in vitro* or *in vivo* experiments, can be reduced to the elastic modulus based on the expressions derived earlier. However, it should be kept in mind that certain assumptions have been made in deriving those expressions. For example, an expression for the elastic modulus was derived based on the thin-walled elastic tube model (Equation 2.29). This expression is applicable only in cases where $t/R < 0.1$. As can be observed from Figure 4.20, the t/R ratio for most blood vessels ranges from 0.105 to 0.15. Hence, the thick-walled formulation may be more appropriate in analyzing the material properties of these vessels. The other important assumptions made in the formulations described earlier are the homogeneity, incompressibility, and isotropic behavior of the material. As already discussed, blood vessels are not homogeneous and actually consist of several layers and components. Expressions for the elastic moduli derived earlier for thick-walled models include information on the Poisson's ratio. It is common to assume that blood vessels, similar to other biological soft tissue, are incompressible and, hence, one can assign a value of 0.5 for ν. This is supported by the observation that volumetric strain computations of the vessel walls of excised dogs indicate that blood vessels are essentially incompressible. Due to the tethering of the blood vessels, it can be expected that the elastic modulus in the longitudinal direction will be larger than those in the circumferential and radial directions. Numerous studies have been reported on the computed elastic modulus in the radial, circumferential, and axial directions with the vessel generally being increasingly stiffer along those directions, respectively.

4.2.2.2 Experimental Results

Mechanical properties of blood vessels were assessed *in vivo* by the simultaneous measurement of intraarterial pressure and the arterial diameter in dogs in the 1960s. The arteries were assumed to be thin-walled and incompressible and the viscoelastic behavior of the vessel was determined by the relationship

$$\sigma_\theta = \frac{pr}{t} = E\frac{\Delta r}{R_2} + E_v\frac{d}{dt}\left(\frac{\Delta r}{R_2}\right) \tag{4.38}$$

A simple viscoelastic model has been assumed in deriving the aforementioned relationship with the circumferential stress σ_θ, the circumferential strain $\Delta r/R_2$, and the rate of strain in the circumferential direction $d/dt(\Delta r/R_2)$. Data for various arterial segments in the systemic circulation from very young to old dogs were presented in this study. The results showed that the viscous component was relatively small compared with the elastic modulus. The *in vivo* elastic moduli of various arterial segments from the thoracic aorta to the femoral arteries ranged from 1,953 to 34,944 Gm/cm^2.

Bergel (1961a,b) has presented data for static and dynamic elastic moduli for the blood vessels based on the thick-walled theory for a homogeneous and isotropic material. The *in vitro* experiments were performed on excised blood vessels from dogs with transmural pressure load of up to 240 mmHg. A nonlinear behavior characterized by stiffening of the vessels with increasing pressure is apparent from the static study results shown in Figure 4.25. Incremental elastic moduli determined for a dog's aorta as well as the femoral and carotid arteries in this study are included in Table 4.4.

Bergel (1961b) also performed dynamic studies by superimposing a sinusoidal variation over a static pressure of 100 mmHg and measuring the diameter changes employing a photo-optical technique. The dynamic elastic moduli computed for the canine arteries at various frequencies are compared with the corresponding static values (0 Hz) in Table 4.5 and the results show that the dynamic incremental modulus is significantly increased even at 2 Hz compared with the corresponding static values.

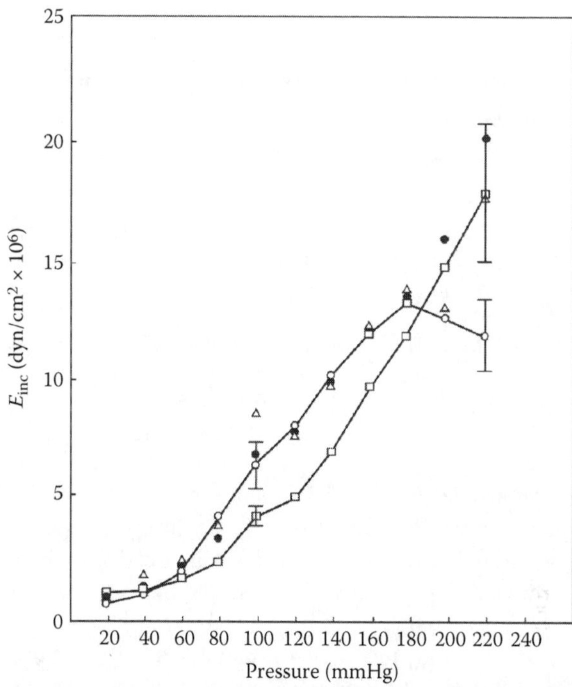

FIGURE 4.25 Incremental static elastic modulus as a function of transmural pressure for dog's arteries. Δ, Thoracic aorta; □, abdominal aorta; ο, femoral artery; •, carotid artery. (Redrawn from Bergel, D.H., *J. Physiol.*, 156, 445, 1961. With permission from the Physiological Society.)

TABLE 4.4
Incremental Static Elastic Moduli (×10⁶ dyn/cm²) for the Arterial Wall

Pressure (mmHg)	Thoracic Aorta	Abdominal Aorta	Femoral Artery	Carotid Artery
40	1.2 ± 0.1 (6)	1.6 ± 0.4 (4)	1.2 ± 0.2 (6)	1.0 ± 0.2 (7)
100	4.3 ± 0.4 (12)	8.9 ± 3.5 (8)	6.9 ± 1.0 (9)	6.4 ± 1.0 (12)
160	9.9 ± 0.5 (6)	12.4 ± 2.2 (4)	12.1 ± 2.4 (6)	12.2 ± 2.7 (7)
220	18.2 ± 2.8 (5)	18.0 ± 5.5 (3)	20.4 ± 4.4 (6)	12.2 ± 1.5 (7)

Source: From Bergel, D.H., *J. Physiol.* 156, 445, 1961. With permission from the Physiological Society.
Note: Figures in parentheses refer to the number of specimens in the experiments.

At higher frequencies, the dynamic modulus does not show further changes. The dynamic elastic moduli computed at mean arterial pressures ranging from 87 to 130 mmHg and pulse frequencies ranging from 1.1 to 2.8 Hz in the dog arteries *in vivo* showed a monotonic increase from the thoracic aorta to the femoral arteries. The viscous modulus ranged from 9% to 12% of the corresponding dynamic modulus. Effect of age on the viscoelastic properties of the human arterial wall have also been investigated and the results showed that the viscous component of the elastic modulus was

TABLE 4.5
The Dynamic Elastic Moduli (×10⁶ dyn/cm²) for the Canine Arteries at Various Frequencies

Vessel/Frequency	0 Hz	2 Hz	5 Hz	18 Hz
Thoracic aorta	4.4 ± 0.40 (10)	4.7 ± 0.42 (10)	4.9 ± 0.45 (10)	5.3 ± 0.80 (4)
Abdominal aorta	9.2 ± 0.94 (7)	10.9 ± 0.88 (7)	11.0 ± 0.82 (7)	12.2 ± 0.46 (4)
Femoral artery	9.0 ± 1.15 (5)	12.0 ± 0.81 (5)	12.0 ± 0.82 (5)	10.6 ± 1.39 (5)
Carotid artery	6.9 ± 0.48 (6)	11.0 ± 1.00 (6)	11.3 ± 0.99 (6)	11.5 ± 1.03 (6)

Source: From Bergel, D.H., *J. Physiol.* 156, 458, 1961. With permission from the Physiological Society.

Note: Figures in parenthesis show the number of specimens used in the experiments.

larger in the femoral arteries and can be attributed to higher muscular content in the wall. In the "young" group, the wall stiffness was observed to increase toward the peripheral vessels and in the "old" group, the opposite trend was observed. Such studies indicate the presence of regional variation in the mechanical properties of arteries. Studies have also been reported on the anisotropic behavior of the arterial wall. Mean values for the incremental moduli in the radial, circumferential, and longitudinal directions of 5,480, 7,510, and 10,100 Gm/cm^2, respectively, at a mean arterial pressure of 154 cm H_2O have been reported from data obtained *in vivo* in dogs. These studies also showed that the elastic moduli increased with increased mean arterial pressure. Moreover, the longitudinal elastic modulus measured on the same vessels *in vitro* showed a decrease after the removal of tethering of the vessels *in situ*.

The viscoelastic behavior of arteries is usually assessed by experiments on specimens obtained from healthy animals of various species and the results obtained have suggested an anisotropic, nonlinear stress–strain relationship under a transmural load from 0 to about 240 mmHg. It can be anticipated that vascular disease would alter the material behavior. Common vascular diseases in humans include atherosclerosis, high blood pressure (hypertension), and diabetes. Atherosclerosis is the formation of plaques within the artery wall and lumen and is associated with the accumulation of cholesterol combined with LDL that dissolve in plasma. The formation and growth of these lesions and their relationship with the local flow dynamics are further described in Chapter 6. In brief, early atheroma results from abnormal deposition of LDL-cholesterol within the intima, followed by a cellular response, composed of macrophages, lymphocytes, and proliferating vascular smooth muscles. Collagen and elastin fibers eventually replace the cellular constituents, resulting in a changing histological picture with the lesion development. Initially, the arteries respond by remodeling or thinning of the media in order to accommodate the expanding lesion within the arterial wall in order to maintain the lumen cross section for blood flow. With further development of the plaque and as the contents become calcified, the plaques protrude into the lumen and begin occluding the cross section available for blood flow. It can be anticipated that the arterial wall material property is continually altered with the various stages of lesion development and several studies have been reported on the nature of such alterations.

The arterial wall also responds to increased blood pressure by the reorganization and thickening (*hypertrophy*) of the medial wall in the artery. The wall thickening will result in the circumferential stress due to the transmural blood pressure returning to normal levels. Diabetes also affects the material behavior of the arterial wall and studies on the alterations in arterial wall material behavior with these diseases continue to be the subject of ongoing research.

The interaction between stress and strain for an elastic material is the constitutive relationship describing the behavior of the material under external loading. In order to mathematically describe the material behavior for nonlinear material such as blood vessels, exponential, polynomial, or logarithmic relationships between stress and strain have been generally employed. In developing mathematical relationships for nonlinear and anisotropic materials, it is convenient to describe the material behavior in the form of a strain energy function (work done on the material in the deformation process) and to express the relationship in terms of material constants. A best curve fit of the force-deformation experimental data is employed for determining the material constants for the mathematical relationship being employed. Further details on such material behavior descriptions for biological soft tissues including blood vessels can be found in Fung (1981) and other similar more recent publications.

4.2.3 Residual Stress on Blood Vessels

In engineering materials, a component that is not subjected to an external load will not have any deformation and no internal stresses will develop in the material. The arteries are subject to external loads through the transmural blood pressure and, hence, using the same analogy as for general engineering materials, it can be expected that arteries will be stress-free at zero transmural load. In the last couple of decades, several studies have demonstrated that the arterial wall tissue is not stress-free at zero transmural loads. This fact can be demonstrated as follows. A small segment of an artery is excised into a ring-shaped element and, subsequently, a radial cut is made on the ring-shaped segment. Should the artery be stress-free, the artery will maintain its circular shape even after the radial cut. However, it has been demonstrated that the arterial segment opens to a sector (a horseshoe shape) within a few minutes after the longitudinal cut as schematically shown in Figure 4.26 with the arterial wall

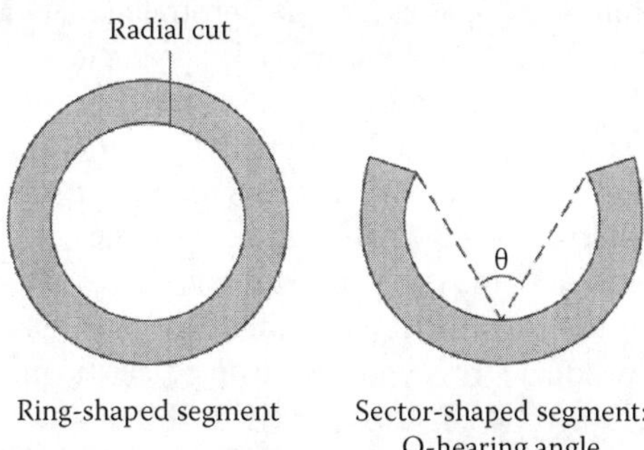

FIGURE 4.26 Schematic of a ring-shaped arterial segment and the open sector (horseshoe-shaped) stress-free state of the segment after a radial cut.

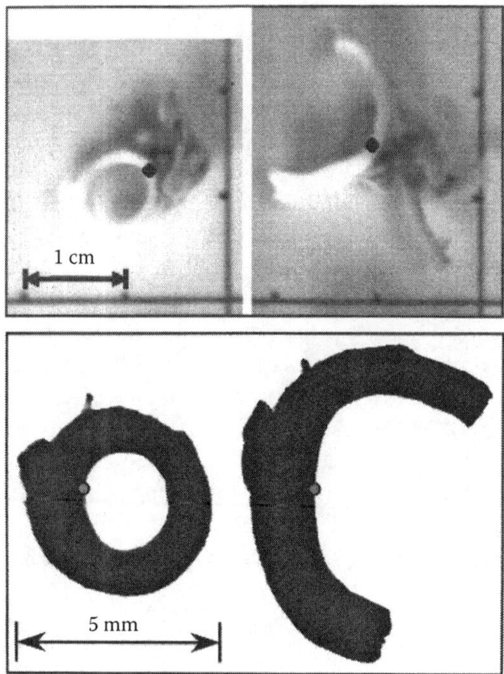

FIGURE 4.27 A photograph of an excised ring-shaped pig's femoral arterial segment and the open-sector-shaped stress-free state of the artery with an additional radial cut.

being stress-free in this open segment. The artery is assumed to be stress-free in the sector-shaped configuration because an additional radial cut will result in two pieces that do not result in noticeable additional strains or change in shape. A photograph of an excised pig's femoral artery in the ring-shaped configuration and in the sector-shaped stress-free state after a radial cut is shown in Figure 4.27.

It is evident, then, that the ring-shaped arterial segment is subjected to a prestress (or residual stress) even with no load (zero transmural pressure). The magnitude of the prestress has been generally described in terms of the opening angle of the sector shape as shown in Figure 4.26. Studies have demonstrated that the residual stress is a function of the anatomical location of the arterial segment (e.g., carotid artery versus femoral artery), and the species from which the segments are obtained. The opening angle also varies depending upon the location of the radial cut of the ring-shaped segment. By measuring the circumferential lengths of the intimal and adventitial boundaries in the uncut (ring-shaped) configuration and the corresponding lengths in the open sector configuration, the residual strains at zero load can be computed and have been shown to be compressive in the intimal layer and tensile in the adventitial layer. The computed residual stress with an assumed elastic modulus demonstrates that the magnitudes of the residual stress are about 10% of the estimated circumferential stress in the arterial wall under physiological transmural load. Under normal physiological loading neglecting the residual stress, it has been shown that circumferential stress is generally larger in the intimal border and decreases toward the adventitial border. Thus, the inclusion of a residual stress that is compressive in the intimal border and tensile in the adventitial border will result in a circumferential stress distribution across the arterial wall thickness which is more uniform under physiological loading. The presence of residual strain and stress has been implicated in the remodeling of the arterial wall. Finite element studies indicate that the distribution of the circumferential stress throughout the wall thickness is more uniform if the residual strain effect is included in the analysis.

4.2.4 Material Characterization of Cardiac Muscle

As was described in Chapter 3, the cardiac muscles constantly contract and relax in order to develop blood pressure and maintain adequate circulation to the various organs in the body. The basic structure of the cardiac muscle is a fiber that is arranged in columns that are roughly cylindrical in shape with a diameter of 10–20 μm and a length of 50–100 μm. The fibers are oriented nearly vertically in the inner (*endocardium*) and outer (*epicardium*) layers of the muscle. The fiber orientation undergoes a gradual change through the myocardium such that the fibers in the middle third of the wall thickness are oriented circumferentially. Individual muscle fibers are surrounded by a surface-limiting membrane called the *sarcolemma*. Within the sarcolemma, each fiber contains rodlike structures called the *fibrils*. The fibrils run the length of the fiber and contain serially repeating structures called the *sarcomeres*. Mitochondria are interspersed within the fibrils while the sarcotubular system surrounds the fibrils and connects with the sarcolemma. The sarcomeres are the fundamental functional units of cardiac contraction.

In order to describe the behavior of cardiac muscles, both the passive elastic characteristics (during the diastolic phase) and the active contractile properties (during the early systolic phase) of the cardiac muscle need to be analyzed. The cardiac muscles are at least orthotropic with the force-deformation behavior being stiffer along the direction of the fibers compared with that in the transverse direction. Since the fiber orientation gradually changes along the thickness of the muscle, passive elastic deformation tests are usually performed on strips of papillary muscle since the fibers are oriented along the longitudinal direction in these muscles. Just as with other biological soft tissue, the passive stress–strain behavior of cardiac muscles is also nonlinear and an exponential stress–strain relationship is generally employed to describe the rheological properties of the cardiac muscle. The contractile properties of the cardiac muscle (and skeletal muscle) are generally described using the force-velocity relationship that is typically obtained using the following steps. Strips of isolated papillary muscles are stretched with a preload and temporarily fixed at this length. An after load is then attached in this configuration and the muscle is stimulated. The peak velocity of contraction for the given total load (preload and after load) is measured as the muscle contracts under the stimulation. By varying the initial length of contraction as well as the preload, a family of force-velocity curves is obtained. In the case of cardiac muscle, the data extrapolated to obtain the velocity at no load from the set of curves converge to a single point referred to as the maximum velocity of shortening. The passive elastic properties as well as the maximum velocity of shortening can be altered if the cardiac muscles are diseased due to myocardial infarction or *cardiomyopathy*.

4.3 SUMMARY

In this chapter, the rheological behavior of blood was considered. The basic relationships for viscometry were developed and the application of viscometry to measure the viscosity of blood and plasma was discussed. The importance of understanding the rheological behavior of blood and its changes with diseased states was briefly discussed. A study of the arterial wall material behavior is important for a basic understanding of the physiology of blood vessels. The arteries serve as a pressure reservoir in the circulation. As blood is ejected from the left ventricle during systole, the vessel walls distend as the arterial pressure rises. Later, during diastole, the passive arterial wall tension maintains a force to drive the blood through the peripheral capillaries. Assessment of mechanical properties of the blood vessels in various segments of the peripheral circulation is important in the understanding of the propagation of pressure pulses and the pressure–flow relationship in the circulation under normal and diseased states. It is also important to understand the interaction between blood flowing through the lumen and the vessel wall. Knowledge of the behavior of the normal artery will also be helpful in early detection of any diseases of the blood vessels such as atherosclerosis. Study of the material characterization of the cardiac muscles is also important in our understanding of normal physiological behavior and various alterations that occur with the onset of diseases.

PROBLEMS

4.1 Derive the relationship for the torque developed in a Couette viscometer (Equation 4.4). A typical Couette viscometer with a 4.0 cm inner diameter, 4.2 cm outer diameter, and 6 cm height is used to measure the viscosity of blood. If the angular velocity is 50 rpm, compute the torque required to rotate the outer cylinder. Also plot the distribution of the rate of shear between the inner and the outer cylinder. Use a whole blood viscosity of 3.5 cP.

4.2 For a typical red blood cell, the intracellular fluid volume is 87 μm^3 and the surface area of the cell is 163 μm^2. If the red blood cell had a spherical shape with the same intracellular fluid volume, compute the surface area for the same. What is the advantage of the biconcave shape for the red blood cell?

4.3 Plot apparent viscosity as a function of shear rate for the relationship given by Equation 4.6 for a range of shear rates from 1 to 500 s^{-1}. Compute the apparent viscosity of blood at a rate of shear of 230 s^{-1}. Use a plasma viscosity of 1.2 cP.

4.4 For a normal hematocrit of 43% and fibrinogen concentration of 0.3 g/100 mL, compute the yield stress for blood employing the empirical formulae given in Equation 4.8. In a capillary with a diameter of 5 μm and a length of 1 mm, estimate the minimal pressure gradient required for the blood to overcome the computed yield stress and induce flow through the vessel.

4.5 Derive the expression for the flow rate and the apparent viscosity for the cell-free boundary layer model described in the text.

4.6 For human blood, assuming values of plasma viscosity of 1.2 cP and whole blood viscosity of 3.3 cP at 37°C, compute the apparent viscosity of blood flowing through a tube of 100 μm diameter using both the cell-free marginal layer and the sigma effect theories. Assume a cell-free layer thickness of 3 μm and a mean thickness of unsheared laminae of 15 μm. Compare the values from both the theories.

4.7 Assume that whole blood with a hematocrit of 45% flows through a small diameter tube. The total flow rate is 16 cc/s, although in the core region it is 12 cc/s and in the peripheral region it is 4 cc/s. The blood cells accumulate in the core region with a volume of 10 mm^3 and there are no blood cells present in the cell-free peripheral region which has a volume of 6 mm^3. By performing a mass balance on the red blood cells, determine the hematocrit in the core region and the average hematocrit in the whole tube. What is the effect on apparent viscosity of the blood in the tube?

4.8 In an artery of an animal with an internal diameter of 1 cm and a wall thickness of 0.75 mm at an end diastolic pressure of 85 mmHg, an 8% increase in the diameter was measured for a pulse pressure of 45 mmHg. Compute the circumferential stress in the wall of the artery as well as the elastic modulus of the vessel at the mean arterial pressure assuming that the arterial wall is thin-walled and made of linear isotropic elastic material.

4.9 For the data given in Problem 4.8, compute the elastic modulus at the mean arterial pressure and compare the results from using the thin-walled artery model. Also compute the incremental elastic modulus employing $\Delta p = 45$ mmHg. (Assume $\nu = 0.5$.)

4.10 In an experiment with a canine femoral artery, the following stress–strain relationship was obtained. Using the data, compute the incremental elastic modulus at a strain of 0.15.

Strain	**0.0**	**0.03**	**0.05**	**0.07**	**0.09**	**0.10**	**0.12**	**0.15**	**0.17**	**0.19**	**0.21**	**0.23**	**0.25**	**0.27**	**0.28**
Stress ($\times 10^5$ dyn/cm^2)	0.0	0.3	1	2	5	10	15	31	48	66	83	102	121	119	102

4.11 A ring-shaped specimen of an animal artery was radially cut and the horseshoe-shaped geometry of the specimen after the cut is shown in the figure. The coordinates of several anatomical points in the stress-free state geometry of the specimen are also indicated in the figure. Compute the opening angle as a measure of the prestress of the arterial specimen.

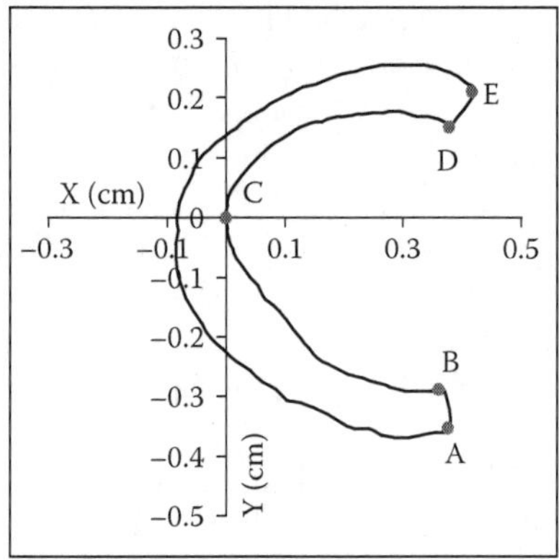

Key Point Coordinates (cm)		
A	0.381	−0.351
B	0.369	−0.291
C	0	0
D	0.38	0.151
E	0.422	0.207

REFERENCES

Bergel, D. H. (1961a) The static elastic properties of the arterial wall. *J. Physiol.* 156: 445–457.

Bergel, D. H. (1961b) The dynamic elastic properties of the arterial wall. *J. Physiol.* 156: 458–469.

Burton, A. C. (1971) *Physiology and Biophysics of the Circulation*, Year Book Medical Publishers, Chicago, IL.

Cooney, D. O. (1976) *Biomedical Engineering Principles: An Introduction to Fluid, Heat and Mass Transport Processes*, Marcel Dekker, New York.

Copley, A. L. and Stainsby, G., eds. (1960) *Flow Properties of Blood*, Pergamon Press, Oxford, U.K.

Dinsdale, A. and Moore, F. (1962) *Viscosity and Its Measurement*, Reinhold Publishing Corporation, New York.

Fung, Y. C. (1981) *Biomechanics: Mechanical Properties of Living Tissues*, Springer-Verlag, New York.

Holzapfel, G. A., Gasser, T. C., and Ogden, R. W. (2000) A new constitutive framework for arterial wall mechanics and a comparative study of material models. *J. Elasticity* 61: 1–48.

Merrill, E. W., Margetts, W. G., Cokelet, G. R., and Gilliland, E. R. (1965) The Casson equation and rheology of blood near zero shear. In *Proceedings of the Fourth International Congress on Rheology*, Copley, A. L., ed., Wiley-Interscience, New York, pp. 135–143.

Whitmore, R. L. (1968) *Rheology of Circulation*, Pergamon Press, New York.

5 Static and Steady Flow Models

5.1 INTRODUCTION

In this chapter, we will discuss some applications of hydrostatics and steady flow models to describe blood flow in arteries. Even though the flow in the human circulatory system is unsteady, particularly at the pre-capillary level, steady flow models do provide some insight into the aspects of flow through the arteries and some useful applications can be found using the steady flow models. As would be expected, steady flow models are also simpler to use because of the absence of time variations in the governing equations (cf. the equations of motion, Equations 1.43a through 1.43c). Steady flow models also avoid the complexity of having a moving interface between the blood and the vessel wall as the artery distends in response to pulsatile pressure.

5.2 HYDROSTATICS IN THE CIRCULATION

For a typical adult, the mean arterial pressure at the level of the heart is about 100 mmHg. In the supine (i.e., lying down) position, pressures in the blood vessels of the head and legs would be ~95 mmHg (Figure 5.1). However, when a person is standing up, the hydrostatic effects that were discussed in Section 1.3 must be taken into account.

In order to assess the pressure differences due to gravitational effects, the force balance of Equation 1.12 can be applied as

$$\Delta p = \rho g h \tag{1.12}$$

Using the previous equation and knowing the density of blood, the pressures in the blood vessels can be estimated as shown in the figure. Since arteries are relatively stiff vessels, the increase in pressure due to hydrostatic effects will only cause minimal alterations in the blood volume since the vessel cross section remains nearly constant. However, in the veins, the blood volume will be greatly affected because they are much thinner and can expand significantly (see Section 3.4). In fact, if the venous tone is low and a person suddenly stands up, they may actually faint because of the increased pooling of blood in the lower extremities which reduces blood flow back to the heart and, thus, flow to the brain. Moreover, due to the corresponding decrease of pressure in the head due to further increases in elevation, the veins in that region may be in a partially collapsed state. Typically, the veins take on an elliptical or dumb bell shape in which flow of blood still persists but against a much

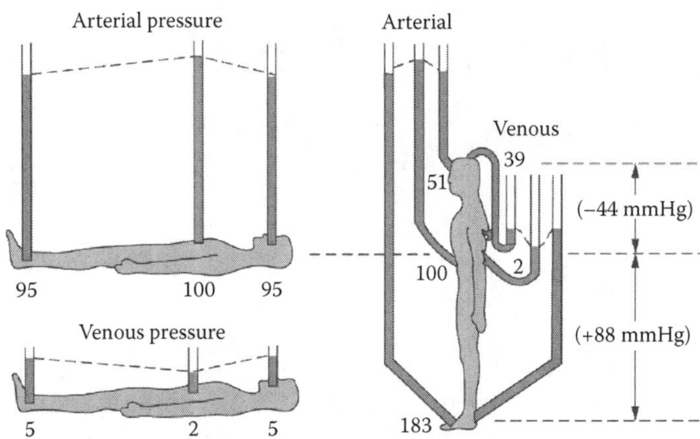

FIGURE 5.1 Hydrostatic pressure differences in the circulation. (Redrawn from Burton, A.C., *Physiology and Biophysics of the Circulation*, Year Book Medical Publishers, Chicago, IL, Copyright 1971, Elsevier.)

higher resistance. A good way to prevent this is by flexing the muscles in the leg calf so as to effectively pump the blood out of the lower veins and back to the heart. In the event of fainting, however, the resultant change in posture from standing to supine is the ideal "remedy" for the effects of *cerebral hypotension*.

5.3 APPLICATIONS OF THE BERNOULLI EQUATION

The *Bernoulli equation*, derived in Section 1.6, was based upon the assumption of steady flow along a streamline in an incompressible, inviscid fluid (Figure 1.9) and is given by the relationship

$$p+\rho\frac{V^2}{2}+\rho gz=H \tag{1.62}$$

where H is a constant and is referred to as the "total head" or total energy per unit volume of fluid.

This equation can be applied to several disease conditions in the circulatory system such as flow through constrictions and across orifices, keeping in mind the assumptions used in deriving the equation.

5.3.1 Total versus Hydrostatic Pressure Measurement

The most common method for measuring intravascular blood pressure clinically is to insert a fluid-filled catheter into a vessel then externally connecting the catheter to a pressure transducer. The pressure measured is then that sensed at the tip of the catheter and transmitted along the fluid channel to the manometer (this device is known as a "*fluid-filled catheter manometer*"). In addition to the pressure energy, however, the effect of kinetic energy on the pressure measurement must also be taken into account, as seen in Equation 1.62.

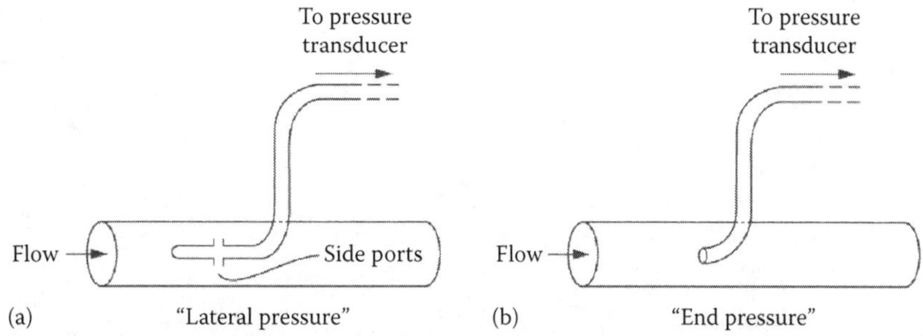

FIGURE 5.2 Schematic for the measurement of lateral and end pressure: (a) lateral opening in the catheter and (b) opening at the end of the catheter.

The hydrostatic pressure, p, would be best measured by the catheter shown in the configuration with a lateral port (Figure 5.2a). However, when the catheter opening faces the flow as shown in the configuration Figure 5.2b, the fluid that impinges against the catheter opening slows to zero velocity. When that happens, the kinetic energy in the fluid will be converted into pressure and will introduce a difference between the end pressure and the lateral pressure:

$$p_e - p_1 = p_k = \frac{\rho V^2}{2} \tag{5.1}$$

In this equation and in subsequent discussions on the application of Bernoulli equation in biological flows, V will refer to the mean velocity over the cross section of the artery/conduit. This difference can be significant, especially in segments of narrowed vessels where velocities, and thus, the kinetic energy, become considerable. Thus, for normal physiological pressure measurements, openings are located at the sides of the catheter such that lateral pressures are measured. In the case of catheter-tipped pressure transducers where a sensor is directly placed on the catheter, these pressure-sensing elements are also mounted on the side of the catheter.

5.3.2 Arterial Stenoses and Aneurysms

In patients with vascular disease, segments of an artery may become narrowed due to fatty deposits and atherosclerosis, resulting in a *stenosis*. Here, the Bernoulli equation can be applied to the flow conditions to estimate the effects of this narrowing. If, for example, a cross section of an artery is stenosed such that the diameter at that cross section is less than its normal value (Figure 5.3), then from the principle of conservation of mass

$$A_1V_1 = A_2V_2$$

where

subscript 1 denotes a cross section upstream to the stenosis
subscript 2 at the narrowest site of the stenosis

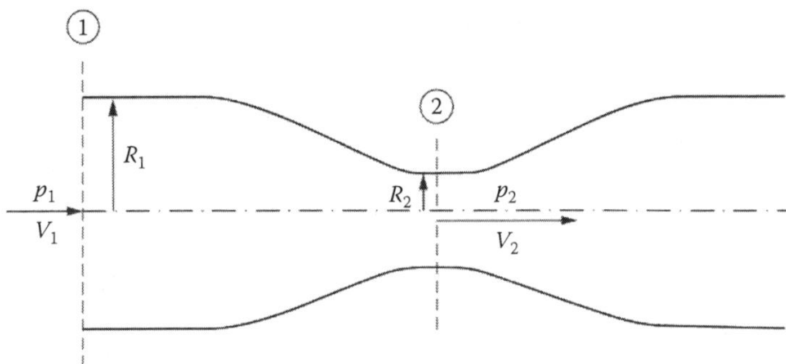

FIGURE 5.3 Application of Bernoulli equation to an arterial stenosis.

If the cross sections under consideration are relatively close to each other, we can neglect the effect of viscous dissipation and apply the Bernoulli equation. Over a short distance, the gravitational changes will also be negligible and the relationship in Equation 1.62 will reduce to

$$p_1 + \frac{\rho V_1^2}{2} = p_2 + \frac{\rho V_2^2}{2} \tag{5.2}$$

Since p_1, V_1, and V_2 are known, the pressure at the site of constriction, p_2, can be computed. To express the kinetic energy per unit volume (also in terms of mmHg), the conversion factor $1\ \text{g/cm}\cdot\text{s}^2 = 7.5 \times 10^{-4}$ mmHg can be used.

Example 5.1

Consider a case where there is a focal stenosis of a 6 mm diameter femoral artery in which its cross-sectional diameter is reduced to one-third of normal. Then, the velocity at the stenosis, V_2, will be nine times the upstream velocity, V_1. Furthermore, if the flow rate through the artery were 50 cm³/min, then the velocities, V_1 and V_2, are

$$V_1 = (50\ \text{cm}^3/\text{min})/(60 \cdot \pi(0.6\ \text{cm})^2/4) = 2.95\ \text{cm/s}$$

$$V_2 = 9 \cdot V_1 = 26.5\ \text{cm/s}$$

Therefore, if the pressure at the upstream is 100 mmHg, then the pressure at the stenosis will be reduced by

$$\rho/2\ \left[V_2^2 - V_1^2\right] = 9300\ \text{g/(cms}^2) = 0.29\ \text{mmHg}$$

One result of a lower pressure at a constriction is that under severe conditions, the vessel walls may actually cave in under sufficient external pressure, even to the point of complete occlusion. In this case, the flow velocity will slow down due to frictional resistance and the kinetic energy will be converted to pressure. Then, the pressure at the constriction will once again increase, reopening the artery. This phenomenon will repeat itself cyclically, resulting in the phenomenon of arterial flutter. This is actually the mechanism behind the *Korotkoff sounds* that are used with the traditional blood pressure measurement made with an inflated cuff around the arm and sensed by a stethoscope.

A converse condition can occur where there is a weakening of the arterial wall and a corresponding increase in the lumen cross section which causes a bulge or an *aneurysm* to occur. It is thought that an aneurysm forms due to a weakening of the vessel wall, possibly because of an excess of a degradation enzyme known as *elastase* which acts to break down *elastin*, a normal load-bearing fiber in the artery wall. It is commonly seen in the distal, or abdominal, aorta where it is referred to as an *abdominal aortic aneurysm* (AAA). Analysis performed on the energy present in the flow similar to that mentioned earlier shows that the flow velocity is reduced at the cross section of the aneurysm and that some of the kinetic energy will, thus, be converted into pressure at that site. Although the increase in pressure may not be significant in the resting state (<5 mmHg), the corresponding conversion from kinetic energy to pressure may be substantial under *exercise* conditions when aortic velocity increases several fold. The increase in pressure will lead to a corresponding increase in wall stress (see Section 2.2), which may be sufficient to cause further expansion of the aneurysm cross section. This sequence of events acts as a positive feedback loop in that further enlargement of the artery reduces velocity and, again, increases static pressure. Ultimately, this process may result in the bursting of the vessel at that site. Obviously, this is never a desirable outcome, but when it occurs in the major outlet vessel from the heart, it is particularly critical, being fatal in ~50% of cases.

5.3.3 Cardiac Valve Stenoses

Another application of the Bernoulli equation is in the analysis of natural and prosthetic heart valves. In traditional engineering applications, this analysis is based on flow through an orifice as used for flow meters placed in internal flows. An example of this is flow through a nozzle as shown schematically in Figure 5.4. As the fluid passes through the sharp edges of the nozzle, flow separation causes a recirculation region immediately downstream of the nozzle. The fluid in the core region continues to accelerate to form a contracted cross section (denoted by 2 in the figure) referred

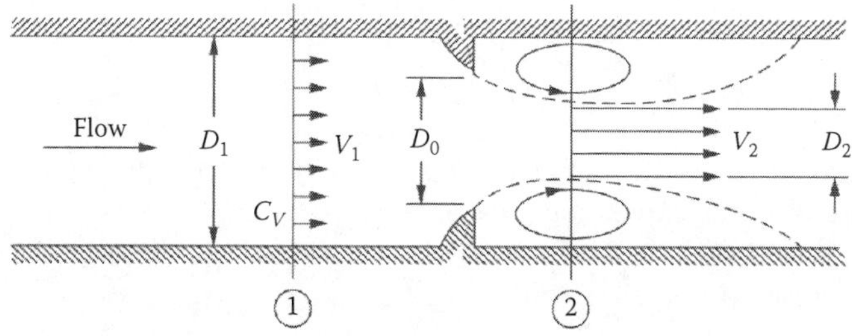

FIGURE 5.4 Schematic of the flow through a nozzle.

to as the *vena contracta*. At this cross section, the streamlines are parallel to the axis of the tube and the pressure over the cross section is uniform.

Keeping in mind the assumptions used in deriving the Bernoulli equation and also neglecting the effect of gravity, the Bernoulli equation can be written as

$$p_1 - p_2 = \frac{\rho}{2}\left(V_2^2 - V_1^2\right) = \frac{\rho V_2^2}{2}\left(1 - \frac{V_1^2}{V_2^2}\right)$$

Also, from the continuity equation, we have

$$\left(\frac{V_1}{V_2}\right)^2 = \left(\frac{A_2}{A_1}\right)^2$$

Substituting this relation, we get

$$p_1 - p_2 = \frac{\rho V_2^2}{2}\left[1 - \left(\frac{A_2}{A_1}\right)^2\right]$$

Solving the previous equation, we can express the ideal velocity, V_{2ideal}, as

$$V_{2ideal} = \sqrt{\frac{2(p_1 - p_2)}{\rho\left[1 - (A_2/A_1)^2\right]}}$$

The velocity computed using the previous expression is "ideal" because we used the Bernoulli equation and, thus, have neglected the effect of fluid viscosity. As can be observed from Figure 5.4, the area at position 2 where the streamlines are essentially parallel to the axis is smaller than that at the throat of the orifice. The area A_2 can be related to the throat area A_0 by introducing a *contraction coefficient*, C_c, such that

$$C_c = \frac{A_2}{A_0}$$

Then the expression for V_{2ideal} becomes

$$V_{2ideal} = \sqrt{\frac{2(p_1 - p_2)}{\rho\left[1 - C_c^2(A_0/A_1)^2\right]}}$$

Due to frictional losses, the velocity at position 2 will be less than the ideal value given by the previous expression. Hence, a *velocity coefficient*, C_V, is introduced such that

$$C_V = \frac{V_{2actual}}{V_{2ideal}}$$

Then, the actual volume flow rate can be computed as

$$Q = A_2 V_{2actual} = C_c A_0 C_V V_{2ideal}$$

or

$$Q = A_0 C_c C_V \sqrt{\frac{2(p_1 - p_2)}{\rho\left[1 - C_c^2 (A_0/A_1)^2\right]}}$$

Squaring the expression and rewriting, we obtain

$$p_1 - p_2 = \frac{\rho Q^2}{2}\left[\frac{1 - C_c^2 (A_0/A_1)^2}{A_0^2 C_c^2 C_V^2}\right]$$

or

$$p_1 - p_2 = \frac{\rho Q^2}{2}\frac{1}{A_0^2 C_d^2}$$

where $C_d = C_c C_V \Big/ \sqrt{1 - C_V^2 (A_0/A_1)^2}$ is defined as the *discharge coefficient.*

The discharge coefficient C_d depends upon the geometry of the nozzle as well as the dimensions of the tube and the throat of the nozzle. In flow meter applications, the discharge coefficient is determined experimentally. In clinical practice, this expression is applied to determine the *effective orifice area* (EOA) of heart valves in the fully open position. In terms of the area at the throat, we get

$$\text{EOA} = A_0 = \frac{Q_m}{C_d}\sqrt{\frac{\rho}{2\Delta p}} \tag{5.3}$$

where

Q_m is the mean flow rate

$\Delta p = p_1 - p_2$

In the case of the EOA for aortic valves, Q_m is replaced by the mean systolic flow (MSF) rate (as opposed to the cardiac output). Equation 5.3 was employed in the 1950s to estimate the orifice area of human heart valves and is commonly referred to as the *Gorlin equation* in the clinical literature. For the *aortic valve*, the Gorlin equation is given by

$$AVA = \frac{MSF}{44.5\sqrt{\Delta p_m}} \tag{5.4}$$

where

AVA is the aortic valve area

Δp_m is the mean pressure drop across the valve

The constant 44.5 (cm/s)/(mmHg)$^{1/2}$) takes into account the conversion of units between the MSF (mL/s) and the mean systolic pressure drop (mmHg) and it also includes an assumed discharge coefficient to compute the orifice area in cm^2. The corresponding Gorlin equation for the *mitral valve* is given by

$$MVA = \frac{MDF}{31.0\sqrt{\Delta p_m}} \tag{5.5}$$

where the mean diastolic flow (MDA) rate (mL/s) and the mean diastolic pressure gradient (mmHg) are used.

Measurements of the flow rate and the pressure drop across the valves can be used to predict the effective valve orifice areas of the natural valves suspected of being stenotic. Such information is useful for cardiac surgeons in deciding when to replace diseased valves. For normal aortic and mitral valves, a discharge coefficient close to unity is assumed. In the case of natural heart valves with centralized flow and no obstructions, the analogy with the flow through a nozzle may be reasonable. This formula is also extensively used to predict the effective valve orifice area of prosthetic valves. However, due to obstruction of the leaflets, especially with mechanical valves, the discharge coefficient can be expected to be significantly different from that of natural valves. The common practice is to perform *in vitro* experiments in which the actual EOA can be measured and to determine the discharge coefficient for each type of prosthetic valve.

The expression for the EOA derived earlier is based on steady flow across a nozzle and is thus applied assuming constant systolic flow conditions. In reality, however, even during this period when the valve is fully open, the blood flow goes through acceleration and deceleration phases so that the flow is time dependent. Therefore, a more rigorous analysis should include the acceleration of the fluid as well as viscous dissipation. In one-dimensional analysis, the pressure drop across an orifice can be written as (Young, 1979)

$$\Delta p = A\frac{dQ}{dt} + BQ^2 + CQ \tag{5.6}$$

where

Q is the flow rate
dQ/dt represents the temporal acceleration
BQ^2 represents the convective acceleration
CQ represents the viscous dissipation

The inertial term (time dependence) can be eliminated by averaging Equation 5.6 over the forward flow interval (time during which the valve is open), resulting in

$$\Delta p_m = BQ_m^2 + CQ_m \tag{5.7}$$

or by taking the measurements at the time of peak flow when dQ/dt will be identically equal to zero, which results in

$$\Delta p_p = BQ_p^2 + CQ_p \tag{5.8}$$

In this relationship, the subscript "p" denotes that the values are measured at the instant of peak flow through the orifice. Performing a dimensional analysis on the important parameters for flow through an orifice—pressure p, flow rate Q, orifice area A, density ρ, and viscosity μ—shows that the constants B and C can be related to

$$B = \frac{\rho}{A^2}$$

and

$$C = \frac{\mu}{A^{3/2}}$$

respectively. Hence, the relationships for the peak and mean pressure drops can be rewritten as

$$\Delta p_m = k_1 \frac{\rho}{A^2} Q_m^2 + k_2 \frac{\mu}{A^{3/2}} Q_m \tag{5.9}$$

and

$$\Delta p_p = k_1 \frac{\rho}{A^2} Q_p^2 + k_2 \frac{\mu}{A^{3/2}} Q_p \tag{5.10}$$

Substituting typical physiological values for ρ, μ, A, and Q into the previous equations and performing an order of magnitude study, it can be observed that the inertial term in both the equations (first term on the RHS) is three orders of magnitude larger than the viscous effect (second term on the RHS). Thus, the viscous effects can indeed be neglected in flow through the valves. By computing the mean values during the forward flow duration, the EOA relationship (Equation 5.3) will reduce to the form

$$EOA = KQ_{rms}\sqrt{\frac{\rho}{\Delta p_m}} \tag{5.11}$$

The difference between the previous relationship and the Gorlin equation derived earlier is the root mean square flow rate used here instead of the mean flow rate used in the Gorlin equation. The relationship using the peak flow will be given by

$$EOA = KQ_p\sqrt{\frac{\rho}{\Delta p_p}} \tag{5.12}$$

where
Q_p is the peak flow rate
Δp_p is the pressure drop across the valve at the *instant of peak flow rate*

The use of the previous two relationships rather than the Gorlin equation provides more accurate values for the valve orifice area from the rigorous fluid mechanical analysis discussed earlier.

A dimensional analysis of steady flow through an orifice has shown that

$$C_d = f\left(\frac{d}{D}, Re\right)$$

where
d is the orifice diameter
D is the diameter of the pipe
Re is the Reynolds number ($=\rho VD/\mu$)

For a given valve geometry, the only variable in the aforementioned relationship is the flow rate and, hence, it has been proposed that

$$EOA = \frac{kQ}{C_d(Q)\sqrt{\Delta p}} \tag{5.13}$$

where $C_d(Q)$ is the discharge coefficient as a function of flow rate Q. Using an *in vitro* experimental setup in which the orifice areas of prosthetic valves of various geometries were measured using planimetry over a range of flow rates, studies have demonstrated that when the discharge coefficient was expressed as a linear function of flow rate such as

$$C_d(Q) = C_1Q + C_2 \tag{5.14}$$

the prediction capability of the effective valve orifice areas was significantly improved.

5.4 RIGID TUBE FLOW MODELS

The simplest model for blood flow through a vessel would be steady, fully developed flow of a Newtonian fluid through a straight cylindrical tube of constant circular cross section. Such flows are characterized as *Poiseuille* flow in the honor of J.L.M. Poiseuille (1799–1869) who performed experiments relating pressure gradient, flow, and tube geometry in such a model. From his experiments, he empirically derived the relationship given as follows:

$$Q = \frac{K \Delta p D^4}{L} \tag{5.15}$$

where
- Q is the flow rate
- Δp is the drop in pressure in a tube of length L and diameter D

K denotes a constant that was found to be independent of the other variables. Hagenbach, working independently, arrived at the theoretical solution for the aforementioned problem that introduced fluid viscosity as follows

$$Q = \frac{\pi R^4 (p_1 - p_2)}{8 \mu L} \tag{5.16}$$

where
- μ is the coefficient of viscosity
- R is the tube radius

From Equations 5.15 and 5.16, it can be observed that $K = \pi/128\mu$. Thus, the relationship in Equation 5.2 is also referred to as the *Hagen–Poiseuille* law. We have already derived the aforementioned relationship in Chapter 1 from the *Navier–Stokes* equation (Equation 1.53). We also utilized this relationship considering the forces acting on a volume element of the fluid in Chapter 4 in our discussions on the principles of the capillary viscometer. Several assumptions were made in deriving the relationship for the flow rate given in Equation 5.16 and we should critically examine the validity of these assumptions in models describing blood flow in arteries. The assumptions are as follows:

1. *Newtonian fluid*: The governing equations used in deriving the expression for the velocity profile assumed that the fluid is Newtonian with a constant viscosity coefficient. When we discussed the viscous behavior of blood in Section 4.1.3, we concluded that the rheology of blood can best be described by *Casson relationship* and that blood exhibits nonlinear shear stress versus rate of shear characteristics, especially at low rates of shear. However, it was also determined that at relatively high rates of shear, the viscosity coefficient asymptotically approaches a constant value. Thus, for flow in

large blood vessels, where relatively large shear rates can be expected during systole, a Newtonian description appears to be reasonable.

2. *Laminar flow*: The governing equations also assume that the flow regime is laminar. For steady flow in cylindrical pipes, we can define a critical Reynolds number, Re_c, beyond which the flow can be considered to be turbulent. In a typical human aorta, one can estimate the Reynolds number assuming a diameter at the root of the aorta of 2.5 cm and a mean time–averaged flow velocity of 20 mL/s (based on a cardiac output of 6 Lpm) and compute a magnitude of about 1500. Whole blood density of 1.056 g/cc and a viscosity coefficient of 0.035 P were used in this computation. Thus, the time-averaged Reynolds number is observed to be well below the critical value of about 2100. If a peak flow rate of 20 L/m is assumed during systole, then the Reynolds number during that part of the cardiac cycle is about 5100. However, the human aorta is a distensible vessel with a complex geometry so the critical Reynolds number determined from experiments in rigid straight cylindrical pipes is not applicable in this situation. *In vivo* velocity measurements using hot film anemometry have indicated disturbed flow during the deceleration phase of the cardiac cycle although there is no experimental evidence of *sustained turbulence* in the human circulation (in the absence of any diseased states such as valvular or arterial stenoses). Thus, the assumption of laminar flow in the model also appears to be reasonable.
3. *No slip at the vascular wall*: The innermost lining of the arterial wall in contact with the blood is a layer of firmly attached endothelial cells and it appears to be reasonable to assume no slip at the interface.
4. *Steady flow*: As pointed out earlier, the steady flow model is the simplest to deal with mathematically and, therefore, was used in deriving the aforementioned relationship. Based on this assumption, we neglected the inertial forces in the simplifications of the governing equations. However, as discussed in the review of cardiovascular physiology (Chapter 3), flow through human arteries is clearly pulsatile, consisting of systolic and diastolic phases; therefore, the assumption of steady flow is *not* valid in the major part of the circulatory system.
5. *Cylindrical shape*: The tube model discussed earlier assumed a circular cross section and axisymmetry. Even though this geometry may be a good approximation for most of the arteries in the systemic circulation, the veins and the pulmonary arteries are more elliptical in shape. The arteries also have a taper with their cross sections narrowing with distance downstream. Thus, the general assumption of a circular cross section without taper is a deviation from reality.
6. *Rigid wall*: As was discussed in Section 3.4, the arterial walls are viscoelastic and distend with the pulse pressure. The interaction between the flowing blood and the distensible arterial wall is an important factor in the description of the flow dynamics. Thus, the assumption of rigid walls in the model is also *not* valid. However, for the special case of steady flow models in the circulatory system, distensibility of the vessels will not affect the solution.

7. *Fully developed flow*: The model described earlier also assumes that the flow is fully developed, which implies that the velocity profile remains the same at any cross section with distance downstream. However, as the blood leaves the ventricle through the aortic valve, the velocity profile in the aorta is relatively flat and a finite length is needed before the flow may become fully developed (as described in the next section). Similarly, even in the distal arteries, flow passes through several branching points and curved arterial sections. At each location where the cross-sectional geometry deviates from a straight arterial segment, the flow will also be appropriately altered. Thus, the assumption of fully developed flow is also *not* valid.

It can be observed that in applying the steady flow models to describe blood flow in the circulation, the assumptions of steady flow, wall rigidity, cylindrically shaped lumens, and fully developed flow are all clearly *violated*. We will discuss unsteady flow models in distensible vessels in the next chapter. In order to analyze the effect of complex noncylindrical geometry as well as the developing nature of flow, experimental measurements or use of computational fluid dynamic (CFD) simulations are necessary (see Chapter 11). At this point, however, we will use the basic relationship obtained with this simplified steady flow model in order to introduce some applications in the flow through the arterial system.

5.4.1 Vascular Resistance

We introduced the concept of resistance to flow in the chapter on cardiovascular physiology (Chapter 3). The vascular resistance is given by the relationship

$$R_s = \frac{\Delta p}{Q} \tag{3.3}$$

This expression is analogous to the electrical resistance given by

$$R_s = \frac{E}{I} \tag{5.17}$$

where

I is the current

E is the voltage across a segment of a circuit

If the pressure drop is measured in terms of mmHg and the flow rate in terms of mL/s, then the resistance is expressed as mmHg · s/cm^3 or a peripheral resistance unit (PRU) and it is used in physiological literature. From the Poiseuille expression for flow rate through a tube (Equation 1.53), we obtained the relationship

$$R_s = \frac{8\mu L}{\pi R^4} \tag{3.4}$$

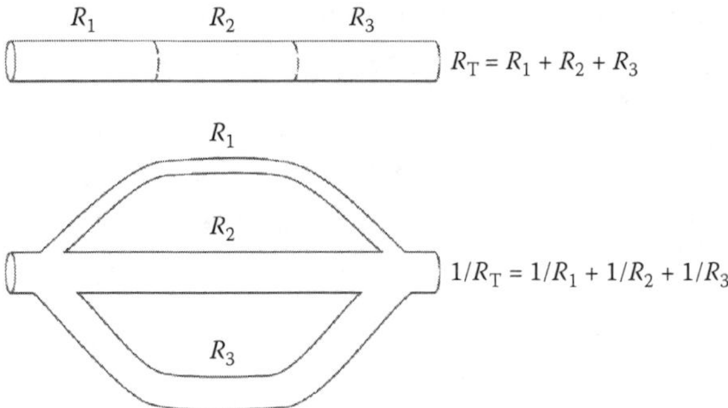

FIGURE 5.5 Total resistance with tubes in series or parallel configuration.

When the vessels are in series, the total resistance will be the sum of the individual resistances. When the vessels are in parallel, the total resistance across the vessels can be computed using the relationship shown in Figure 5.5.

This formula for the vascular resistance, derived from the steady, fully developed flow relationship can be used to estimate the resistance in segments of the vascular system. For example, the mean pressures at the aortic root and at the terminal end of the vena cava can be measured along with the time-averaged flow rate through the systemic circulation. These data can be used to compute the resistance in the systemic circulation as a measure of the functioning of the circulatory system. Similarly, the pulmonary vascular resistance can also be determined by measurement of the corresponding pressures. The expression for the resistance (Equation 3.4) shows that it is inversely proportional to the fourth power of the radius, and thus, a small change in the radius of the vessel will considerably affect the resistance to flow. The implication of this is that the autonomic nervous system in the body controls the tension of the smooth muscles in the vessel wall in the arterioles. Thus, with the alteration of the muscle tension, the arterioles can be distended or contracted selectively to control the amount of blood flow into the various segments of the body.

Even though the measurement of vascular resistance yields information about the state of the circulatory system and, hence, can be used as a diagnostic parameter, several limitations must be kept in mind on the information provided: (1) It does *not* indicate which pathway between the two points of measurement is constricted or dilated; (2) it does *not* indicate the cause for the change (due to nervous stimulation, increased transmural pressure, or other causes); (3) it yields information *only* on net changes and does *not* indicate local changes; and (4) it does *not* provide information to distinguish between dilation of the vessels or the opening of new vessels (*angiogenesis*).

5.4.2 Regional Alterations in Vascular Resistance

Due to the powerful effect of vessel radius upon flow ($Q \propto R^4$ under constant pressure drop), the body has the capability of widely altering the blood flow to various regions in the circulatory system by appropriate increases or decreases in the diameter of the arterioles supplying those regions. A typical example of such selective regional alterations is that of heavy exercise when blood flow to the skeletal muscles can increase by as much as 20 times the baseline blood flow (see Problem 5.9). The effects of exercise on the circulatory system are (1) increase in mean arterial pressure and (2) increase in the cardiac output. These occur because the sympathetic nervous system stimulates the heart to increase the heart rate and the cardiac contraction forces in order to increase the cardiac output to several times the normal level. The muscles in the systemic veins are also contracted in order to increase the mean systemic filling pressure. Simultaneously, the arterioles of most of the peripheral circulation are contracted, thereby increasing the resistance to flow in those regions of the circulatory system, while the arterioles supplying the active muscles are dilated in order to decrease their resistance to blood flow, thereby providing increased perfusion to those muscles. In general, blood flow through the coronary arteries and the cerebral circulation are maintained at adequate rates since the arterioles in these regions are not subjected to vasoconstriction (Guyton and Hall, 2000).

Another example of regional alterations in blood flow is the decrease of flow experienced in vessels close to the skin surface on a cold day. This happens in order to reduce body heat loss and to sustain perfusion to the visceral organs such as the heart, liver, kidney, lungs, and the brain at a constant body temperature. Constriction of the arterioles near the skin increases the resistance to flow at the body surface and also causes blood flow to be diverted to the core region of the body.

5.5 ESTIMATION OF ENTRANCE LENGTH AND ITS EFFECT ON FLOW DEVELOPMENT IN ARTERIES

As pointed out in Section 1.8.1.3, as fluid enters a pipe from a reservoir, the velocity profile will be relatively flat and the fluid must pass through a finite length of the tube before the velocity profile attains a final shape. This observation is represented in Figure 5.6.

At the tube entrance, the fluid coming in contact with the tube wall will be forced to have zero velocity—that is, the "no slip" condition, due to frictional forces and a gradient in velocity is established in the radial direction. Further downstream, more and more fluid is retarded due to the radial penetration of shearing effects of fluid adjacent to the wall. At the same time, the fluid in the core region is actually accelerated by the unbalanced pressure and viscous forces which then maintains a constant flow rate at all cross sections in the tube (i.e., satisfies the continuity requirement). Consequently, the initially blunt profile is progressively modified and, ultimately, a parabolic velocity profile is established further downstream. Thus, very near the

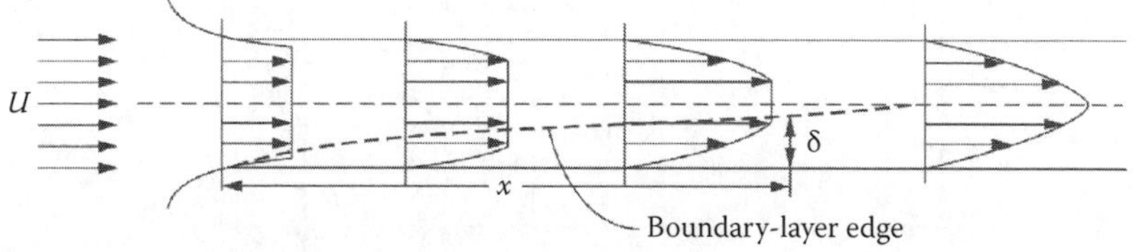

FIGURE 5.6 Concept of entry length before the flow becomes fully developed.

entrance, the radial distance in the fluid over which the viscous effects are present is very small. However, as we proceed downstream, the viscous effects have diffused further in the radial direction. The "thickness" within which this diffusion has occurred is referred to as the *boundary layer.* At some location downstream, the boundary layer grows to the point where it reaches the centerline of the tube and, at this point, the flow is said to become *fully developed.* In Chapter 1, we presented a relationship for the entrance length (Equation 1.78) in terms of tube diameter and the Reynolds number for laminar flow. We will now show the basis for such a relationship based on the effect of inertial and viscous drag forces within the boundary layer.

A small fluid element within the boundary layer is considered in Figure 5.7. Let the area A_1 and A_2 be equal to A. The tangential shear stresses in those areas are $\mu(du/dy)|_1$ and $\mu(du/dy)|_2$, respectively. The net viscous force on the element will be the area times the change in stress with the distance y from the wall and will be given by

$$\mu\frac{d}{dy}\left(\frac{du}{dy}\right)A(y_2-y_1)$$

In the absence of flow acceleration, the viscous forces must be balanced by the inertial forces acting on the element. However, a solution of the governing equations in the boundary layer is too complicated to be solved analytically. By assigning suitable scales to the variables representing the two forces, an estimate of the entrance length can be obtained. To estimate the viscous forces, we use the boundary layer thickness δ at a distance X from the entrance and the free stream velocity U in the previous equation. Then the viscous force is proportional to

$$\frac{\mu U}{\delta^2}A(y_2-y_1)$$

The inertial force acting on the element is given by

$$\rho(\text{Convective acceleration})(\text{Volume of the element})$$

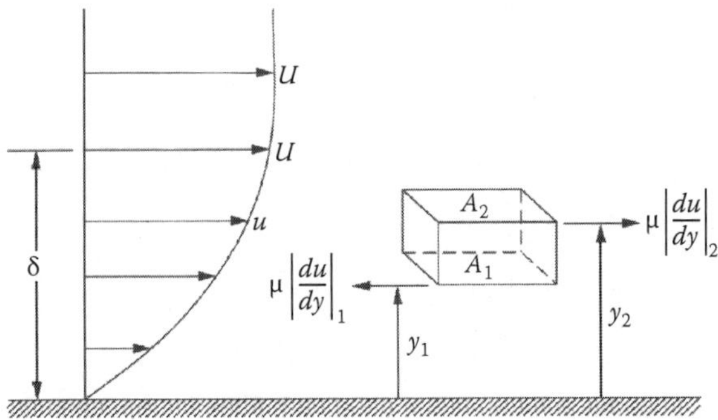

FIGURE 5.7 A force balance on a fluid element in the boundary layer.

If the boundary layer thickness is considered at a distance X from the entrance of the tube, then the time scale for the fluid to reach that distance (the convection time) is X/U. The convective acceleration at this location is then proportional to $U/(X/U)$, or, U^2/X. Thus, the inertial force on the element will be given by

$$\rho \frac{U^2}{X} A(y_2 - y_1)$$

Equating these two forces, we obtain

$$\rho \frac{U^2}{X} = k\mu \frac{U}{\delta^2}$$

where k is the proportionality constant that can be determined from experiments. Thus, the boundary layer thickness at any axial location can be written as

$$\delta \propto \sqrt{\frac{\mu X}{\rho U}}$$

From the previous relationship, we can see that the boundary layer grows in proportion to the square root of the distance. Also, the boundary layer thickness decreases at any given location as the flow rate through the tube increases, producing a corresponding increase in the free stream velocity. The boundary layer will fill the tube and the flow will become fully developed (i.e., with no further convective acceleration in the fluid) when the boundary layer thickness equals the radius, or $\delta = D/2$, where D is the diameter of the tube. Then, the entrance length will be given by

$$X_e = kD^2 \frac{U}{\nu}$$

or

$$X_e = kD\left(\frac{UD}{\nu}\right) \tag{5.18}$$

where the terms in the parenthesis represent the Reynolds number. In this relationship, $\nu = \mu/\rho$ is referred to as the kinematic viscosity. Equation 5.18 can be used to predict the entrance length for steady laminar flow through a straight pipe of circular cross section. The magnitude for the constant k has been experimentally determined to be ~0.06. Thus, if an artery were assumed to be a straight cylindrical tube with steady and laminar flow, we would be able to estimate the distance at which the flow would become fully developed using the expression given in Equation 5.18. Note that this relationship is valid only for flows with Reynolds numbers greater than 50.

In cases where the Reynolds number is close to zero (e.g., in capillaries where the Reynolds number is ≤0.01), the entrance length becomes a constant of 0.65 D.

In arterial flow, flow development is affected by a number of factors. First, in large arteries, for example, the entrance length is relatively long since it depends not only on vessel diameter but also on the Reynolds number (Equation 5.18), both of which are large. This produces a situation in which a large portion of most major arteries is exposed to developing flow with higher velocity gradients near the wall. Second, the axial velocity profile becomes skewed at sites of curvature and bifurcation of the arteries (see Section 6.6) with higher velocity (and, thus, a higher velocity gradient) toward one wall and a lower velocity toward the opposite wall. One of the implications of this is that the intimal lining of arteries is exposed to higher shear forces proximally, and lower shear forces distally. Also, there is a general tendency for higher shear forces on the outer wall of curvatures and branch inlets and on the flow divider of bifurcations. In terms of the boundary layer, it will be thinner in regions of high velocity compared with regions with a low velocity. The size of the boundary layer is also important in terms of mass transport of molecules (i.e., gas and nutrient) between the blood and artery wall since diffusive effects are more important than convective effects in large boundary layer regions. This is the basis for one theory of atherosclerosis (see Section 6.4) in that certain molecules, such as LDL, may accumulate within regions of thicker boundary layers and tend to stay in that region for longer time, enhancing their diffusive transport to the subendothelial region and initiating atherosclerotic lesions.

5.6 FLOW IN COLLAPSIBLE VESSELS

In the relationship derived for flow through conduits (Section 1.5.3.2), we observed that the flow through an individual conduit is proportional to the pressure drop across the system when the flow is laminar. Even when the flow is turbulent, the flow rate will monotonically increase with an increase in pressure drop but not in a linear fashion. In the circulatory system, however, the conduits are flexible and, in some instances, the transmural (i.e., across the vessel wall) pressure can cause significant collapse of the conduit. This is especially true downstream of a stenosis where the pressure in the conduit can drop below that of the extramural (i.e., outside the vessel wall) pressure. In such cases, the flow through the conduit is no longer dependent upon the upstream, p_1, and downstream, p_2, pressure difference, but rather on the difference between the upstream pressure and the pressure surrounding the conduit, p_e. When that happens, flow through the conduit can remain relatively constant even though the downstream pressure, p_2, varies widely. This phenomena is variously described as *flow limitation*, *Starling resistor phenomenon*, *sluice effect*, and *waterfall effect*. It has been observed in blood flow situations such as from extrathoracic to intrathoracic veins, diseased coronary arteries, pulmonary blood flow, and flow through cerebral vessels and in urine flow.

Let us consider a system of blood vessels as shown in Figure 5.8 where all the vessels are assumed to be rigid. Pressure at the inlet of the channel is assumed to be 12 mmHg and the pressure drop across the arteries, capillaries, and veins is assumed to be 3, 6, and 3 mmHg, respectively. These pressure drops are due to viscous

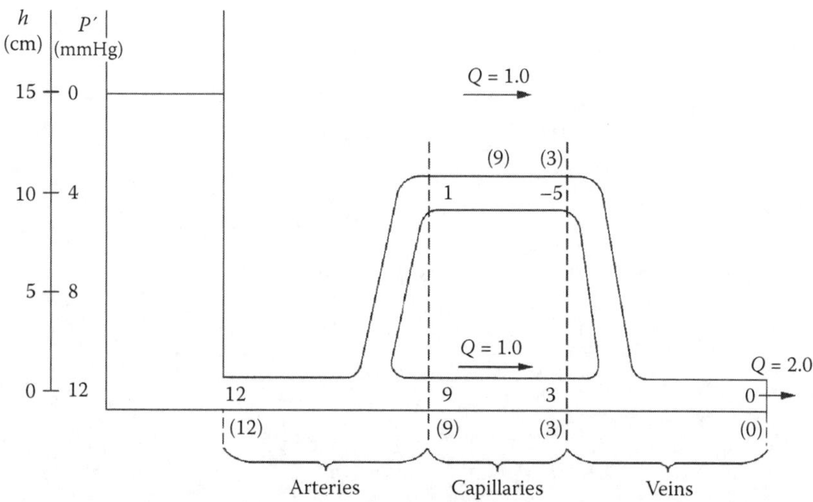

FIGURE 5.8 Pressure and flow through rigid pipe segments. (Redrawn from Milnor, W.R., *Hemodynamics*, Williams & Wilkins, Baltimore, MD, 1989.)

dissipation as the fluid flows across the vessel. A total flow rate of 2 mL/s is assumed to be evenly divided between the two segments. The vertical distance between the vessels and the corresponding hydrostatic pressure difference are also shown on the scale on the left of the figure. The resulting pressures that include the hydrostatic effect are given inside the vessels and the pressures due to the effects of viscous losses alone are given at the outside. If the vessel in the upper segment is not rigid but is made of a thin elastic material, it will collapse due to the low transmural pressure and, thus, the flow would cease in the upper segment. However, as soon as the flow ceases, the pressure would rise to 4 mmHg due to the static conditions and the vessel would once again open. Thus, this sequence of events will be repeated continuously and has been demonstrated in *in vitro* experiments. However, *in vivo*, thin-walled vessels will tend to attain an equilibrium state as shown in Figure 5.9 (Milnor, 1989). Assume here that the capillary segments collapse to a narrow lumen at a transmural pressure of 0.2 mmHg and completely collapse at 0 mmHg. Pressure and flow through the upper channel will reach a state of equilibrium at about 0.1 mmHg transmural pressure with a lower flow through the upper segment as shown in Figure 5.9.

The phenomenon described earlier can be used to explain flow through the lung capillaries. When a person is standing, little flow occurs through the capillaries in the apices of the lung due to the collapse of the blood vessels. As discussed earlier, the flow rate through a rigid tube is dependent on the distal pressure which is not necessarily true in a collapsed vessel as discussed in the following. Figure 5.10 shows two rigid vessels connected by a collapsible vessel. The collapsible vessel is enclosed in a box so that the pressure outside the vessel can be independently set. This arrangement is also referred to as *Starling's resistor*. The collapsible segment is assumed to be fully open at a transmural pressure of 0.2 mmHg and to be completely closed at 0 mmHg. The pressures at various points in the system (in mmHg) are included in the figure. The flow through the vessel will reach equilibrium when

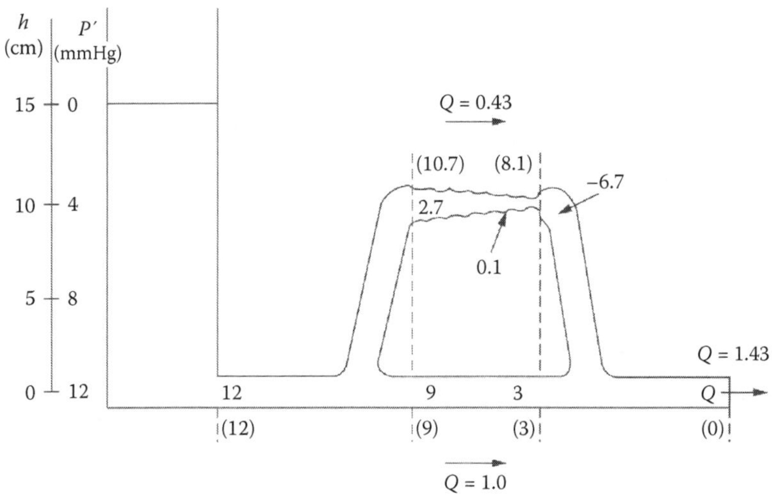

FIGURE 5.9 Effect of vessel collapsibility on the pressure and flow. (Redrawn from Milnor, W.R., *Hemodynamics*, Williams & Wilkins, Baltimore, MD, 1989.)

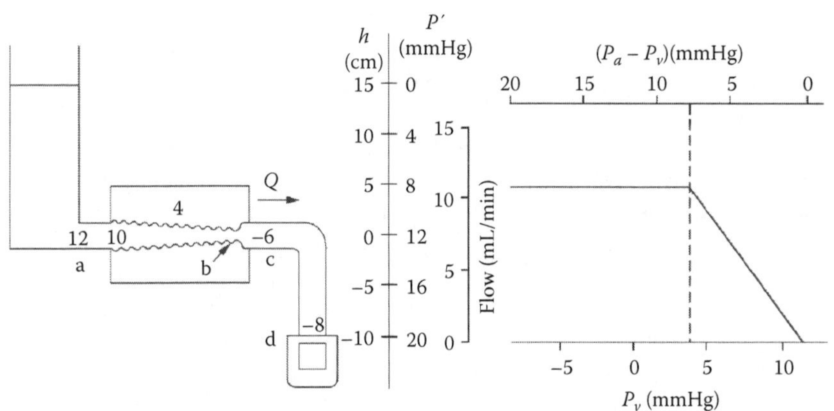

FIGURE 5.10 Pressure and flow through a collapsible tube. (Redrawn from Milnor, W.R., *Hemodynamics*, Williams & Wilkins, Baltimore, MD, 1989.)

the pressure inside the vessel is 4.1 mmHg representing a transmural pressure of 0.1 mmHg. Changing the distal pressure at point "c" by raising or lowering the outflow beaker will not alter the flow through the vessel provided it is not raised above 4.2 mmHg. However, changing the pressure within the box will affect the flow. The interaction between the variables is represented in the curve shown on at the right half part of the figure.

When the outlet pressure P_v is equal to the inlet pressure P_a, there is no flow through the vessel. Gradually decreasing the outlet pressure results in a linear increase in the flow through the vessel until the outlet pressure equals the pressure in the box surrounding the vessel. Further decrease in the outlet pressure does not increase the flow through the vessel even though the gradient $P_a - P_v$ continues to increase.

The model described earlier is similar to that occurring in the lungs. Here, the pressure in the box would depict the alveolar pressure and, due to the low pressure in the vessels in the lung circulation combined with the hydrostatic effects, the capillary acts like a sluice gate controlled by the arterial pressure and the alveolar pressure. Such a phenomenon where the flow is independent of the downstream pressure is also described as the "vascular waterfall." The physics of this phenomenon, in which the mechanism by which the flow becomes independent of the variation in the downstream pressure, is explained by the "inertial" and "frictional" mode of flow limitation. In the "inertial" mode explanation, the upstream and downstream pressure is assumed to be decoupled at a point in the converging (collapsed) conduit at which the flow has accelerated to a velocity that exceeds the pressure wave propagation velocity of the system at that point. Pressure disturbances distal to the "choke point" cannot be propagated upstream since the medium is moving in the opposite direction with a velocity greater than the pressure wave propagation velocity. In the mechanism due to the "frictional" mode of flow limitation, it is suggested that changes in the upstream pressure alter the pressure distribution in the adjacent segment of the conduit to cause a compensatory change in the flow resistance in a direction to maintain a constant flow through the conduit.

5.7 SUMMARY

In this chapter, we used simple steady flow models to derive some relationships between the flow and pressure in the circulatory system and discussed some clinical applications based on the simplified models. We will now consider the effect of unsteady flow and the distensibility of the blood vessels as we proceed on to more realistic models to describe blood flow dynamics in the arterial system.

PROBLEMS

5.1 For a typical human, the diameter at the root of the aorta is 2.5 cm, the time-averaged flow rate (cardiac output [CO]) is 5.5 Lpm and the peak flow rate during systole is 20 Lpm.

a. Calculate the Reynolds number based on the time-averaged flow rate as well as the peak flow rate assuming a Poiseuille flow relationship.
b. Compute the corresponding wall shear stress in the aorta.
c. Assuming time-averaged flow rates of 0.6 L/min in the carotid artery (diameter ≈ 0.8 cm) and a flow rate of 0.3 L/min for a femoral artery (diameter ≈ 0.5 cm), calculate the Reynolds number and wall shear rate in these vessels also.
d. Do you think that the flow in the aorta becomes turbulent based on the calculated Reynolds numbers?

5.2 Assume that the blood is flowing through an aorta of 1.0 cm in diameter at an average velocity of 50 cm/s. Let the mean pressure in the aorta be 100 mmHg. If the blood were to enter a region of stenosis where the diameter of the aorta is only 0.5 cm, what would be the approximate pressure at the site of narrowing? (Assume blood density to be 1.056 g/cm^3: 1 g/cm $\cdot$ s^2 = 7.5 × 10^{-4} mmHg.)

5.3 Reconsider the aforementioned problem where the blood enters an aneurysm region with a diameter of 3.0 cm.

a. Determine the pressure in the aneurysm.

b. If for conditions of vigorous exercise, the velocity of blood upstream of the aneurysm were four times the normal value (200 cm/s), what pressure would develop at the aneurysm? (Assume blood density to be 1.056 g/cm^3: 1 g/cm $\cdot$ s^2 = 7.5×10^{-4} mmHg.)

c. If the wall thickness of the aneurysm is 0.15 cm and the effective Young's modulus is 10^8 dyn/cm^2, what would be the increase in aortic diameter under the exercise condition?

d. Review the assumptions that you made in this analysis and discuss their effect on the solution.

5.4 Estimate the pressure difference between the inlet and outlet of a capillary that would be needed if blood is flowing through the capillary with a velocity of 0.2 cm/s. Assume that (1) the capillary diameter is 8 μm, (2) the capillary length is 200 μm, and (3) the apparent viscosity of blood is 2.5 cP. The friction factor for laminar flow in tubes can be expressed as $f = 16/Re$, where Re is the Reynolds number and $f = R\Delta p/\rho V^2 L$.

5.5 A patient with a stenosed aortic valve has a pressure drop of 30 mmHg at a CO of 4.5 L/min and a HR of 72 bpm. Using the Gorlin equation, determine the effective valve orifice area. What percentage is this of a normal valve orifice area with a diameter of 1.5 cm?

5.6 At resting conditions, a person has an average aortic pressure of 100 mmHg and a CO of 5 L/min. Upon exercise, these values rise to 120 mmHg and 7.5 L/min, respectively.

a. What is the total peripheral resistance (TPR) in each case (in PRUs)?

b. Assuming that the outflow vessel is effectively a long, straight tube under steady flow conditions, what increase in average vessel radius would occur?

5.7 Assume that blood entering the aorta from the left ventricle has a steady state mean velocity of 30 cm/s. If the diameter of the aorta at the entry is 1.2 cm, estimate the distance in the aorta that the blood has to travel before the flow becomes fully developed. What are the assumptions made in the formula used in computing this entry length which is not realistic in the human circulation?

5.8 Consider a simple network of blood vessels shown in the figure. Segments 1 has a diameter of 1 cm whereas segments 2, 3, and 4 have a diameter of 0.25 cm. All the segments have a length of 10 cm. (a) If the total pressure drop Δp between the inlet and outlet is 100 mmHg, compute the blood flow rates in each segment assuming representative values for whole blood viscosity and density and (b) if the diameter of the segment 2 is reduced to 0.22 cm, compute the new flow rates through each of the segments.

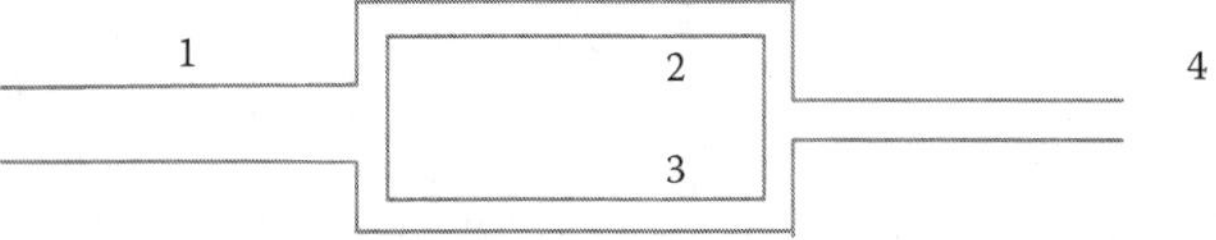

5.9 The figure illustrates the flow of blood through various segments in the systemic circulation as well as to the lung. The table includes the blood flow rate through each of those organs at rest. Under acute exercise conditions, the resistance to the flow is altered (through vasoconstriction or vasodilation) through each of the segments as indicated in the table. The normal Δp at rest for the systemic circulation of 100 mmHg also increases to 130 mmHg while the Δp for the pulmonary circulation remains unchanged at 10 mmHg. Determine the blood flow through each of the vascular beds under acute exercise conditions.

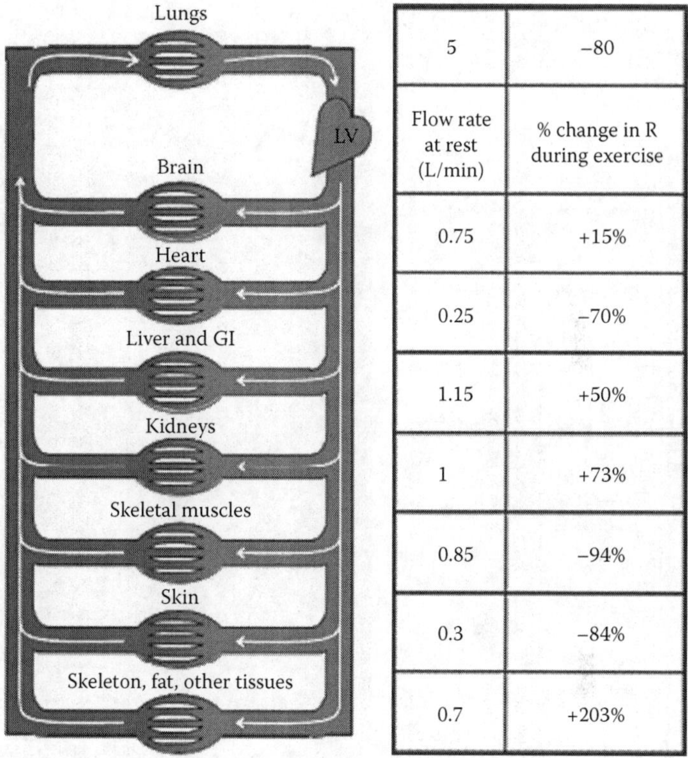

5	−80
Flow rate at rest (L/min)	% change in R during exercise
0.75	+15%
0.25	−70%
1.15	+50%
1	+73%
0.85	−94%
0.3	−84%
0.7	+203%

REFERENCES

Burton, A. C. (1971) *Physiology and Biophysics of the Circulation*, Year Book Medical Publishers, Chicago, IL.

Guyton, A. C. and Hall, J. E. (2000) *A Textbook of Medical Physiology*, 10th edn., W.B. Saunders Company, Philadelphia, PA.

Milnor, W. R. (1989) *Hemodynamics*, Williams & Wilkins, Baltimore, MD.

Young, D. F. (1979) Fluid mechanics of arterial stenosis. *J. Biomech. Eng*. 101: 157–173.

6 Unsteady Flow and Nonuniform Geometric Models

6.1 INTRODUCTION

Even though the steady flow models considered in the previous chapter provided us with some insight on the flow through arteries and we considered some applications using the same, more realistic models need to take into account the unsteady nature of flow through the circulatory system. In the unsteady models, the effect of pressure pulse propagation through the arterial wall, the effect of inertial forces due to the acceleration and deceleration of blood, and the effect of distensibility of the arteries on blood flow will be considered. Some applications of the unsteady flow models on the understanding of the blood flow dynamics in the circulatory system will be discussed.

6.2 WINDKESSEL MODELS FOR THE HUMAN CIRCULATION

Early theories to describe the blood flow in circulation considered the arterial system to be elastic storage vessels, which transformed the discontinuous flow due to the pumping of the heart into steady flow in the peripheral organs. The theory based on the concept that the blood vessels act as elastic storage vessels is referred to as the Windkessel model. This name arose from the analogy of early fire engines where the repeated strokes of the water pump were smoothed out to provide a nearly continuous flow by an air compression chamber (Windkessel, in German).

The *Windkessel theory* considers the arteries as a system of interconnected tubes with a storage capacity. A schematic representation of the Windkessel model for blood flow is shown in Figure 6.1. The fluid is pumped into the Windkessel chamber intermittently by the ventricular ejection and the outflow at the other end is based on the pressure gradient and the resistance to flow based on the Poiseuille theory. The storage capacity of the elastic blood vessels will be given by the distensibility D_i, such that

$$D_i = \frac{dV}{dp} \tag{6.1}$$

where

V is the volume

p is the pressure

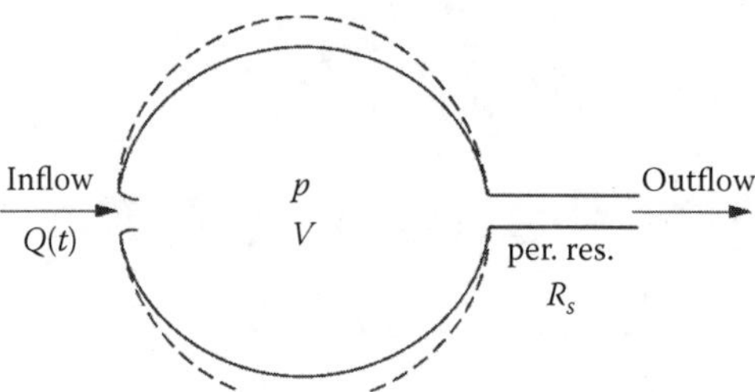

FIGURE 6.1 Schematic representation of blood flow in the circulation based on the Windkessel theory.

The *bulk modulus* or the modulus of volume elasticity, k (see Chapter 1), is related to distensibility by the relationship

$$k = \frac{Vdp}{dV} = \frac{V}{D_i}$$

The rate of storage of volume in the elastic chamber dV/dt can be written as

$$\frac{dV}{dt} = \left(\frac{dV}{dp}\right)\frac{dp}{dt}$$

or

$$\frac{dV}{dt} = D_i \frac{dp}{dt}$$

A mass balance can be written for the fluid in the elastic chamber as

$$\text{Inflow} - \text{outflow} = \text{rate of storage}$$

that is,

$$Q(t) - \frac{p}{R_s} = D_i \frac{dp}{dt}$$

The outflow is represented by the drop in pressure $(p - p_V)$ over the peripheral resistance R_s, and when the venous pressure, p_V, is assumed to be close to zero, this reduces to p/R_s.

The simplest assumption on the inflow is

$$Q(t) = Q_0 \quad 0 \le t \le t_s$$

and

$$Q(t) = 0 \quad t_s \le t \le T$$

where

t_s is the time at end systole
T is the duration of the cardiac cycle
Q_0 is a constant

Then the equation for systole can be written as

$$\frac{dp}{dt} + \frac{p}{R_s D_i} = \frac{Q_0}{D_i}$$

with the initial condition $p = p_0$ at $t = 0$.

Integrating the previous equation, we obtain

$$p(t) = R_s Q_0 - (R_s Q_0 - p_0)e^{-(t/R_s D_i)} \tag{6.2}$$

During diastole, the equation reduces to the form

$$\frac{dp}{dt} = -\frac{p}{R_s D_i}$$

with the condition that $p = p_T$ at $t = T$.

Integration of the previous equation yields

$$p(t) = p_T e^{-(t-T)/R_s D_i} \tag{6.3}$$

where

p_T is the pressure at the end of diastole
T is the duration of the cycle

Figure 6.2 shows a typical pressure pulse curve using the Windkessel theory and an arterial pressure pulse curve is shown in the inset. With the assumption of constant inflow, the stroke volume V_s will be given by

$$V_s = Q_0 t_s$$

Other patterns of inflow conditions with Q as a function of time (e.g., a half sine wave) have also been considered using this Windkessel theory. Then, the stroke volume during a cardiac cycle will be given by

$$V_s = \int_0^{t_s} Q(t)dt$$

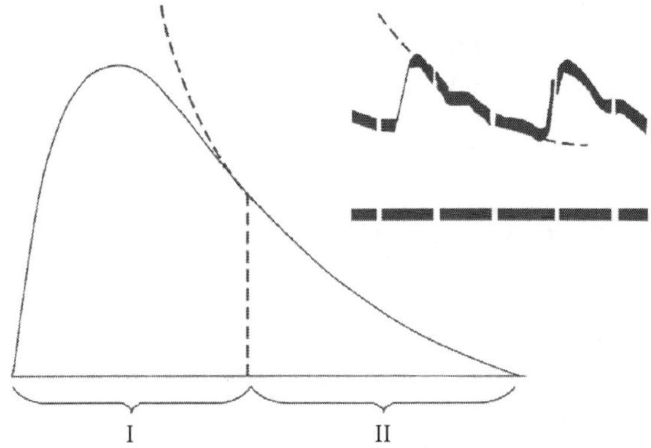

FIGURE 6.2 Pressure pulse plot from the Windkessel theory. I represents the pressure as a function of time during the forward flow phase of the cardiac cycle. II represents the time interval in which the inflow stops and the pressure decays exponentially given by the relationship in Equation 6.3. An actual pressure recording is displayed in the insert. (Redrawn from Noordergraaf, A., *Circulatory Systems Dynamics*, Academic Press, New York, Copyright 1978, with permission from Elsevier.)

The stroke volume determined using this theory could also be used to estimate the cardiac output. Even though Windkessel theory is able to estimate the pressure changes in the arterial system, there are several drawbacks in applying this theory for understanding the flow dynamics in circulation. The Windkessel theory assumes that the pressure pulse wave propagates instantly throughout the arterial system and neglects the finite time needed for the pulse wave transmission, as we will see later. Several improved models using the Windkessel theory incorporating traveling waves and wave reflections have also been considered. However, even with such models, details of the velocity profiles and mechanical forces due to the blood flowing at various segments in the circulatory system cannot be studied.

6.3 CONTINUUM MODELS FOR PULSATILE FLOW DYNAMICS

6.3.1 Wave Propagation in the Arterial System

In order to describe the mechanical events due to pulsatile blood flow through a segment of an artery, the laws of classical mechanics need to be applied and solutions obtained from the governing equations describing the motion. A number of theoretical and experimental studies have appeared in attempting to describe pulsatile flow through the arterial system. We will attempt to develop some of the basic models describing the pulsatile flow in elastic vessels and discuss some of the applications to understand the flow through the human circulatory system under normal states and in the presence of arterial disease.

The pressure pulse, generated by the contraction of the left ventricle, travels with a finite speed through the arterial wall and the speed of transmission is dependent on the wall elastic properties as well as the interaction between the wall and the blood contained within. The pressure pulse also changes shape as it travels downstream due to the interaction between the forward moving waves and the waves reflected at discontinuities in the arterial system such as branching and curvature sites. We will develop some relationships for the speed of wave propagation in the arterial system.

6.3.1.1 Moens–Korteweg Relationship

Consider an infinitely long, thin-walled elastic tube of circular cross section as shown in Figure 6.3. We will consider the governing equations for the fluid and the elastic tube in deriving the relationship for the wave propagation. Since the flow is axisymmetric, the velocity component in the ϕ-direction as well as the change of other variables in the ϕ-direction will be equal to zero. Then the continuity equation in the cylindrical coordinate system (see (b) in Table 1.1) will reduce to the form

$$\frac{1}{r}\frac{\partial}{\partial r}(rV_r)+\frac{\partial V_z}{\partial z}=\frac{\partial V_r}{\partial r}+\frac{V_r}{r}+\frac{\partial V_z}{\partial z}=0 \tag{6.4}$$

The momentum equations in the r- and z-directions can be rewritten as

$$\rho\left(\frac{\partial V_r}{\partial t}+V_r\frac{\partial V_r}{\partial r}+v_z\frac{\partial V_r}{\partial z}\right)=F_r-\frac{\partial p}{\partial r}+\mu\left(\frac{\partial^2 V_r}{\partial r^2}+\frac{1}{r}\frac{\partial V_r}{\partial r}-\frac{V_r}{r^2}+\frac{\partial^2 V_r}{\partial z^2}\right)$$

$$\rho\left(\frac{\partial V_z}{\partial t}+v_r\frac{\partial V_z}{\partial r}+v_z\frac{\partial V_z}{\partial z}\right)=F_z-\frac{\partial p}{\partial z}+\mu\left(\frac{\partial^2 V_z}{\partial r^2}+\frac{1}{r}\frac{\partial V_z}{\partial r}+\frac{\partial^2 V_z}{\partial z^2}\right)$$

In these equations, the dependent variables (velocity components and the pressure) are a function of r, z, and t. We will neglect the body forces (gravitational force) in the horizontal segment of the artery under consideration.

Initially, we will assume that the fluid is *inviscid* and hence the viscous force terms will drop out from the previous equations. However, the momentum equations will still contain the nonlinear convective acceleration terms and we will perform an assessment of the contributions due to the nonlinear terms in our analysis. We will write the estimated magnitude of each term below the corresponding term in the continuity and momentum equations. In the momentum equations, we will assume that the leading temporal acceleration term to have the predominant effect and compare the relative magnitudes of the nonlinear convective acceleration terms with

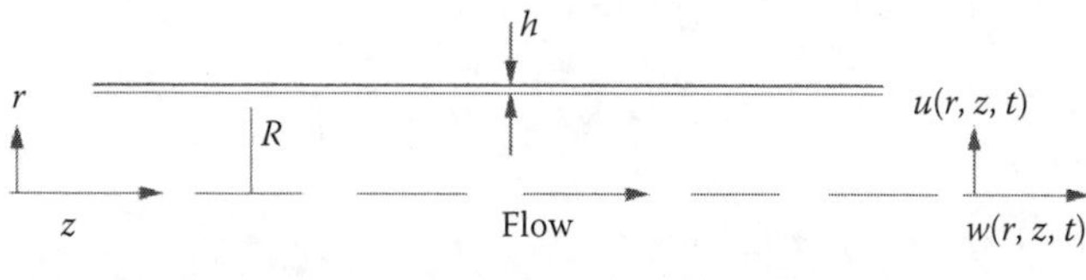

FIGURE 6.3 Schematic diagram of a model for wave propagation in a thin-walled elastic tube.

respect to the leading term. We will scale the magnitude of the dependent variables in order to determine the magnitude of each term as follows:

$$V_r \rightarrow u, \quad V_z \rightarrow w, \quad r \rightarrow R, \quad z \rightarrow \lambda, \quad \text{and} \quad t \rightarrow \tau$$

If λ is the wavelength and τ is the period of the pulse wave through the elastic tube, then the wave speed c will be given by

$$c = \frac{\lambda}{\tau}$$

We will also assume that the ratio of fluid velocity to the pulse wave velocity is much smaller than unity, that is, $w/c \ll 1$.

The magnitudes of the terms in the continuity equation with V_φ neglected will be

$$\frac{\partial V_r}{\partial r} + \frac{V_r}{r} + \frac{\partial V_z}{\partial z}$$

$$\sim \frac{u}{R} \quad \frac{u}{R} \quad \frac{w}{\lambda}$$

Multiplying each term with R/w, we have

$$\sim \frac{u}{w} \quad \frac{u}{w} \quad \frac{R}{\lambda}$$

We observe that the ratio u/w, which is the same order as that of R/λ, can also be assumed to be much less than unity. Hence, the radial velocity induced by the tube displacement in the radial direction can be expected to be much smaller than the axial velocity magnitudes.

Let us consider the magnitude of the inertial terms in the r-direction momentum equation

$$\frac{\partial V_r}{\partial t} + V_r \frac{\partial V_r}{\partial r} + V_z \frac{\partial V_r}{\partial z}$$

$$\sim \frac{u}{\tau} \quad \frac{u^2}{R} \quad \frac{wu}{\lambda}$$

Multiplying each term with τ/u, we get

$$1 \quad \frac{\tau u}{R} \quad \frac{w\tau}{\lambda}$$

$$1 \quad \frac{u}{w}\frac{w}{R/\tau} \quad \frac{w}{\lambda/\tau}$$

Since $u/w \sim R/\lambda$ and $R/\tau \sim \lambda/\tau \sim c$, we have

$$1 \quad \frac{R}{\lambda}\frac{w}{c} \quad \frac{w}{c}$$

Similarly, in the z-direction momentum equation, comparing the magnitudes of the inertial terms,

$$\frac{\partial V_z}{\partial t} + V_r\frac{\partial V_z}{\partial r} + V_z\frac{\partial V_z}{\partial z}$$

$$\sim \frac{w}{\tau} \quad \frac{uw}{R} \quad \frac{w^2}{\lambda}$$

Multiplying each term with τ/w, we get

$$1 \quad \frac{u}{w}\frac{w}{R/\tau} \quad \frac{w}{\lambda/\tau}$$

and hence,

$$1 \quad \frac{R}{\lambda}\frac{w}{c} \quad \frac{w}{c}$$

Comparing the order of magnitude of the convective acceleration terms with the temporal acceleration term, we can neglect the nonlinear terms as a first approximation since $R/\lambda \ll 1$ and $w/c \ll 1$. Thus, we conclude that the nonlinear convective acceleration terms have a smaller effect on the flow dynamics compared with the temporal acceleration term and, thus, can be neglected as a first approximation. Then, the momentum equations in the r- and z-directions reduce to the form

$$\rho\frac{\partial u}{\partial t} = -\frac{\partial p}{\partial r} \tag{6.5}$$

and

$$\rho\frac{\partial w}{\partial t} = -\frac{\partial p}{\partial z} \tag{6.6}$$

If we assume that the pressure gradient in the axial direction ($\partial p/\partial z$) is the dominant driving force inducing the flow, we can assess the magnitude of the radial pressure gradient, $\partial p/\partial r$ with respect to the axial pressure gradient. In Equation 6.4, the LHS term is $-(\rho u/\tau)$ and the RHS term is $-(p/R)$. In the axial direction, the LHS term of Equation 6.5 is $-(\rho w/\tau)$ and the RHS term is $-(p/\lambda)$.

Taking the ratio of magnitudes of these two equations, we get

$$\frac{\rho u/\tau}{\rho w/\tau}=\frac{p/R}{p/\lambda}$$

Since the axial pressure gradient is the most important term, we assign a value of unity for that term and get

$$\frac{\rho u/\tau}{\rho w/\tau}=\frac{p/R}{1}$$

or

$$\frac{p}{R}=\frac{u}{w}\sim\frac{R}{\lambda}$$

Since $R/\lambda \ll 1$, we can neglect the gradient of pressure in the radial direction. In other words, the pressure is assumed to be a constant in a cross section from the order of magnitude study. Thus, p is a function of z and t only.

The flow rate through the tube will be given by

$$A\bar{w}(z,t)=\pi R^2\bar{w}(z,t)=2\pi\int_0^R wr\,dr$$

where $\bar{w}$ is the mean velocity over the cross section.

Integrating the continuity equation over the cross section, we have

$$\int_0^R \frac{\partial w}{\partial z}2\pi r\,dr+\int_0^R \frac{1}{r}\frac{\partial}{\partial r}(ur)2\pi r\,dr=0$$

Combining the previous two equations, we get

$$\frac{\partial}{\partial z}[\pi R^2\bar{w}(z,t)]+2\pi ur\Big|_0^R=0$$

Due to axisymmetry, we have $u\big|_{r=0}=0$. Also $u\big|_{r=R}=u_R$ where u_R is the radial velocity magnitude at the wall. Thus, we obtain

$$u_R(z,t)=-\frac{R}{2}\frac{\partial\bar{w}}{\partial z} \tag{6.7}$$

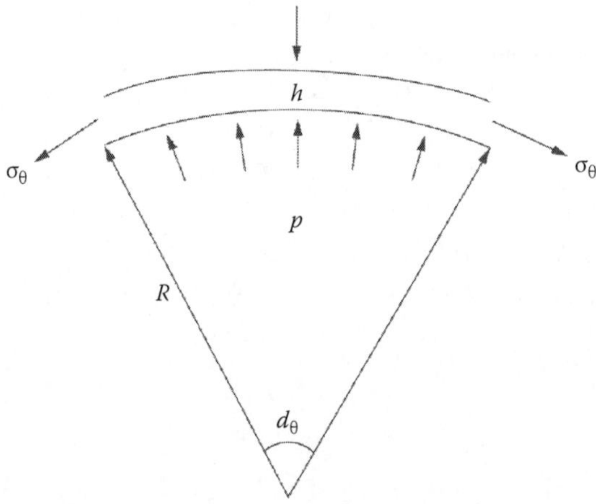

FIGURE 6.4 An element of the tube wall with the forces acting on the same.

Thus, with the simplifying assumptions and the order of magnitude study, the two reduced governing equations for the fluid motion are 6.6 and 6.7.

Let us now consider the equations of motion for the tube wall. We will assume that the tube is *thin-walled* and, hence, neglect the bending stresses and the stress variation in the radial direction. Let $\eta(z,t)$ be the displacement of the tube in the radial direction. Figure 6.4 represents a segment of the tube wall with the forces acting on the element shown. The length of the segment along the axial direction is assumed to be unity.

The circumferential strain can be computed as

$$\varepsilon_\theta = \frac{2\pi(R+\eta)-2\pi R}{2\pi R} = \frac{\eta}{R}$$

The hoop stress (stress in the wall along the circumferential direction) will be given by

$$\sigma_\theta = E\varepsilon_\theta = E\frac{\eta}{R}$$

Applying the Newton's law in the radial direction, we have

$$\rho_t hR\,d\theta\frac{d^2\eta}{dt^2} = pR\,d\theta - \sigma_\theta h\,d\theta$$

In this equation, the term on the LHS represents the inertial force and the terms on the RHS represent the forces due to the internal pressure and the hoop stress in the membrane, respectively, and ρ_t is the density of the tube wall material. As an initial approximation, if we *neglect the inertial forces* using the same reasoning as that for neglecting $\partial p/\partial r$, the equation of motion for the tube reduces to

$$p(z,t) = \frac{hE\eta}{R^2} \tag{6.8}$$

Finally, the boundary condition at the interface equates the fluid velocity in the radial direction at the wall with the rate of the tube displacement in the radial direction and is given by the equation

$$\frac{d\eta}{dt} = \dot{\eta} = u_R$$

Using Equation 6.7, we have

$$\dot{\eta} = -\frac{R}{2}\frac{\partial \bar{w}}{\partial z}$$

Differentiating Equation 6.8 and substituting,

$$\dot{\eta} = \frac{R^2}{hE}\frac{\partial p}{\partial t} = -\frac{R}{2}\frac{\partial \bar{w}}{\partial z}$$

and rewriting the same, we obtain

$$-\frac{\partial \bar{w}}{\partial z} = \frac{2R}{hE}\frac{\partial p}{\partial t}$$

Differentiating with respect to time, we get

$$-\frac{\partial}{\partial t}\frac{\partial \bar{w}}{\partial z} = \frac{2R}{hE}\frac{\partial^2 p}{\partial t^2}$$

Since the pressure is a constant over a cross section and, hence, independent of the r-coordinate, integrating Equation 6.6 over the cross section, we get

$$\frac{\partial \bar{w}}{\partial t} = -\frac{1}{\rho}\frac{\partial p}{\partial z}$$

Differentiating with respect to z and substituting, we get

$$\frac{2R}{hE}\frac{\partial^2 p}{\partial t^2} = -\frac{\partial}{\partial t}\left(\frac{\partial \bar{w}}{\partial z}\right) = -\frac{\partial}{\partial z}\left(\frac{\partial \bar{w}}{\partial t}\right) = \frac{\partial}{\partial z}\left(\frac{1}{\rho}\frac{\partial p}{\partial z}\right)$$

and hence,

$$\frac{\partial^2 p}{\partial z^2} = \frac{1}{hE/2R\rho}\frac{\partial^2 p}{\partial t^2} = \frac{1}{c_0^2}\frac{\partial^2 p}{\partial t^2}$$

The previous equation is the wave equation from which we obtain the relationship for the velocity of wave propagation, c_0 as

$$c_0^2 = \frac{hE}{2R\rho} \tag{6.9}$$

The previous equation is known as the *Moens–Korteweg* relationship and expresses the speed of a pressure pulse wave propagation through a thin-walled elastic tube containing an incompressible, inviscid fluid. The wave speed is directly proportional to the modulus of elasticity of the tube and to the ratio of tube thickness and the radius. However, this expression yields a constant value for the wave speed whereas experimental measurements have shown that the pulse wave speed in the arteries is a function of the frequency.

Hence, going back to the derivation of the tube equations, we will retain the inertial force term that we neglected earlier. Then the equation of motion for the tube segment will be

$$p = \frac{Eh}{R^2}\eta + \rho_t h\frac{d^2\eta}{dt^2}$$

where the inertial term has been retained in the last term. To obtain the solution of this second-order differential equation, we will assume that the pulse pressure is sinusoidal of the form

$$p = A\sin(kz - \omega t)$$

where

$k = 1/\lambda$, λ being the wave length
ω is the circular frequency of oscillation

We will assume that the tube displacement will also follow the same form and hence

$$\eta = B\sin(kz - \omega t)$$

Substituting the relationship for the pressure, radial displacement of the tube, and its derivative into the differential equation, we obtain

$$A\sin(kz - \omega t) = \left[\frac{Eh}{R^2} - \rho_t h\omega^2\right]B\sin(kz - \omega t)$$

or

$$p = \left[\frac{Eh}{R^2} - \rho_t h \omega^2 \right] \eta$$

Differentiating with respect to time and using the continuity equation relationship, we get

$$\frac{\partial p}{\partial t} = \left[\frac{Eh}{R^2} - \rho_t h \omega^2 \right] \frac{\partial \eta}{\partial t} = -\frac{R}{2} \left[\frac{Eh}{R^2} - \rho_t h \omega^2 \right] \frac{\partial \overline{w}}{\partial z}$$

This equation can be rewritten as

$$-\frac{\partial \overline{w}}{\partial z} = \frac{2R}{hE^*} \frac{\partial p}{\partial t}$$

where

$$E^* = E \left[\frac{h}{R^2} - \frac{\rho_t h \omega^2}{E} \right]$$

Differentiating once again with respect to time, we get

$$\frac{2R}{hE^*} \frac{\partial^2 p}{\partial t^2} = -\frac{\partial}{\partial t} \left[\frac{\partial \overline{w}}{\partial z} \right] = -\frac{\partial}{\partial z} \left[\frac{\partial \overline{w}}{\partial t} \right]$$

Thus,

$$\frac{\partial^2 p}{\partial z^2} = \frac{1}{hE^*/2R\rho} \frac{\partial^2 p}{\partial t^2}$$

The aforementioned relationship is the wave equation, and thus, the wave speed is given by

$$c_0^2(\omega) = \frac{hE}{2R\rho} \left[1 - \frac{\omega^2 \rho_t R^2}{E} \right] \qquad (6.10)$$

Even though Equation 6.10 includes the frequency in the relationship, in magnitude, the second term in parenthesis is much smaller than unity and hence the computed wave speed will be essentially a constant for a wide range of frequencies. A plot of

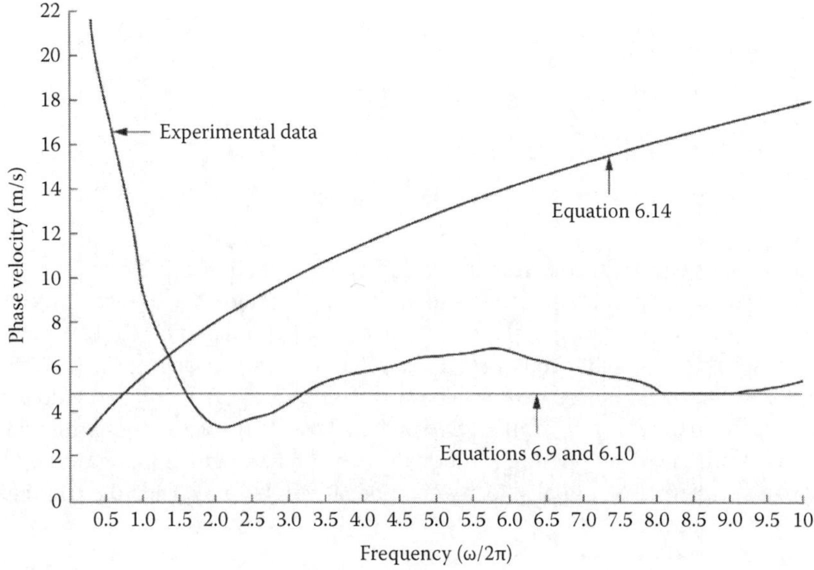

FIGURE 6.5 Pulse wave velocity plotted as a function of frequency from the theoretical models compared with experimental data. (Experimental curve redrawn from Noordergraaf [1978]. With permission from Elsevier.)

Equations 6.9 and 6.10 along with experimentally measured wave speed as a function of frequency are included in Figure 6.5. As can be observed, the theoretical computation essentially predicts a constant wave speed in variation with the experimentally observed values. We will now consider the effect of the inclusion of the viscosity on our analysis.

6.3.1.2 Womersley Model for Blood Flow Including Viscosity Effects

Womersley (1955a,b, 1957a,b) published an extensive treatise on theoretical analysis of blood flow through arteries. Earlier, Morgan and Kiely (1954) among others have also reported on models of blood flow through the arteries. These models considered unsteady flow of incompressible, Newtonian fluid through elastic tubes and obtained expressions for the velocity profiles in the cross section of the tube. Once again, we will consider an axisymmetric elastic tube of circular cross section as shown in Figure 6.3. Due to axisymmetric flow, the tangential velocity component V_θ will be equal to zero in the governing equations and the variation with respect to θ can also be neglected. As before, performing an order of magnitude study on the nonlinear terms in the radial and axial momentum equations (see (b) in Table 1.1), we can show that the nonlinear terms can be neglected in comparison with the leading temporal acceleration terms. Thus, the simplified continuity and momentum equations, including viscous effects, will be

$$\frac{\partial V_r}{\partial r} + \frac{V_r}{r} + \frac{\partial V_z}{\partial z} = 0$$

$$\frac{\partial V_r}{\partial t} = -\frac{1}{\rho}\frac{\partial p}{\partial r} + \frac{\mu}{\rho}\left[\frac{\partial^2 V_r}{\partial r^2} + \frac{1}{r}\frac{\partial V_r}{\partial r} + \frac{\partial^2 V_r}{\partial z^2} - \frac{V_r}{r^2}\right]$$

$$\frac{\partial V_z}{\partial t} = -\frac{1}{\rho}\frac{\partial p}{\partial z} + \frac{\mu}{\rho}\left[\frac{\partial^2 V_z}{\partial r^2} + \frac{1}{r}\frac{\partial V_z}{\partial r} + \frac{\partial^2 V_z}{\partial z^2}\right]$$

In the previous equations, the gravitational forces have been neglected by assuming that the artery is horizontal. For a solution for flow through elastic tubes, we need to develop the governing equations for the elastic tube in addition to the previous equations and then simultaneously solve the equations with the appropriate interface boundary conditions. Before we consider the effect of wall elasticity on the flow, we will initially assume that the wall is *rigid* and analyze for the velocity distribution in the fluid. With the assumption of rigidity, there will be no radial motion of the wall and with symmetry; the radial velocity component will be zero. Then the continuity equation will reduce to

$$\frac{\partial V_z}{\partial z} = \frac{\partial^2 V_z}{\partial z^2} = 0$$

The momentum equation in r-direction will reduce to

$$\frac{\partial p}{\partial r} = 0$$

From the aforementioned relationship, we observe that the pressure is a function of axial distance and time alone (being constant over the cross section) and the axial velocity component is a function of radius and time alone. Or in other words, $p(z, t)$ and $w(r, t)$.

The momentum equation in the z-direction will reduce to

$$\frac{\partial V_z}{\partial t} = -\frac{1}{\rho}\frac{\partial p}{\partial z} + \frac{\mu}{\rho}\left[\frac{\partial^2 V_z}{\partial r^2} + \frac{1}{r}\frac{\partial V_z}{\partial r}\right]$$

Since p is a function of z and t, dp/dz will be a function of time only. For a sinusoidal variation in the pressure gradient, we will assume a relationship

$$\frac{dp}{dz} = Ae^{i\omega t}$$

where A is a constant representing the amplitude of the pressure gradient pulse.

Then, it follows that the velocity will also be of similar form and hence we have

$$V_z = w(r)e^{i\omega t}$$

Substituting these equations into the governing equation in the z-direction, we have

$$i\omega w e^{i\omega t} = -\frac{A}{\rho} e^{i\omega t} + \frac{\mu}{\rho}\left[\frac{d^2 w}{dr^2} + \frac{1}{r}\frac{dw}{dr}\right] e^{i\omega t}$$

which can be rewritten as

$$\frac{d^2 w}{dr^2} + \frac{1}{r}\frac{dw}{dr} - \frac{i\omega\rho}{\mu} w = \frac{A}{\mu}$$

We will normalize the radius in the equation by the relationship

$$r' = \frac{r}{R}$$

Then the differential equation will reduce to the form

$$\frac{d^2 w}{dr'^2} + \frac{1}{r'}\frac{dw}{dr'} - i\alpha^2 w = \frac{A}{\mu} R^2 \qquad (6.11)$$

where

$$\alpha^2 = R^2 \frac{\omega\rho}{\mu}$$

or

$$\alpha = \frac{d}{2}\sqrt{\frac{\rho\omega}{\mu}} \qquad (1.82)$$

where d is the diameter of the tube.

The term α is a nondimensional parameter known as the unsteady Reynolds number and also is referred to in the literature as the unsteadiness parameter or the Womersley parameter. α can be rewritten as

$$\alpha^2 = R^2 \frac{\omega\rho}{\mu} \propto \frac{\rho R v/\tau}{\mu v/R}$$

The numerator represents the inertial forces and the denominator represents the viscous forces similar to the Reynolds number defined earlier. Table 6.1 gives the typical values for the radius of the aorta as well as the femoral artery for various

TABLE 6.1
Radius of the Vessel, Heart Rate, and the Womersley Parameter for the Various Species

Species	Weight (kg)	Vessel	Radius (cm)	Heart Rate (bpm)	α[a]
Mouse	0.017	*Aorta*	0.035	500	1.4
Rat	0.6		0.13	350	4.3
Cat	3		0.21	140	4.4
Rabbit	4		0.23	280	6.8
Dog	20		0.78	90	13.1
Man	75		1.5	70	22.2
Ox	500		2.0	52	25.6
Elephant	2000		4.5	38	49.2
Rat	0.6	*Femoral*	0.04	350	1.5
Rabbit	4		0.08	280	2.4
Dog	20		0.23	90	3.9
Man	75		0.27	70	4.0

Source: From Milnor, W.R., *Hemodynamics*, 2nd edn., Williams & Wilkins, Baltimore, MD, 1989.

[a] At fundamental frequency.

species and the corresponding Womersley parameter values. As can be observed, even though the radius and heart rate vary over a wide range among the species, the variation in Womersley parameter for the various species is within one order of magnitude.

The differential equation given in Equation 6.11 is of the form

$$z^2 \frac{d^2w}{dz^2} + z\frac{dw}{dz} + (z^2 - \gamma^2)w = 0$$

and is known as the Bessel's equation of the first kind and γth order. The solution for the equation is the Bessel function of the first kind and γth order is J_γ. With the appropriate boundary conditions, the solution for the Equation 6.10 is

$$w = \frac{AR^2}{i\mu\alpha^2}\left[1 - \frac{J_0(\alpha r' i^{3/2})}{J_0(\alpha i^{3/2})}\right]$$

and hence,

$$V_z = \frac{AR^2}{i\mu\alpha^2}\left[1 - \frac{J_0(\alpha r' i^{3/2})}{J_0(\alpha i^{3/2})}\right]e^{i\omega t} \tag{6.12}$$

In these equations, i is the imaginary number $\sqrt{-1}$.

To obtain an expression for the instantaneous flow rate in any given cross section, the aforementioned relationship can be integrated over the cross section to obtain

$$Q = 2\pi\int_0^1 wr'\,dr' = \frac{\pi R^2 A e^{i\omega t}}{i\omega\rho}\left[1 - \frac{2J_1(i^{3/2}\alpha)}{i^{3/2}\alpha J_0(i^{3/2}\alpha)}\right] \tag{6.13}$$

The results given earlier for the axial velocity and the instantaneous flow rate are complex functions and can be separated into the real and imaginary parts. They can also be expressed in terms of the modulus and phase and the phase angle will represent the phase lag or lead with respect to the applied harmonic pressure gradient. Womersley (1955a and b) expressed the complex expressions in terms of modulus and phase angle by using the relationship

$$M_0' e^{i\varepsilon_0} = \left[1 - \left\{\frac{J_0(i^{3/2}\alpha r')}{J_0(i^{3/2}\alpha)}\right\}\right]$$

and

$$M_{10}' e^{i\varepsilon_{10}} = \left[1 - \left\{\frac{2J_1(i^{3/2}\alpha)}{i^{3/2}J_0(i^{3/2}\alpha)}\right\}\right]$$

In these expressions, M' represents the modulus and ε represents the phase angle. Thus, the expressions for the velocity and the instantaneous flow rate were given by

$$V_z = \left\{\frac{Ae^{i\omega t}}{i\omega\rho}(M_0' e^{i\varepsilon_0})\right\}$$

and

$$Q = \left\{\frac{\pi R^2 A e^{i\omega t}}{i\omega\rho}(M_{10}' e^{i\varepsilon_{10}})\right\}$$

The solution will be the real part of the previous equation corresponding to the real part of the applied complex pressure gradient, and, after replacing $1/\omega\rho$ with $R^2/\mu\alpha^2$, can be expressed using trigonometric functions as

$$V_z = -\frac{|A|R^2}{\mu}\frac{M_0'}{\alpha^2}\sin(\omega t - \phi + \varepsilon_0)$$

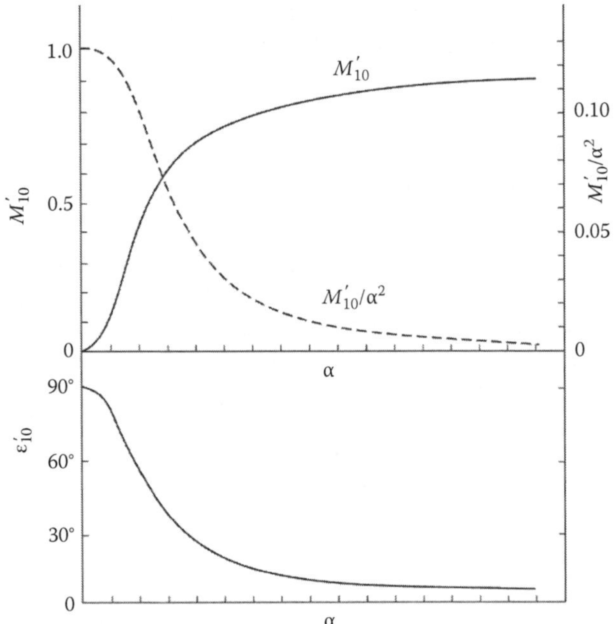

FIGURE 6.6 M'_{10}, M'_{10}/α^2, and ε'_{10} as a function of α. (Redrawn from Milnor, W.R., *Hemodynamics*, 2nd edn., Williams & Wilkins, Baltimore, MD, 1989.)

and

$$Q = \frac{|A|\pi R^4}{\mu}\frac{M'_{10}}{\alpha^2}\sin(\omega t - \phi + \varepsilon'_{10})$$

The relationship for the instantaneous flow rate can be rewritten as

$$Q = \frac{|A|\pi R^4}{\mu}\frac{M'_{10}}{\alpha^2}\cos(\omega t - \phi + [90^\circ - \varepsilon'_{10}])$$

Thus, for a given applied sinusoidal pressure gradient, the results shown earlier describe the velocity profile over a cross section as well as the instantaneous flow rate. Figure 6.6 shows a plot of M'_{10}, M'_{10}/α^2, and ε'_{10} as a function of a. It can be observed from the figure that as α approaches 0, M'_{10}/α^2 approaches 1/8, which is the constant for Poiseuille flow relationship in steady flow (zero frequency) and ε'_{10} approaches 90. It can be observed that the phase lag is zero when ε'_{10} is 90. Thus, with α equal to 0, we have steady flow with maximum flow rate and zero phase lag between the applied pressure gradient and flow. With increasing frequency of oscillation, the flow rate decreases and the phase lag between the pressure gradient and the flow increases. Figure 6.7 shows a measured pressure gradient from the main pulmonary artery of a human subject. This pressure gradient pulse, which repeats

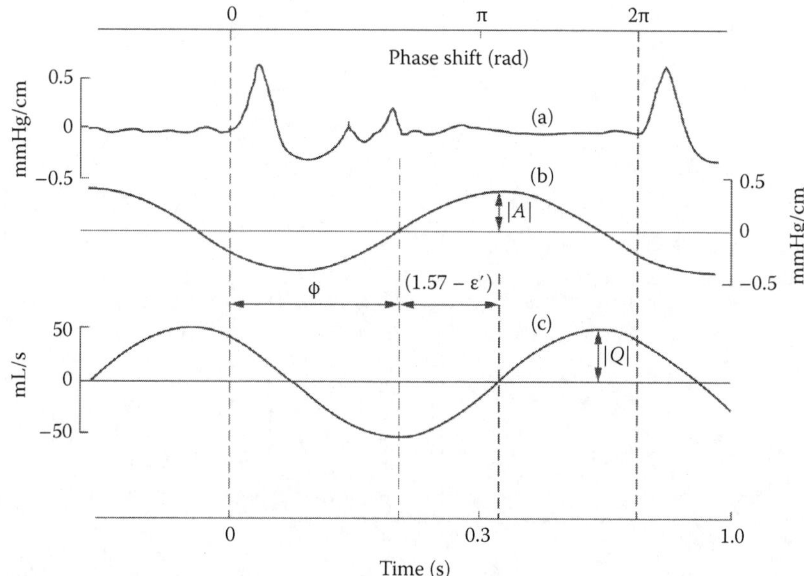

FIGURE 6.7 Pressure gradient, $\Delta p/\Delta z$, measured from the main pulmonary artery of a human (a), the first harmonic of the pressure gradient (b), and the first harmonic of the computed instantaneous flow rate (c) curves. (Redrawn from Milnor, W.R., *Hemodynamics*, 2nd edn., Williams & Wilkins, Baltimore, MD, 1989.)

itself for every cycle, can be resolved into various harmonics using the Fourier series expansion. The middle panel shows the first harmonic of the pressure gradient pulse and the bottom panel shows the instantaneous flow rate computed. The modulus and amplitude of the first harmonic of the pressure gradient and the computed flow rate are also shown in the figure. It can also be observed that the flow lags behind the pressure gradient. Since the applied pressure gradient and the computed flow rate are sinusoidal, averaging the flow rate over a cycle will yield a zero flow rate.

Figure 6.8 shows the synthesis of a measured pressure gradient (panel (d)) into four harmonics. Panel (a) shows the first two harmonics and panels (b), (c), and (d) show the consecutive addition of the other two harmonics to obtain the resulting pressure gradient. The computation of the corresponding instantaneous flow rate for each of the harmonics is shown superimposed with the corresponding pressure gradient in Figure 6.9. Note the phase difference between the pressure gradient and the flow rate in each of the harmonics.

As pointed out earlier, when the flow rate curves are time averaged over a cardiac cycle, zero net flow will be the result. However, we know that the arteries have a net positive flow (cardiac output) and this is incorporated by the addition of a steady or dc component of flow as shown in Figure 6.10. In this figure, the addition of the four harmonics of the flow is shown and in the last panel, the x-axis is shifted down to include a steady flow component. The time average of this flow rate curve in a cycle will give the stroke volume and multiplied by the heart rate will give the cardiac output.

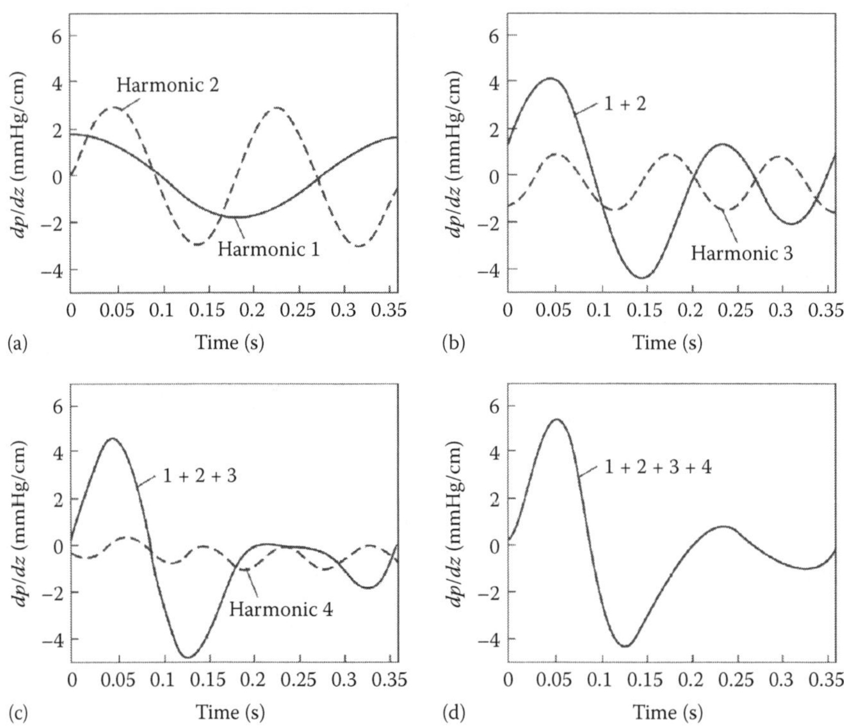

FIGURE 6.8 The first four harmonics of the pressure gradient measured in the dog's femoral artery: (a) plots of first and second harmonic; (b) addition of the first two harmonics and plot of the third harmonic; (c) addition of first three harmonics and the plot of the fourth harmonic; and (d) the resultant plot with the addition of the first four harmonics. (From Nichols, W.W. and O'Rourke, M.F., *McDonald's Blood Flow in Arteries*, 3rd edn., Lea & Febiger, Philadelphia, PA, 1990.)

Figure 6.11a shows a mean velocity curve computed from the theory. The measured pressure gradient curve used in the computations is included in Figure 6.11b. A comparison between the computed mean velocity curve and the measured curve (McDonald, 1974) shows good agreement in spite of the assumptions used in deriving the expression for the theoretical flow rate.

Equation 6.11 gives the expression for the velocity profile in the lumen using the aforementioned theory and once again, the velocity profiles can be computed for the various harmonics of the pressure gradient and plotted for various times during the cardiac cycle. Figure 6.12 shows velocity profiles plotted as a function of the nondimensional radius for the first four harmonics, the angle in the y-axis representing the time in the cardiac cycle (ωt). Panel (a) represents the fundamental frequency with $\alpha = 3.34$ and panels (b), (c), and (d) represent the next three harmonics with values of 4.72, 5.78, and 6.67, respectively.

It can be noted that the profiles are plotted only for one-half of the cardiac cycle. Since the velocity varies as a sinusoidal function, the profiles for the other half will be a mirror image of the first half. Several interesting features can be

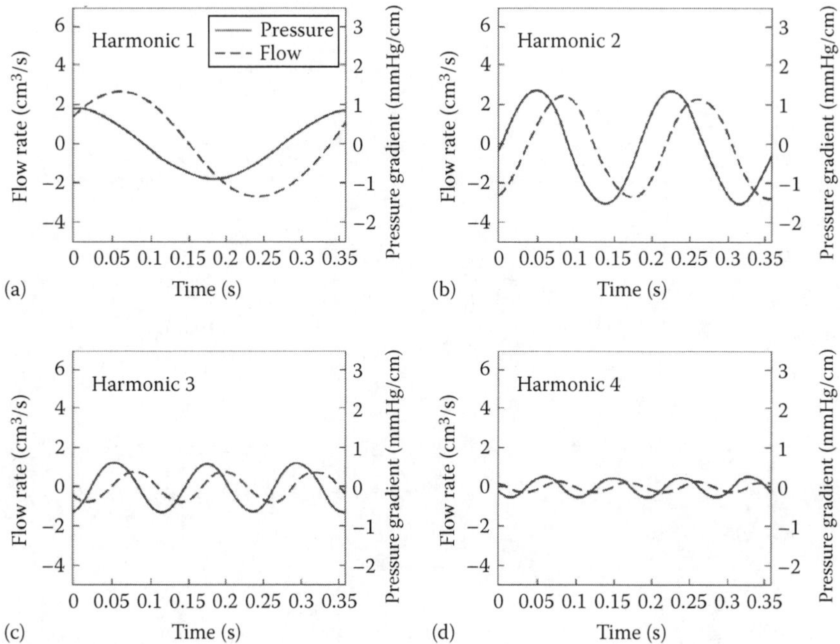

FIGURE 6.9 The first four harmonics of the pressure gradient are plotted along with the corresponding flow rate computed using Equation 6.13: (a) first harmonic; (b) second harmonic; (c) third harmonic; and (d) fourth harmonic. The radius of the femoral artery was assumed to be 0.15 cm and a for the first harmonic was assumed to be 3.34.

noted from this figure. It can be observed that the profiles do not become completely parabolic at any time during the cardiac cycle. Since the velocity of the fluid at the wall is zero, the laminae near the wall are slowed down first due to the viscous forces and the fluid motion near the wall are slower. Thus, when the pressure gradient reverses, the fluid near the wall tends to reverse direction easily. Also, some time must elapse before the viscous diffusion occurs toward the core region. Hence, as the frequency increases in the subsequent harmonics, the viscous effects are not felt in the core region and the velocity profile is relatively flat during most of the cardiac cycle. Figure 6.13 shows the computed velocity profile in the femoral artery of a dog from the measured pressure gradient and with an addition of a steady flow component (a parabolic velocity profile with an axial velocity of 22.65 cm/s). Once again, it can be observed that the velocity profile reversal occurs first near the wall.

6.3.1.3 Wave Propagation in an Elastic Tube with Viscous Flow

In the relationships derived in the previous section, we assumed that the tube is rigid and that assumption implies an infinite wave speed. However, we know that the pulse wave propagates through the arteries with a finite speed and so we will now introduce the effect of tube elasticity. Hence, we need to derive the governing equations of motion for the elastic tube. We will assume that the tube is homogeneous, isotropic,

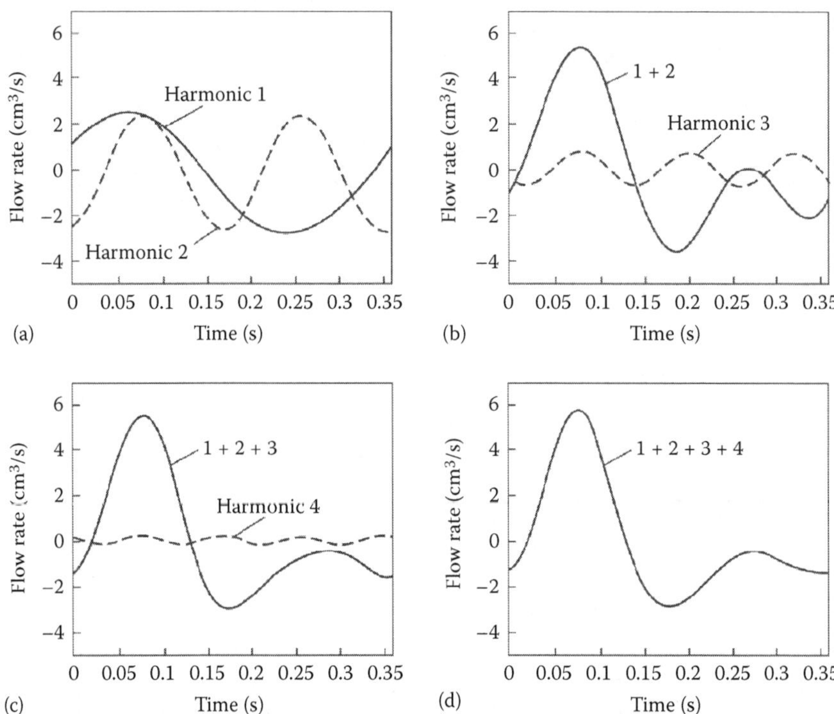

FIGURE 6.10 The addition of the first four harmonics of the computed flow rate to yield the flow rate through the femoral artery: (a) plots of first and second harmonic; (b) addition of the first two harmonics and plot of the third harmonic; (c) addition of first three harmonics, and the plot of the fourth harmonic; and (d) the resultant plot with the addition of the first four harmonics. The plot on the bottom right shows an offset in which a steady flow component with a mean velocity of 22.65 cm/s has been added. The mean velocity was computed based on the Poiseuille flow relationship with the steady flow component of the measured pressure drop.

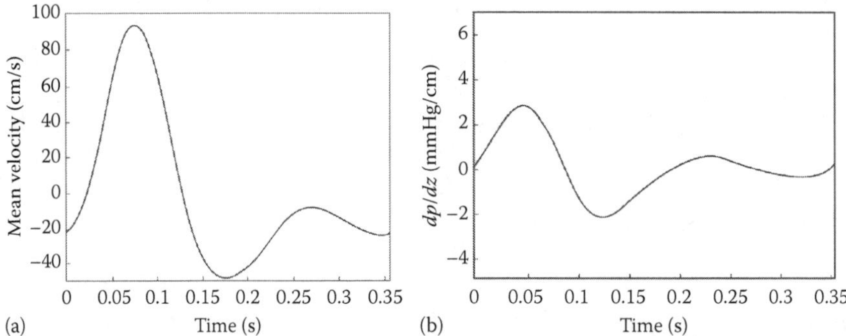

FIGURE 6.11 Plots of (a) the computed flow rate (steady flow component and the first four harmonics) and (b) measured pressure gradient through the femoral artery of a dog. The agreement between the computed and the measured flow rate profiles is very good. (From Nichols, W.W. and O'Rourke, M.F., *McDonald's Blood Flow in Arteries*, 3rd edn., Lea & Febiger, Philadelphia, PA, 1990.)

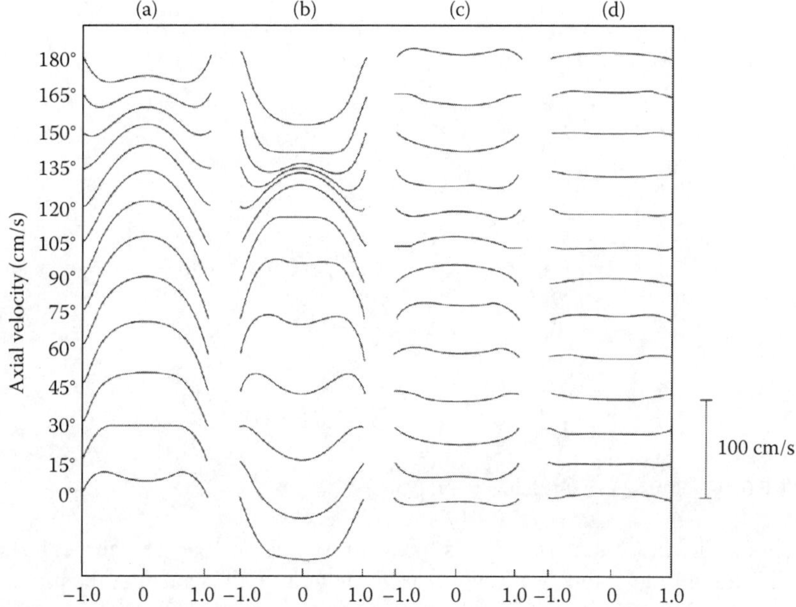

FIGURE 6.12 Velocity profiles plotted as a function of nondimensional radius in the femoral artery of a dog computed using the relationship given in Equation 6.12. (a), (b), (c), and (d) refer to the first four harmonics with $\alpha = 3.34$, 4.72, 5.78, and 6.67, respectively.

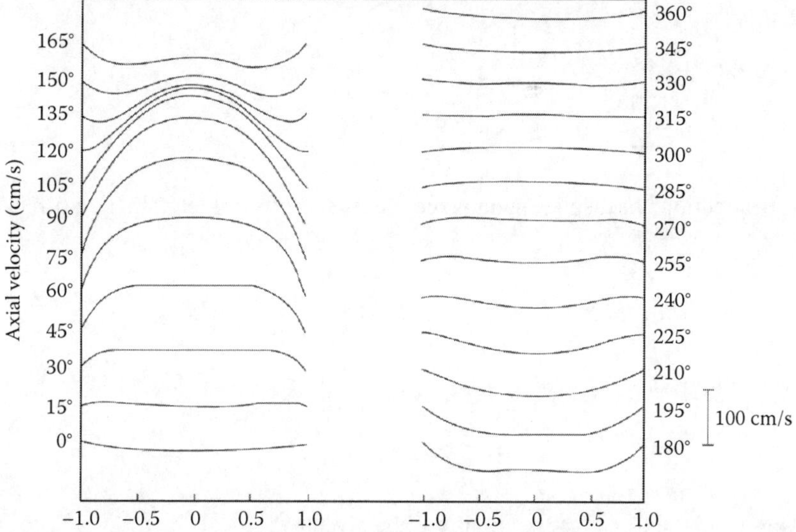

FIGURE 6.13 Computed velocity profiles plotted as a function of the nondimensional radius during a cardiac cycle in the femoral artery of a dog. A parabolic velocity profile with a mean axial velocity of 22.65 cm/s has been superposed on the first four harmonics in the plots.

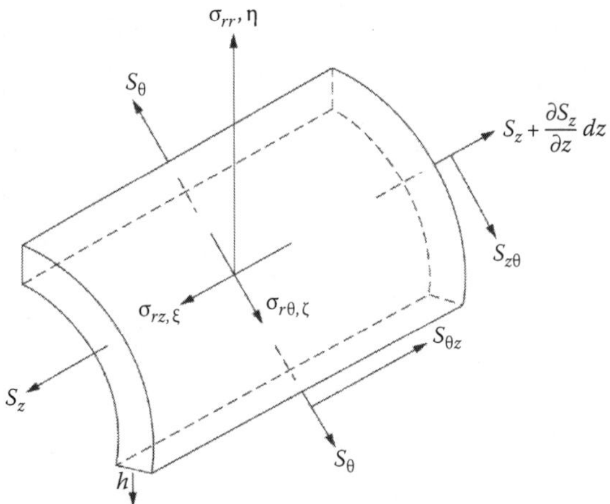

FIGURE 6.14 Stresses on an element of the tube.

with Hookean elastic material and is also thin-walled so that we can neglect the bending stresses in the tube wall. Figure 6.14 shows a small element of the tube with all the stresses represented. σ represents the forces exerted on the tube due to the fluid and S represents the stresses within the tube membrane. Displacements in the r-, θ-, and z-directions are, respectively, η, ζ, and ξ. ρ_t is the tube material density and h is the thickness of the tube.

The equation of motion in the r-direction will be

$$\rho_t hR\, d\theta\, dz \frac{\partial^2 \eta}{\partial t^2} = \sigma_{rr} R\, d\theta\, dz - S_\theta h\, dz\, d\theta$$

and will simplify as

$$\rho_t h \frac{\partial^2 \eta}{\partial t^2} = \sigma_{rr} - S_\theta \frac{h}{R}$$

In the θ-direction, the displacement is zero due to the axisymmetry. In the z-direction, we get

$$\rho_t hR\, d\theta\, dz \frac{\partial^2 \xi}{\partial t^2} = -\sigma_{rz} R\, d\theta\, dz + \frac{\partial S_z}{\partial z} h\, dz R\, d\theta$$

and will simplify as

$$\rho_t h \frac{\partial^2 \xi}{\partial t^2} = -\sigma_{rz} + \frac{\partial S_z}{\partial z}$$

The strains in the θ- and z-directions will be given by

$$\varepsilon_\theta = \frac{2\pi(R+\eta) - 2\pi R}{2\pi R} = \frac{\eta}{R}$$

and

$$\varepsilon_z = \frac{\partial \xi}{\partial z}$$

From the generalized Hooke's law, we can derive the expressions for the tube stresses as follows:

$$E\varepsilon_z = S_z - \nu S_\theta$$

and

$$E\varepsilon_\theta = S_\theta - \nu S_z$$

Solving for the tube stresses in terms of strains, we get

$$S_\theta = E\frac{(\varepsilon_\theta + \nu\varepsilon_z)}{(1-\nu^2)}$$

and

$$S_z = E\frac{(\varepsilon_z + \nu\varepsilon_\theta)}{(1-\nu^2)}$$

Thus,

$$S_\theta = E\frac{\left[(\eta/R) + \nu(\partial\xi/\partial z)\right]}{(1-\nu^2)}$$

and

$$S_z = E\frac{\left[(\partial\xi/\partial z) + \nu(\eta/R)\right]}{(1-\nu^2)}$$

or

$$\frac{\partial S_z}{\partial z} = E\frac{\left[(\partial^2\xi/\partial z^2) + (\nu/R)(\partial\eta/\partial z)\right]}{(1-\nu^2)}$$

The fluid stresses in the cylindrical coordinates are

$$\sigma_{rr} = -p + 2\mu\frac{\partial V_r}{\partial r};\quad \sigma_{r\theta} = \mu\left[\frac{1}{r}\frac{\partial V_r}{\partial \theta} + \frac{\partial V_\theta}{\partial r} - \frac{V_\theta}{2r}\right]$$

$$\sigma_{\theta\theta} = -p + 2\mu\left[\frac{1}{r}\frac{\partial V_\theta}{\partial \theta} + \frac{V_r}{r}\right] \qquad \sigma_{\theta z} = \mu\left[\frac{\partial V_\theta}{\partial z} + \frac{1}{r}\frac{\partial V_z}{\partial \theta}\right]$$

$$\sigma_{zz} = -p + 2\mu\frac{\partial V_z}{\partial z} \qquad \sigma_{rz} = \mu\left[\frac{\partial V_z}{\partial r} + \frac{\partial V_r}{\partial z}\right]$$

Substituting the stress relationships into the equations of motion, we get

$$\rho_t h\frac{\partial^2 \eta}{\partial t^2} = -p + 2\mu\left.\frac{\partial V_r}{\partial r}\right|_{r=R} - \frac{hE}{(1-\nu^2)}\left[\frac{\eta}{R^2} + \frac{\nu}{R}\frac{\partial \xi}{\partial z}\right]$$

and

$$\rho_t h\frac{\partial^2 \xi}{\partial t^2} = -\mu\left[\frac{\partial V_z}{\partial r} + \frac{\partial V_r}{\partial z}\right]_{r=R} + \frac{hE}{(1-\nu^2)}\left[\frac{\partial^2 \xi}{\partial z^2} + \frac{\nu}{R}\frac{\partial \eta}{\partial z}\right]$$

The governing equations of motion for the fluid, along with the previous two equations, must be solved simultaneously to obtain the solutions for the dependent variables (i.e., the velocity components, pressure, and the tube displacements). The boundary conditions at the interface between the fluid and the tube are specified as

$$\frac{\partial \eta}{\partial t} = V_r\Big|_{r=R}$$

and

$$\frac{\partial \xi}{\partial t} = V_z\Big|_{r=R} \quad \frac{\partial \xi}{\partial t} = w\Big|_{r=R}$$

Morgan and Kiely (1954) as well as Womersley (1957a,b) have presented the solutions for the earlier-formulated problem. As before, by performing an order of magnitude study, the equations can be linearized and further simplifications can be made. To obtain the solutions for a harmonic input pressure gradient, the pressure can be assumed to be of the form

$$p = Pe^{i(kz-\omega t)}$$

where $k = k_1 + ik_2$ in which $k_1 = 1/\lambda$ is the wave number and k_2 is the damping constant. Morgan and Kiely (1954) obtained the solutions for the velocity profiles in terms of Bessel functions. They also presented results for specialized cases of small viscosity and large viscosity.

For small viscosity, the wave speed and damping constant were given by the relationship

$$C = \frac{\omega}{k_1} = \pm\left(\frac{Eh}{2R\rho}\right)^{1/2}\left[1 - \left\{1 - \nu + \frac{\nu^2}{4}\right\}\frac{1}{R}\left(\frac{\mu}{2\rho\omega}\right)^{1/2}\right] \tag{6.14}$$

and

$$k_2 = \pm\omega\left(\frac{2R\rho}{Eh}\right)^{1/2}\left(\frac{\mu}{2\rho\omega}\right)^{1/2}\frac{1}{R}\left(1 - \nu + \frac{\nu^2}{4}\right)$$

For large viscosity, the relationships are

$$C = \pm\left(\frac{Eh}{2R\rho}\right)^{1/2} R\left(\frac{\omega\rho}{\mu}\right)^{1/2}\frac{1}{\sqrt{(5-4\nu)}}$$

and

$$k_2 = \pm\left(\frac{2R\rho}{Eh}\right)^{1/2}\frac{1}{R}\left(\frac{\mu}{\omega\rho}\right)^{1/2}\sqrt{(5-4\nu)}$$

The plot of the wave velocity for the low viscosity case as a function of frequency is also shown in Figure 6.5. The theoretical results predict an increase in phase velocity with increase in frequency in contrast to the experimental results. Even though the theoretical models presented earlier appear to yield reasonable results for blood velocity profiles, further improvements are necessary in order to simulate the propagation of pulse waves in the arterial wall as briefly described in the following. In deriving the aforementioned relationships for flow of incompressible viscous fluid through an elastic tube, we made several simplifying assumptions and we will discuss the validity of those assumptions.

1. *Laminar flow*: This condition is generally satisfied in the circulation for most of the time. During peak systole near the aortic root, some disturbance to flow has been measured and also in vessels like the main pulmonary artery. However, sustained turbulent flow may not exist in the circulation under normal conditions. Turbulent or highly disturbed flow may be present distal to the diseased valves, in the presence of stenosis or with implanted prosthetic devices.
2. *Newtonian fluid*: In our discussion of blood rheology, we learned that the blood exhibits a non-Newtonian behavior at low shear rates. However, in relatively large blood vessels, the rates of shear are expected to be high for most of the pulsatile flow cycle and the assumption of a Newtonian fluid appears to be reasonable.
3. *Uniform cylindrical tube*: This assumption is an approximation to formulate the governing equations in the cylindrical coordinate system. The blood vessels are not perfectly cylindrical and also the cross section tapers

in the axial direction and thus the cross-sectional area reduces in the distal portions even though the tapering is very gradual. For a single conduit, the reduction in cross section can be approximated by an exponential form (Li, 1987). For the aorta, the change in cross section can be expressed as

$$A(z) = A_0 e^{-kz/r}$$

where the taper factor k can be expressed as

$$k = \left(\frac{r}{z}\right) \ln\left(\frac{A_0}{A}\right)$$

In the previous equation, A_0 is the cross-sectional area at the proximal site, r is the radius, z is the distance along the axis. For the peripheral vessels, Li (1987) expressed the change in cross sections using a relationship

$$A = A_0 e^{-kz}$$

where the magnitudes for k were computed for each of the vessels from *in vivo* measurements.

4. *Entrance effects*: The derivations given earlier assume a fully developed flow which is a condition that does not exist in the circulation. In order to distribute blood throughout the body, blood vessels branch out very often and their geometry is very irregular and includes some curvature. Hence, fully developed flow cannot be expected in the blood vessels and this assumption is also invalid.
5. *Reflected waves*: The elastic tube was assumed to be infinitely long without the presence of any discontinuities such as curvature or branching where wave reflections can occur. The effect of wave reflections has not been taken into account in our formulation.
6. *Linearization of equations*: Through an order of magnitude study, the equations were linearized with the assumption that the contributions from the nonlinear terms are relatively small. Since the equations were linearized, it was also possible for us to superimpose the solutions for the higher harmonics to obtain the solution for physiological pulsatile flow. Hence, we have neglected the contributions of the nonlinear terms and have also ignored the nonlinear interactions between the harmonics. Womersley (1957a) has shown that neglecting the nonlinear terms in the governing equations for the fluid will result in an error of about 5% in the computed velocity magnitudes.
7. *Thin-walled tube*: As was discussed in a previous chapter, a thick-walled tube model is more appropriate for the blood vessel wall and the thin-walled formulation is again a simplifying approximation.
8. *Homogeneous, isotropic, Hookean material*: The blood vessel has several components and is not homogeneous. It also exhibits at least a transversely orthotropic behavior and a nonlinear load deformation. Hence, this assumption is also an approximation.

In order to remove the restrictions on the assumption of discussed earlier in the blood flow models, several theoretical investigations have been reported in the literature. Typical studies have included wave propagation through an initially stressed elastic tube containing viscous fluid; wave propagation in a tethered, initially stressed orthotropic elastic tube. Experimental studies have included the transmission characteristics of axial waves in blood vessels by superimposing sinusoidal waves in segments of arteries and measuring the wave speed. The dissipation and dispersion properties of small waves in arteries and veins with viscoelastic wall properties have also been analyzed. The wave propagation in a thick-walled viscoelastic tube containing Newtonian fluid as well as the effect of wall compressibility on the transmission characteristics has been analyzed. Experimental measurements of the pressure wave propagation in the canine femoral artery have suggested that linearized wave propagation models are reasonably accurate in predicting the flow and pressure wave propagation. With each complexity introduced in the model for theoretical analysis, the solution procedure becomes complicated because the nonlinear governing equations for the tube and the fluid have to be simultaneously considered with the appropriate interface boundary conditions. Moreover, verification of the results presented from the theoretical analysis is extremely difficult because detailed measurements of wave propagation *in vivo* are exceedingly complex.

6.4 HEMODYNAMIC THEORIES OF ATHEROGENESIS

As discussed earlier (Section 3.10), the development of atherosclerosis in large arteries is the leading cause of cardiovascular mortality in the Western world. Atherosclerosis is a dangerous disease because it not only obstructs the artery lumen, but it also may result in a plaque rupture where the fibrous cap covering the plaque breaks open and exposes a highly thrombogenic surface. The common sites of predilection of atherosclerosis in the human circulation were shown earlier in Figure 3.25. These sites include the coronary arteries, the branching of the subclavian and common carotids in the aortic arch, the bifurcation of the common carotid to internal and external carotids especially in the carotid sinus region distal to the bifurcation, the renal arterial branching in the descending aorta and in the ileofemoral bifurcations of the descending aorta. The common feature in the location for the development of the lesion is the presence of curvature, branching, and bifurcation present in these sites. The fluid dynamics at these sites can be anticipated to be vastly different from other segments of the arteries that are relatively straight and devoid of any branching segments. Hence, several investigators have attempted to link the fluid dynamically induced stresses with the formation of atherosclerotic lesions in the human circulation. The hemodynamic theories for the genesis of atheromatous plaques and the detailed description of the fluid dynamics at corresponding sites in the human circulation will be considered in the following sections.

It has been observed that, coincident with the geometric features, is a deviation of blood flow from simple antegrade, axial path lines to more complex patterns (Figure 6.15). What all of these changes have in common fluid dynamically is the presence of low, and potentially reversed, flow velocities associated with locally altered pressures and shear stresses.

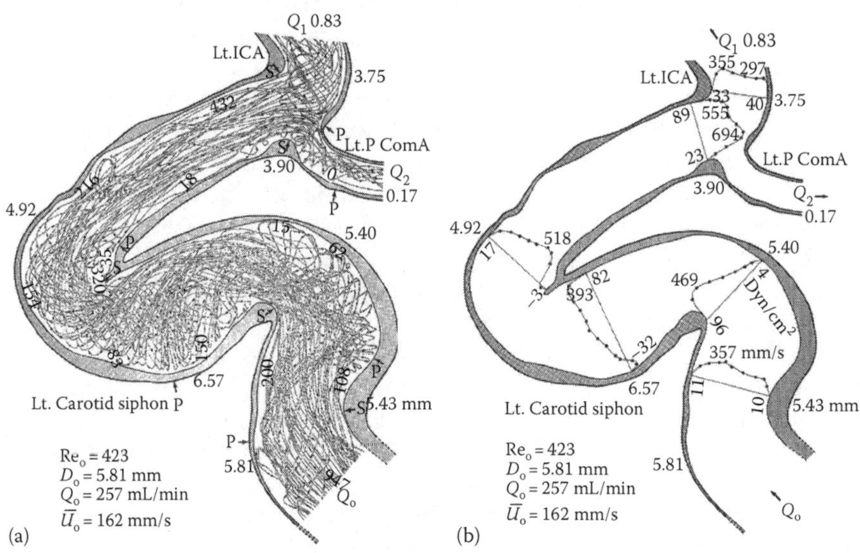

FIGURE 6.15 (a) Detailed flow patterns observed in steady flow in the carotid siphon prepared from a 70-year-old male subject showing the occurrence of flow separation at a proximal portion of the inner wall of each of the curved segments, strong deflection of the main flow at the sites of confrontation with the outer wall of the bends, development of strong secondary flows that resulted in the formation of a helicoidal flow, and formation of slow recirculation flows adjacent to the inner wall of the bends where atherosclerotic wall thickenings were localized. At the branching site of the PComA, formation of spiral secondary flows was observed in the distal portion of the ICA and the PComA due to strong deflection of the main flow at the vessel wall around the flow divider. Solid lines represent the paths of particles located in or close to the median plane; short, dotted lines represent paths far out of the median plane; and long, dotted lines represent particles located between the first two types of paths. The arrows at S and P indicate the points of flow separation and stagnation, respectively. The numbers at the outside of the vessel and along the particle paths indicate inner diameters of the vessel measured at each location and particle translational velocities (mm/s) at the positions shown, respectively. The numbers given under the letters Q_1 and Q_2 indicate the fraction of the flow that entered the particular branch out of the total inflow Q_o. (b) Distributions of fluid axial velocity and wall shear stress in the carotid siphon obtained in a vessel, which is the same as that shown in panel (a) and under the same flow conditions as those presented in panel (a). Atherosclerotic wall thickenings were found mainly along the inner walls of the bends in the carotid siphon and at the outer walls (hips) of the branching site of the PComA where both the fluid velocity and wall shear stress were low. The approaching velocity profile at the branching site of the PComA showed an asymmetrical bipolar shape with a summit having the highest velocity locating on the side of the PComA. Numbers at the outside and inside of the vessel indicate the inner diameter of the vessel and wall shear stress measured at each location, respectively. Numbers on each velocity profile indicate the fluid velocity at that location. (From *World Neurosurg.*, 73, Takeuchi, S. and Karino, T., Aneurysm flow patterns and distributions of fluid velocity and wall shear stress in the human internal carotid and middle cerebral arteries, 174–185, Copyright 2010, with permission from Elsevier.)

6.4.1 Low Pressure, Low and High Wall Shear Stress Theories

One of the earliest theories on the cause of atherosclerosis development was the *low pressure* theory (Texon, 1957). This publication was one of the first attempts to link fluid dynamics with atherogenesis. It was based on the hypothesis that at sites of arterial curvature such as the human aorta, as the blood is forced to turn around the curve, pressure will increase on the outer wall and correspondingly decrease at the inner wall of curvature. It was proposed that the pressure at the inner wall would decrease significantly to become negative and, hence, would literally pull the endothelium into the lumen, initiating the disease process. It was later shown that the radial pressure gradient is very small and that a significant decrease in pressure will not occur; hence, the effect proposed in this theory is not probable. Nonetheless, this publication was important in that it did contribute toward the thought process on hemodynamic effects on the endothelial cells and initiation of atheroma.

Some investigators have also suggested a role for elevated shear stress as an initiating factor in atherosclerosis because it would produce actual physical damage to the endothelial cells and also impair the normal mass transport process. In 1968, Fry published a significant study on the effect of wall shear stresses on the endothelial cells that formed the basis for the *high shear stress* theory. It consisted of *in vivo* canine studies in which he introduced a plug in the descending aorta with known dimensions of an orifice in order to increase the flow rate and wall shear stresses to which the endothelial cells would be exposed. The opening in the plug was eccentric so that part of the luminal circumference was exposed to the endothelial cells. By the analysis of the equations of motion, he justified neglecting the stresses due to local acceleration as well as turbulent stress fluctuations and used the time averaged wall shear stress relationship

$$\tau = \frac{R}{2}\frac{\partial p}{\partial z}$$

By measuring the time averaged pressure at various axial distances along the plug, he was able to calculate a range of wall shear stresses to which the endothelial cells were subjected. The ECs were exposed to known stresses for 1–3 h as Evans blue dye (which tags the diffusion of albumin into the wall) was injected into the bloodstream. The animals were then sacrificed and the tissue subjected to histological study to look at the morphology of the ECs. Fry concluded that ECs appeared to be normal if the time averaged shearing stresses were below $379 \pm 85\,\text{dyn/cm}^2$.

A more widely held hypothesis is that atherosclerosis is correlated with low fluid wall shear stress. The fundamental mechanism cited for this theory is that abnormally low wall shear stresses, τ_w, impair mass transport between blood and the vessel wall, potentially impacting not only the uptake of nutrients and oxygen by the vessel wall from the blood but also the release of waste products and carbon dioxide into the blood from the wall. This latter effect would help explain how material components typically found in atherosclerotic lesions and plaques, such as cholesterol, may build up in the vessel wall near regions with slow or stagnant flow. This *shear-dependent mass transport* theory was proposed by Caro et al. (1971) who like Texon observed differences in the hemodynamics of the aortic arch. Their focus, however, was on wall shear stress which is higher on the outer wall of aortic curvature and lower on the inner wall of curvature. And since atherosclerotic lesions occur along the inner wall of curvature where there is low shear stress, their proposal was that cholesterol is actually synthesized in the arterial wall and diffuses into the lumen where it is washed away by the bloodstream. In the regions of high wall shear stresses (and, hence, velocity gradients), more cholesterol is washed away by the blood flow. On the other hand, where the shear stress is low, excess cholesterol is deposited on the surface of the lumen initiating atheroma development. Thus, it is the shear-dependent mass transport that is responsible for atheroma growth. Furthermore, the endothelium has been shown to "switch" from an *atheroprotective* to an *atherogenic* state when exposed to low wall shear stress (Figure 6.16). Under low and oscillatory shear conditions, endothelial cells exist in a prothrombotic state and secrete more of those agents that promote increased thrombogenicity, vasoconstriction, and cellular proliferation.

Thus, low and high wall shear stress theories were debated for several years. Numerous model studies were performed to determine the velocity profile and shear stress distribution at the curvature and branching sites in the human circulation. Experimental studies included idealized models (2D and 3D) and subsequently castings made from cadaveric specimens. Studies included qualitative flow visualization and velocity measurements using hot-film anemometry and subsequently laser Doppler velocity measurements. Theoretical models were also initially restricted to 2D idealized models and then 3D models with regular geometries. Initially, studies were restricted to steady flow conditions to isolate regions of high and low wall shear stresses and correlate the same with regions of lesion presence *in vivo*. Subsequently, studies were extended to unsteady flow conditions for detailed analysis of time-dependent velocity profiles and wall shear stress distribution. With the development of more sophisticated measurement techniques such as laser Doppler and particle image velocimetry techniques (see Section 10.7), more detailed data analysis became possible. Simultaneously, with computational fluid dynamic algorithm development and the advent of high-speed computers, detailed CFD models were also developed (see Chapter 11). In addition, using sophisticated imaging modalities such as MRI (see Section 10.8), computed tomographic (CT), and ultrasound imaging, morphologically realistic 3D geometrical reconstruction of the segments of interest also became available. Studies on arterial sites of interest resulted in additional theories as well. As a result of this work, the high shear stress theory became less widely supported than the low shear stress theory since the levels of wall stress necessary for cellular erosion to occur were determined to be rarely seen under normal flow conditions.

6.4.2 Time Varying Wall Shear Stress, Oscillatory Shear Index, and Wall Shear Stress Gradients

While several studies have shown modest correlations between anatomic changes in the vessel wall and the mean wall shear stress acting on it, there is insufficient evidence to exclude other factors as well. Thus, additional theories have arisen based on the *rate of change of wall shear* (i.e., *wall shear stress gradients* [WSSG]) with respect to either time or position. This allows for consideration of the pulsatile nature of arterial flow and also the wide range of geometric shapes that exist in the arterial tree. Therefore, the temporal wall shear stress gradient, $\partial\tau_w/\partial t$, and the oscillatory

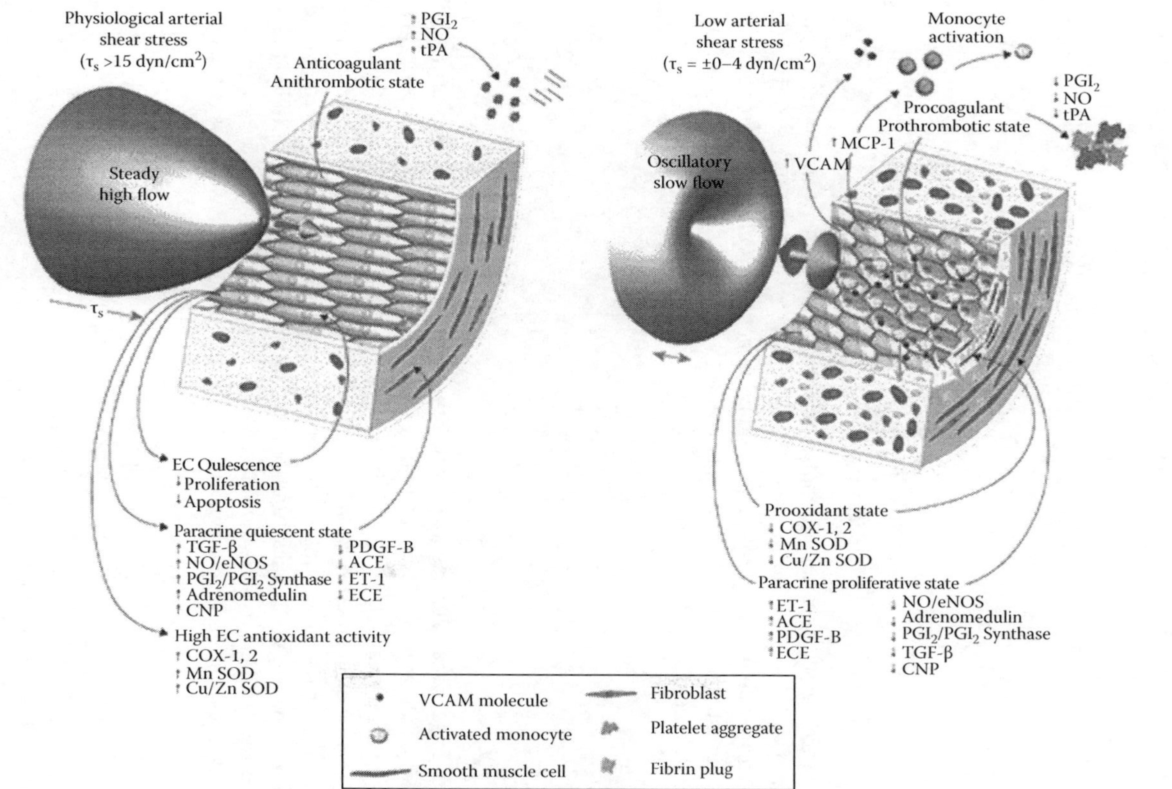

FIGURE 6.16 Effect of shear stress on endothelial cells (EC) and smooth muscle cells (SMC). (From Malek, A.M. et al., *JAMA*, 282, 2035, 1999. With permission from the American Medical Association.)

shear index, OSI, have been investigated to see if rapid changes in wall shear magnitude and/or direction, respectively, correlate with development of atherosclerosis. This could be due, for example, to greater stimulation of growth factors produced by endothelial cells and the consequent thickening of the vessel wall. The *temporal wall shear stress gradient* (TWSSG) is obtained by taking the time derivative to the magnitude of τ_w, and hence,

$$|TWSSG| = \frac{\partial \tau_w}{\partial t}$$

with its mean value calculated as

$$|TWSSG| = \frac{1}{T}\int_0^T |TWSSG|\, dt$$

In addition to regions experiencing pulsatile forward flow, there are many regions where the flow is reversed during part of the cardiac cycle causing the wall shear stress to vary from a large positive magnitude to negative values. Ku proposed an OSI and attempted to show a correlation of that with atheroma development (Ku et al., 1985). As defined,

$$OSI = 0.5\left(1 - \frac{\left|\int_0^T \tau_w\, dt\right|}{\int_0^T |\tau_w|\, dt}\right)$$

the OSI is greater than zero as long as there is some directional change during the flow cycle. The maximum value of OSI is 0.5 in the case of pure oscillatory flow without any net forward flow.

The *spatial wall shear stress gradient* (SWSSG) has been evaluated to determine if local changes in forces acting on the endothelial cells could induce gaps in the intercellular junction where mass transport would proceed in an uncontrolled manner. Since the wall shear stress tensor has two components, one in the mean wall shear stress direction "*m*" and one normal "*n*" to the same, the SWSSG is defined as

$$|SWSSG| = \sqrt{\left(\frac{\partial \tau_m}{\partial m}\right)^2 + \left(\frac{\partial \tau_n}{\partial n}\right)^2}$$

with its mean value being given as

$$|SWSSG| = \frac{1}{T}\int_0^T |SWSSG|\, dt$$

In spite of all these theories, none is able to completely explain the initiation and growth of atherosclerotic plaque. For example, with injury to the endothelium, plaque formation and development will also heavily depend on the transport of LDL-cholesterol and its absorption into the subendothelial region. Furthermore, some evidence has been presented in the literature that regions of hypoxia contribute toward plaque formation. Availability of oxygen is a limiting factor in the ability of cells to metabolize lipids and some models have suggested that in regions of stagnation and recirculation, the concentration of lipid is high (due to large residence time) whereas oxygen concentration is low (due to reduced saturation of oxygen in red blood cells in the region of stagnation and recirculation).

6.5 WALL SHEAR STRESS AND ITS EFFECT ON ENDOTHELIAL CELLS

While the generation of blood flow is provided by the heart, control of the distribution of flow to various organs is determined by changes in the resistance of individual vessels. These changes are dynamic and can be controlled either systemically or locally. Systemic regulation can be accomplished by either neural or hormonal signals. Within a given vessel, however, independent responses can be made to local changes in flow dynamics. In particular, changes in blood pressure and flow rate can be "sensed" by the vessel through a signal transduction process mediated through the endothelial cells. Since the endothelial cells are in direct contact with the blood, they can readily detect changes in flow dynamics by monitoring the forces acting on them, such as the normal force (i.e., pressure) and the longitudinal/axial force (i.e., shear stress). Thus, they become the key mechanosignal transducers of "information" between the blood and the vessel wall.

To accomplish this function, the endothelial cells are equipped with a variety of communication channels attached to the cell membrane which can sense force changes and then transmit corresponding signals to elicit specific responses (Figure 6.17). Some of these sensors are actually embedded in the membrane (e.g., integrins, G-protein and other receptors, specific ion channels, etc.) while others act through structures that are attached to the membrane and extend through the cytoplasm (e.g., actin fibers).

When these sensors are activated, the cell can elicit a number of responses that may involve its morphology, level of mass transport, stimulatory effects, or proliferative state. For example, one of the earliest responses of an endothelial cell to changes in the flow environment, especially to the shear stress acting upon it, is morphological and includes such things as a change in shape, orientation, and amount of its intracellular actin content (Figure 6.18).

Other responses include either increased or decreased passage of charged ions into the cell, changes in actin fiber orientation, and the release of various agents. It is also possible for these membrane-sensed signals to trigger the activity of the endothelial cell's nucleus, resulting in the production of specific proteins that alter the vessel's degree of thrombogenicity, constriction or dilation, or ability to increase

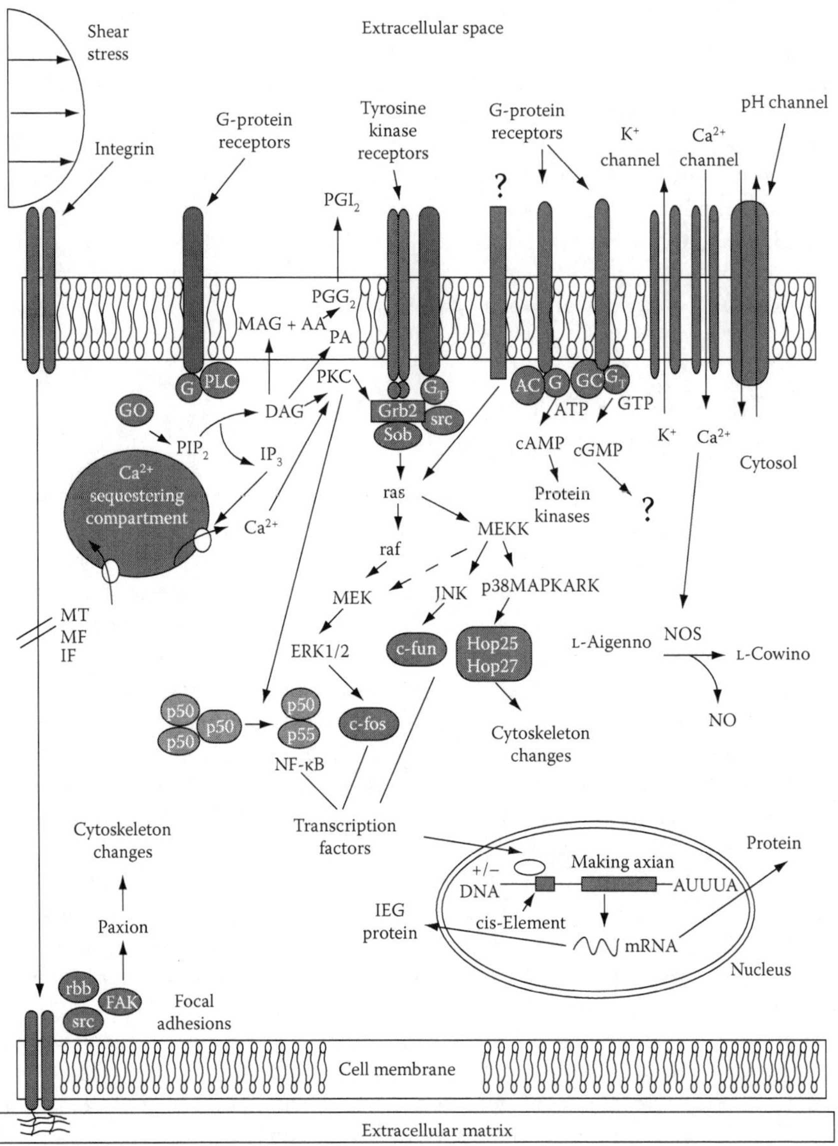

FIGURE 6.17 Schematic representation of the multiple "shear stress–responsive" signaling pathways, their cross talk, and integration. (With permission from Papadaki, M. and Eskin, S.G., Effects of fluid shear stress on gene regulation of vascular cells, *Biotechnol. Prog.*, 13, 209–221. Copyright 1997 American Chemical Society.)

wall thickness. This latter effect is mediated through *growth factors* that generally act upon neighboring subendothelial cells, primarily the smooth muscle cells and fibroblasts in the vessel media. Growth factors have the ability to cause these cells to replicate, migrate or, occasionally, to phenotypically change (i.e., take on new functions).

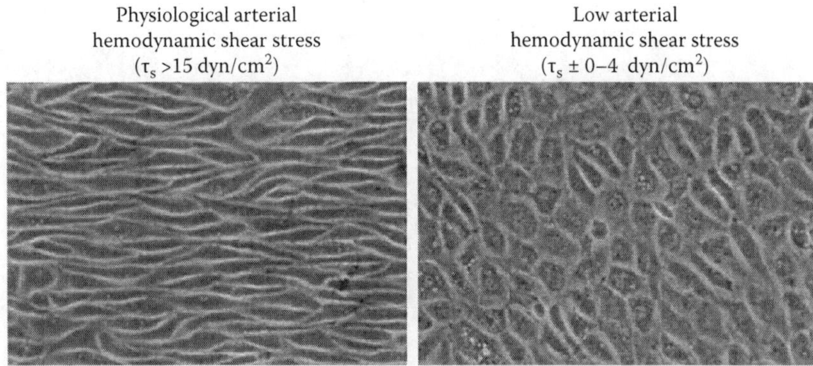

FIGURE 6.18 Transformation of endothelial cell morphology by fluid shear stress. (From Malek, A.M. et al., *JAMA*, 282, 2035, 1999. With permission from the American Medical Association.)

6.6 FLOW THROUGH CURVED ARTERIES AND BIFURCATIONS

Unlike many manmade flow systems that consist of long, straight, and uniformly sized tubes connected at the ends or at right angles to each other, the human arterial vasculature is a complex network of tapered and curved tubes connected at various angles and bifurcations with no distinct end points (Figure 6.19). While these geometric structures are necessary for carrying blood from the heart to other organs, they impose major changes on the patterns of flow through them that, in turn, affect the dynamics of the circulation and the forces acting on the inner lining of the vessels. As discussed in the following, this latter effect is the subject of much research into the possible causes of arterial disease (see Section 6.4).

6.6.1 Curved Vessels

One of the first anatomic features encountered by the blood upon its exit from the heart is the aortic arch (Figure 6.19). This curved shape enables the blood that is being ejected from the heart in a cephalic (i.e., toward the head) direction to reverse and move in a caudal (i.e., toward the feet) direction toward the body. Dean (1927) analyzed fully developed viscous flow in curved tubes with small curvature and since then numerous computational and experimental studies on curved tube flow have been reported in the literature. In brief, as the flow enters a curvature site, the fluid is being forced to change direction to follow the curve and, thus, a radial pressure gradient develops between the outer and inner wall of curvature. The fluid is also subjected to centrifugal force that is proportional to the square of the axial velocity. In the case of *inviscid* flow, these two forces balance each other and hence the axial velocity profile is skewed toward the inner wall of curvature and no secondary flow develops. With *viscous* fluid, the two opposing forces do not balance each other and hence a *secondary flow* develops resulting in two vortices, called "Dean vortices." The axial velocity profile becomes skewed toward the *outer wall of curvature* as shown in Figure 6.20 where higher wall shear stresses are then found.

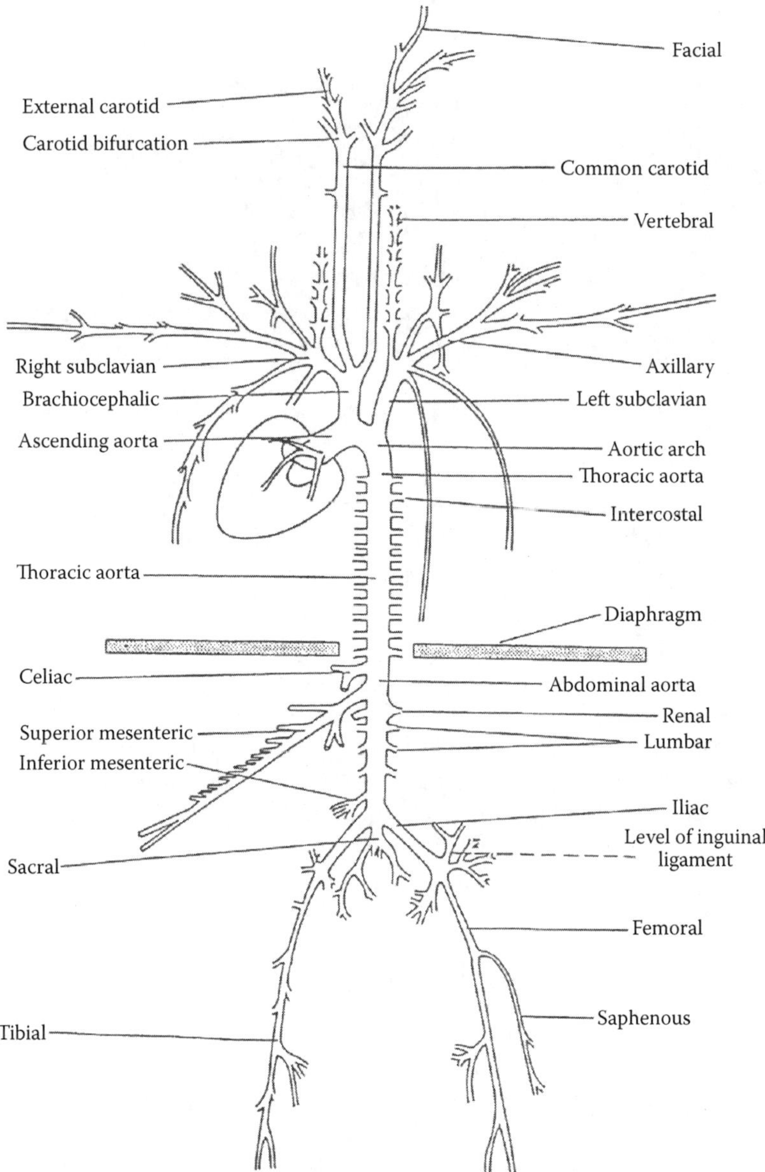

FIGURE 6.19 Anatomy of major systemic arteries (canine). (From Caro, C.G., Fitz-gerald, J.M., Pedley, T.J., and Schroter, R.C., *Proc. Roy. Soc. London B*, 1978 by permission of Oxford University Press.)

As the curvature continues, however, those high velocity regions eventually impact with the outer wall and are deflected in a circumferential direction. The result is that blood with a high axial velocity now acquires a circumferential component as well and is convected around the outer surface of the aorta toward the *inner* curvature of the vessel. The velocity profile at this point takes on a reverse image of the outwardly

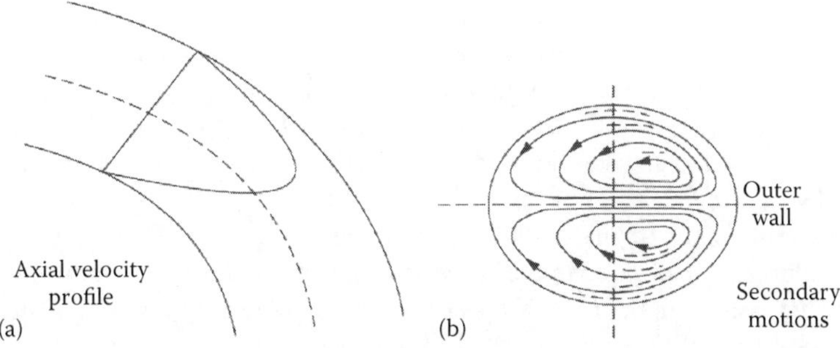

FIGURE 6.20 Schematic of the flow development in a curved vessel with secondary flow: (a) skewed axial velocity profile and (b) the secondary motion plot in a cross section in the curved segment.

skewed profile seen more proximally. The axial locations where these transitions occur vary depending upon the exact geometry of the vessel and the flow rate (i.e., the CO). Superimposed on this is the fact that flow into the aortic arch is a developing flow since the velocity profile at the aortic root past the aortic valve is relatively flat. In developing flow, the viscous effect is confined to the boundary layer region initially and the fluid in the core region acts as inviscid fluid. Hence, the velocity profile is initially skewed toward the inner wall of the tube and slowly moves toward the outer wall in the downstream region. Furthermore, the aortic arch is not only curved in the lateral plane (i.e., left-to-right), but it also has a degree of curvature in the anteroposterior (AP) plane (i.e., front-to-back). Arterial branches from the arch directed toward the head (e.g., the innominate, carotid, and vertebral arteries) also affect these flow patterns as they siphon off about 25% of the cardiac output and the cross section in the descending aorta is reduced by about 40% from that in the ascending aorta.

The classic approach to analyzing *steady* flows in this type of geometry is to apply the Bernoulli equation (see Section 1.6) in a form that also allows for energy losses to occur. This "modified Bernoulli equation"

$$p+\rho\frac{V^2}{2}+\rho gz = H \tag{1.62}$$

includes the term, H, called the "head loss" (in units of pressure), that accounts for the fact that energy is dissipated through frictional and nonaxial flow motion effects. The value of H is obtained by applying an experimental coefficient, K_L, to the term $\rho V^2/2$ where V is the mean velocity in the tube. For a 180° bend, K_L is approximately equal to 0.2.

Further complicating these geometric factors is the high degree of pulsatility of flow in the aorta ($\alpha \approx 20$), which leads to rapid changes in inertia, limited boundary layer development, and more stable (i.e., less turbulent) flow. Analysis of purely oscillatory flow in a curved tube have shown that the viscous effects are confined to the boundary layer region, thus producing four Dean vortices in a cross section where the vortices in the boundary layer region are opposite in direction to the vortices in the core region. During *systole*, the flow is accelerated forward along the curved tube, and secondary flow leads to skewing of the axial velocity profile. During *early diastole*, flow moving along the inner wall of curvature reverses direction; hence, the wall shear stress along the inner wall is reversed whereas slight forward flow persists along the outer wall of curvature. Thus, the axial velocity profile is initially skewed toward the outer wall; the maximum axial velocity then moves toward the inner wall and subsequently moves toward the outer wall again. As a result, the inner wall region is subjected to an oscillating shear stress that is forward in systole but reverse in diastole (Figure 6.21a and b).

The secondary flow consists of a single vortex in the form of a corkscrew that persists below the diaphragm in the descending aorta and this secondary flow affects the flow distribution in the renal arteries as well as in the iliac bifurcation. The secondary flow also reverses direction during diastole.

Due to the importance of vessel curvature upon flow development, a nondimensional parameter known as the *Dean number*, N_D, has been defined as

$$N_D = Re\left(\sqrt{\frac{R_v}{R_c}}\right) \quad (6.15)$$

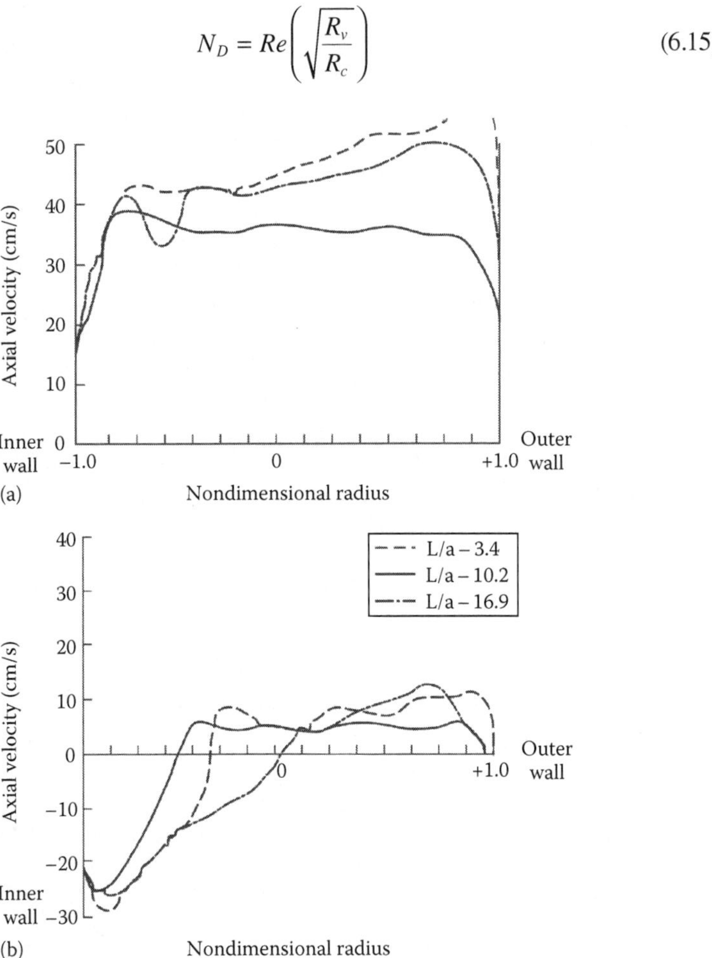

FIGURE 6.21 Axial velocity profiles in (a) systole and (b) diastole at various cross sections in a curved tube. (From Chandran, K.B., *J. Biomech. Eng.*, 115, 611, 1993. With permission from the American Society of Mechanical Engineers.)

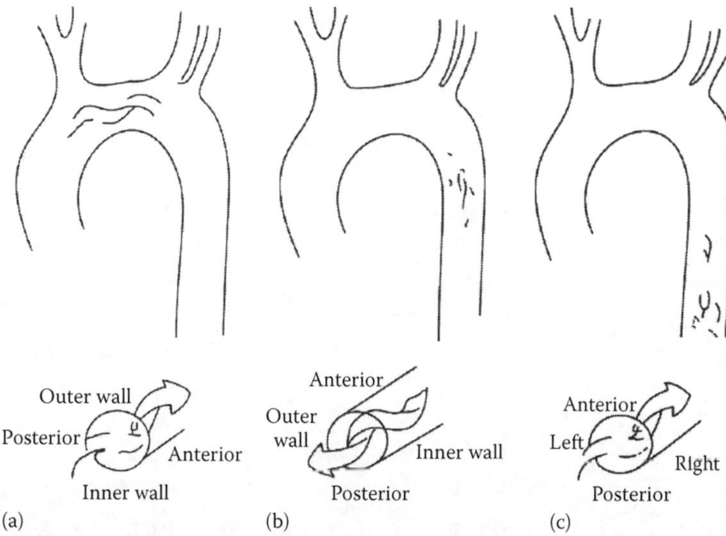

FIGURE 6.22 Forward and backward directed helices in the aorta during: (a) peak systole; (b) end systole; and (c) diastole. (From Frazin, L.J., Lanza, G., Vonesh, M., Khasho, F., Spitzzeri, C., McGee, S., Mehlman, D., Chandran, K.B., Talano, J., and McPherson, D.D., Functional chiral asymmetry in descending thoracic aorta, *Circulation*, 82, 1985–1994, 1990. With permission from W.W. Lippincott Co.)

and can be used for evaluating flow patterns in the aortic arch. This parameter is based on the more familiar Reynolds number, *Re*, which has been modified by the inclusion of the relative size of the vessel, R_v, and its radius of curvature, R_c. As can be seen, a high Dean number indicates significant inertial effects and/or a small radius of curvature resulting in enhanced secondary flow motions. A low Dean number, on the other hand, would indicate relatively unimportant secondary flow effects. In the human aorta, the average Dean number is high (~1500) due to a large *Re* and small R_c. The increased magnitude of the Reynolds number during systole (~8000) also leads to a higher Dean number and, thus, stronger secondary motions. The combination of strong secondary motions and rapid changes in flow rate gives rise to reversals of the helical pattern in the aortic arch as flow first accelerates (systole) and then decelerates (diastole) (Figure 6.22).

Other vascular sites where curvature effects can be important are in the coronary bifurcation (whose geometry varies dynamically with the beating heart) and the aorto-iliac bifurcation which has a slight curvature out of the AP plane.

6.6.2 Bifurcations and Branches

While there are several major bifurcations in the arterial system, there is only one that is nearly symmetrical—the *aorto-iliac bifurcation* (Figure 6.23). This site is distinguished by branch vessels each having cross-sectional areas of about 60% of that of the terminal aorta (i.e., their total branch area = 1.2 times the aortic area) and angles

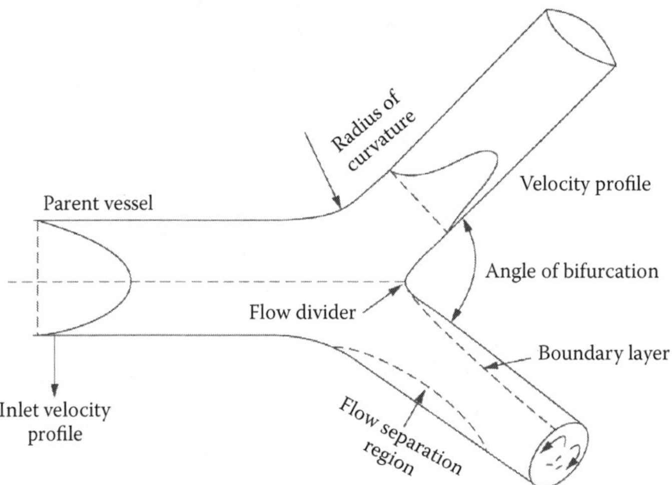

FIGURE 6.23 Schematic of the aorto-iliac bifurcation geometry and the flow development in the branch vessels.

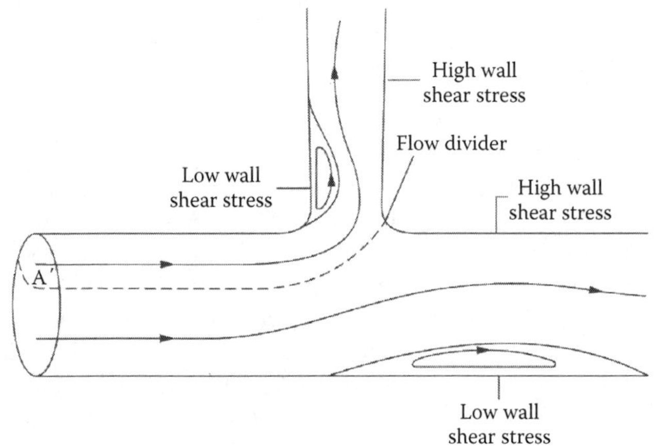

FIGURE 6.24 Schematic of an arterial branching site.

of about 30° from the body axis. Branching of a vessel (Figure 6.24) can originate from a main artery (such as the renal arterial branch from the descending aorta).

As blood enters the bifurcation site, the flow divides into the two daughter vessels at the *flow divider* region (medial junction of the iliac arteries). At the divider walls of bifurcations, the boundary layers are relatively thin with maximum axial velocity outside the boundary layer. As the blood enters the daughter vessel with a finite radius of curvature, the faster moving fluid is found toward the flow divider due to secondary flow development. If the corners of the outer wall are sharp, flow separation may be present along the outer wall of the bifurcation (lateral iliac arteries).

With an asymmetric bifurcation such as the junction of the left main into the left anterior descending (LAD) and circumflex (Cx) coronary arteries, the flow in the

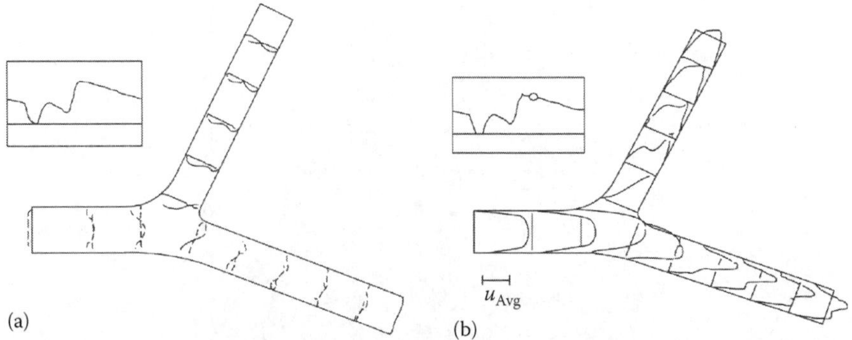

FIGURE 6.25 Axial velocity profiles in the left anterior descending and left circumflex coronary artery during (a) systole and (b) diastole. (From He, X. and Ku, D.N., *J. Biomech. Eng.*, 118, 74, 1996. With permission from the American Society of Mechanical Engineers.)

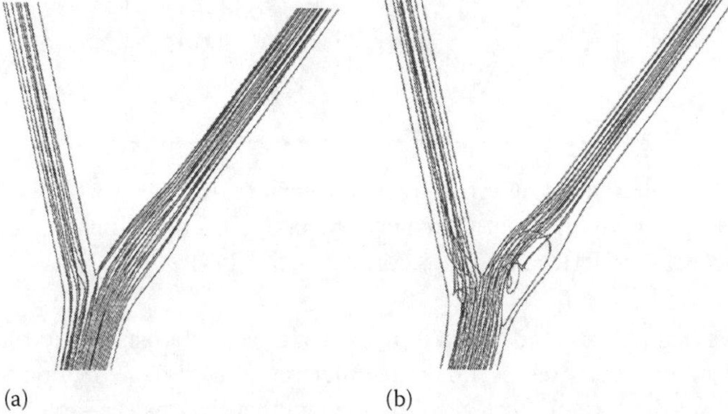

FIGURE 6.26 Streamlines in a model of the carotid bifurcation during: (a) systole and (b) diastole. (From Berger, S.A. and Jou, L.A., *Annu. Rev. Fluid Mech.*, 32, 347, 2000. With permission.)

daughter vessels will not be equal and flow separation may exist in the branch with reduced flow as shown in Figure 6.25. A similar flow distribution would be anticipated in a branch vessel such as a T-junction, roughly corresponding to renal arterial branches off the descending aorta. With an unequal flow distribution, flow separation and low wall shear stresses are found along the outer walls.

Other important arterial bifurcations occur in the carotid (Figure 6.26) and the vertebral basilar (which has a unique converging-diverging configuration) (Figure 6.27) circulations where similar flow effects are seen.

The common carotid artery originates at the aortic arch and bifurcates into the external and internal carotid arteries at the neck level. The external carotid supplies blood to the facial area while the internal carotid provides blood to the brain. A unique feature of the internal carotid artery is that it has a bulge at the bifurcation region, referred to as the *carotid sinus*. Presence of the sinus acts to further accentuate the tendency for flow separation along the outer wall, resulting in a large separation zone that has been widely observed in healthy volunteers. Over time, however, these

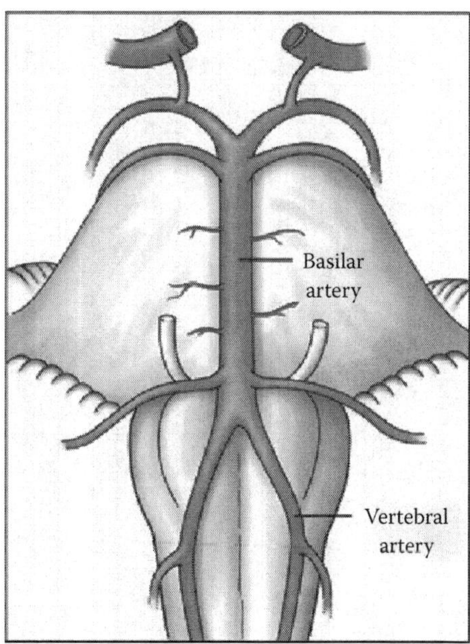

FIGURE 6.27 Depiction of the vertebrobasilar cerebrovasculature. (From University of Illinois, College of Medicine at Chicago, Chicago, IL, http://chicago.medicine.uic.edu/cms/one.aspx?objectId=2862354&contextId=506244)

features have been implicated in the initiation of atherosclerosis due to the resultant low and reversing shear stresses along the outer vessel walls (see Section 6.4).

Arterial branches are characterized by the fact that they have a large discrepancy between the cross-sectional areas of the side branch and the main artery (Figure 6.24). Typical ratios for the total area of the outlet branches to the area of the inlet artery can range from 0.8 to 1.3. There is also a wide variation of takeoff angles for the branches with many of these being large and some approaching 90°, such as the intercostal arteries (branches off the thoracic aorta) and the renal arteries (branches off the abdominal aorta). Due to the large asymmetry at a branch, flow in the branch vessel is characterized by (1) velocity profiles that are highly skewed toward the flow divider, (2) secondary flow motions, and (3) a tendency for flow separation along the outer walls. Distal to the branch point, flow in the main vessel (e.g., the abdominal aorta distal to the mesenteric artery) becomes skewed toward the branch, contains secondary flow, and may demonstrate separated flow along the wall opposite to the branch orifice (Figure 6.28). As a result of these features, wall shear stresses are generally higher along the flow divider and lower along both the outer wall of the branch and the wall opposing the branch. Again, these latter features coincide closely to the observed sites of atherosclerosis development in patients.

It is possible to estimate the changes in energy distribution through a branch section if we apply the "modified Bernoulli equation" to this geometry. Here, the appropriate value of K_L would depend on the degree of corner roundness, the branch angle, and so on, and would typically have a value of ~1.0.

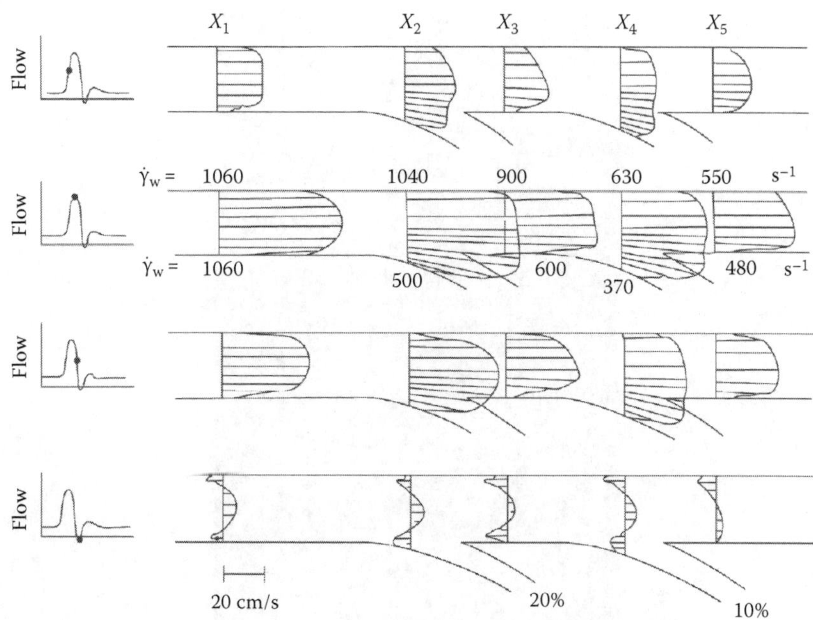

FIGURE 6.28 Composite laser Doppler velocity profiles in flow model at five axial locations and at four times during the flow pulsatile wave. Peak flow rates estimated from slope of velocity profile and the corresponding wall shear rates are shown on second figure from top. (From *J. Biomech.*, 16, Lutz, R.J., Hsu, L., Menawat, A., Zrubek, J., and Edwards, K., Comparison of steady and pulsatile flow in a double branching arterial model, 753–766, Copyright 1983, with permission from Elsevier.)

6.7 FLOW THROUGH ARTERIAL STENOSES AND ANEURYSMS

The result of atherosclerosis is the development of an obstruction, or *stenosis*, within the vessel which eventually either reduces or completely blocks its blood flow. Initially, as the lesion grows, the arterial wall remodels and becomes thinner in order to accommodate the lesion and maintain the lumen cross-sectional area. However, after the limit for remodeling is reached, the lesion starts to protrude into the lumen and occludes the cross-sectional area available for flow of blood. With increasing occlusion and reduced cross-sectional area becoming available for flow of blood, the blood flow dynamics past the stenosis becomes complex (Figure 6.29). Until the lesion is at advanced stages, there are no clinical symptoms and currently there are no reliable methods to detect the lesions in the early stages when appropriate pharmacological or mechanical interventions can be utilized to arrest or reverse the disease process. In general, the atherosclerotic plaque often progresses to a moderate or severe level (e.g., 50%–99% occlusion) and then either a blood clot forms in the remaining vessel lumen which stops flow or a piece of the plaque and/or thrombus breaks off and *embolizes* (i.e., migrates) distally to a small arterial branch causing ischemia or tissue death. Stenoses are characterized by being very *focal* (i.e., they only extend over a short distance) and generally *eccentric* (i.e., asymmetric) in shape.

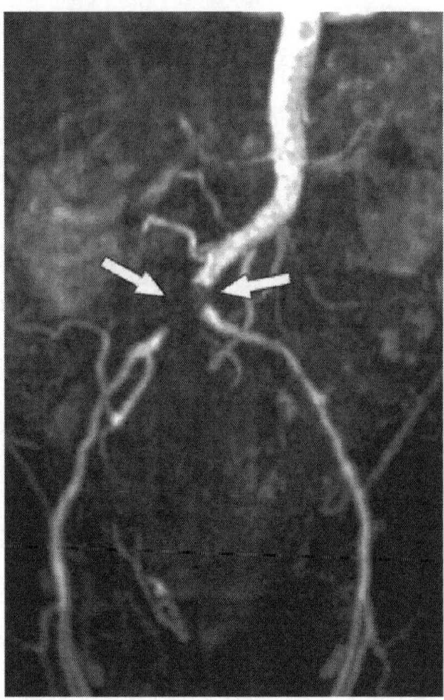

FIGURE 6.29 Contrast-enhanced MR angiography (CE-MRA) with 0.1 mmol/kg of gadobenate dimeglumine displays entire peripheral runoff vasculature to calf arteries. Short segment occlusion of right common iliac artery and high-grade stenosis of left common iliac artery are evident (*arrows*). (From Thurnher, S. et al., *AJR*, 189, 1223. With permission from The American Roentgen Ray Society.)

From a fluid mechanics standpoint, stenoses are sites that can produce relatively large changes in local velocity as governed by the *conservation of mass*

$$V_1A_1 = V_2A_2$$

or

$$V_2 = \left(\frac{A_1}{A_2}\right)V_1$$

where

V_1 and V_2 are the mean velocities
A_1 and A_2 are the areas of cross sections 1 and 2, respectively

Since A_1 is always greater than A_2 (site of stenosis), V_2 will be larger than V_1. This increased velocity is accompanied by formation of a *jet* through the stenosis (Figure 6.30).

Due to the Bernoulli effect, the increased velocity present at the throat of the stenosis also produces a reduced pressure. With increasing degree of stenosis, the pressure at the throat can decrease significantly and may even cause the vessel to collapse.

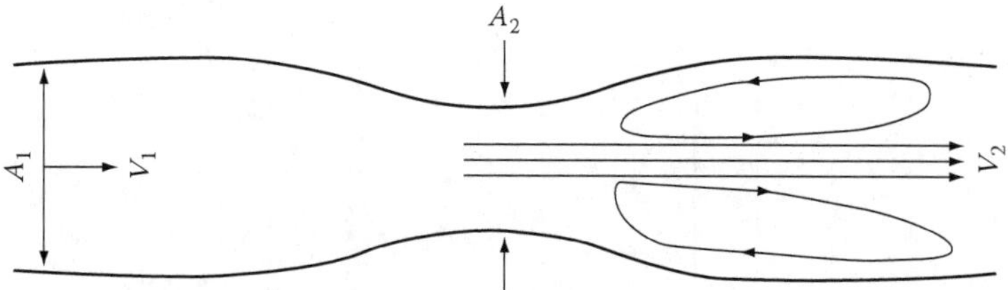

FIGURE 6.30 Schematic of flow through a stenosis.

Distal to the stenosis, vortices may be present and the flow may become turbulent with more severe degrees of stenosis. In these cases of advanced stenosis, autopsy results have shown that the plaques actually rupture, producing thrombus deposition at this site that induces a sudden occlusion of the vessel. Hence, research studies are also being performed to characterize unstable plaques in order to better predict rupture of the plaques.

Upon exit into the undiseased artery downstream, the high jet momentum causes it to persist for a finite distance before expanding to fill the normal vessel cross-sectional area. In this distal region, the flow is said to separate from the vessel wall before eventually reattaching. This *separated flow region* between the jet and the vessel wall contains slower moving and recirculating (i.e., reversing) flow. Studies have shown that flow separation and reattachment generally start with stenoses having 40% occlusion and that the region of separation increases with increasing flow rate. Formation of multiple vortices is seen with higher area occlusion. As can be observed, flow separation distal to the stenosis is not observed with the asymmetric stenosis. Further growth in the lesion is probably required for flow separation to be induced with asymmetric stenosis. These simulations are all based on steady flow analysis in rigid stenoses of regular geometry, whereas actual stenoses will have an irregular 3D geometry. With further growth in stenosis, flow separation, pressure fluctuations, and turbulent stresses may induce rupture at the distal site resulting in thrombus growth and occlusion of the vessel or emboli lodging in the distal flow field creating cardiac arrest or neurological deficit.

In some cases, blood in the jet may accelerate to velocities where the Reynolds number may be in the *turbulent range*. One consequence of this is the production of heat and diagnostically useful sounds. In stenosed heart valves, these sounds are called "*murmurs*" while in stenosed arteries they are referred to as "*Bruits*." Due to the complex flow patterns observed, there is a measurable pressure drop across a stenosis due to energy losses associated with recirculating and nonaxial flow movement and the possible onset of turbulence. This pressure drop may be approximated by considering the stenosis as a sudden contraction/expansion combination similar to the "modified Bernoulli equation" used earlier in the analysis of curves and branches to obtain

$$\Delta p = K_L\left(\rho\frac{V^2}{2}\right)$$

where K_L for a rounded entrance would be ~0.04 and K_L for a rounded exit would be ~1.0.

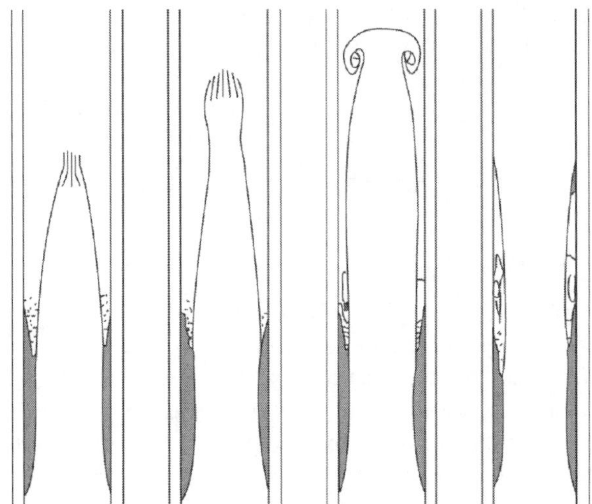

FIGURE 6.31 Flow patterns through symmetric stenoses of 20% diameter reduction. (From *J. Vasc. Surg.*, 12, Rittgers, S.E. and Shu, M.C.S., Doppler color-flow images from a stenosed arterial model: Interpretation of flow patterns, 511–522, Copyright 1990, with permission from Elsevier.)

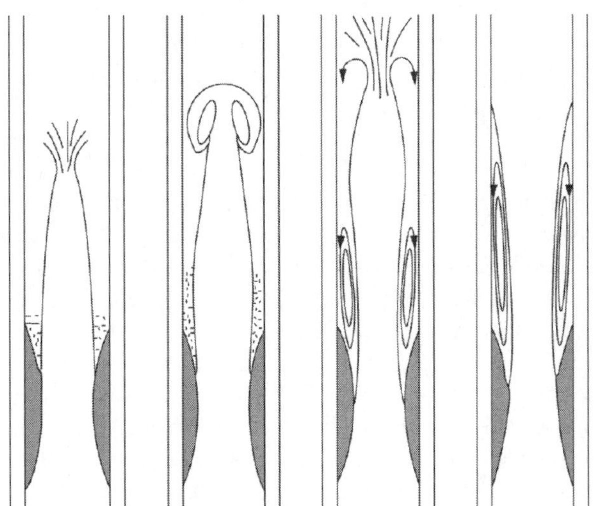

FIGURE 6.32 Flow patterns through symmetric stenoses of 40% diameter reduction. (From *J. Vasc. Surg.*, 12, Rittgers, S.E. and Shu, M.C.S., Doppler color-flow images from a stenosed arterial model: Interpretation of flow patterns, 511–522, Copyright 1990, with permission from Elsevier.)

Examples of pulsatile flow through a series of symmetric stenoses are shown in Figures 6.31 through 6.34. The diagrams illustrate flow patterns at and downstream of *symmetrical* stenoses of 20%, 40%, 60%, and 80% diameter reduction under flow conditions simulating those in a carotid artery. As can be seen, a jet is formed through the stenosis that reaches a maximum length for 40% and 60% cases.

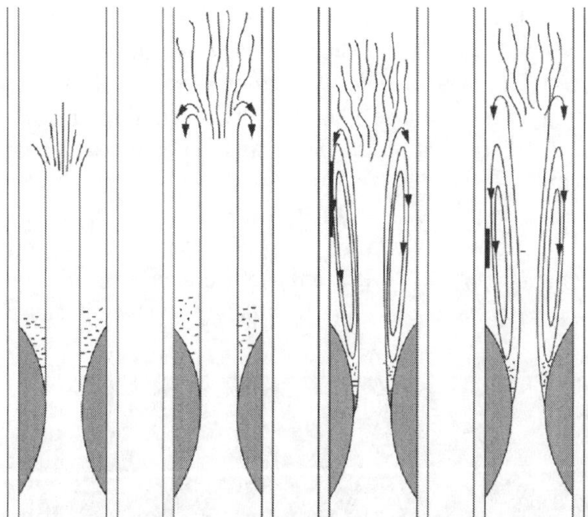

FIGURE 6.33 Flow patterns through symmetric stenoses of 60% diameter reduction. (From *J. Vasc. Surg.*, 12, Rittgers, S.E. and Shu, M.C.S., Doppler color-flow images from a stenosed arterial model: Interpretation of flow patterns, 511–522, Copyright 1990, with permission from Elsevier.)

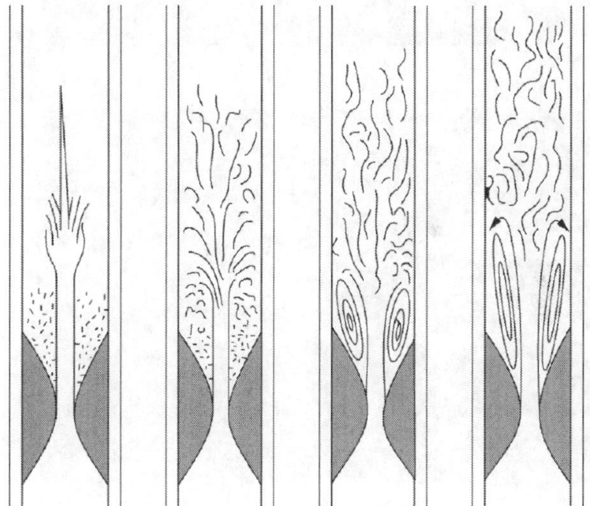

FIGURE 6.34 Flow patterns through symmetric stenoses of 80% diameter reduction (From *J. Vasc. Surg.*, 12, Rittgers, S.E. and Shu, M.C.S., Doppler color-flow images from a stenosed arterial model: Interpretation of flow patterns, 511–522, Copyright 1990, with permission from Elsevier.)

With further stenosis (80% case), the jet shortens and becomes turbulent. In all cases, a separation zone is seen outside the jet in which flow recirculation occurs across a region proportional in size to the degree of stenosis. It can further be seen that these patterns fluctuate during the flow cycle, with the jet being most pronounced at either peak systole or during the deceleration phase. Flow separation zones are generally larger and more stable during the late diastolic phase. The presence of a severe stenosis (Figure 6.34) may cause a reduced flow rate through the artery and then a lack of oxygen (*ischemia*) and nutrients to tissues downstream. Mild to moderate stenoses, however, often do not produce a significant reduction in blood flow because of the vascular bed dilatation that occurs downstream, compensating for the increased resistance upstream.

Stenosis eccentricity produces a further elevation of the wall shear stresses, especially along the crown, or cap, of the plaque as well as enlarging the size of the separation zone (Figure 6.35). It is easy to see from these data how wall shear stresses might cause *plaque cap rupture* in which the connective tissue covering the

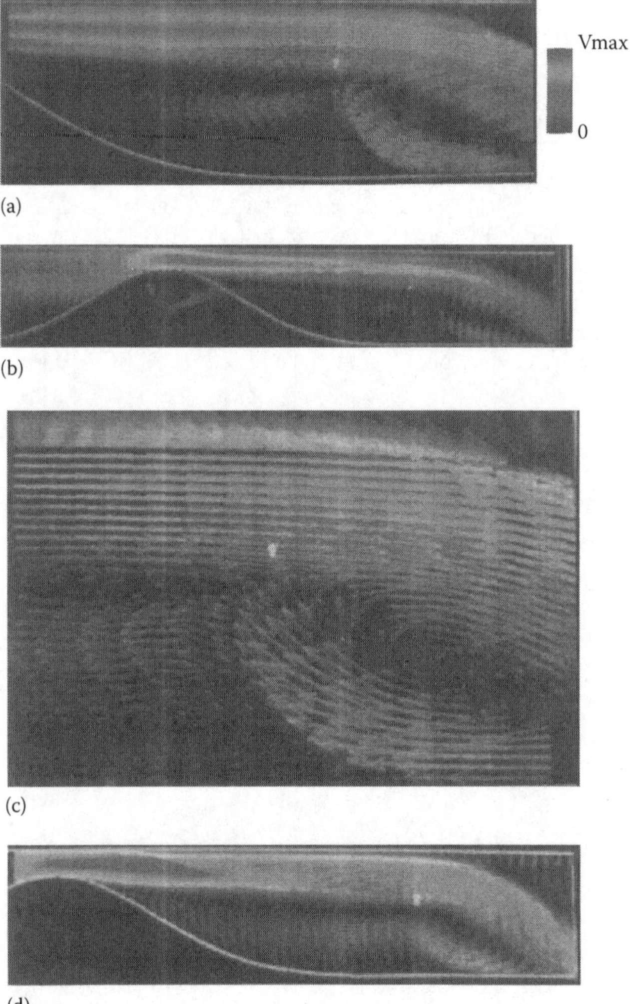

FIGURE 6.35 Flow simulation in a 95% eccentric arterial stenosis. (a) Acceleration phase; (b) peak systole; (c) detail of separation zone during peak systole; and (d) deceleration phase.

atherosclerotic plaque is removed, exposing the highly thrombogenic plaque contents to the bloodstream and inducing rapid thrombosis.

Model results such as those shown earlier are very useful in identifying the most relevant parameters to measure for diagnostic purposes and also for determining the potential for clinical consequences (i.e., thrombosis formation) by studying the high shear levels in the jet and the long residence times in the recirculation zones. If the flow is turbulent, it may be severe enough to cause hemolysis of red blood cells or activation of platelets. This latter effect is an important consequence since, once activated, platelets may enter the recirculation zones and reside long enough to attach to the vessel wall and stimulate other platelets to become activated. If the resultant platelet aggregation proceeds to a critical mass, a thrombus may form and grow to occlude the entire vessel.

Another important clinical problem involves the abnormal dilation of major arteries, called *aneurysm formation* (see Section 5.3.2). *Abdominal aortic aneurysms* (AAA) are by far the most common sites while aneurysms of the descending thoracic aorta, transverse aortic arch, thoraco-abdominal aorta, and popliteal artery are also seen, often in conjunction with AAAs (Figure 6.36). Less frequently, aneurysms

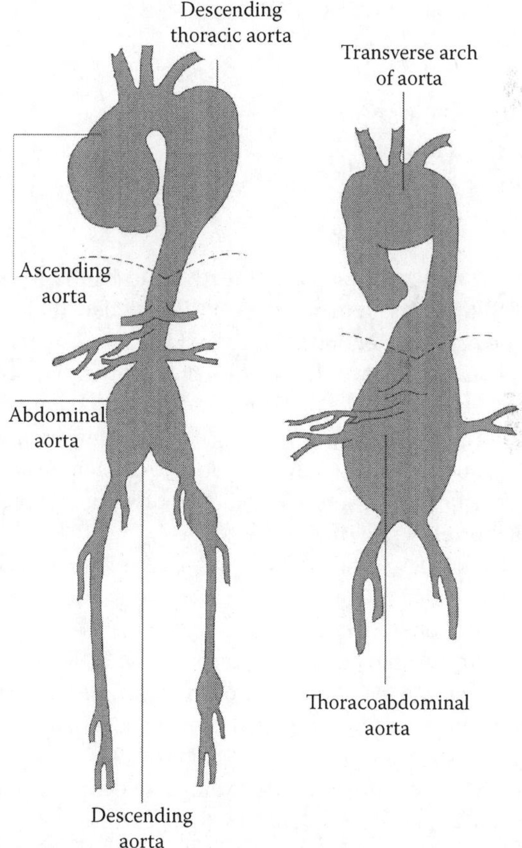

FIGURE 6.36 Patterns of aneurysmal vascular disease. (From Gotto, A.M. et al., *Atherosclerosis*, Upjohn, Pfizer, Inc., New York, 1977. With permission.)

may also form intracranially within one of the vessels making up the Circle of Willis or adjacent arteries. This condition is particularly critical since rupture of an artery within the brain would lead to ischemia and elevated pressure on the surrounding tissues which cannot be relieved by expansion of the skull. Geometrically, aneurysms generally fall into one of the two categories: (1) symmetrical or "fusiform" aneurysms where the expansion occurs uniformly around the circumference of the vessel and (2) asymmetrical or "saccular" aneurysms where the expansion is restricted only to part of the circumference.

There are several biomechanical implications of this disease. One is that the vessel will experience increased wall stresses which, if allowed to progress, will eventually rupture the vessel. For the case of a fusiform aneurysm, the level of wall stresses can be approximated by using *LaPlace's equation* for a symmetric, thin-walled cylinder. Summing the forces acting on the upper half of the vessel and setting them equal to zero give

$$\sigma_\theta = \frac{pR}{t} \tag{2.24}$$

where

σ_θ is the circumferential wall stress (N/m^2)
t is the wall thickness (m)
p is the internal pressure (N/m^2)
R is the cylinder radius (m)

Thus, the stress in the wall will increase directly with its diameter, assuming that the pressure and wall thickness remain constant (in practice, the wall also thins due to *conservation of mass* and continued enzymatic activity). This, in turn, further increases the vessel diameter until it reaches a size and wall stress beyond which rupture is imminent. From clinical experience, an abdominal aorta of 5 cm diameter (compared with a normal diameter of $\leq$2 cm) has a rupture risk of about 5% per year and is, therefore, used as a value for initiating treatment (usually placement of a bypass graft). It is critical to diagnose patients by this time since those aneurysms that rupture have a mortality rate of about 50%.

From a fluid mechanics viewpoint, this large expansion of the vessel produces unusual flow characteristics that include large vortices near the vessel walls and a central stream whose dimensions depend on the size and eccentricity of the AAA. Vortices form in the bulge region of an aneurysm and, due to the Bernoulli effect, the pressure at the bulged cross section increases. Due to the stagnant blood in the bulge, thrombus deposition and growth can also occur in this region. Detailed computational analysis of the hemodynamics within aneurysms will be presented in Sections 11.3.2 and 11.3.4.

Conservation of mass requires that the average velocity through the aneurysm must decrease and since blood has a tendency to clot when moving slowly or when static, most aneurysms develop thrombus within the dilated pockets. Some may then form a pseudo flow channel similar in size to that of the undiseased (normal) vessel. This can be quite dangerous because the aorta may appear normal on radiographic arteriography when, in fact, the vessel wall is highly stretched and weakened. In some cases, thrombus from an AAA may embolize to distal sites such as the foot, producing an ischemic condition known as a "blue toe" syndrome. Surgical treatment of AAA involves exposure of the aorta, removal of the diseased segments, and placement of a graft (typically *Dacron*) and this also has an associated risk to the patient. Since not all AAAs larger than 5 cm rupture and some smaller aneurysms do, biomechanical studies are ongoing in order to study their fluid dynamics and effects upon the wall to better predict wall stress distributions in the AAA and the possible potential for rupture.

6.8 SUMMARY

In this chapter, some of the unsteady flow models to simulate blood flow in arteries were presented. Even though the wave propagation through the elastic tube was included in the models, more emphasis was put on the nature of blood flow through the arteries. Description of the various hemodynamic theories correlating flow dynamics in curved arterial segments, as well as in regions of bifurcations and branches with the genesis and growth of atheroma in these regions has been included. The nature of unsteady flow dynamics in arterial curvature and bifurcation sites, as well as in the region of stenosis and aneurysm is also discussed.

PROBLEMS

6.1 Show that the Womersley parameter is analogous to the Reynolds number for unsteady flow.

6.2 For a typical human aorta, the diameter of the lumen is 30 mm and the thickness of the wall is 4 mm. Assuming a blood density of 1.056 g/cm^3 and a viscosity of 0.035 P, calculate the Womersley number if the heart rate is 72 bpm. Diameters for the carotid and femoral arteries of a typical human are about 0.8 and 0.5 cm, respectively. Compute the Womersley numbers for each of these arterial segments for the same heart rate.

6.3 In an experiment on an exposed abdominal aorta of a dog, the pulse wave speed is determined to be 1.5 m/s. The wall thickness of the artery was measured to be 5% of the diameter. Estimate the Young's modulus for the aorta. In another segment of the same artery, the pulse wave speed was double the previous value. What can you conclude from this?

6.4 List the assumptions made in deriving the Moens–Korteweg relationship for wave propagation.

6.5 In deriving the relationship for the velocity profiles for oscillatory motion in an elastic tube, Morgan and Kiely assumed that the pressure gradient followed the relationship

$$p = Pe^{i(kz-\omega t)} \quad \text{where } k = k_1 + ik_2$$

Under these conditions, show that k_2 represents a damping constant.

6.6 In the derivations of velocity profiles for oscillatory flow of viscous fluid through an elastic tube assuming axisymmetric flow (Figure 6.3), list the boundary conditions used in obtaining the solution. Here, u and w are the velocity components while η and ξ are the tube displacements in the radial and axial directions, respectively.

6.7 The pressure gradient and flow rate measured in the femoral artery of a dog are shown in Figure 6.11. Resolve them into their first four harmonics and plot them. Also, plot the sum of the four harmonics and compare this with the measured signals.

REFERENCES

Berger, S. A. and Jou, L. A. (2000) Flow in stenotic vessels. *Annu. Rev. Fluid Mech.* 32: 347–382.

Caro, C. G., Fitz-gerald, J. M., Pedley, T. J., and Schroter, R. C. (1971) Atheroma and arterial wall shea. Observation, correlation and proposal of a shear dependent mass transfer mechanism for atherogenesis. *Proc. Roy. Soc. London B* 177: 109–159.

Chandran, K. B. (1993) Flow dynamics in the human aorta. *J. Biomech. Eng.* 115: 611–615.

Dean, W. R. (1927) Note on the motion of fluid in a curved pipe. *Phil. Mag.* 20: 208–223.

Frazin, L. J., Lanza, G., Vonesh, M., Khasho, F., Spitzzeri, C., McGee, S., Mehlman, D., Chandran, K. B., Talano, J., and McPherson, D. D. (1990) Functional chiral asymmetry in descending thoracic aorta. *Circulation* 82: 1985–1994.

Fry, D. L. (1968) Acute vascular endothelial changes associated with increased blood velocity gradients. *Circ. Res.* 22: 165–197.

Gotto Jr., A. M., Robertson Jr., A. L., Epstein, S. E., DeBakey, M. E., and McCollum III, C. H. (1977) *Atherosclerosis*, Upjohn, Pfizer, Inc., New York.

He, X. and Ku, D. N. (1996) Pulsatile flow in the human left coronary artery bifurcation: Average conditions. *J. Biomech. Eng.* 118: 74–82.

Ku, D. N., Giddens, D. P., Zarins, C. K., and Glagov, S. (1985) Pulsatile flow and atherosclerosis in the human carotid bifurcation. Positive correlation between plaque location and low oscillating shear stress. *Arteriosclerosis* 593: 293–302.

Li, J. K.-J. (1987) *Arterial System Dynamics*, New York University Press, New York.

Lutz, R. J., Hsu, L., Menawat, A., Zrubek, J., and Edwards, K. (1983) Comparison of steady and pulsatile flow in a double branching arterial model. *J. Biomech.* 16: 753–766.

Malek, A. M., Alper, S. L., and Izumo, S. (1999) Hemodynamic shear stress and its role in atherosclerosis. *JAMA* 282: 2035–2042.

McDonald, D. A. (1974) *Blood Flow in Arteries*, Williams & Wilkins, Baltimore, MD.

Milnor, W. R. (1989) *Hemodynamics*, 2nd edn., Williams & Wilkins, Baltimore, MD.

Morgan, G. W. and Kiely, J. P. (1954) Wave propagation in a viscous liquid contained in a flexible fluid. *J. Acoust. Soc. Am.* 26: 323–328.

Nichols, W. W. and O'Rourke, M. F. (1990) *McDonald's Blood Flow in Arteries*, 3rd edn., Lea & Febiger, Philadelphia, PA.

Noordergraaf, A. (1978) *Circulatory Systems Dynamics*, Academic Press, New York.

Papadaki, M. and Eskin, S. G. (1997) Effects of fluid shear stress on gene regulation of vascular cells. *Biotechnol. Prog.* 13: 209–221.

Rittgers, S. E. and Shu, M. C. S. (1990) Doppler color-flow images from a stenosed arterial model: Interpretation of flow patterns. *J. Vasc. Surg.* 12: 511–522.

Takeuchi, S. and Karino, T. (2010) Aneurysm flow patterns and distributions of fluid velocity and wall shear stress in the human internal carotid and middle cerebral arteries. *World Neurosurg.* 73: 174–185.

Texon, M. (1957) A hemodynamic concept of atherosclerosis, with particular reference to coronary occlusion. *Arch. Intern. Med.* 99: 418–427.

Thurnher, S. et al. (2007) Diagnostic performance of gadobenate dimeglumine—Enhanced MR angiography of the iliofemoral and calf arteries: A large-scale multicenter trial. *AJR* 189: 1223–1237.

Womersley, J. R. (1955a) Method for the calculation of velocity, rate of flow and viscous drag in arteries when the pressure gradient is known. *J. Physiol.* 127: 553–563.

Womersley, J. R. (1955b) Oscillatory motion of a viscous liquid in a thin-walled elastic tube. I. The linear approximation for long waves. *Phil. Mag.* 46: 199–221.

Womersley, J. R. (1957a) The mathematical analysis of arterial circulation in a state of oscillatory motion, Wright Air Development Center, Technical Report WADC-TR-56–614.

Womersley, J. R. (1957b) Oscillatory flow in arteries: The constrained elastic tube as a model of arterial flow and pulse transmission. *Phys. Med. Biol.* 2: 178–187.

7 Native Heart Valves

7.1 INTRODUCTION

The heart has four valves whose main function is to control the direction of blood flow through the heart, permitting forward flow and preventing back flow. On the right side of the heart, the *tricuspid* and *pulmonary* valves regulate the flow of blood that is returned from the body to the lungs for oxygenation. The *mitral* and *aortic* valves control the flow of oxygenated blood from the left side of the lungs back to the body. The aortic and pulmonary valves allow blood to be pumped from the ventricles into arteries on the left and right sides of the heart, respectively. Similarly, the mitral and tricuspid valves lie between the atria and ventricles of the left and right sides of the heart, respectively. The aortic and pulmonary valves open during systole when the ventricles are contracting and close during diastole when the ventricles are filling with blood that enters through the open mitral and tricuspid valves. During isovolumic contraction and relaxation, all four valves are closed (Figure 7.1a). In Figure 7.1b and c, the pressure and volume information for the left heart is shown to illustrate the timings of a normal cardiac cycle. The details of the cardiac events and the opening of the valves are included in Section 3.3.

When closed, the pulmonary and tricuspid valves must withstand a pressure of ~30 mmHg. The closing pressures on the left side of the heart, however, are much higher. Specifically, the aortic valve withstands pressure of ~100 mmHg while the mitral valve resists pressure up to 150 mmHg. Since diseases of the valves on the left side of the heart are more prevalent than those on the right side, most of this chapter will focus on the aortic and mitral valves. Where pertinent, reference will be made to the pulmonary and tricuspid valves, which tend to be impacted more by congenital heart disease.

7.2 AORTIC AND PULMONARY VALVES

The *aortic valve* is composed of three semilunar cusps, or leaflets, contained within a connective tissue sleeve (Figure 7.2). The valve cusps are attached to a fibrous ring embedded in the fibers of the ventricular septum and the anterior leaflet of the mitral valve. Each of the leaflets is lined with endothelial cells and has a dense collagenous core adjacent to the high pressure aortic side (Figure 7.3). The side adjacent to the aorta is termed the *fibrosa* and is the major fibrous layer within the belly of the leaflet. The layer covering the ventricular side of the valve is called the *ventricularis* and is composed of both collagen and elastin. The ventricularis is thinner than the fibrosa and presents a very smooth surface to the flow of blood. The central portion of the valve, called the *spongiosa*, contains variable loose

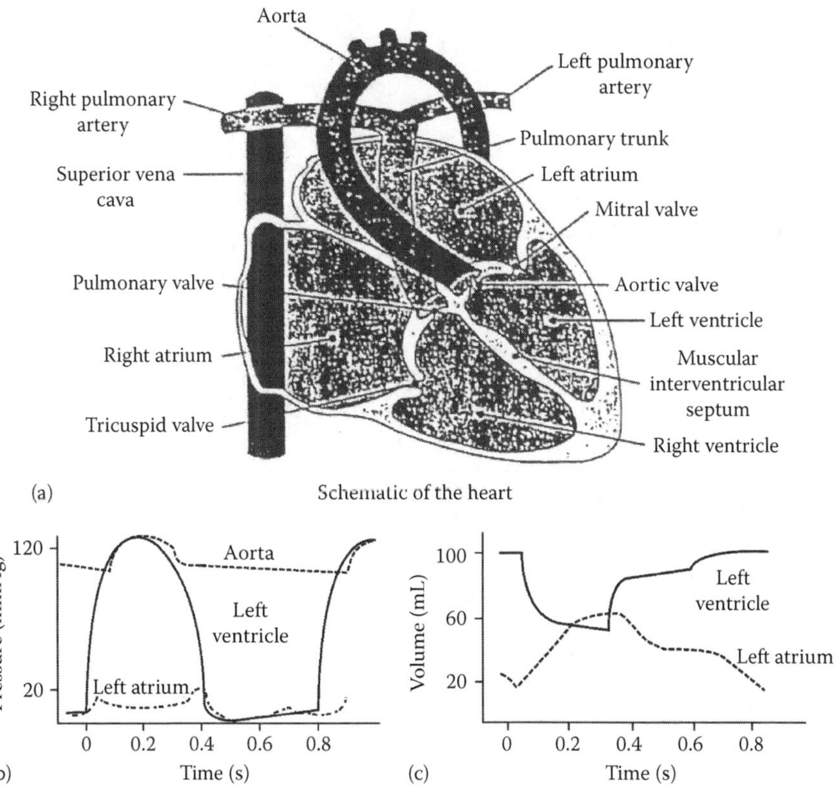

FIGURE 7.1 (a) A schematic of the four chambers of the heart with the valves. (b and c) Typical pressure and flow curves for the left heart.

connective tissue, proteins, and glycosaminoglycans (GAG) and is normally not vascularized. The collagen fibers within the fibrosa and ventricularis are not organized in the unstressed state but when a stress is applied, they become oriented primarily in the circumferential direction with a lower concentration of elastin and collagen in the radial direction.

The fibrous annular ring of the aortic valve separates the aorta from the left ventricle. Superior to this ring is a structure called the *sinus of Valsalva* or the aortic sinus. The sinus comprises three bulges at the root of the aorta, with each bulge aligned with the belly or central part of the specific valve leaflet. Each valve cusp and corresponding sinus is named according to its anatomical location within the aorta. Two of these sinuses give rise to coronary arteries that branch off the aorta, providing blood flow to the heart itself. The right coronary artery is based at the right or right anterior sinus, the left coronary artery exits the left or left posterior sinus, and the third sinus is called the noncoronary or right posterior sinus. Figure 7.2 shows the configuration of the normal aortic sinuses and valve in the closed position.

Because the length of the aortic valve cusps is greater than the annular radius, a small overlap of tissue from each leaflet protrudes and forms a coaptation surface within the aorta when the valve is closed. This overlapped tissue, called the *lunula*,

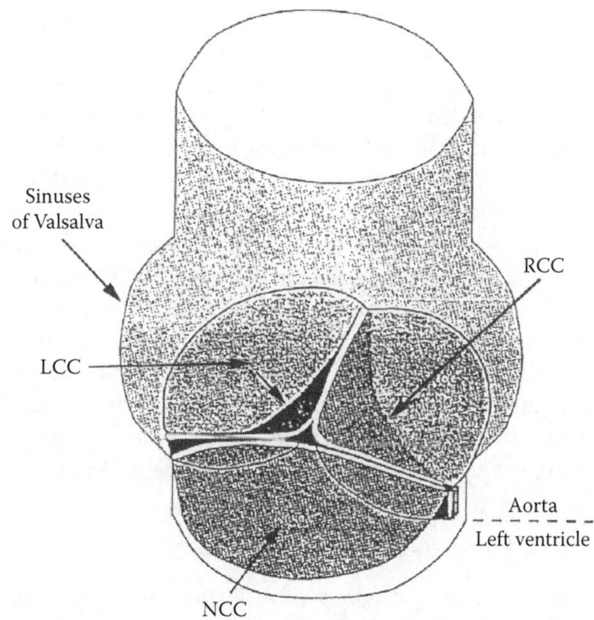

FIGURE 7.2 The aortic sinuses and valve in the closed position. The noncoronary cusp (NCC) is in front. The left and right coronary cusps (LCC and RCC) are positioned as marked. The aorta is above the closed valve in this orientation and the left ventricle is below the dashed line. (From Yoganathan, A.P. et al., Heart valve dynamics, in *The Biomedical Engineering Handbook*, 2nd edn., Bronzino, J.D., ed., CRC Press, Boca Raton, FL, 2000. With permission.)

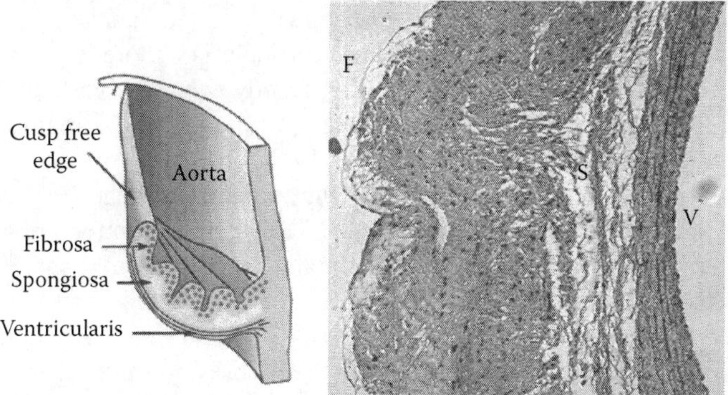

FIGURE 7.3 Schematic and histological section of an aortic valve leaflet showing the fibrosa, spongiosa, and ventricularis layers.

may help to ensure that the valve is sealed. When the valve is in the open position, the leaflets extend to the upper edge of the sinuses of Valsalva. The anatomy of the pulmonary valve is similar to that of the aortic valve, but the surrounding structure is slightly different. The main differences are that the sinuses are smaller in the pulmonary artery and the pulmonary valve annulus is slightly larger than that of the aortic valve.

The dimensions of the aortic and pulmonary valves and their leaflets have been measured in a number of ways. Before noninvasive measurement techniques such as echocardiography became available, valve measurements were recorded from autopsy specimens. An examination of 160 pathological specimens revealed the aortic valve diameter to be 23.2 ± 3.3 mm, whereas the diameter of the pulmonary valve was measured at 24.3 ± 3.0 mm. However, according to M-mode echocardiographic measurements, the aortic root diameter at end systole was 35 ± 4.2 mm and 33.7 ± 4.4 mm at the end of diastole. The differences in these measurements reflect the fact that the autopsy measurements were not performed under physiological pressure conditions and that intrinsic differences in the measurement techniques exist. On average, pulmonary leaflets are thinner than aortic leaflets—0.49 mm versus 0.67 mm—although the leaflets of the aortic valve show variable dimensions depending on the respective leaflet. For example, the posterior leaflet tends to be thicker, have a larger surface area, and weigh more than the right or left leaflet; and the average width of the right aortic leaflet is greater than that of the other two.

7.2.1 Mechanical Properties

Like most biological tissues, the aortic valve leaflets are anisotropic, inhomogeneous, and viscoelastic. The variation in thickness and composition across the leaflets is responsible for their inhomogeneous material properties. The aortic valve leaflet has numerous circumferentially aligned collagen fiber bundles, providing local stiffness to the regions where they traverse. Between the fiber bundles, the valve leaflet is less stiff.

The fiber structure of the valve leaflets accounts for the anisotropy. The collagen fibers within leaflets are mostly aligned along the circumferential direction and the leaflets are stiffer in the circumferential direction than in the radial direction (Vesely and Noseworthy, 1992; Yap et al., 2010). The ventricularis is more extensible radially than circumferentially while the fibrosa is uniformly extensible in both directions. The basal region tends to be relatively isotropic while the central region shows the greatest degree of anisotropy (Lo and Vesely, 1995).

Elastin fibers are present at a lower concentration than collagen, and are mostly oriented radially. Elastin in the ventricularis consists of continuous amorphous sheets or compact meshes while elastin in the fibrosa consists of complex arrays of large tubes that extend circumferentially across the leaflet (Scott and Vesely, 1996). These tubes may surround the large circumferential collagen bundles in the fibrosa. Mechanical testing of elastin structures from the fibrosa and ventricularis separately have shown that elastin structures impose tensile forces on collagen fibers during valve unloading, leading to the conclusion that the purpose of elastin in the aortic valve leaflet is to maintain a specific collagen fiber configuration and return the fibers to the resting unloaded configurations between loading cycles (Vesely, 1998).

Billiar and Sacks (2000) tested porcine aortic valve leaflets and found that their response curve was similar to those of collagen fibers, where stress increases exponentially with strain. With increasing stress, the leaflets exhibit three distinct responses consecutively: starting a low stiffness "toe" region, moving on to a transitional "heel" region, and a high stiffness "linear" region (Figure 7.4). This is in

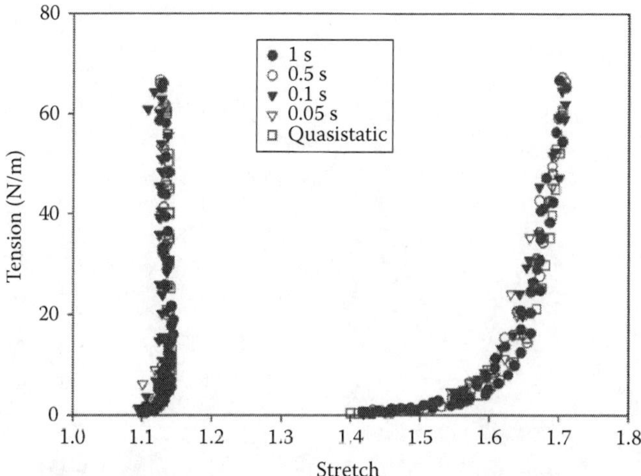

FIGURE 7.4 Mechanical response of fresh aortic valve leaflet to equibiaxial stress at different loading rates, demonstrating the anisotropy of the tissue as well as the insensitivity of the tissue to loading rates. (Adapted from Stella, J.A. et al., *J. Biomech.*, 40, 3169, 2007.)

accordance to the fiber architecture of the valve leaflet: the "toe" region represents the uncrimping of the collagen fiber curls and the elastic response of elastins while the "linear" region represents the stretching of already straightened collagen fibers (Sacks et al., 1998). As expected, the leaflet as a whole was found to have higher stiffness in the circumferential direction than in the radial direction. Further dynamic testing revealed that, at physiological loading rates, the leaflet material behaves elastically, although the leaflets are viscoelastic in nature (Doehring et al., 2004; Stella et al., 2007). The leaflet is capable of undergoing large, rapid anisotropic strains in response to transvalvular pressures, and returns to its original configuration when unloaded with little hysteresis and creep. This leads to the leaflet being described as "quasielastic." Performing engineering analysis of the valve structures, Christie (1992) concluded that the primary load bearing elements in the valve leaflet are circumferential in direction. This conclusion is in line with the presence of collagen fiber bundles oriented circumferentially. Radial stress was found to be small compared with circumferential stress in the closed valve.

In addition to the collagen and elastin, clusters of lipids have been observed in the central spongiosa of porcine aortic valves. Vesely et al. (1994) have shown that the lipids tend to be concentrated at the base of the valve leaflets while the coaptation regions and free edges of the leaflets tend to be devoid of these lipids. In addition, the spatial distribution of the lipids within the spongiosa layer of the aortic leaflets corresponds to areas in which calcification is commonly observed on bioprosthetic valves, suggesting that these lipid clusters may be potential nucleation sites for calcification. In contrast, pulmonary leaflets showed a substantially lower presence of lipids (Dunmore-Buyze et al., 1995).

The pulmonary valve leaflet has similar mechanical properties as the aortic valve, as shown in Figure 7.5. While the pulmonary valve leaflet is less stiff than the aortic valve in the radial direction, its circumferential direction stiffness is similar to that

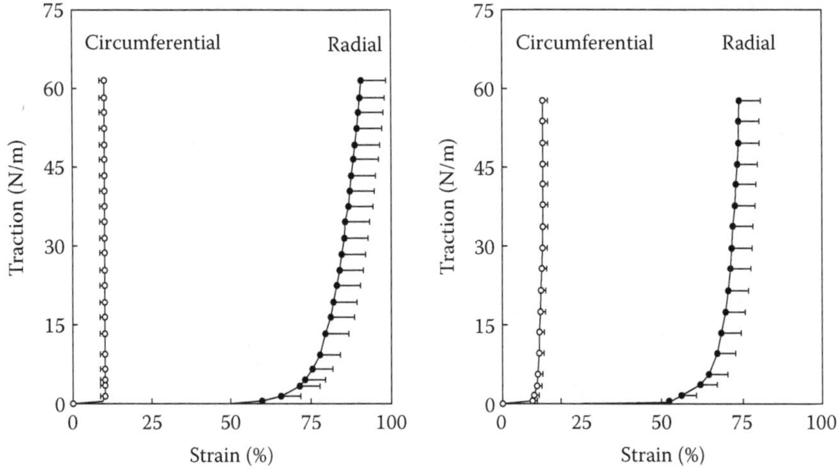

FIGURE 7.5 The mechanical properties of fresh pulmonary valve leaflet (left) versus the aortic valve leaflet (right), from equibiaxial stress mechanical tests. (Adapted from Christie, G.W. and Barratt-Boyes, B.G., *Ann. Thorac. Surg.*, 60, S195, 1995.)

of the aortic valve, indicating a more pronounced anisotropy (Christie and Barratt-Boyes, 1995). However, the pulmonary valve leaflet has similar extensibilities as the aortic valve leaflet, as well as similar viscoelastic material parameters (Leeson-Dietrich et al., 1995).

7.2.2 Valve Dynamics

7.2.2.1 Aortic Root Dynamics

During the cardiac cycle, the heart undergoes translation and rotation due to its own contraction pattern. As a result, the base of the aortic valve varies in size, translates, and rotates. The dynamics of the aortic root are a result of the combination of passive response to pressures on both sides of the valve, as well as active contractions of the muscular shelf on the anteriomedial segment of the annulus. Using marker fluoroscopy in sheeps, Dagum et al. characterized the aortic root motion. During isovolumetric contraction, the annulus and sino-tubular junction undergo rapid circumferential expansion and the aortic root increases in longitudinal length without shear or torsion. During ejection phase, the annulus undergoes circumferential contraction whereas the sino-tubular junction continues to expand, and the aortic root undergoes nonuniform shearing which results in torsional deformation. During the isovolumetric contraction, the aortic root undergoes further circumferential contraction at both the annulus and the sino-tubular junction, and experiences further shearing and torsional deformation, as well as longitudinal compression. During early diastole, the annulus and sino-tubular junction recoils from its dynamically loaded configuration by expanding, and the root is elongated and untwisted from its motion during other phases. Torsional deformation has been described to be nonuniform over the three sinus segments (Dagum et al., 1999).

7.2.2.2 Aortic Valve Leaflet Dynamics

The systolic motion of the aortic valve can be described in three phases: the rapid opening phase, the slow closing phase, and the rapid closing phase. The rapid opening phase lasts for about 60 ms. When leaflets rapidly open at an average speed of 20 cm/s, the valve opens to the fullest extent and blood accelerates through the valve. The slow closing phase, which lasts for 330 ms, is when the bulk of ejection occurs, and valve leaflets move ~13 mm. The rapid closing phase occurs during late systole, lasts for 40 ms, and experiences leaflet speed of 26 cm/s (Leyh et al., 1999).

Earlier experiments in measuring the physiological deformations of the aortic valve leaflets involves using marker fluoroscopy, in which the aortic valve leaflets were surgically tagged with radiopaque markers and imaged with high-speed x-rays (Thubrikar, 1990). The leaflets were found to be longer during diastole than systole in both the radial and circumferential directions, as is expected due to the high transvalvular pressure across the closed aortic valve stretching the leaflets. Yap et al. (2010) characterized the deformational dynamics of the aortic valve leaflets *in vitro* at high spatial and temporal resolution, and showed that average diastolic stretch ratio of the valve to be 15%–18% in the circumferential direction and 45%–54% in the radial direction at the base and belly regions of the valve. It was found that during diastole, the leaflets rapidly reach the peak stretch ratios and stay at approximately the same stretch ratio until the rapid unloading phase at end diastole. During systole, however, the valve stretches slightly in the radial direction (to a lesser extent than during diastole) due to drag forces induced by forward flow. The valve compresses slightly in the circumferential direction due to Poisson's effect of radial stretch. It has been reasoned that the stretching of the valve leaflets during diastole is useful in allowing leaflets to come together and achieve proper coaptation. Additionally, the shortening of the leaflets during systole reduces obstruction of the aorta during the ejection of blood (Christie, 1992).

Drastic changes in the valve area described earlier are results of the valve reacting to the stresses in a passive manner. It is currently unclear if active contractions of aortic valve cells play a role in the deformation dynamics of the leaflets. Active contractions of aortic valve cells were studied and found to be able to impart very small forces at physiological biochemical stimulations (Kershaw et al., 2004). On the other hand, stimulants such as serotonin and endothelin were found to significantly alter the stiffness of valve leaflets at the posttransitional zone of the response curve (high stiffness zone) (El-Hamamsy et al., 2009). It is unclear if the stiffness of the pretransitional zone (low stiffness zone) is altered, which is the main determinant of the amount of stretch suffered by the leaflets under physiological loads. Active cell contraction has also been observed to impart additional bending stiffness to the valve leaflet (Merryman et al., 2006). This is an important consideration that the aortic valve leaflet experiences substantial bending during the cardiac cycle: valve leaflet is convex, bulging toward the ventricle during diastole, and bulging toward the sinus when open, with the base of the valve leaflet bent to allow the opening. It is hypothesized that leaflet cell contractions is a regulatory mechanism of leaflet kinematics, and that biochemical cues are used to control leaflet stiffness tone to influence function.

7.2.2.3 Aortic Valve Fluid Dynamics

During systole, vortices develop in all three sinuses behind the leaflets of the aortic valve. The function of these vortices was first described by Leonardo da Vinci in 1513, and they have been researched extensively in this century primarily through the use of *in vitro* models. It has been hypothesized that the vortices help to close the aortic valve so that blood is prevented from returning to the ventricle during the closing process. These vortices create a transverse pressure difference that pushes the leaflets toward the center of the aorta and each other at the end of systole, thus minimizing any possible closing volume. However, as shown *in vitro* by Reul et al. (1981) and Talukdar, the axial pressure difference alone is enough to close the valve. Without the vortices in the sinuses, the valve still closes but its closure is not as quick as when the vortices are present. The adverse axial pressure difference within the aorta causes the low inertia flow within the developing boundary layer along the aortic wall to be the first to decelerate and reverse direction. This action forces the belly of the leaflets away from the aortic wall and toward the closed position. When this force is coupled with the vortices that push the leaflet tips toward the closed position, a very efficient and fast closure is obtained. Closing volumes have been estimated to be <5% of the forward flow.

The parameters that describe the normal blood flow through the aortic valve are the velocity profile, time course of the blood velocity or flow, and magnitude of the peak velocity. These are determined in part by the pressure difference between the ventricle and aorta and by the geometry of the aortic valve complex. As seen in Figure 7.6, the velocity profile at the level of the aortic valve annulus is relatively flat. However, there is usually a slight skew toward the septal wall (<10% of the centerline velocity) which is caused by the orientation of the aortic valve relative to the long axis of the left ventricle. This skew in the velocity profile has been shown by many experimental techniques, including hot film anemometry, Doppler ultrasound, and MRI. In healthy individuals, blood flows through the aortic valve at the beginning of systole and then rapidly accelerates to its peak value of 1.35 ± 0.35 m/s; for children, this value is slightly higher at 1.5 ± 0.3 m/s. At the end of systole, there is a very short period of reverse flow that can be measured with Doppler ultrasound. This reverse flow is probably either a small closing volume or the velocity of the valve leaflets as they move toward their closed position. In the presence of aortic stenosis, peak velocities through the valve could be as high as 5 m/s and large magnitudes of turbulent shear stresses that could induce hemolysis. The flow patterns just downstream of the aortic valve are of particular interest because of their complexity and relation to arterial disease. Highly skewed velocity profiles and corresponding helical flow patterns have been observed in the human aortic arch using magnetic resonance phase velocity mapping (see Section 10.8.4).

Flow through the pulmonary valve behaves similarly to that of the aortic valve but the magnitude of the velocity is not as great. Typical peak velocities for healthy adults are 0.75 ± 0.15 m/s; again, these values are slightly higher for children at 0.9 ± 0.2 m/s (Weyman, 1994). As seen in Figure 7.7, the spatial velocity profile is relatively flat, with only a slight skew to the velocity profile.

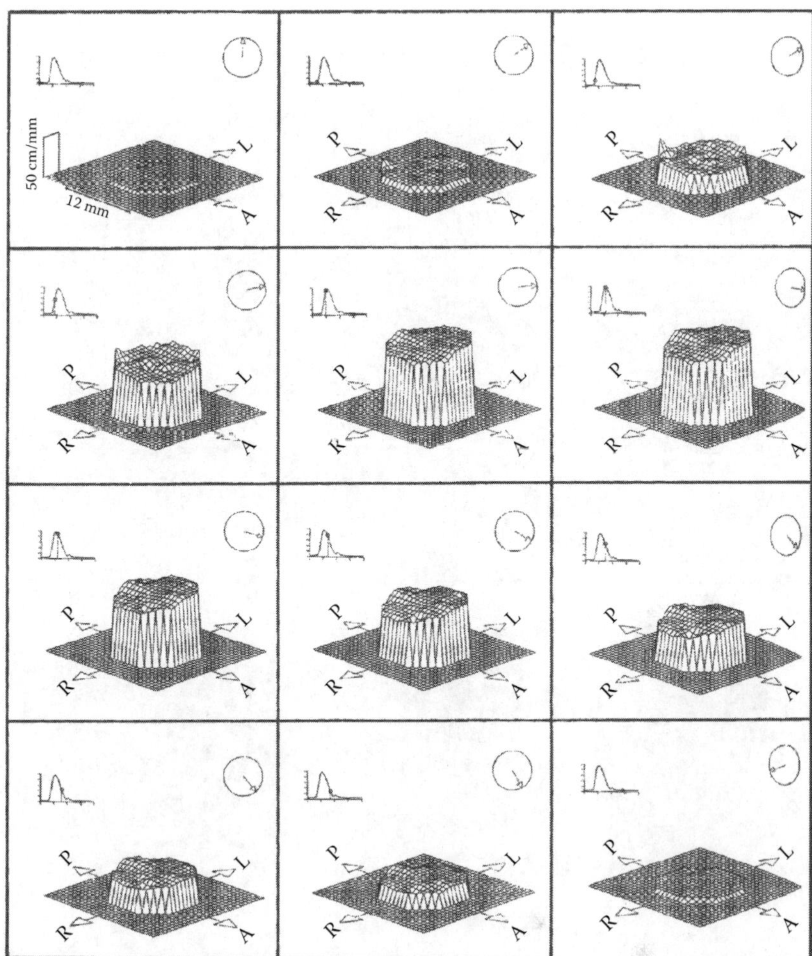

FIGURE 7.6 Velocity profiles measured 2 cm downstream of the aortic valve with hot film anemometry in dogs. The timing of the measurements during the cardiac cycle is shown by the marker on the aortic flow curve. (From *J. Biomech.*, 16, Paulsen, P.K. and Hansenkam, J.M., 201–210, Copyright (1983), with permission from Elsevier.)

The point of peak velocity can be discerned, and is near to the inferior wall of the pulmonary trunk artery. The peak velocity is generally within 20% of the spatial mean throughout the cardiac cycle. This point can be observed to move along the wall toward the left wall during the ejection phase. There is a region of reverse flow that occurs in late systole, which may be representative of flow separation. Secondary flow patterns can also be observed in the pulmonary artery and its bifurcation. *In vitro* laser Doppler anemometry experiments have shown that these flow patterns are dependent on the valve geometry/degree of stenosis and thus can be used to evaluate function and fitness of the heart valve (Sung and Yoganathan, 1990).

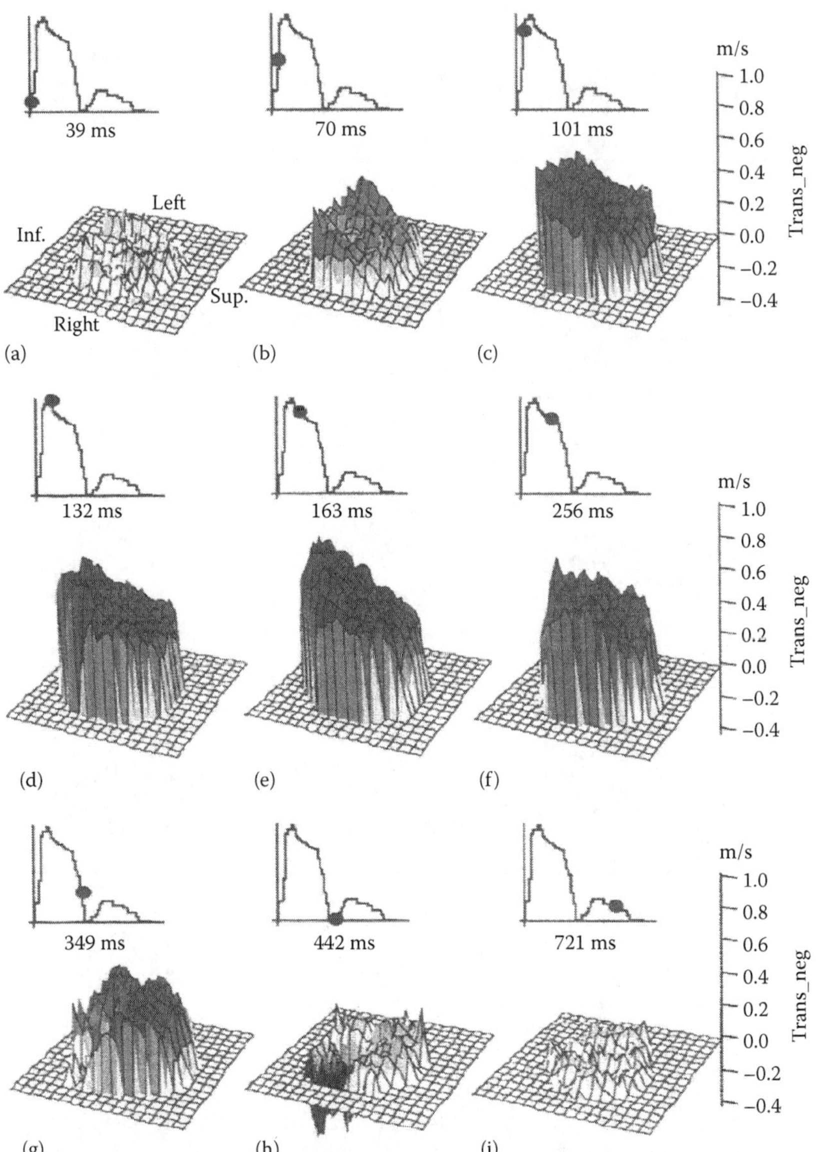

FIGURE 7.7 Velocity profiles downstream of the human pulmonary valve obtained with magnetic resonance phase velocity mapping. The timing of the measurements is shown by the marker on the flow curve. Figures (a) to (i): different time points within the cardiac cycle. (From *Am. Heart J.*, 128, Sloth, E. et al., 1130–1138, Copyright (1994), with permission from Elsevier.)

7.3 MITRAL AND TRICUSPID VALVES

The mitral (Figure 7.8) and tricuspid valves are similar in structure with both valves composed of four primary elements: the *valve annulus*, the *valve leaflets*, the *papillary muscles* (PMs), and the *chordae tendineae*. The base of the mitral leaflets forms the mitral annulus, which attaches to the atrial and ventricular walls, and aortic root. At the free edge of the leaflets, the chordae tendineae insert at multiple locations and extend to the tips of the PMs. This arrangement provides continuity between the valve and ventricular wall to enhance valvular function. The valvular apparatus, or complex, requires an intricate interplay between all components throughout the cardiac cycle.

The mitral annulus is an elliptical ring composed of dense collagenous tissue surrounded by muscle. It goes through dynamic changes during the cardiac cycle by not only changing in size, but also by moving three-dimensionally. The circumference of the mitral annulus ranges from 8 to 12 cm during diastole. Recent studies involving the measurement of annular shape have also shown that the mitral annulus is not planar, but instead has a 3D form. The annulus actually forms a saddle, or ski-slope, shape. This 3D shape must be taken into account when noninvasively evaluating valvular function.

The mitral valve is a bileaflet valve comprising an anterior and posterior leaflet. The leaflet tissue is primarily collagen-reinforced endothelium, but also contains striated muscle cells, nonmyelinated nerve fibers, and blood vessels. The anterior and posterior leaflets of the valve are actually one continuous piece of tissue, as shown in Figure 7.9. The free edge of this tissue shows several indentations, two of which are regularly placed, called the *commisures*. The commisures separate the tissue into the anterior and posterior leaflets. The location of the commisures can be identified by the fan-like distribution of chordae tendineae and the relative positioning of the PMs.

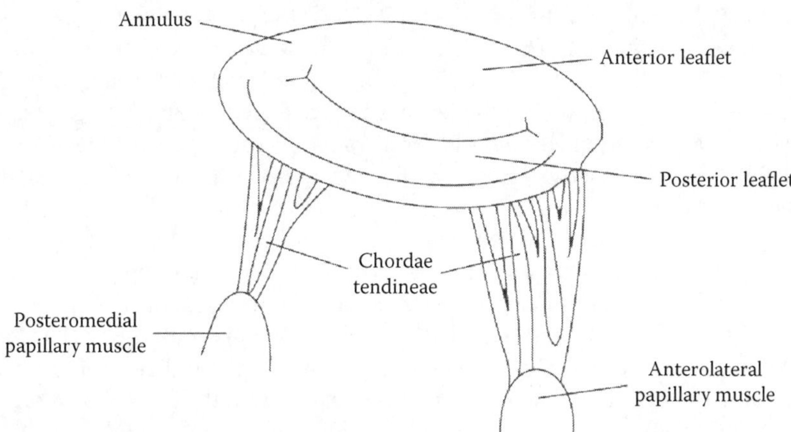

FIGURE 7.8 Schematic of the mitral valve showing the valve leaflets, papillary muscles, and chordae tendineae. (From Yoganathan, A.P. et al., Heart valve dynamics, in *The Biomedical Engineering Handbook*, 2nd edn., Bronzino, J.D., ed., CRC Press, Boca Raton, FL, 2000. With permission.)

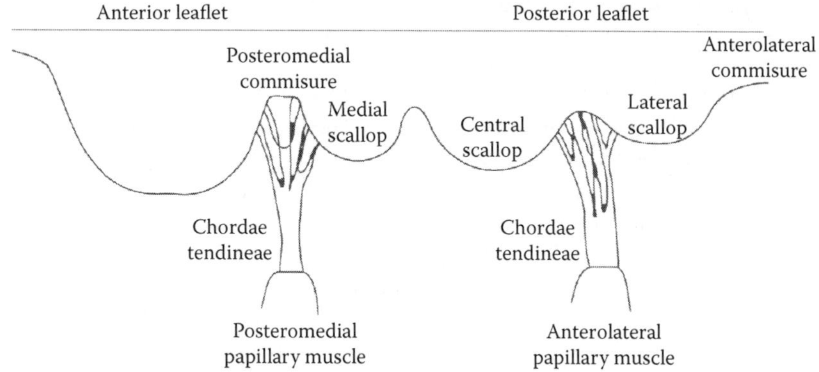

FIGURE 7.9 Diagram of the mitral valve as a continuous piece of tissue. The posterior and anterior leaflets are indicated, as are the scallops, chordae tendineae, and papillary muscles. (From Yoganathan, A.P. et al., Heart valve dynamics, in *The Biomedical Engineering Handbook*, 2nd edn., Bronzino, J.D., ed., CRC Press, Boca Raton, FL, 2000. With permission.)

The combined surface area of both leaflets is approximately twice the area of the mitral orifice. This extra surface area permits a large line of coaptation and ample coverage of the mitral orifice during normal function and provides compensation in cases of disease. The posterior leaflet encircles roughly two-thirds of the mitral annulus and is essentially an extension of the mural endocardium from the free walls of the left atrium. The anterior leaflet portion of the annulus is a line of connection for the leaflet, the wall of the ascending aorta, the aortic valve, and the atrial septum. The anterior leaflet is slightly larger than the posterior leaflet and is roughly semilunar in shape as opposed to the quadrangular-shaped posterior leaflet. The normal width and height of the anterior leaflet are ~3.3 and 2.3 cm, respectively. The height of the posterior leaflet is 1.3 cm while the commisure height is <1.0 cm. The posterior leaflet typically has indentations, called *scallops*, that divide the leaflet into three regions—the medial, central, and lateral scallops.

The mitral leaflet tissue can be divided into both rough and clear zones. The rough zone is the thicker part of the leaflet and is defined from the free edge of the valve to the valve's line of closure. The term "rough" is used to denote the texture of the leaflet due to the insertion of the chordae tendineae in this area. The clear zone is thinner and translucent and extends from the line of closure to the annulus in the anterior leaflet and to the basal zone in the posterior leaflet. Unlike the mitral valve, the tricuspid valve has three leaflets—an anterior leaflet, a posterior leaflet with a variable number of scallops, and a septal leaflet. The tricuspid valve is larger and structurally more complicated than the mitral valve and the separation of the valve tissue into distinct leaflets is less pronounced than with the mitral valve. The surface of the leaflets is similar to that of the mitral valve; however, the basal zone is present in all of the leaflets.

Chordae tendineae from both leaflets attach to each of the PMs (anterior and posterior). The chordae tendineae consist of an inner core of collagen surrounded by loosely meshed elastin and collagen fibers with an outer layer of endothelial cells. In the mitral complex structure, there are marginal and basal chordae that insert into the mitral leaflets. From each PM, several chordae originate and branch into the marginal and basal chordae. The thinner marginal chordae insert into the leaflet free edge at multiple insertion points, while the thicker basal chordae insert into the leaflets at a higher level toward the annulus. The marginal chordae function to keep the leaflets stationary while the basal chordae seem to act more as supports.

The left side of the heart has two PMs, called anterolateral and posteromedial, that attach to the ventricular free wall and tether the mitral valve in place via the chordae tendineae. This tethering prevents the mitral valve from prolapsing into the left atrium during ventricular ejection. On the right side of the heart, the tricuspid valve has three PMs. The largest one, the anterior PM, attaches to the valve at the commisure between the anterior and posterior leaflets. The posterior PM is located between the posterior and septal leaflets. The smallest PM, called the septal muscle, is sometimes not even present. Improper tethering of the leaflets will result in valve prolapse during ventricular contraction, permitting the valve leaflets to extend into the atrium. This incomplete apposition of the valve leaflets can cause regurgitation, which is leaking of the blood being ejected back into the atrium.

The tricuspid valve annulus is lined with the septal wall and the right free wall of the heart. The tricuspid valve has three leaflets instead of two, which are named according to their position in the heart: anterior, posterior, and septal leaflet. The septal leaflet is located along the septal wall and is attached to the wall with short chordae (Silver et al., 1971). The anterior and posterior leaflets are located along the free wall with the anterior leaflet reported to be the largest (Skwarek et al., 2006; Anwar et al., 2007a,b; Shah and Raney, 2008). While it is typically accepted that the tricuspid valve has three main leaflets, numerous studies have reported there to be a variable number of leaflets ranging from 2 up to 7 leaflets (Silver et al., 1971; Victor and Nayak, 2000). The septal leaflet is always present but the number of leaflets along the free wall can vary. Figure 7.10 shows the explanted porcine tricuspid valve, demonstrating the relevant structures.

The annulus is a fibrous ring located on the perimeter of the valve and connects the leaflets to the myocardial wall. The annulus has a complex 3D geometry, as seen in Figure 7.11 (Silver et al. 1971; Hiro et al., 2004; Fukuda et al., 2006; Anwar et al., 2007a,b; Jouan et al., 2007; Kwan et al., 2007). While some studies

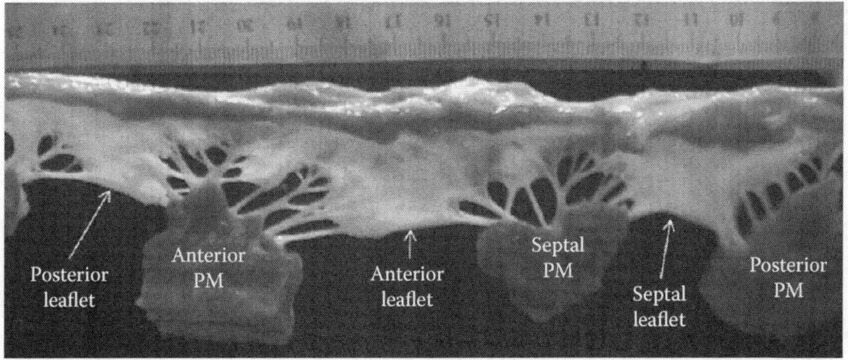

FIGURE 7.10 Explanted porcine valve, showing leaflet and PM locations relative to another.

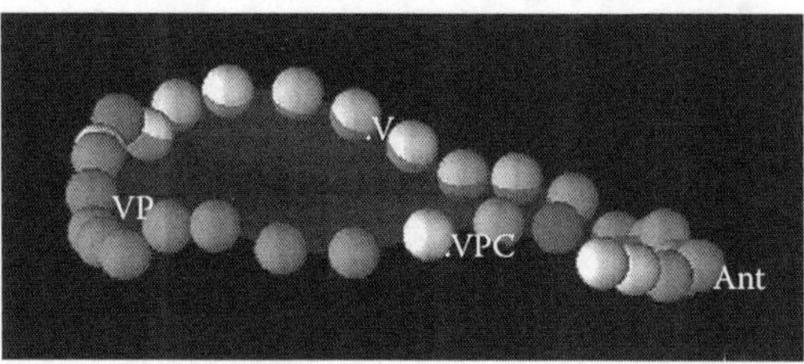

FIGURE 7.11 3D representation of the complex shape of the tricuspid annulus using 3D echocardiography and 3D in house software. (From Kwan, J. et al., *Eur. J. Echocardiogr.*, 8, 375, 2007.)

have reported the annulus to be oval (Anwar et al., 2007a,b), others report that it is triangular (Silver et al., 1971). Annulus areas range from 7.6 to 11.2 cm^2 during systole and 11.3 to 18.35 cm^2 during diastole (Tei et al., 1982; Anwar et al., 2007a,b; Kwan et al., 2007).

There are three PMs located in the right ventricle which connect to the leaflets via chordae tendineae. The PMs on the right side of the heart are not as well-defined as those seen on the left side of the heart, as with the mitral valve (Joudinaud et al., 2006). The PMs are named according to their location in the ventricle: septal, anterior, and posterior. The septal PM is located on the anterior side of the septum between the septal and anterior leaflets. The posterior PM is located on the posterior side between the septal and posterior leaflets. The anterior PM is located on the free wall between the anterior and posterior leaflets. The PMs exist in multiple geometric morphologies and are classified into three groups based upon their structure: fingerlike, with the muscle protruding; tethered, with the muscle embedded in the myocardial wall; and vestigial, with the chords attaching directly to the well (Joudinaud et al., 2006) (Figure 7.12).

Each PM has several chords that attach to the two corresponding leaflets. For example, the anterior PM has chords that insert into the anterior and posterior leaflets. The chords insert into different locations on the leaflet, including the free edge, base, and belly of the leaflet. Chords are classified as marginal/primary, inserting into the free edge of the leaflet; rough zone/supplemental, inserting between

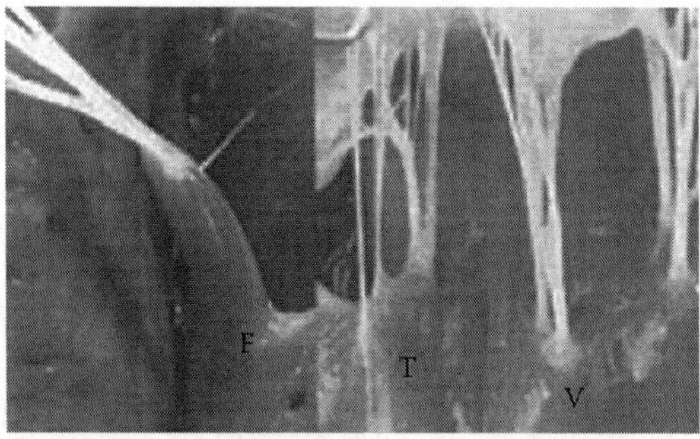

FIGURE 7.12 Classification of the three groups of papillary muscles. F, Fingerlike; T, tethered; and V, vestigial. (As classified using excised porcine hearts from Joudinaud, T.M. et al., *J. Heart Valve Dis.*, 15, 382, 2006.)

the marginal and intermediate chords; and deep/intermediate, inserting into the belly of the leaflet. Silver et al. (1971) report the deep/strut chordae to be the longest (1.7 ± 0.4 cm). All chords have similar thickness ranging from 0.8 ± 0.3 cm to 1.1 ± 0.4 cm (Silver et al., 1971).

7.3.1 Mechanical Properties

Studies on the mechanical behavior of the mitral leaflet tissue have been conducted to determine the key connective tissue components that influence the valve function. Histological studies have shown that the tissue is composed of three layers that can be identified by differences in cellularity and collagen density. Analysis of the leaflets under tension indicated that the anterior leaflet would be more capable of supporting larger tensile loads than the posterior leaflet, since the anterior leaflet has a thicker collagen-rich fibrosa layer. This is confirmed by uniaxial tensile testing (Kunzelman and Cochran, 1992). The differences in the mechanical properties between the two leaflets may require different material selection for repair or replacement of the individual leaflets. Grashow et al. (2006) performed equibiaxial mechanical testing of the anterior leaflet. The leaflet was found to exhibit a mechanical response curve similar to that of collagen, with a very long toe region of large strain and slow loading followed by a region of small strain and rapid loading (Figure 7.13). The leaflet exhibits no hysteresis in the circumferential direction, and a very small amount in the radial direction. The valve leaflet was found to be strain rate–insensitive over a range of loading rates from 0.07 to 20 Hz, maintaining the same mechanical response and hysteresis.

Studies have also been done on the strength of the chordae tendineae. The tension of chordae tendineae in dogs was monitored throughout the cardiac cycle by Salisbury et al. (1963). They found that the tension only paralleled the left ventricular pressure tracings during isovolumic contraction, indicating slackness at other times in the cycle. Investigation of the tensile properties of the chordae

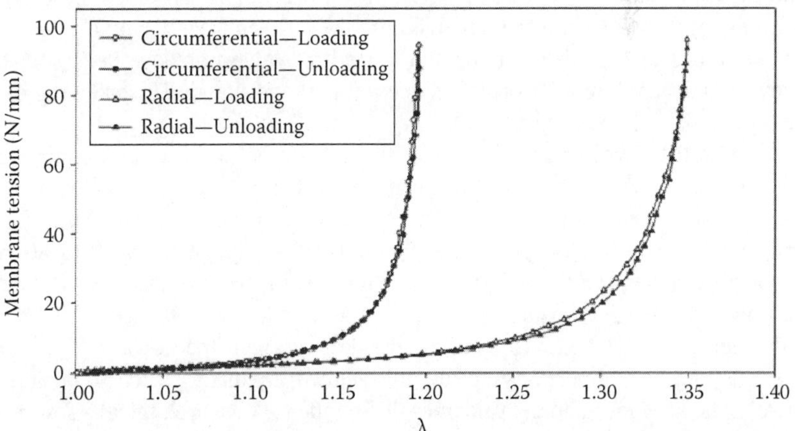

FIGURE 7.13 Mechanical response of the mitral valve anterior leaflet to equibiaxial tensile testing. (Adapted from Grashow, J.S. et al., *Ann. Biomed. Eng.*, 34, 315, 2006.)

tendineae at different strain rates by Lim et al. (1975) found that the chordae had a nonlinear stress–strain relationship. They found that the size of the chordae had a more significant effect on the development of the tension than did the strain rate. The smaller chordae with cross-sectional areas of 0.001–0.006 cm^2 had a modulus of 2×10^9 dyn/cm^2, while larger chordae of cross-sectional areas of 0.006–0.03 cm^2 had a modulus of 1×10^9 dyn/cm^2.

A theoretical study of the stresses sustained by the mitral valve was performed by Ghista et al. (1973). This study determined that the stress level can reach as high as 2.2×10^6 dyn/cm^2 just prior to the opening of the aortic valve, with the left ventricular pressure rising to 150 mmHg. A mathematical model has also been created for the mechanics of the mitral valve. It incorporates the relationship between chordae tendineae tension, left ventricular pressure, and mitral valve geometry. This study examined the force balance on a closed valve and determined that the chordae tendineae force was always more than half the force exerted on the mitral valve orifice by the transmitral pressure gradient. During the past 10 years, computational models have been developed of mitral valve mechanics, with the most advanced modeling being 3D finite element models (FEM) of the complete mitral apparatus. Kunzelman et al. (2007) has developed a model of the mitral complex that includes the mitral leaflets, chordae tendineae, contracting annulus, and contracting PMs. From these studies, the maximum principal stresses found at peak loading (120 mmHg) were 5.7×10^6 dyn/cm^2 in the annular region, while the stresses in the anterior leaflet ranged from 2×10^6 to 4×10^6 dyn/cm^2. This model has also been used to evaluate mitral valve disease, repair in chordal rupture, and valvular annuloplasty.

7.3.2 Valve Dynamics

The valve leaflets, chordae tendineae, and PMs all participate to ensure normal functioning of the mitral valve. During isovolumic relaxation, the pressure in the left atrium exceeds that of the left ventricle, and the mitral valve cusps open. Blood flows through the open valve from the left atrium to the left ventricle during diastole. The velocity profiles at both the annulus and the mitral valve tips have been shown to be skewed and therefore are not flat as is commonly assumed. This skewing of the inflow profile is shown in Figure 7.14.

The initial filling is enhanced by the active relaxation of the ventricle, maintaining a positive transmitral pressure. The mitral velocity flow curve shows a peak in the flow curve, called the E-wave, which occurs during the early filling phase. Normal peak E-wave velocities in healthy individuals range from 50 to 80 cm/s. Following active ventricular relaxation, the fluid begins to decelerate and the mitral valve undergoes partial closure. Then, the atrium contracts and the blood accelerates through the valve again to a secondary peak, termed the A-wave. The atrium contraction plays an important role in additional filling of the ventricle during late diastole. In healthy individuals, velocities during the A-wave are typically lower than those of the E-wave, with a normal E-wave/A-wave velocity ratio ranging from 1.5 to 1.7. Thus, normal diastolic filling of the left ventricle shows two distinct peaks in the flow curve with no flow leaking back through the valve during systole.

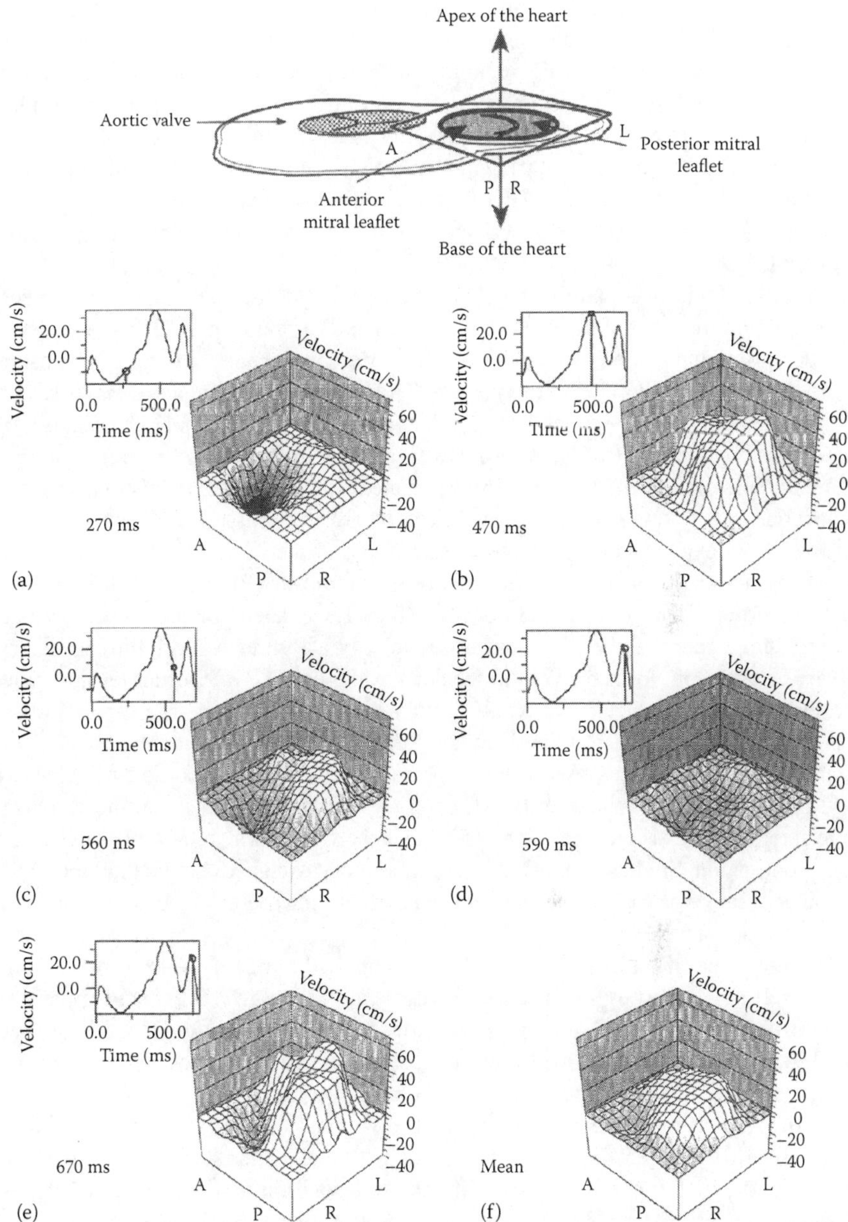

FIGURE 7.14 Two-dimensional transmitral velocity profiles recorded at the level of the mitral annulus in a pig. (a) Systole; (b) peak E-wave; (c) deceleration phase of early diastole; (d) mid-diastolic period (diastasis); (e) peak A-wave; and (f) time-averaged diastolic cross-sectional mitral velocity profile. (From *J. Am. Coll. Cardiol.*, 24, Kim, W.Y., Bisgaard, T., Nielsen, S.L., Poulsen, E.M., Pedersen, E.M., Hasenkam, J.M., and Yoganathan, A.P., Two-dimensional mitral flow velocity profiles in pig models using epicardial Doppler echocardiography, 532–545, Copyright 1994, with permission from Elsevier.)

The tricuspid flow profile is similar to that of the mitral valve although the velocities in the tricuspid valve are lower because it has a larger valve orifice. In addition, the timing of the valve opening is slightly different. Since the peak pressure in the right ventricle is less than that of the left ventricle, the time for right ventricular pressure to fall below the right atrial pressure is less than the corresponding time period for the left side of the heart. This leads to a shorter right ventricular isovolumic relaxation and, thus, an earlier tricuspid opening. Tricuspid closure occurs after the mitral valve closes since the activation of the left ventricle precedes that of the right ventricle.

A primary focus in explaining the fluid mechanics of mitral valve function has been understanding the closing mechanism of the valve. Bellhouse in 1972 first suggested that the vortices generated by ventricular filling were important for the partial closure of the mitral valve following early diastole. Their *in vitro* experiments suggested that without the strong outflow tract vortices, the valve would remain open at the onset of ventricular contraction, thus resulting in a significant amount of mitral regurgitation before complete closure. Later, *in vitro* experiments by Reul et al. (1981) in a left ventricle model made from silicone suggested that an adverse pressure differential in mid-diastole could explain both the flow deceleration and the partial valve closure, even in the absence of a ventricular vortex. Thus, the studies by Reul et al. (1981) suggest that the vortices may provide additional closing effects at the initial stage; however, the pressure forces are the dominant effect in valve closure. A more unified theory of valve closure put forth by Yellin includes the importance of chordal tension, flow deceleration, and ventricular vortices, with chordal tension being a necessary condition for the other two. Their animal studies indicated that competent valve closure can occur even in the absence of vortices and flow deceleration. Recent studies using MRI to visualize the 3D flow field in the left ventricle showed that in normal individuals a large anterior vortex is present at initial partial closure of the valve, as well as following atrial contraction. Studies conducted in our laboratory using MRI of healthy individuals clearly show vortices in the left ventricle, which may be an indication of normal diastolic function.

Another area of interest has been the motion of the mitral valve complex. The heart itself moves throughout the cardiac cycle and, similarly, the mitral apparatus also moves and changes shape. Recent studies have been conducted that examined the 3D dynamics of the mitral annulus during the cardiac cycle. These studies have shown that, during systole, the annular circumference decreases from the diastolic value due to the contraction of the ventricle and this reduction in area ranges from 10% to 25%. This result agrees with an animal study of Tsakiris that looked at the difference in the size, shape, and position of the mitral annulus at different stages in the cardiac cycle. They noted an eccentric narrowing of the annulus during both atrial and ventricular contractions that reduced the mitral valve area by 10%–36% from its peak diastolic area. This reduction in the annular area during systole is significant, resulting in a smaller orifice area for the larger leaflet area to cover. The annulus not only changes size, but also translates during the cardiac cycle. The movement of the annulus toward the atrium has been suggested to play a role in ventricular filling, possibly increasing the efficiency of blood flow into the ventricle. During ventricular contraction, there is a shortening of the left ventricular chamber along its longitudinal axis, and also the mitral and tricuspid annuli move toward the apex.

The movement of the PMs is also important in maintaining proper mitral valve function. The PMs play an important role in keeping the mitral valve in position during ventricular contraction. Abnormal strain on the PMs could cause the chordae to rupture, resulting in mitral regurgitation. It is necessary for the PMs to contract and shorten during systole to prevent mitral prolapse; therefore, the distance between the apex of the heart to the mitral apparatus is important. The distance from the PM tips to the annulus was measured in normal individuals during systole and was found to remain constant. In patients with mitral valve prolapse, however, this distance decreased, corresponding to a superior displacement of the PM toward the annulus.

The normal function of the mitral valve requires a balanced interplay between all of the components of the mitral apparatus, as well as the interaction of the atrium and ventricle. The *in vitro* engineering studies of mitral valve function have provided some insight into its mechanical properties and dynamics. Further fundamental and detailed studies are needed to aid surgeons in the repair of diseased mitral valves and in understanding the changes in function due to mitral valve pathologies. In addition, these studies are crucial for improving the design of prosthetic valves that more closely replicate native valve function (see Chapter 8). The main function of the tricuspid valve is to prevent the backflow of blood from the ventricle to the atrium during systole, when blood is being pumped from the right ventricle to the pulmonary artery. The typical pressures on the right side of the heart range from 0 to 5 mmHg for the atrium and 5 to 40 mmHg for the ventricle as reported using catheter measurements (Hurst et al., 2004). The tricuspid valve closes with the initiation of isovolumetric contraction and remains closed throughout systole and isovolumetric relaxation. Once the pressure in the right ventricle is lower than that in the atrium, the valve opens. The valve remains closed for approximately one-third of the cardiac cycle.

The tricuspid valve annulus area significantly increases from early to late systole in healthy subjects by 5.4% ± 1.6% (Kwan et al., 2007) and experiences differences ranging from 28% to 48% from its minimum to maximum area throughout the cardiac cycle (Tei et al., 1982; Fukuda et al., 2006; Jouan et al., 2007). The area of the tricuspid valve annulus is at its maximum during diastole increasing the efficiency of filling by providing a larger orifice (Jouan et al., 2007) and minimum during systole aiding coaptation of the leaflets. In addition to changes in area throughout the cardiac cycle, the annulus changes its shape as well. As seen in Figure 7.11, the annulus of the tricuspid valve has a 3D saddle (Hiro et al., 2004; Fukuda et al., 2006; Kwan et al., 2007), with the annulus becoming more planar during diastole (Hiro et al., 2004). Figure 7.15 shows that the PMs move in a clockwise manner during systole. The anterior PM experiences the greatest movement during the cardiac cycle due to the contraction of the myocardium since the PM is located on the free wall. The motion of the PMs has been observed to twist, shift, and bend in relation to the annulus plane, while the distance from the PMs to the annulus plane remains relatively constant (Jouan et al., 2007).

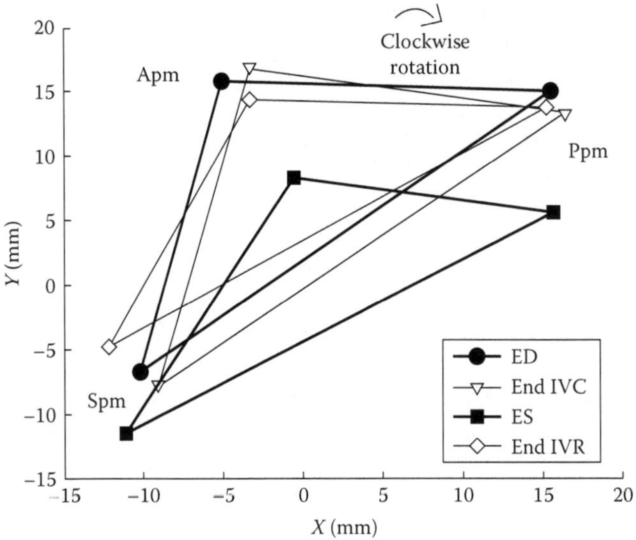

FIGURE 7.15 Results from an *in vivo* sonomicrometry study on sheep show the clockwise rotation motion of the papillary muscles over the cardiac cycle. (From Jouan, J. et al., *J. Heart Valve Dis.*, 16(5), 511, 2007.)

PROBLEMS

7.1 Gorlin equation was derived in Chapter 5 for the orifice area as

$$A_0 = \frac{Q_m}{C_d}\sqrt{\frac{\rho}{2\Delta p}}$$

Assuming a specific value for the discharge coefficient, the Gorlin equations for the aortic (AVA) and mitral (MVA) valve area are given by

$$AVA = \frac{MSF}{44.5\sqrt{\Delta p}} \quad \text{and} \quad MVA = \frac{MDF}{31.0\sqrt{\Delta p}}$$

MSF and MDF are mean systolic and diastolic flow rates, respectively (mL/s). The pressure drop is expressed as mmHg. The constants are derived to incorporate unit conversions and with assumed discharge coefficients for the aortic and mitral valve orifices in order to compute the orifice area in units of cm^2. Determine the discharge coefficients used for the aortic and mitral valves used in the aforementioned relationships.

7.2 Upon examination of a 43 year old patient with a history of rheumatic fever at 7 years of age, the following data were obtained.

Left ventricular pressure (systolic/end diastolic) (mmHg)	182/24
Cardiac output (L/min)	3.4
Aortic pressure (mmHg)	118/74
Mean left atrial pressure (mmHg)	36
Heart rate (bpm)	90
Systole as a percentage of cardiac cycle	40
Diastole as a percentage of cardiac cycle	60
LV–Aorta mean pressure difference (mmHg)	64
LA–LV mean pressure difference (mmHg)	12

Calculate the aortic and mitral valve orifice areas for the patient using the equations from Problem 7.1.

Hint:

Flow through the valve
= [{Cardiac output (mL/min)}]/[{systolic/diastolic period (s)} × heart rate (bpm)]

7.3 The pressure drop across the aortic valve can be computed by the application of Bernoulli equation given below where subscript 1 stands for the left ventricular outflow tract and subscript 2 stands for the aortic root. The viscous losses are assumed to be negligible as the blood travels across the valve orifice.

$$p_1 + \frac{\rho V_1^2}{2} = p_2 + \frac{\rho V_2^2}{2}$$

Assuming that the velocity in the outflow tract is negligible compared with that in the aortic root when the aortic valve is fully open, the pressure drop across the valve can be computed using the previous equation. If the average velocity of the blood in the aortic root distal to the valve is measured by a Doppler probe in m/s, show that the pressure drop in mmHg can be expressed as

$$p_1 - p_2 = 4V_2^2 \qquad (1.65)$$

REFERENCES

Anwar, A. M., Geleijnse, M. L., Soliman, O. I. I., McGhie, J. S., Frowijn, R., Nemes, A., van den Bosch, A. E., Galema, T. W., and ten Cate, F. J. (2007a) Assessment of normal tricuspid valve anatomy in adults by real-time three-dimensional echocardiography. *Int. J. Cardiovasc. Imaging* 23(6): 717–724.

Anwar, A. M., Soliman, O. I. I., Nemes, A., van Geuns, R. J. M., Geleijnse, M. L., and ten Cate, F. J. (2007b) Value of assessment of tricuspid annulus: Real-time three-dimensional echocardiography and magnetic resonance imaging. *Int. J. Cardiovasc. Imaging* 23(6): 701–705.

Bellhouse, B. J. (1972) Fluid mechanics of a model mitral valve and left ventricle. *Cardiovasc. Res.* 6(2): 199–210.

Billiar, K. L. and Sacks, M. S. (2000) Biaxial mechanical properties of the natural and glutaraldehyde treated aortic valve cusp—Part I: Experimental results. *J. Biomech. Eng.* 122(1): 23–30.

Christie, G. W. (1992) Anatomy of aortic heart valve leaflets: The influence of glutaraldehyde fixation on function. *Eur. J. Cardiothorac. Surg.* 6(Suppl. 1): S25–S32; discussion S33.

Christie, G. W. and Barratt-Boyes, B. G. (1995) Mechanical properties of porcine pulmonary valve leaflets: How do they differ from aortic leaflets? *Ann. Thorac. Surg.* 60(2 Suppl.): S195–S199.

Dagum, P., Green, G. R., Nistal, F. J., Daughters, G. T., Timek, T. A., Foppiano, L. E., Bolger, A. F., Ingels, N. B., Jr., and Miller, D. C. (1999) Deformational dynamics of the aortic root: Modes and physiologic determinants. *Circulation* 100(19 Suppl.): II54–II62.

Doehring, T. C., Carew, E. O., and Vesely, I. (2004) The effect of strain rate on the viscoelastic response of aortic valve tissue: A direct-fit approach. *Ann. Biomed. Eng.* 32(2): 223–232.

Dunmore-Buyze, J., Boughner, D. R., Macris, N., and Vesely, I. (1995) A comparison of macroscopic lipid content within porcine pulmonary and aortic valves. Implications for bioprosthetic valves. *J. Thorac. Cardiovasc. Surg.* 110(6): 1756–1761.

El-Hamamsy, I., Balachandran, K., Yacoub, M. H., Stevens, L. M., Sarathchandra, P., Taylor, P. M., Yoganathan, A. P., and Chester, A. H. (2009) Endothelium-dependent regulation of the mechanical properties of aortic valve cusps. *J. Am. Coll. Cardiol.* 53(16): 1448–1455.

Fukuda, S., Saracino, G., Matsumura, Y., Daimon, M., Tran, H., Greenberg, N. L., Hozumi, T., Yoshikawa, J., Thomas, J. D., and Shiota, T. (2006) Three-dimensional geometry of the tricuspid annulus in healthy subjects and in patients with functional tricuspid regurgitation—A real-time, 3-dimensional echocardiographic study. *Circulation* 114: I492–I498.

Ghista, D. N. and Rao, A. P. (1973) Mitral-valve mechanics—stress/strain characteristics of excised leaflets, analysis of its functional mechanics and its medical application. *Med. Biol. Eng. Comput.* 11(6): 691–702, DOI: 10.1007/BF02478657.

Grashow, J. S., Yoganathan, A. P., and Sacks, M. S. (2006) Biaxial stress–stretch behavior of the mitral valve anterior leaflet at physiologic strain rates. *Ann. Biomed. Eng.* 34(2): 315–325.

Hiro, M. E., Jouan, J., Pagel, M. R., Lansac, E., Lim, K. H., Lim, H. S., and Duran, C. M. G. (2004) Sonometric study of the normal tricuspid valve annulus in sheep. *J. Heart Valve Dis.* 13(3): 452–460.

Hurst, J. W. and O'Rourke, R. A. (2004) *The Heart*, McGraw-Hill Professional, New York.

Hurst, J. W. and O'Rourke, R. A. (2004) *The Heart: Manual of Cardiology*, McGraw-Hill Professional, New York.

Jouan, J., Pagel, M. R., Hiro, M. E., Lim, K. H., Lansac, E., and Duran, C. M. G. (2007) Further information from a sonometric study of the normal tricuspid valve annulus in sheep: Geometric changes during the cardiac cycle. *J. Heart Valve Dis.* 16(5): 511–518.

Joudinaud, T. M., Flecher, E. M., and Duran, C. M. G. (2006) Functional terminology for the tricuspid valve. *J. Heart Valve Dis.* 15(3): 382–388.

Kershaw, J. D., Misfeld, M., Sievers, H. H., Yacoub, M. H., and Chester, A. H. (2004) Specific regional and directional contractile responses of aortic cusp tissue. *J. Heart Valve Dis.* 13(5): 798–803.

Kim, W. Y., Bisgaard, T., Nielsen, S. L., Poulsen, E. M., Pedersen, E. M., Hasenkam, J. M., and Yoganathan, A. P. (1994) Two-dimensional mitral flow velocity profiles in pig models using epicardial Doppler echocardiography. *J. Am. Coll. Cardiol.* 24(2): 532–545.

Kunzelman, K. S. and Cochran, R. P. (1992) Stress/strain characteristics of porcine mitral valve tissue: Parallel versus perpendicular collagen orientation. *J. Card. Surg.* 7(1): 71–78.

Kunzelman, K. S., Einstein, D. R., and Cochran, R. P. (2007) Fluid-structure interaction models of the mitral valve: Function in normal and pathological states. *Phil. Trans. R. Soc. B* 362(1484): 1393–1406.

Kwan, J., Kim, G. C., Jeon, M. J., Kim, D. H., Shiota, T., Thomas, J. D., Park, K. S., and Lee, W. H. (2007) 3D geometry of a normal tricuspid annulus during systole: A comparison study with the mitral annulus using real-time 3D echocardiography. *Eur. J. Echocardiogr.* 8(5): 375–383.

Leeson-Dietrich, J., Boughner, D., and Vesely, I. (1995) Porcine pulmonary and aortic valves: A comparison of their tensile viscoelastic properties at physiological strain rates. *J. Heart Valve Dis.* 4(1): 88–94.

Leyh, R. G., Schmidtke, C., Sievers, H. H., and Yacoub, M. H. (1999) Opening and closing characteristics of the aortic valve after different types of valve-preserving surgery. *Circulation* 100(21): 2153–2160.

Lim, K. O. and Boughner, D. R. (1975) Mechanical properties of human mitral valve chordae tendineae: Variation with size and strain rate. *Can. J. Physiol. Pharmacol.* 53(3): 330–339, 10.1139/y75-048.

Lo, D. and Vesely, I. (1995) Biaxial strain analysis of the porcine aortic valve. *Ann. Thorac. Surg.* 60(2 Suppl.): S374–S378.

Merryman, W. D., Huang, H. Y., Schoen, F. J., and Sacks, M. S. (2006) The effects of cellular contraction on aortic valve leaflet flexural stiffness. *J. Biomech.* 39(1): 88–96.

Paulsen, P. K. and Hasenkam, J. M. (1983) Three dimensional visualization of velocity profiles in the ascending aorta of dogs, measured with a hot-film anemometer. *J. Biomech.* 16: 201–210.

Reul, H., Talukder, N., and Müller, E. W. (1981) Fluid mechanics of the natural mitral valve. *J. Biomech.* 14(5): 361–372.

Sacks, M. S., Smith, D. B., and Hiester, E. D. (1998) The aortic valve microstructure: Effects of transvalvular pressure. *J. Biomed. Mater. Res.* 41(1): 131–141.

Salisbury, P. F., Cross, C. E., and Rieben, P. A. (1963) Chorda tendinea tension. *AJP—Legacy Content* 205(2): 385–392.

Scott, M. J. and Vesely, I. (1996). Morphology of porcine aortic valve cusp elastin. *J. Heart Valve Dis.* 5(5): 464–471.

Shah, P. M. and Raney, A. A. (2008) Tricuspid valve disease. *Curr. Probl. Cardiol.* 33(2): 47–84.

Silver, M. D., Lam, J. H. C., Ranganat, N., and Wigle, E. D. (1971) Morphology of human tricuspid valve. *Circulation* 43(3): 333–348.

Skwarek, M., Hreczecha, J., Dudziak, M., and Grzybiak, M. (2006) The morphology of the right atrioventricular valve in the adult human heart. *Folia Morphol.* 65(3): 200–208.

Sloth, E., Houlind, K. C., Oyre, S., Kim, W. Y., Pedersen, E. M., Jorgensen, H.S., and Hasenkam, J. M. (1994) Three-dimensional visualization of velocity profiles in the human main pulmonary artery with magnetic resonance phase-velocity mapping. *Am. Heart J.* 128: 1130–1138.

Stella, J. A., Liao, J., and Sacks, M. S. (2007) Time-dependent biaxial mechanical behavior of the aortic heart valve leaflet. *J. Biomech.* 40(14): 3169–3177.

Sung, H. W. and Yoganathan, A. P. (1990) Secondary flow velocity patterns in a pulmonary artery model with varying degrees of valvular pulmonary stenosis: Pulsatile *in vitro* studies. *J. Biomech. Eng.* 112(1): 88–92.

Tei, C., Pilgrim, J. P., Shah, P. M., Ormiston, J. A., and Wong, M. (1982) The tricuspid-valve annulus—Study of size and motion in normal subjects and in patients with tricuspid regurgitation. *Circulation* 66(3): 665–671.

Thubrikar, M. (1990) *The Aortic Valve*, CRC Press, Boca Raton, FL.

Vesely, I. (1998) The role of elastin in aortic valve mechanics. *J. Biomech.* 31(2): 115–123.

Vesely, I. and Noseworthy, R. (1992) Micromechanics of the fibrosa and the ventricularis in aortic valve leaflets. *J. Biomech.* 25(1): 101–113.

Vesely, I., Macris, N., Dunmore, P. J., and Boughner, D. (1994) The distribution and morphology of aortic valve cusp lipids. *J. Heart Valve Dis.* 3(4): 451–456.

Victor, S. and Nayak, V. M. (2000) Tricuspid valve is bicuspid. *Ann. Thorac. Surg.* 69(6): 1989–1990.

Weyman, A. E. (1994) *Principles and Practices of Echocardiography*. Lea & Febiger, Philadelphia, PA.

Yap, C. H., Kim, H. S., Balachandran, K., Weiler, M., Haj-Ali, R., and Yoganathan, A. P. (2010) Dynamic deformation characteristics of porcine aortic valve leaflet under normal and hypertensive conditions. *Am. J. Physiol. Heart Circ. Physiol.* 298(2): H395–H405.

Yoganathan, A. P., Lemmon, J. D., and Ellis, J. T. (2000) Hard tissue replacement. In *The Biomedical Engineering Handbook*, 2nd edn., Bronzino, J. D., ed., CRC Press LLC, Boca Raton, FL.

Part III

Cardiovascular Implants, Biomechanical Measurements, and Computational Simulations

8 Prosthetic Heart Valve Dynamics

8.1 INTRODUCTION

Heart valve disease is one of the main afflictions of the cardiovascular system and can be caused by rheumatic fever, ischemic heart disease, bacterial or fungal infection, connective tissue disorders, trauma, and malignant carcinoid. In advanced form, it leads to various disabilities and, ultimately, to death. The valves that are most commonly affected are the mitral, aortic, and tricuspid valves. Malfunction of the valves affects their hemodynamic (i.e., fluid dynamic) performance in two primary ways:

1. *Stenosis*: narrowing of the valve, which results in a greater resistance to blood flow and, therefore, a greater pressure drop across the valve
2. *Incompetence*: failure of the valve to close completely, allowing blood to flow in the reverse direction (also called "regurgitation") when the valve should be shut

Both of these conditions reduce the efficiency of the heart and place additional stresses and strains upon it.

The decision to perform corrective surgery on the natural valve or to replace it with a prosthetic valve is often made on the basis of an evaluation of the functional impairment of the natural valve. A classification for such an evaluation as proposed by the New York Heart Association is utilized and surgery is usually limited to patients belonging to Classes III and IV.

The first clinical use of a cardiac valvular prosthesis took place in 1952 when Dr. Charles Hufnagel implanted an artificial caged ball valve to treat aortic insufficiency. The Plexiglas cage contained a ball occluder, and was inserted into the *descending* aorta without the need for cardiopulmonary bypass. It did not cure the underlying disease, but it did relieve regurgitation from the lower two-third of the body.

The first implant of a replacement valve in the actual anatomic position took place in 1960 along with the advent of cardiopulmonary bypass. Since that time, the achievements in valve design and the success of artificial heart valves as replacements have been remarkable with >50 different cardiac valves having been introduced over the past 35 years. Unfortunately, after many years of experience and success, not all problems associated with heart valve prostheses have been eliminated. The most serious current problems and complications are

- Thrombosis and thromboembolism
- Anticoagulant-related hemorrhage

- Tissue overgrowth
- Infection
- Paravalvular leaks due to healing defects
- Valve failure due to material fatigue or chemical change

While new valve designs continue to be developed, it is important to understand their history in order to be able to improve their future effectiveness.

8.2 BRIEF HISTORY OF HEART VALVE PROSTHESES

This section on replacement valves highlights only a relatively small number of the many designs that have been tried, but includes those that are either the most commonly used today or those that have made notable contributions to the advancement of replacement heart valves.

8.2.1 Mechanical Valves

The use of the caged ball valve in the descending aorta became obsolete with the development of what today is referred to as the *Starr-Edwards ball-and-cage* valve in 1960. Similar in concept to the original Hufnagel valve, it was designed to be inserted in place of the excised diseased natural valve. This form of intracardiac valve replacement was used in the mitral position, and for aortic and multiple valve replacements. Since 1962, the Starr-Edwards valve has undergone many modifications in order to improve its performance in terms of reduced hemolysis and thromboembolic complications. However, the changes have focused on materials and techniques of construction and have not altered the overall concept of the valve design in any way (Figure 8.1a).

Other manufacturers have produced variations of the ball-and-cage valve, notably the *Smeloff-Cutter valve* and the *Magovern prosthesis*. In the case of the former, the ball is slightly smaller than the orifice. A subcage on the proximal side of the valve retains the ball in the closed position with its equator in the plane of the sewing ring. A small clearance around the ball ensures easy passage of the ball into the orifice. This clearance also gives rise to a mild regurgitation which is felt, but not proven, to be beneficial in preventing thrombus formation. The Magovern valve consists of a standard ball-and-cage format that incorporates two rows of interlocking mechanical teeth around the orifice ring. These teeth are used for inserting the valve and are activated by removing a special valve holder once the valve has been correctly located in the prepared tissue annulus. Dislocation of this valve due to imperfect placement in a calcified annulus has been observed and, thus, the Magovern valve is no longer in use.

Due to the high profile design characteristics of the ball valves, low profile–caged disc valves were developed in the mid-1960s, especially for the mitral position. Examples of the caged disc designs are the *Kay-Shiley* and *Beall* prostheses, which were introduced in 1965 and 1967, respectively (Figure 8.1b). Caged disc valves were used exclusively in the atrioventricular position, but, due to their inferior hemodynamic characteristics, are rarely used today.

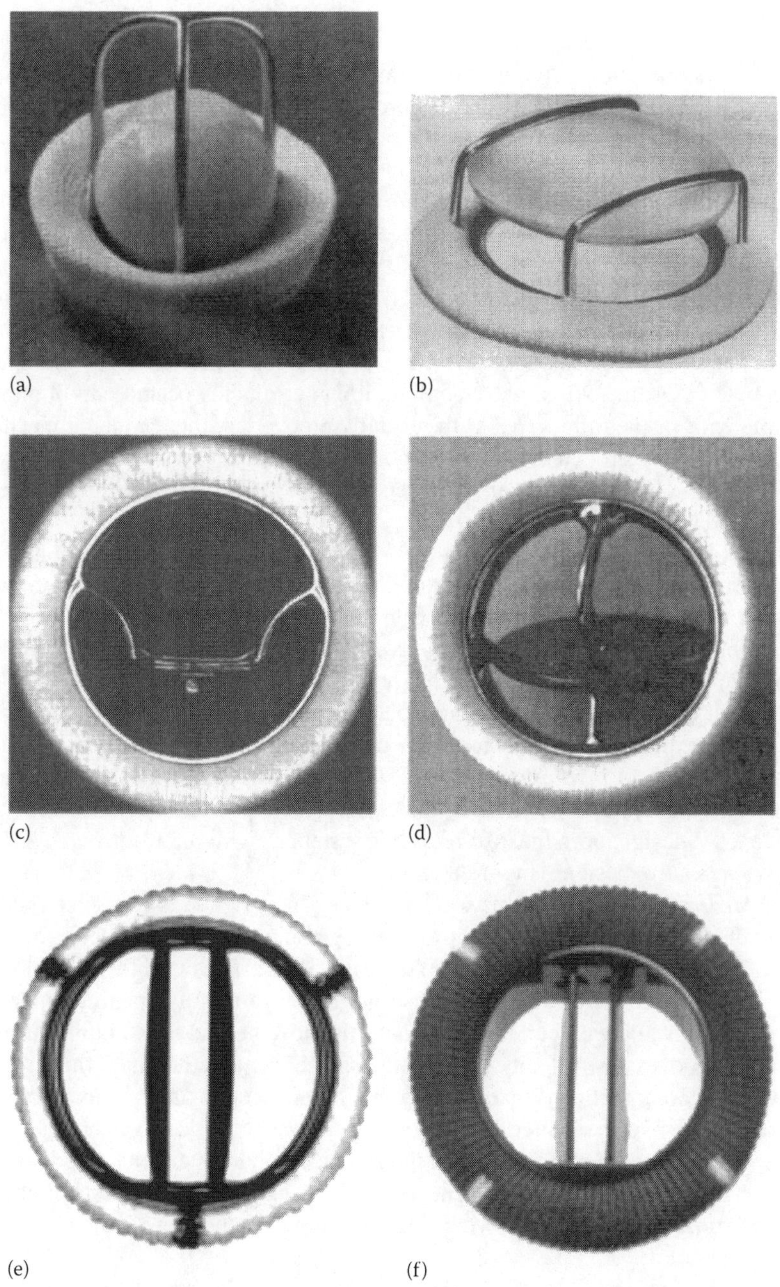

FIGURE 8.1 Photographs of various mechanical heart valves: (a) Starr-Edwards Caged ball valve; (b) caged disc heart valve; (c) Bjork-Shiley tilting-disc valve; (d) Medtronic Hall tilting-disc valve; (e) St. Jude Medical bileaflet valve; and (f) CarboMedics bileaflet valve. (From Yoganathan, A.P., Cardiac valve prostheses, in *The Biomedical Engineering Handbook*, Bronzino, J.D., ed., CRC Press, Boca Raton, FL, 1995. With permission.)

Currently, the ball-and-cage valve is no longer the most popular mechanical valve, having been superseded, to a large extent, by *tilting-disc* and *bileaflet* valve designs. These designs overcome two major drawbacks of the ball valve—namely, high profile configurations and excessive occluder-induced turbulence in the flow through and distal to the valve.

The most significant developments in mechanical valve design occurred in 1969 and 1970 with the introduction of the *Bjork-Shiley* and *Lillehei-Kaster* tilting-disc valves (Figure 8.1c). Both prostheses involve the concept of a "free" floating disc that, in the open position, tilts to an angle that depends on the design of the disc-retaining struts. In the original Bjork-Shiley valve, the angle of the tilt was 60° for the aortic and 50° for the mitral model. The Lillehei-Kaster valve has a greater angle of tilt of 80°, but in the closed position is preinclined to the valve orifice plane by an angle of 18°. In both cases, the closed valve configuration permits the occluder to fit into the circumference of the inflow ring with virtually no overlap, thus reducing mechanical damage to erythrocytes. A small amount of regurgitation backflow induces a "washing-out" effect of debris and platelets and theoretically reduces the incidence of thromboemboli.

The main advantage of the tilting-disc valve is that in the open position it acts like an aerofoil in the blood flow where induced flow disturbances are substantially less than those obtained with a ball occluder. Although the original Bjork-Shiley valve employed a Delrin® occluder, all present-day tilting-disc valves use pyrolytic carbon (PYC) for these components. It should also be noted that the "free" floating disc can rotate during normal function, thus preventing excessive contact wear from the retaining components on one particular part of the disc. Various improvements to this form of mechanical valve design have been developed but have tended to concentrate on alterations either to the disc geometry, as in the Björk-Shiley convexo-concave design, or to the disc-retaining system as with the *Medtronic Hall* and *Omniscience* valve designs (Figure 8.1d).

The *Medtronic Hall* prosthesis was introduced in 1977 and is characterized by a central, disc-control strut, with a mitral opening angle of 70° and an aortic opening angle of 75°. An aperture in the flat, PYC-coated disc affixes it to the central guide strut. This strut not only retains the disc but also controls its opening angle and allows it to move downstream 1.5–2.0 mm; this movement is termed disc "translation" and improves flow velocity between the orifice ring and the rim of the disc. The ring and strut combination is machined from a single piece of titanium for durability. All projections into the orifice (pivot points, guide struts, and disc stop) are open-ended, streamlined, and are placed in the region of highest velocity to prevent the retention of thrombi by valve components. The sewing ring is of knitted Teflon. The housing is rotatable within the sewing ring for optimal orientation of the valve within the tissue annulus.

Most recent mechanical valve designs are based on the bileaflet all-PYC valve designed by *St. Jude Medical, Inc.* introduced in 1978 (Figure 8.1e). This design incorporates two semicircular hinged PYC occluders (leaflets) that, in the open position, are intended to provide minimal disturbance to flow. The leaflets pivot within grooves made in the valve orifice housing. In the fully open position, the flat leaflets are designed to open to an angle of 85°.

The *CarboMedics bileaflet prosthesis* gained FDA approval in 1993 (Figure 8.1f). It is also made of Pyrolite, which is known for its durability and thromboresistance. The valve has a recessed pivot design and is rotatable within the sewing ring. The two leaflets are semicircular, radiopaque, and open to an angle of 78°. A titanium stiffening ring is used to lessen the risk of leaflet dislodgment or impingement. The CarboMedics Top Hat—an aortic version of this prosthesis was designed for implantation in the supra-annular position. This allows for an increase in the size of the implanted valve, thus improving forward flow hemodynamics of the valve.

Improving bulk flow hemodynamics of the bileaflet valve type has been a recent design goal for St. Jude Medical as well. The St. Jude Medical HP valve, introduced in 1993, features a decrease in thickness from the sewing cuff design of the original St. Jude Medical valve. This modification allows the placement of a proportionally larger housing within the cuff for a given tissue annulus diameter, thus increasing the orifice area available for flow. The *St. Jude Medical Regent* valve offers a further improvement in bulk flow hemodynamics over the original St. Jude Medical valve. This improvement is created by structurally reinforcing the housing of the St. Jude Medical HP, allowing a decrease in its thickness that further increases the internal orifice area available for flow.

The *Sorin Bicarbon* valve, marketed by Sorin Biomedica of Italy, is popular outside the United States. The curvature of the leaflets of the Bicarbon valve reduces pressure loss caused by the small central orifice of the original bileaflet valve design. The pivots of this valve are made up of two spherical surfaces of different radii of curvature. This design may reduce wear because the leaflet projection rolls across the housing, instead of sliding against it, when the valve opens and closes.

The *ATS Open Pivot* valve also features a change in the pivot design. Traditional bileaflet valve pivots are made up of an extension of the leaflet fitting into a recess in the housing where thrombus then has a tendency to form. The Open Pivot design inverts this traditional pivot mechanism, exposing the pivot to bulk forward flow. Exposure to high-velocity flow may then remove the protein and cell deposition on the pivot surface that leads to thrombus formation.

The *On-X* valve, marketed by the Medical Carbon Research Institute, is the most recent design introduction to the United States. Some of the innovative features of this valve are a length-to-diameter ratio close to that of native heart valves, a smoothed pivot recess that allows the leaflets to open at an angle of 90° relative to the valve housing, and a two-point landing mechanism during valve closure. The first two features result in improved bulk flow hemodynamics, while the latter may result in a more even distribution of stresses during valve closure, a quiet closure event, and a reduced cavitation potential.

The majority of valve replacements today utilize mechanical valves and the most popular design is the bileaflet with ~80% of the mechanical valves implanted today being bileaflet prostheses.

8.2.2 Tissue Valves

Two major disadvantages with the use of mechanical valves are (1) the need for lifelong anticoagulation therapy and (2) the accompanying problems of bleeding.

Furthermore, the hemodynamic function of even the best-designed valve differs significantly from that of the natural healthy heart valve. An obvious step forward in the development of heart valve substitutes was the use of naturally occurring heart valves. This lead to the approach of using antibiotic or cryo-treated human aortic valves (called *homografts*) removed from cadavers for implantation in place of a patient's own diseased valve.

The first of these homograft procedures was performed by Ross in 1962, and the overall results so far have been satisfactory. This is, perhaps, not surprising since the homograft replacement valve is optimum both from the point of view of structure and function. In the open position, these valves provide unobstructed central orifice flow and also have the ability to respond to deformations induced by the surrounding anatomical structure. As a result, such substitutes are less damaging to the blood when compared with the rigid mechanical valve. The main problem with these cadaveric allografts is that they are no longer living tissue and, therefore, lack the unique quality of cellular regeneration typical of normal living systems which makes them more vulnerable to long-term damage. Furthermore, they are available in very limited quantities.

An alternative approach is to transplant the patient's own pulmonary valve into the aortic position. This operation was also first carried out by Ross in 1967, and his study of 176 patients followed up over 13 years showed that such transplants continued to be viable in their new position with no apparent degeneration. This transplantation technique, however, is limited in that it can only be applied to one site.

The next stage in the development of tissue valve substitutes was the use of autologous fascia lata (a wide layer of membrane that encases the thigh muscles) either as free or frame-mounted leaflets. The former approach for aortic valve replacement was reported by Senning in 1966 and details of a frame-mounted technique were published by Ionescu and Ross in 1969. The approach combined the more natural leaflet format with a readily available living autologous tissue. Although early results seemed encouraging, even Senning expressed doubt about the value of this approach in 1971, and by 1978, fascia lata was no longer used in either of the aforementioned, or any other, form of valve replacement. The failure of this technique was due to the inadequate strength of this tissue when subjected to long-term cyclic stressing within the heart.

Alternative forms of tissue leaflet valves were being developed in parallel with the work on fascia lata valves. In these designs, however, more emphasis was placed on optimum performance characteristics than on the use of living tissue. In all these cases, the configuration involved a three-leaflet format that was maintained by the use of a suitably designed mounting frame. It was realized that naturally occurring animal tissues would be rejected by the host if used in an untreated form. Consequently, a method of chemical treatment had to be found, which prevented this antigenic response but which did not degrade the mechanical strength of the tissue.

Formaldehyde has been used by histologists for many years to arrest autolysis and to "fix" tissue in the state in which it was removed. It had been used to preserve biological tissues in cardiac surgery but, unfortunately, was found to produce shrinkage and also increase the "stiffness" of the resulting material. For these reasons, formaldehyde was not considered ideal as a method of tissue treatment. Glutaraldehyde is another histological fixative that has been used especially for preserving fine detail for electron microscopy. It is also used as a tanning agent by the leather industry. In addition to arresting autolysis, glutaraldehyde produces a more flexible material due to increased collagen cross-linking. Glutaraldehyde has the additional ability of reducing the antigenicity of xenograft tissue to a level at which it can be implanted into the heart without significant immunological reaction.

Clinical experience with different tissue valve designs has increasingly indicated time-dependent (i.e., 5 to 7 year) structural changes such as calcification and leaflet wear, leading to valve failure and subsequent replacement. Valve leaflet calcification is more prevalent in children and young adults, and, therefore, tissue valves are rarely used in those cases at the present time. While such problems have not been eliminated by fixation with glutaraldehyde, new technologies are promising. For example, α-amino oleic acid and an ethanol treatment for glutaraldehyde-fixed tissue are currently approved by the FDA for fixing tissue valves. α-Amino oleic acid reduces calcification by shielding negatively charged aldehyde groups that could attract positively charged calcium ions with amino groups on adjacent molecules. Treatment with ethanol extracts negatively charged lipids from aldehyde-fixed tissue. The anti-mineralization qualities of these fixatives have been shown *in vivo*, but long-term results of their clinical performance have yet to be seen.

In 1969, Kaiser et al. described a valve substitute using an explanted glutaraldehyde-treated porcine aortic valve that was mounted on a rigid support frame. Following modification in which the frame was replaced by one having a rigid base ring with flexible posts, this valve became commercially available as the *Hancock porcine xenograft* in 1970 (Figure 8.2a). It remains one of the three most popular valve substitutes of this type. One of the other two valves is the *Carpentier-Edwards bioprosthesis*, introduced commercially by Edwards Laboratories in 1976, which uses a totally flexible support frame.

In 1977, production began of the *Hancock modified orifice* (MO) valve, which is a refinement of the Hancock Standard valve. The Hancock MO represents a composite

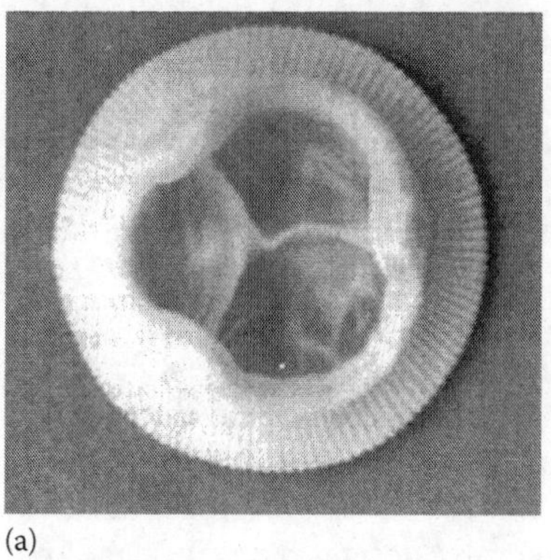
(a)

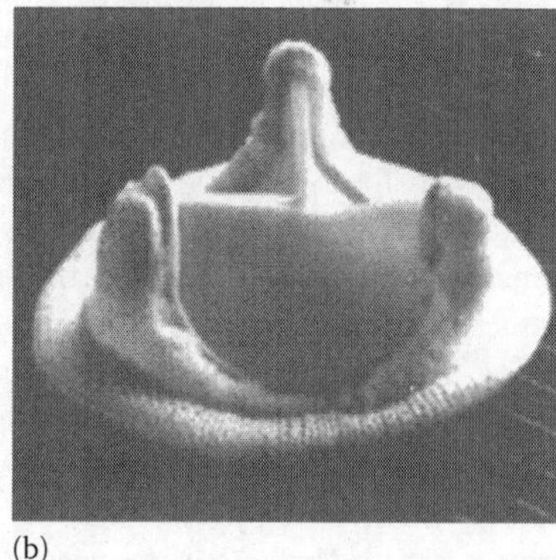
(b)

FIGURE 8.2 Photographs of biological leaflet valves: (a) a Hancock porcine bioprosthetic valve and (b) a Carpentier-Edwards pericardial valve prosthesis. (From Yoganathan, A.P. Cardiac valve prostheses, in *The Biomedical Engineering Handbook*, Bronzino, J.D., ed., CRC Press, Boca Raton, FL, 1995. With permission.)

nature wherein the right coronary leaflet containing the muscle shelf is replaced by a noncoronary leaflet of the correct size from another porcine valve. The valve is then mounted into a Dacron-covered polypropylene stent. The Hancock II and Carpentier-Edwards supra-annular porcine bioprostheses are second-generation bioprosthetic valve designs that were introduced in the early 1980s. The porcine tissue used in these valves is initially fixed at 1.5 mmHg and then again at high pressure which is a fixation method designed to ensure good tissue geometry. Both valves are treated with anti-mineralization solutions and have obtained FDA approval.

In porcine prostheses, the use of the intact biologically formed valve makes it unnecessary to manufacture individual valve cusps. While this has the obvious advantage of reduced complexity of construction, it does require a facility for harvesting an adequate quantity of valves so that an appropriate range of valve sizes with suitable quality can be made available. This latter problem was not an issue in the production of the three-leaflet calf pericardium valve developed by Ionescu et al. since this valve involved the molding of fresh tissue to a tricuspid configuration around a support frame. As the tissue is held in this position, it is treated with a glutaraldehyde solution. The valve, marketed in 1976 as the *Ionescu-Shiley pericardial xenograft*, was discontinued in the mid-1980s due to structural failure problems.

Early clinical results obtained with tissue valves indicated their superiority to mechanical valves with respect to a lower incidence of thromboembolic complications. For this reason, the use of tissue valves increased significantly during the late 1970s.

The *Carpentier-Edwards pericardial valve* consists of three pieces of pericardium mounted completely within an Elgiloy wire stent to reduce potential abrasion between the Dacron-covered frame and the leaflets. The pericardium is retained inside the stent by a Mylar button rather than by holding sutures (Figure 8.2b).

The *Medtronic Mosaic* valve, approved by the FDA in 2000, is the successor to the Hancock II porcine bioprosthesis. This valve features a compliant sewing ring that seals tightly in a valve annulus, a thin stent design, and a zero pressure fixation technique. The first two of these features improve bulk flow hemodynamics of the valve while the latter prevents tissue from being fixed in a prestressed state and may improve its longevity.

The most recent major change in heart valve design is the introduction of the stentless bioprosthesis by Dr. Tirone David. Dr. David hypothesized that fixing prosthesis leaflets to the aortic root would distribute mechanical stresses into the aortic tissue instead of focusing them on the leaflet tissue near the stents of traditional bioprostheses. In 1980, Dr. Yoganathan and collaborators stated that the absence of the stent was also thought to improve hemodynamics as there is less obstruction to flow. Dr. David collaborated with St. Jude Medical to produce the Toronto SPV aortic valve, which was approved by the FDA in 1997. Hemodynamic tests of this valve showed very little resting pressure gradient and clinical results of resistance to wear are very promising. Two other stentless aortic valve designs have since been brought to the market: the *Medtronic Freestyle* and *Edwards Prima* valves. The Prima valve allows full root or subcoronary implantation and removes the coronary arteries from the root while the Freestyle offers implantation by a variety of surgical techniques and offers ligated coronary arteries.

Stentless bioprostheses are only currently approved for aortic valve replacements in the United States. Stentless mitral valves have been under development for a number of years as clinical trials with these valves were first reported in 1992. Clinical and *in vitro* studies of stentless mitral valves have shown that they have superior hemodynamics but the questionable durability of these valves and complexity of the implantation technique have delayed their approval for the U.S. market.

8.2.3 Summary of Mechanical versus Tissue Valves

The clear advantage of mechanical valves is their long-term durability. Current mechanical valves are manufactured from a variety of materials, such as PYC and titanium. Although structural failure of mechanical valves is rare, it is usually catastrophic when it occurs. One major disadvantage of the use of mechanical valves is the need for continuous, lifelong anticoagulation therapy to minimize the risk of thrombosis and thromboembolic complications. Unfortunately, the anticoagulation therapy may lead to bleeding problems; therefore, careful control of anticoagulation medication is essential for the patient's well-being and quality of life. Another concern is the hemodynamic performance of the prosthesis. The function of even the best mechanical valve designs differs significantly from that of normal heart valves.

The major advantage of tissue valves compared with mechanical valves is that tissue valves have a lower incidence of thromboembolic complications. Therefore, most patients receiving tissue valves are not required to take anticoagulants long term. The major disadvantages to tissue valves are material fatigue and/or wear of valve leaflets, and calcification of valve leaflets, especially in children and young adults. Valve deterioration, however, usually takes place slowly with these valves, and thus, patients can be monitored by echocardiography and other noninvasive techniques.

8.2.4 Transcatheter Valves

Apart from mechanical heart valves (MHVs) and the bioprosthetic xeno/homografts, transcatheter valves have emerged more recently, arguably, as a separate category of replacement valve, due to its different means of implantation and target patient population. The traditional method for valve replacement is the open heart surgery procedure that involves opening up the chest and heart, excising the diseased valve and suturing the replacement valve in place. The transcatheter valve features a treated bioprosthetic valve mounted onto a collapsible stent and is delivered to the heart and implanted with a catheter, and thus no open heart procedures are required. At present, the procedure is targeted at patients who have high mortality risk in an open heart surgery due to age or other comorbidities such as diabetes or coronary diseases, and also for patients who would be denied conventional valve replacement therapy. It can be noted that as much as 33% of severe aortic stenosis patients fall within this category (Iung et al., 2005). The alternative options currently available for these patients, such as pharmacological treatment and percutaneous valvuloplasty, are much less effective than transcatheter valve replacement (Kapadia et al., 2009).

Transcatheter valves can be delivered in the transfemoral or transapical manner. In the former, the catheter gains access to the diseased valve by entering through the femoral artery and backtracking through the aorta to the heart. In the latter, the catheter enters the left ventricle directly from the apex of the heart. Balloon valvuloplasty is first performed to the calcified aortic valve to open it. The ventricle is temporarily induced into a state of rapid pacing with a pacemaker so as to reduce blood outflow through the aortic valve to facilitate valve deployment. Then, the valve is deployed by expanding a second balloon from within the valve. Due to the complicated implantation procedure, the outcome from transcatheter valve replacement therapy showed the presence of a learning curve, where intraoperative mortality decreased with increasing experience of the surgeon (Webb et al., 2007). Nonetheless, the outcomes were considered satisfactory by most clinical researchers (Bleiziffer et al., 2009; Webb et al., 2009).

The two well-known transcatheter valves are the Edwards SAPIEN® and Medtronic CoreValve® (Figure 8.3a and b, respectively). The Edwards SAPIEN valve is composed of three leaflets derived from bovine pericardium which are sewn onto a frame, known as a stent, and placed on a 22–24 Fr catheter for delivery either transapically or transfemorally. Lower mortality rates have been reported for minimally invasive surgical PHV replacements compared with open heart surgery, with mortality rates of about 10% and 30%, respectively. The clinical trial for the SAPIEN valve, the PARTNER (Placement of AoRTic traNscatheterER valves) trial, is underway in North America, results of which are expected in the upcoming years. The Medtronic CoreValve uses a slightly different technology for valve deployment and uses a different xenograft material. Instead of relying on the deformation of the

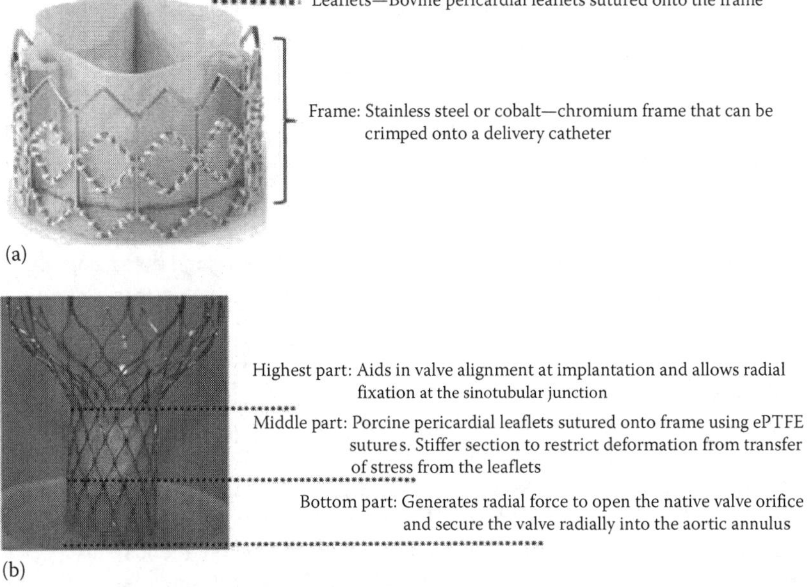
Leaflets—Bovine pericardial leaflets sutured onto the frame
Frame: Stainless steel or cobalt—chromium frame that can be crimped onto a delivery catheter
(a)
Highest part: Aids in valve alignment at implantation and allows radial fixation at the sinotubular junction
Middle part: Porcine pericardial leaflets sutured onto frame using ePTFE sutures. Stiffer section to restrict deformation from transfer of stress from the leaflets
Bottom part: Generates radial force to open the native valve orifice and secure the valve radially into the aortic annulus
(b)

FIGURE 8.3 Structural features of the (a) Edwards SAPIEN® valve and (b) the Medtronic CoreValve®.

stainless steel stent for valve placement such as in the case of the SAPIEN valve, the CoreValve uses a shape memory material, Nitinol® (a nickel-titanium alloy) for the stent. During deployment, the stent self-expands when exposed to physiological temperatures. Three porcine pericardium leaflets are sutured onto the Nitinol frame and crimped onto a 18 Fr catheter. Unlike the SAPIEN valve, the CoreValve is primarily delivered transfemorally and has similar survival rates as the CoreValve.

Several other designs of transcatheter valves are currently being developed. The Sadra Lotus® valve is made of bovine tissues on a Nitinol stent that allows surgeons to resheath and redeploy the valve in case the first deployment resulted in a nonideal valve position. Direct Flow Technologies® have developed a polymeric stent bovine tissue-derived valve that is partially deployed below the aortic annulus, and then moved up into place. The polyester polymeric stent is then filled with a solidifying medium to cure it, and set it in place. A similar Nitinol stent–based technology developed by Ventor Technologies® (now owned by Medtronic®) uses a transapical approach. The JenaValve™ by JenaValve™ Technology utilizes a Nitinol stent that differs in construction from the other valves; it has two layers of clips that anchor the valve to the inside of the aortic annulus and behind the diseased leaflets.

8.2.5 Current Types of Prostheses

At present, over 180,000 prosthetic valves are implanted each year throughout the world. The five most commonly used basic types of prostheses can be grouped as

- Caged ball
- Tilting disc
- Bileaflet
- Stented bioprosthesis
- Stentless bioprosthesis

Valve manufacturers continue to develop new designs of mechanical and tissue valves. While the ideal heart valve prosthesis does not yet exist, and may never be realized, the characteristics of the "perfect" prostheses should be noted. Specifically, the ideal heart valve should

- Be fully sterile at the time of implantation and be nontoxic
- Be surgically convenient to insert at or near the normal location of the heart
- Conform to the heart structure rather than the heart structure conforming to the valve (i.e., the size and shape of the prosthesis should not interfere with cardiac function)
- Show a minimum resistance to flow so as to prevent a significant pressure drop across the valve
- Only have a minimal reverse flow necessary for valve closure so as to keep incompetence of the valve at a low level
- Demonstrate resistance to mechanical and structural wear
- Be long-lasting (≥25 years) and maintain its normal functional performance (i.e., it must not deteriorate over time)

- Cause minimal trauma to blood elements and the endothelial tissue of the cardiovascular structure surrounding the valve
- Show a low probability for thromboembolic complications without the use of anticoagulants
- Be sufficiently quiet so as not to disturb the patient
- Be radiographically visible
- Have an acceptable cost

In terms of specific issues related to heart valve design, the basic engineering considerations are

- Flow dynamics
- Durability (structural mechanics and materials)
- Biological response to the prosthetic implant

8.3 HEMODYNAMIC ASSESSMENT OF PROSTHETIC HEART VALVES

Many of the basic principles of fluid mechanics that we have discussed in earlier chapters can be applied to the design and evaluation of prosthetic heart valves. Considerations that are of particular importance to this analysis are (1) transvalvular pressure drop, (2) effective valve orifice area, (3) regurgitant flow rate, and (4) local flow patterns.

8.3.1 Pressure Drop

Pressure drop and pressure recovery through prosthetic valves can be significant factors affecting the pressure within the left ventricle. A larger pressure drop across a prosthetic valve demands that a larger systolic pressure be generated in the left ventricle to drive flow through the circulation. Since it has been shown that the level left ventricular pressure produced is the primary determinant of myocardial oxygen consumption, it is imperative that the LV pressure be minimized when dealing with prosthetic valves. This continues to be an area of active research as there have been numerous publications detailing the effects of recovery on pressure drop measurements for both natural and prosthetic heart valves. The pressure drop (Δp) across a prosthetic valve is related to the energy losses caused by the valves' presence. Pressure drops across natural valves can be measured with invasively performed catheter techniques. However, it is both difficult and dangerous to pass a catheter through a prosthetic valve. Fortunately, the Bernoulli equation (see Section 1.6) can provide a noninvasive estimate of the pressure drop across prosthetic, and also, natural valves. Neglecting viscous effects under mean conditions, we obtain

$$p_1 - p_2 = \frac{1}{2}\rho(V_2^2 - V_1^2) \tag{1.63}$$

where Position 1 is proximal to the valve and Position 2 is at the orifice. If the velocity upstream of the valve is much smaller than at the valve, V_1 can be neglected and we obtain

$$p_1 - p_2 = 4V_2^2 \tag{1.65}$$

where the constant has units of (mmHg)/(m²/s²). Thus, if the velocity (m/s) is measured with *continuous wave Doppler ultrasound velocimetry* (see Section 10.6), the pressure drop (mmHg) can be obtained *noninvasively* using Equation 1.65.

When measuring pressure distal to prosthetic valves, it is important to note whether or not the recovered pressure is measured. This is especially important when using continuous wave Doppler ultrasound to evaluate prosthetic heart valves. Due to its large sample volume size, continuous wave Doppler ultrasound measures the highest flow velocity that occurs at the *vena contracta*. Consequently, the Doppler-derived pressure drops are always based on the pressure at the *vena contracta*, which is at a site proximal to where pressure recovery occurs. Thus, one is likely to overestimate the transvalvular pressure drop with this method because pressure recovery is not considered. However, even though Doppler ultrasound may overestimate transvalvular pressure drops, they are extremely useful in patient diagnosis. A recent study has shown that Doppler-derived pressure drops measured across small diameter prosthetic mechanical valves (e.g., Medtronic Hall & St. Jude) correlate just as strongly with fluid mechanical energy losses as the recovered pressure drops measured by catheterization.

Due to the larger separation region inherent in flow over bluff bodies, configurations such as the caged disc and caged ball have notably large pressure gradients. Tilting-disc and bileaflet valve designs present a more streamlined configuration to the flow, and, while separation regions may exist in these designs, the pressure gradients are typically smaller than for the bluff shapes. Stented bioprostheses have relatively acceptable pressure gradients for larger diameter valves because they more closely mimic natural valve geometry and motion than mechanical valves, but the smaller sizes (<23 mm) generally have higher pressure gradients than their mechanical valve counterparts, as shown in Figure 8.4. Stentless bioprostheses, in contrast, have comparable or lower pressure drops than mechanical prostheses. The clinical importance of pressure gradients in predicting long-term performance is not clear. The fact that these gradients are a manifestation of energy losses resulting from viscous-related phenomena makes it intuitive that minimizing pressure gradients across an artificial valve is highly desirable, in order to reduce the workload of the pump (i.e., left ventricle).

8.3.2 Effective Orifice Area

Cardiologists have used a variety of methods to determine the forward flow cross-sectional area of a valve. Due to acoustic anomalies caused by prosthetic valves and the limited spatial resolution of echocardiography, it is often impossible to measure the valve area directly. However, applying a control volume analysis to a prosthetic

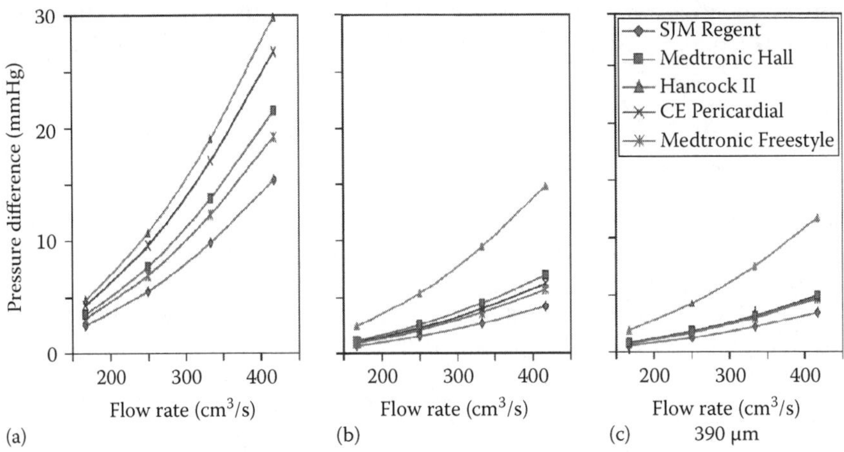

FIGURE 8.4 Comparison of transvalvular pressure drop as a function of root mean square flow rate across various mechanical and biological valve prostheses with tissue annulus diameter of (a) 19/20 mm, (b) 25 mm, and (c) 27 mm. (Note that the pressure drop decreases with larger tissue annulus diameters due to decrease in resistance of flow across the valve.)

valve in the aortic position allows for estimation of the mean area over which fluid flows as shown as follows:

$$A_2 = \int_T \frac{V_1(t)A_1}{V_2(t)}\,dt \tag{8.1}$$

where

A_2 is the area of the *vena contracta* or the effective valve area

A_1 is the area at the upstream face of the control volume, measured by echocardiography

The integral is taken with respect to time over the systolic flow period, V_1 is the velocity upstream of the aortic valve and V_2 is the velocity at the *vena contracta*. Inherent to Equation 8.1 is the assumption that the spatial velocity profile is uniform over the entire orifice area, but because the velocity profile is nonuniform in mechanical prostheses, it is difficult to apply this equation accurately in that case.

By extending the control volume from the left ventricular outflow tract to encompass the entire left ventricle, it is possible to use this technique to determine the mean mitral valve area. The time-velocity integral of both the mitral and the left ventricular outflow tract positions must be calculated over the entire cardiac cycle. It is only necessary to integrate the velocity at the mitral valve during diastole and the velocity of the aortic valve during systole, because these are the only times in which there is flow through the valves. If regurgitation is not present in either valve, Equation 8.1 can be applied and the effective area of the mitral valve can be obtained. When aortic regurgitation is present, the velocity and area at the right ventricular outflow tract can be used instead for calculation of effective mitral orifice area.

Another method of determining valve area can be derived using the Bernoulli equation and conservation of mass. A contraction coefficient (C_d) can be defined as the area of the *vena contracta* divided by the area of the valve orifice (A_0). The continuity equation for flow through an orifice, including the contraction coefficient, appears in Equation 8.2 where Q is the flow rate and V is the velocity at the *vena contracta*:

$$Q = A_0 V C_d \tag{8.2}$$

Solving for V_2 in Equation 1.64, substituting into Equation 8.2 and rearranging, yields an equation that can be used to determine the *effective orifice area* (EOA) of a cardiac valve

$$EOA\,(\mathrm{cm}^2) = \frac{Q_{rms}}{51.6\sqrt{\Delta\bar{p}}} \tag{8.3}$$

where

Q_{rms} is the root mean square systolic/diastolic flow rate (mL/s)
$\Delta\bar{p}$ is the mean systolic/diastolic pressure drop (mmHg)

The nondimensional constant, C_d, was determined by using the density of blood (ρ = 1050 kg/m³) and converting the units to those convenient for biomedical use. The effective area will be in cm² if the root mean square systolic or diastolic flow rate (Q_{rms}) is in mL/s and the mean systolic or diastolic pressure drop (Δp) is measured in mmHg. Similar relationships were derived earlier in Equations 5.4 and 5.5 through the application of Bernoulli's equation where the magnitude of the constants employed depends upon the discharge coefficient for a particular valve. Table 8.1 lists EOAs obtained *in vitro*, for mechanical and tissue valve designs in clinical use today. These results illustrate the fact that the newer mechanical valve designs have better pressure gradient characteristics than porcine bioprostheses in current clinical use.

Another method that has been developed to estimate the orifice area involves measuring the *pressure half time* of an orifice. The pressure half-time ($p_{t/2}$) is the time required for left ventricular pressure to fall to one-half of its peak value. An empirical relation has been established between the area of the mitral valve ($Area_{MV}$) and $p_{t/2}$ as

$$Area_{MV} = \frac{220}{p_{t/2}} \tag{8.4}$$

Equation 8.4 was based on observations that changes in the mitral pressure drop with time were constant for a particular orifice area. The constant in the equation, 220 (cm²·s), was empirically determined. Unfortunately, this equation has been shown to be dependent on a number of factors other than the valve area, including the severity of aortic regurgitation and ventricular wall properties. Furthermore, this equation is ineffective for prosthetic heart valves, thus limiting its application.

TABLE 8.1
Test Data for 27 mm Tissue Annulus Diameter Size Valves with Measurements Obtained Using an *In Vitro* Pulse Duplicator with a Heart Rate of 70 bpm and a Cardiac Output of 5.0 L/min

Valve Type	EOA[a] (cm^2)	*PI*	Regarding Volume (mL/beat)	Peak Turbulence SS[b] (dyn/cm^2)	ΔP (mmHg)
Caged ball	1.75	0.30	5.5	1850	13.6
Tilting disc[c]	3.49	0.61	9.4	1800	3.4
Bileaflet[c]	3.92	0.68	9.15	1940	2.7
Porcine (stented)[c]	2.30	0.40	<2	2980	7.9
Pericardial (stented)[c]	3.70	0.64	<3	1000	3.1
Stentless BHV	3.75	0.65	<4	N/A	3.0

Source: Values compiled from Yoganathan, A., Cardiac valve prostheses, in *The Biomedical Engineering Handbook*, Bronzino, J.D., ed., CRC Press, Boca Raton, FL, pp. 127.1–127.23, 2000.

[a] Effective orifice area (EOA) computed by the application of Gorlin equation (Equation 8.3).

[b] Turbulent stresses were measured at variable distances from the valve seat.

[c] Values reported are mean values from several valve models of the same type.

8.3.3 Regurgitation

Since mechanical prosthetic valves are fairly rigid, they are unable to form tight seals between the occluder and supporting ring when closed. Consequently, regurgitant jets are present in the resultant gaps in the prosthetic valves under normal conditions, although the amount of regurgitation is usually small. Normal regurgitant flow is characterized by having a *closing volume* during valve closure and *leakage* after closure. These parameters are illustrated in Figure 8.5. Regurgitant flow is often characterized by the *regurgitant volume.* The regurgitant volume is the total volume of fluid through the valve per beat due to the retrograde flow and is

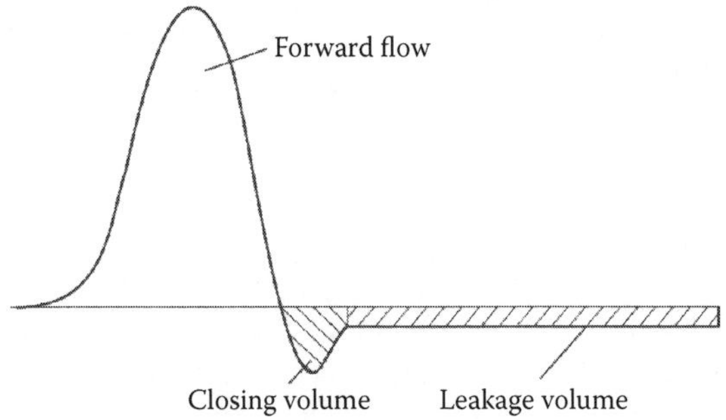

FIGURE 8.5 Schematic illustrating the closing and leakage volume across valve prosthesis. (From Yoganathan, A.P. Cardiac calve prostheses, in *The Biomedical Engineering Handbook*, Bronzino, J.D., ed., CRC Press, Boca Raton, FL, 1995. With permission.)

equal to the sum of the closing volume and the leakage volume. The closing volume is the volume of fluid flowing retrograde through the valve during valve closure. Any fluid volume accumulation after valve closure is due to leakage and is referred to as the *leakage volume*.

Closing regurgitation is related to the valve shape and closing dynamics and the percentage of stroke volume that succumbs to this effect is in the range of 2.0%–7.5% for mechanical valves and is typically less for tissue valves, ranging from 0.1% to 1.5%. Leakage, which depends upon how well the orifices are "sealed" upon closure, has a reported incidence of 0%–10% in mechanical valves and 0.2%–3% in bioprosthetic valves. The overall tendency is for regurgitation to be less for the bioprosthetic heart valves than for mechanical valve designs (see Table 8.1). To distinguish normal from abnormal valve function, it is important to differentiate between normal regurgitant volume and additional regurgitation due to disease. Fluid mechanical analysis of this problem has provided two different techniques—*turbulent jet theory* and *proximal flow convergence* that at least partially fulfill this requirement.

8.3.3.1 Turbulent Jet Theory

Using free turbulent jet theory, relations were derived for the regurgitant flow rate based solely on Doppler ultrasound measurements. Turbulent jets have a number of unique characteristics. Upon entering a chamber, they spread radially, pulling or entraining stationary fluid with them. Initially though, the jet has a core of fluid that is not affected by the stationary fluid. This *potential core* has the same velocity as the jet at the orifice and persists for a few orifice diameters downstream. Once the core vanishes, the jet reaches a state that is amenable to theoretical analysis. However, it is important to recognize the assumptions inherent in this theoretical analysis. One of these is that unsteady flow effects are neglected, and the analysis assumes that the jet enters a stationary fluid and does not impinge on solid boundaries. In the heart, regurgitant jets are unsteady, often impinge on the walls of the heart, and always encounter incoming forward flow. Additional work has been performed, which treats jets in confined and impinging geometries; these geometries more closely resemble the chambers of the left heart. A dimensional analysis model of valvular regurgitation has been reported based on the centerline velocity decay of the jet and the width and length of the receiving chamber and this equation has been shown to be accurate for a number of *in vitro* geometries and conditions.

8.3.3.2 Proximal Flow Convergence

The principle of conservation of mass was also applied in the region proximal to the valvular orifice to measure regurgitant volume. When fluid enters a regurgitant orifice, it must accelerate to reach a peak velocity at the throat of the orifice. If the orifice is circular, this acceleration region should be axisymmetric about the center of the orifice. Thus, upstream of the regurgitant orifice, a series of concentric isovelocity contours can be defined within the flow field which is hemispherical in shape. This physical argument is the basis for the *proximal flow convergence method* of quantifying regurgitant flow rate. If a control volume is constructed to coincide with a hemispherical contour and the regurgitant orifice, the same amount of fluid that enters the volume from an isovelocity contour will exit the control volume through the regurgitant orifice. The control volume statement is represented mathematically in Equation 8.5:

$$Q_0 = (4\pi r^2)V_r \tag{8.5}$$

where

Q_0 is the flow rate at the regurgitant orifice and the term within parentheses is the surface area of the hemispherical surface
V_r is the velocity measured with the color Doppler echocardiography
r is the radial distance at which the velocity is measured

Due to its simplicity and ease of application, this technique has received a great deal of attention, especially for mitral regurgitation. The effects of regurgitant orifice motion, orifice geometry variation, and ultrasound machine settings have all been addressed with both *in vitro* and *in vivo* investigations. In addition, its application to prosthetic valve regurgitation has also been considered. Recent studies have found that isovelocity contours from regurgitant orifices can be described better by a hemielliptical shape than a hemispherical shape, yielding more accurate estimations of regurgitant flow rate *in vitro*. Unfortunately, rigorous *in vivo* validation of the proximal flow convergence technique is difficult.

8.3.4 Flow Patterns and Shear Stresses

The potential of nonphysiological blood flow patterns to promote detrimental changes in the cardiovascular system has long been recognized. The German pathologist Virchow, in 1856, recognized that altered blood flow was one of the three general causes of thrombosis. Nonphysiological blood flow can initiate thrombus formation by imposing forces on blood elements or by changing their frequency of contact. Forces imposed by nonphysiological flow on blood cells can damage their structure or change their conformation, acting as a signal to promote coagulation. Blood flow patterns dictate how often cells and proteins contact the vessel walls and each other. A localized increase in this amount of contact can promote thrombus formation.

Therefore, recirculation zones and stagnation points are flow patterns, which can be detrimental to the healthy circulation. Recirculation zones are vortical regions in which activated platelets and coagulation inducing proteins can concentrate. Since these flow patterns often occur just distal to regions of high shear, they receive more of the coagulating agents than other areas of the flow field. All platelets within a fluid path line leading to a stagnation point are directed toward a vessel wall, and, thus, the stagnation point is a likely area for platelet adhesion, also being dependent on the magnitude of flow normal to the wall. Platelet aggregation in recirculation zone structures and adhesion to a vessel wall has been linked with platelet collision frequency, which is influenced by the speed of the flow.

Peak arterial viscous shear stresses within the normal circulation are between 50 and 200 dyn/cm^2. In valvular flow fields, the shear stresses platelets experience can be an order of magnitude higher than normal physiological values, increasing the likelihood of cell damage. Several studies have been carried out to determine the effects of viscous stresses on blood cells. Results from these studies have shown that (1) the threshold for cell damage by viscous stress occurs at a lower magnitude in the presence of foreign surfaces, (2) cell damage or activation depends on the time which the cells are exposed to a viscous stress as well as the stress magnitude, and (3) platelets are far more sensitive to a viscous stress stimulus than red cells. These studies suggest that the threshold for procoagulant platelet activity initiated by viscous shear stresses during flow across heart valve prostheses lies between 500 and 5000 dyn/cm^2. The effects of the presence of a prosthetic valve surface on this threshold, however, are currently unknown.

Turbulence rarely occurs in the circulation of a healthy human, but when it does, it increases the likelihood of cell damage. Information about the effects of turbulent shear stresses on blood cells is not as abundant as information about the effects of viscous shear stresses. The turbulent shear stress threshold for hemolysis during a 1 ms exposure time has recently been measured at 8000 dyn/cm^2, but sublethal damage to red cells has been observed at turbulent shear stress levels of 500 dyn/cm^2. An earlier study showed a linear correlation between the turbulent intensity within an arterial shunt and the weight of thrombus formed in this shunt, demonstrating that platelets are affected by turbulent shear stresses. However, thus far no attempts have been made to characterize a turbulent shear stress threshold for procoagulant platelet activity, despite the fact that this threshold is likely lower than the threshold for red cell damage. The turbulent shear stress threshold for procoagulant platelet activity is currently thought to be similar to the threshold for platelet activity induced by viscous stresses. These two forms of stresses could act differently, however. Turbulent stresses, unlike viscous stresses, act on a length scale much larger than the molecular scale. If the length scale over which a turbulent stress acts is much larger than the diameter of a blood cell, the cell may not experience the turbulent stress.

Thrombosis and embolism, tissue overgrowth, hemolysis, energy loss, and damage to endothelium adjacent to the heart valve are directly related to the velocity and turbulence fields created by various valve designs, and have been addressed in detail during the past three decades by investigators studying cardiovascular fluid mechanics.

In order to illustrate the abnormal flow fields and elevated levels of turbulent shear stresses created by prosthetic valves, *in vitro* forward flow measurements conducted on valve designs in current clinical use in the United States (i.e., FDA approved) are presented for typical valves in each of five categories—caged ball, tilting-disc, bileaflet, porcine, and pericardial valves. These measurements were obtained on size 27 mm aortic valves in a pulse duplicator that simulated physiological pulsatile flow using the laser Doppler technique described in Section 10.7. The details of the pulse duplicators used for such measurements in various laboratories can be found in publications describing such measurements comparing various mechanical and biological heart valve prostheses. Figures of the *in vitro* flow field studies are presented as schematic diagrams, and represent velocity and turbulence profiles obtained at peak systole, with a cardiac output of 5.0 L/min and a heart rate of 70 beats/min. All downstream distances are measured from the valve sewing ring. Table 8.1 lists peak turbulent shear stress levels measured downstream of the common 27 mm valve prostheses.

8.3.4.1 Caged Ball Valve

Flow emerging from the valve forms a circumferential jet that separates from the ball, hits the wall of the flow chamber, and then flows along the wall. It has very

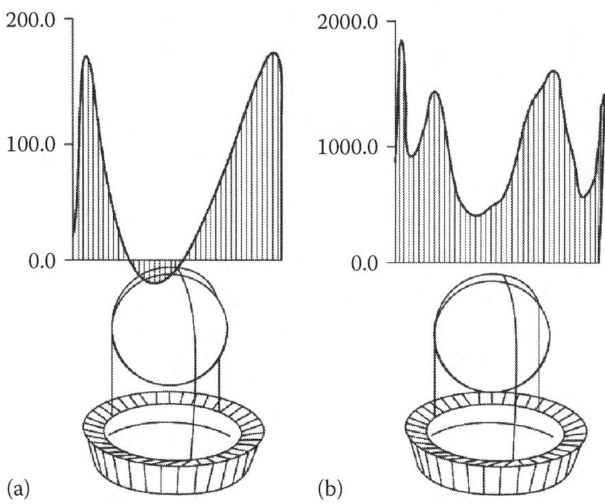

FIGURE 8.6 (a) Velocity profile distal to a caged ball valve in cm/s; (b) Turbulent shear stress in dynes/cm^2 distal to the valve. (From Yoganathan, A.P., Cardiac valve prostheses, in *The Biomedical Engineering Handbook*, Bronzino, J.D., ed., CRC Press, Boca Raton, FL, 1995. With permission.)

high velocities in the annular region. The maximum velocity, measured 12 mm downstream of the valve, is 220 cm/s at peak systole. The peak systolic velocity, measured 30 mm downstream of the valve, is 180 cm/s, as shown in Figure 8.6. High-velocity gradients are observed at the edges of the jet and the maximum velocity gradient (1700 cm/s/cm) is detected in the annular region adjacent to the surface of the ball during peak systole. A large velocity defect is also seen in the central part of the flow chamber as a wake develops distal to the ball. A region of low velocity, reverse flow is observed at peak systole and during the deceleration phase immediately distal to the apex of the cage which has a diameter of about 8 mm. A maximum reverse velocity of −25 cm/s occurs at peak systole 30 mm downstream of the valve. The intensity of the reverse flow during the deceleration phase is not as high as that observed at peak systole and no reverse flow is observed during the acceleration phase. The velocity in the central part of the flow channel, however, is low.

High turbulent shear stresses are present at the edges of the jet. The maximum turbulent shear stress measured is 1850 dyn/cm^2, which occurs at the location of the highest velocity gradient. The intensity of turbulence during peak systole does not decay very rapidly downstream of the valve and elevated turbulent shear stresses occur during most of systole. Turbulent shear stresses as high as 3500 dyn/cm^2 are estimated in the annular region between the flow channel wall and the ball.

8.3.4.2 Tilting-Disc Valve

High-velocity jetlike flows are observed from both the major and minor orifice outflow regions. The orientation of the jets with respect to the axial direction changes as the valve opens and closes. The major orifice jet is larger than the minor orifice jet and has a slightly higher velocity. The peak velocities measured 7 mm downstream of the valve are 210 and 200 cm/s in the major and the minor orifice regions,

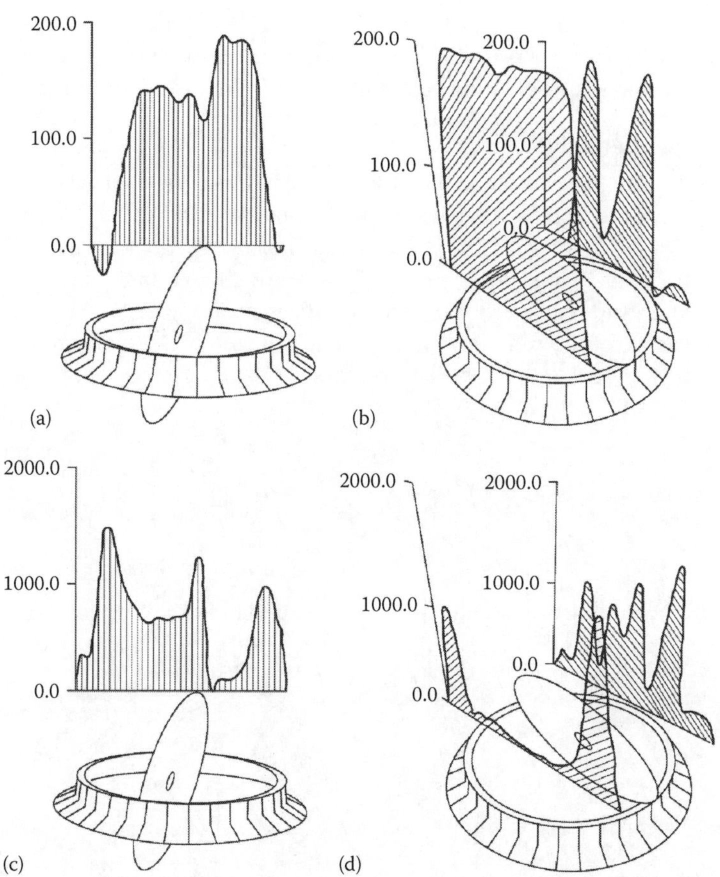

FIGURE 8.7 (a, b) Velocity profile distal to a tilting-disc mechanical valve in cm/s on three different planes; (c, d) Turbulent shear stress in dynes/cm^2 on the same planes. (From Yoganathan, A.P., Cardiac valve prostheses, in *The Biomedical Engineering Handbook*, Bronzino, J.D., ed., CRC Press, Boca Raton, FL, 1995. With permission.)

respectively (Figure 8.7). A region of reverse flow is observed adjacent to the wall in the minor orifice region at peak systole, which extends 2 mm from the wall with a maximum reverse velocity of −25 cm/s. The size of this region increases to 8 mm from the wall during the deceleration phase. A small region of flow separation is observed adjacent to the wall in the major orifice region. In the minor orifice region, a profound velocity defect is observed between 7 and 11 mm distal to the minor orifice strut. Furthermore, the region adjacent to the wall immediately downstream of the minor orifice is stagnant during the acceleration and deceleration phases and has very low velocities (<15 cm/s) during peak systole.

In the major orifice region, high turbulent shear stresses are confined to narrow regions at the edges of the major orifice jet. The peak turbulent shear stresses measured at peak systole are 1200 and 1500 dyn/cm^2, at 7 and 13 mm downstream of the valve, respectively. During the acceleration and deceleration phases, the turbulent shear stresses are relatively low. High turbulent shear stresses are more dispersed in the minor orifice than those in the major orifice region. The turbulent shear stress profiles across the major and minor orifices 15 mm downstream of the valve show a maximum turbulent shear stress of 1450 dyn/cm^2 at the lower edge of the minor orifice jet.

8.3.4.3 Bileaflet Valve

The bileaflet valve has two semicircular leaflets that divide the area available for forward flow into three regions—two lateral orifices and a central orifice. The major part of the forward flow emerges from the two lateral orifices. The measurements along the centerline plane 8 mm downstream of the valve show a maximum velocity of 220 and 200 cm/s for the lateral and central orifice jets, respectively, at peak systole. The velocities of the jets remain about the same as the flow travels from 8 to 13 mm downstream (Figure 8.8). The velocity profiles show two defects that corresponded

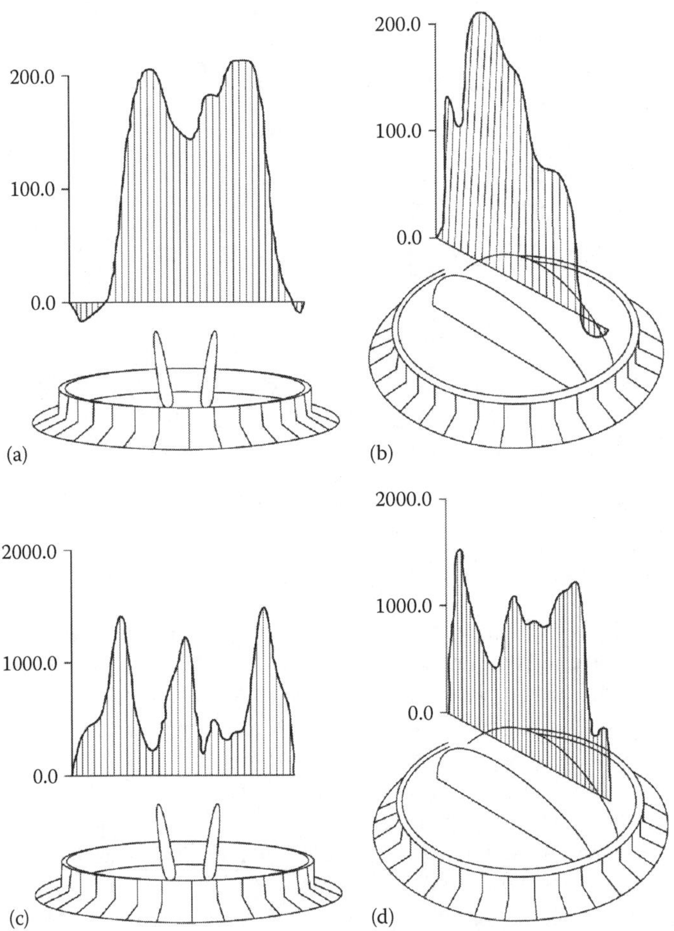

FIGURE 8.8 (a, b) Velocity profile distal to a bileaflet mechanical valve in cm/s on two different planes; (c, d) Turbulent shear stress in dynes/cm^2 on the same planes. (From Yoganathan, A.P., Cardiac valve prostheses, in *The Biomedical Engineering Handbook*, Bronzino, J.D., ed., CRC Press, Boca Raton, FL, 1995. With permission.)

to the location of the two leaflets. The velocity measurements indicate that the flow is more evenly distributed across the flow chamber during the deceleration phase than during the acceleration phase. Regions of flow separation are observed around the jets adjacent to the flow channel wall as the flow separates from the orifice ring. The measurements across the central orifice show that the maximum velocity in the central orifice is 220 cm/s. Small regions of low velocity reverse flow are observed adjacent to the pivot/hinge mechanism of the valve. More flow emerges from the central orifice during the deceleration phase than during the acceleration phase.

High turbulent shear stresses occur at locations of high-velocity gradients and at locations immediately distal to the valve leaflets. The flow along the centerline plane becomes more disturbed as the flow travels from 8 to 13 mm downstream of the valve. The peak turbulent shear stresses measured along the centerline plane at peak systole are 1150 and 1500 dyn/cm^2 at 8 and 13 mm downstream of the valve, respectively. The profiles across the central orifice show that the flow is very disturbed in this region. The maximum turbulent shear stress measured in the central orifice (1700 dyn/cm^2) occurs at peak systole. Since these high turbulent shear stresses across the central orifice are measured 11 mm downstream, it is probable that even higher turbulent shear stresses occur closer to the valve.

8.3.4.4 Porcine Valve

The velocity profiles for an atypical porcine valve taken 10 mm downstream of the valve, along the centerline plane, show that the peak velocity of the jetlike flow emerging from the valve is as high as 220 cm/s at peak systole (Figure 8.9). The peak velocities measured during the acceleration and deceleration phases are about the same—175 and 170 cm/s, respectively. However, the flow is much more evenly distributed during the acceleration phase than during the deceleration phase. No regions of flow separation are observed throughout the systolic period in this plane of measurement. However, the annular region between the outflow surfaces of the leaflets and the flow chamber wall is relatively stagnant throughout systole. The velocity of

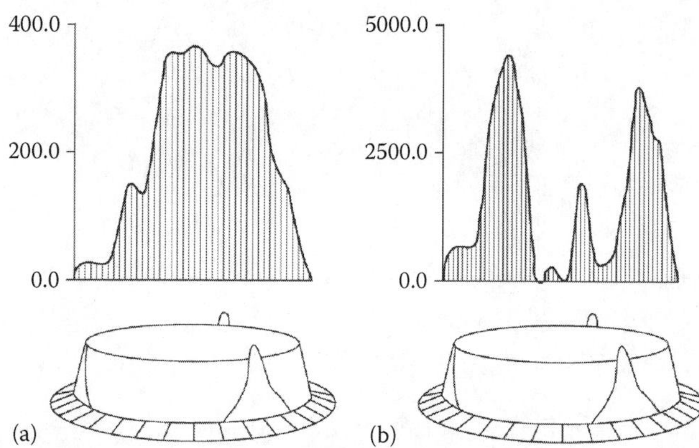

FIGURE 8.9 (a) Velocity profile distal to a porcine bioprosthetic valve in cm/s; (b) Turbulent shear stress in dynes/cm^2 distal to the valve. (From Yoganathan, A.P., Cardiac valve prostheses, in *The Biomedical Engineering Handbook*, Bronzino, J.D., ed., CRC Press, Boca Raton, FL, 1995. With permission.)

the jet increases to about 370 cm/s at peak systole as the flow travels from 10 to 15 mm downstream of the valve. This indicates that the flow tends to accelerate toward the center of the flow channel. High turbulent shear stresses occur at the edge of the jet. The maximum turbulent shear stress is 2750 dyn/cm^2 and is measured 10 mm downstream of the valve along the centerline plane at peak systole. The turbulent shear stresses at the edge of the jet increase as the flow travels from 10 to 15 mm downstream of the valve. The mean and maximum turbulent shear stress measured at peak systole increase to 2000 and 4500 dyn/cm^2, respectively.

8.3.4.5 Pericardial Valve

The velocity profiles obtained distal to a typical pericardial valve along the centerline plane 17 mm downstream of the valve at peak systole show a maximum velocity of 180 cm/s. The maximum velocities measured during the acceleration and deceleration phases are 120 and 80 cm/s, respectively. A region of flow separation that extends about 6 mm from the wall is observed at peak systole and during the deceleration phase. This region is relatively stagnant during the acceleration phase. The maximum velocity of the jet at peak systole does not change as the flow field travels from 17 to 33 mm downstream of the valve (Figure 8.10). However, the size of the region of flow separation decreases and extends only 1 mm from the wall.

Turbulent shear stress measurements taken along the centerline plane 17 mm downstream of the valve show that, during the deceleration phase, elevated turbulent shear stresses are spread out over a wide region (with a maximum value of 1200 dyn/cm^2). At peak systole, the high turbulent shear stresses are confined to a narrow region, with a maximum value of 850 dyn/cm^2. The intensity of turbulence at peak systole increases as the flow travels from 17 to 33 mm downstream of the valve.

8.3.4.6 Transcatheter Valve

In vitro testing of the transcatheter valves showed that they have an EOA of about 1.8 cm^2 and a mean pressure gradient of 8.3 mmHg, which is comparable with stented

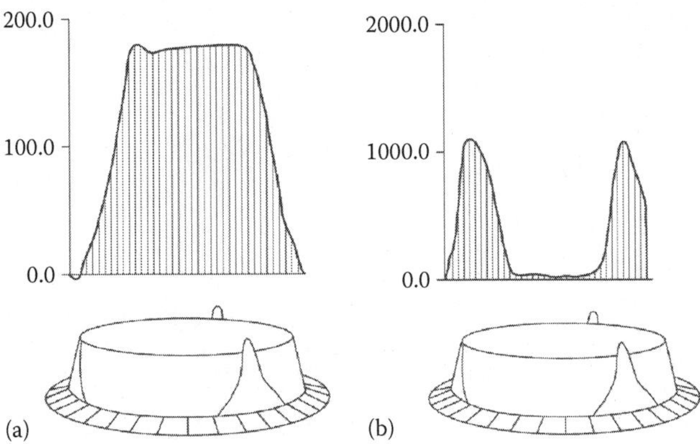

FIGURE 8.10 (a) Velocity profile distal to a pericardial bioprosthetic valve in cm/s; (b) Turbulent shear stress in dynes/cm^2 distal to the valve. (From Yoganathan, A.P., Cardiac valve prostheses, in *The Biomedical Engineering Handbook*, Bronzino, J.D., ed., CRC Press, Boca Raton, FL, 1995. With permission.)

bioprosthesis (Yoganathan et al., 2004; Azadani et al., 2009). The same data gathered from the clinical setting showed that the EOA of transcatheter valves is between 1.5 and 1.8 cm^2, and the corresponding pressure gradient is about 10 mmHg (Webb et al., 2007; Vahanian et al., 2008).

Unlike bioprosthetic valves, regurgitation in transcatheter valves is very common. Mild to moderate regurgitation occurs in >50% of the cases, while severe regurgitation occurs in 5% of the cases (Webb et al., 2007; Grube et al., 2008; Vahanian et al., 2008; Clavel et al., 2009). Regurgitation in transcatheter valves is mostly perivalvular, occurring between the valve and the native tissues rather than through the valve orifice. Since the implanted valve is merely pressed onto native tissues due to pressure exerted by the stents, a complete seal cannot be achieved in majority of the cases, especially when the native aortic valve is heavily calcified and presents a very uneven surface for the transcatheter valve to fit onto. Perivalvular leakage can exert high shear stress on regurgitating blood and cause clots, which may explain the high incidence of vascular complication (10%–15% of cases) (Vahanian et al., 2008).

8.3.5 Leakage Flow through Heart Valve Prostheses

Retrograde flow in mechanical prostheses is composed of the *squeeze flow*, which occurs during valve closure, and the *leakage flow*, which occurs after valve closure. The former, which can be observed in bileaflet and tilting-disc prosthetic designs, is a result of the rising fluid pressure across the valve and the closing occluder. These conditions "squeeze" blood through the interstitial gap between the closing occluder and the valve housing. The latter flow comprises the flow through the hinge region, which is found in the bileaflet designs only, and the leakage flow that can be observed through the perimeter of the closed occluder. Hinge flow is rapidly constricted from a large chamber to the small area of the hinge region and is driven by the elevated transvalvular pressure after valve closure. These retrograde flow phenomena are characterized by elevated fluid velocities (2–3 m/s) and high turbulent shear stresses (150–800 N/m^2) through gaps with an average of 0.5 mm in width.

"Squeeze" flow is closely related to cavitation. Numerical and *in vitro* experiments have shown that the pattern of "squeeze" flow is related to the moving boundaries, that is, the approaching leaflets and the valve housing, and to the velocity of the closing leaflets. Typical closing velocities at the occluder tips range from 1 to 3 m/s. With a gap width of ~50 μm, the peak squeeze-flow velocity has been estimated as high as 30–40 m/s with corresponding negative pressures of ~15 MPa. With a gap width of 48 μm and a high occluder tip velocity of 4 m/s, a peak squeeze flow of ~30 m/s has been reported. It has also been demonstrated that a peak squeeze-flow velocity as high as 150 m/s can exist with gap width of only 0.3 μm. On the other hand, a peak squeeze flow of <10 m/s has been measured through a gap width of ~100 μm. The broad range observed in the measurement of the gap width can be attributed to the difficulties of determining the exact location of the moving occluder with respect to the valve housing, different valve designs, and their manufacturing tolerances.

It has only recently been recognized that *hinge flow* is potentially damaging to the blood. Subsequent studies have shown that hinge geometry design is capable of influencing retrograde flow characteristics. With the myriad of bileaflet

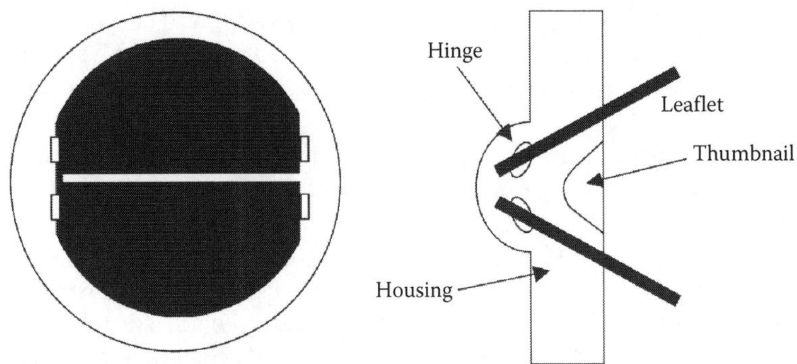

FIGURE 8.11 Schematic of the hinge for one bileaflet valve model. (From *J. Thorac. Cardiovasc. Surg.*, 124, Leo et al., Title of article/title of chapter, 561–574, Copyright (2002), with permission from Elsevier.)

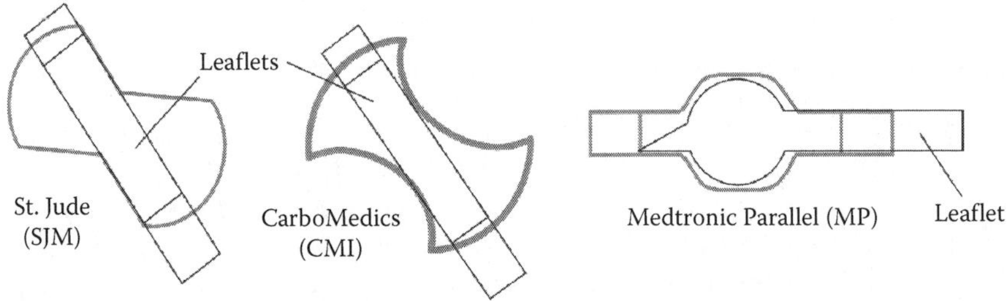

FIGURE 8.12 Comparison of hinge geometry for two commercially available bileaflet valve designs. (From *J. Thorac. Cardiovasc. Surg.*, 124, Leo et al., 561–574, Copyright (2002), with permission from Elsevier.) Structural features of (a) the Edwards SAPIEN® valve and (b) the Medtronic CoreValve®. (Obtained from Padala, M. et al., *Cardiovasc. Eng. Technol.*, 1(1), 77, 2010.)

valve designs currently available, it is important to compare the merits of various hinge designs to assess their potential for thrombogenesis (Figures 8.11 and 8.12). A certain degree of regurgitant flow is usually incorporated into the design of a bileaflet MHV to ensure the washout of critical areas of the valve such as hinges and regions between the leaflet edges and housing. This washout is intended to prevent flow stasis that may be created in the vicinity of these regions, and therefore minimize, if not eliminate, the formation of thrombosis. A properly conducted hinge flow study should compare the flow in both the leakage and forward flow phases to assess stresses on the blood cells and the degree of washout in that particular valve design.

Leakage can also exit the narrow spaces between occluder and housing just upstream of mechanical valves in the form of high speed jets. The pattern of these *leakage jets* is particular to the valve design. Figure 8.12 shows the results of a laser Doppler velocimetry experiment designed to measure velocity and turbulence within half the leakage jets of a bileaflet valve *in vitro* under aortic flow conditions. The lengths and directions of the arrows in this figure are representative of the jet velocity magnitude and direction. The valve diagram in the upper right-hand corner

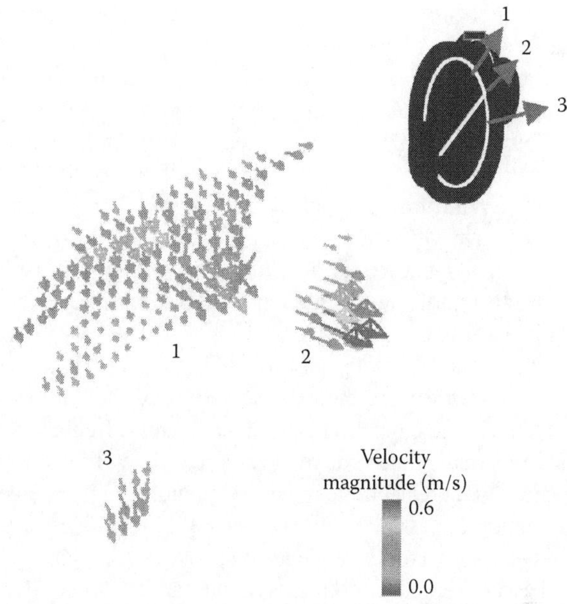

FIGURE 8.13 Laser Doppler measurement of leakage jets in a bileaflet valve near to the leaflet hinges (1, 3), and on the B-datum gap line (2). (From Travis, B., The effects of bileaflet valve pivot geometry on turbulence and blood damage potential, PhD thesis, Georgia Institute of Technology, Atlanta, GA, 2001.)

of this figure shows the relative positions of the leakage jets with respect to the valve. Two of these jets exit the valve from pivots, while the remaining jet appears to exit from the intersection of the two leaflets and the valve housing. The largest velocity magnitude measured in these jets was 0.6 m/s, and the largest turbulent shear stress magnitude measured was 28.9 N/m^2.

A glance at Figure 8.13 shows that the jets exiting from the valve are asymmetric, though the valve itself is symmetric. This is likely due to the small differences in leakage gap widths created by manufacturing tolerances. These tolerances may have a significant effect on the character of the leakage flow. Velocities as high as 3.7 m/s and Reynolds shear stresses as high as 1000 N/m^2 have been reported within mechanical valve leakage jets. If Reynolds shear stresses of these magnitudes occur, the size of the smallest turbulent length scale is about 7 μm. Since this is nearly the same size as the blood cells, it is possible that the turbulence would dissipate its energy directly on them.

8.3.6 Cavitation and HITS

The sudden stop and rebound of a mechanical valve occluder creates high magnitude negative pressure transients. If the magnitudes of these transients are strong enough, local pressures in the vicinity of the valve may drop below the vapor pressure of blood, which may result in the formation of small vapor bubbles.

The implosions of such *cavitation bubbles* generate small, high-velocity jets, and large oscillations in pressure. Severe cavitation phenomena in industry have been shown to damage stainless steel turbine blades. In patients with mechanical valves, cavitation may cause damage to the blood and possibly to the valve structure itself. Cavitation has been suggested as a possible reason for the incidents of leaflet fracture in patients with Edwards-Duromedics bileaflet valves. Bubbles created by cavitation may act as nucleation sites for the formation of gaseous emboli. A form of gaseous emboli, dubbed *high-intensity transient signals* (HITS) due to its nature as detected by Doppler ultrasound, has been observed in examinations of the middle cerebral and carotid arteries of patients with mechanical prostheses.

Many *in vitro* studies have directly visualized the formation and collapse of cavitation bubbles near heart valve prostheses, and have used the number and density of observed bubbles to estimate cavitation intensity. The high-frequency pressure oscillations that occur immediately after valve closure have been linked to cavitation, and have been suggested as a more accurate means of quantifying its intensity. This would enable the quantification of cavitation *in vivo* because fluctuations of pressure can be measured via a catheter with a high-frequency response. Such high-frequency pressure fluctuations have been observed in both sheep and patients with MHVs. In an effort to develop pressure fluctuations as a means of quantifying cavitation, recent work has successfully separated fluctuations resulting from mechanical resonance of the valve structure from other, higher-frequency components representative of cavitation.

Most cavitation studies have been carried out on valves in the mitral position, which has the harshest closure conditions of the four valve positions. During valve closure, the leaflets of a resting human mitral valve are driven shut by a loading condition that is estimated to lie between 750 and 2000 mmHg/s. This causes a prosthetic valve occluder to move from the fully open position to the closed position in a time varying between 20 and 30 ms.

Cavitation potential has been linked to the severity of the closure conditions and to valve design. An early study found that pitting—a sign of wear indicative of cavitation—was noted on valves implanted in sheep forced to exercise, but not on valves implanted in resting sheep. Both *in vitro* and *in vivo* studies have found stronger signs of cavitation, as the loading condition during closure is increased. Increased cavitation potential has been hypothesized for valve designs that feature an occluder rim, which overlaps the annular rim of the valve housing. A dimensional analysis of factors affecting cavitation in tilting-disc valves has linked cavitation potential with several aspects of occluder design and material.

The detection of HITS in the arteries of patients with mechanical prostheses has prompted studies into the nature of these emboli. While vaporous cavitation bubbles implode within a few milliseconds, microbubbles created from gasses dissolved in the blood may remain in the circulation much longer. The inhalation of pure oxygen significantly reduces the number of HITS in the circulation of patients with mechanical prostheses, suggesting that HITS are gaseous in nature, and that these emboli are composed primarily of nitrogen and/or carbon dioxide. An *in vitro* study performed using porcine blood has shown that gaseous emboli are likely to occur when the partial pressure of carbon dioxide exceeds 100 mmHg.

8.4 *IN VITRO* STUDIES OF COAGULATION POTENTIAL AND BLOOD DAMAGE

Results from clinical studies on the blood of patients with MHVs have shown elevated levels of hemolysis, P-selectin, platelet factor 4, and other biochemical markers of blood damage and platelet procoagulant activity. Some of these markers have been used *in vitro* to quantify the effects of controlled flow conditions across a prosthetic valve upon changes in the condition of the blood.

Initial *in vitro* studies used plasma-free hemoglobin as a marker of blood damage. Some of these studies have linked hemolysis of porcine blood to severity of leakage and closure flow conditions. A recent study has found that much more flow energy is dissipated across platelets than erythrocytes in humans, and suggests that markers of platelet procoagulant activity are more sensitive to flow stimuli than plasma-free hemoglobin. Leakage gap width has been linked to an increase in the expression of plasma platelet factor 4 activity and Annexin V binding to platelet surfaces. The relationship between plasma lactate dehydrogenase activity, turbulent shear stress, and exposure of platelets to such a stress has been mathematically modeled and used to compare the potentials of several valve designs to stimulate platelets during forward and leakage flow.

The clotting of milk has been suggested as an analog to the formation of thrombus, as the biochemical mechanisms for milk clot and thrombus formation are similar, and because milk clots and thrombus tend to occur under similar flow conditions. A few studies have attempted to develop *in vitro* systems that initiate milk clotting as a useful tool for predicting locations where thrombus is likely to occur on heart valve prostheses. Though results from these experiments are encouraging, milk coagulation has not yet developed into a tool that is considered predictive of thrombus formation.

8.4.1 Implications for Thrombus Deposition

In the vicinity of mechanical aortic heart valves where peak turbulent shear stresses can easily exceed $150\,N/m^2$, mean turbulent shear stresses are frequently in the range of $20–60\,N/m^2$, and cavitation is possible, platelet activation and aggregation can readily occur. Data indicating that shear-induced platelet damage is cumulative are particularly relevant to heart valves. During an individual excursion through the replacement valve, the combination of shear magnitude and exposure time may not induce platelet aggregation. However, as a result of multiple journeys though the artificial valve, shear-induced damage may accumulate to a degree sufficient to promote thrombosis and subsequent embolization.

All of the aortic and mitral valve designs (mechanical and tissue) studied created mean turbulent shear stress in excess of $20\,N/m^2$ during the major portion of systole and diastole, a level that could lead to damage to blood elements. In the case of mechanical prostheses, the chances for blood cell damage are increased due to the presence of foreign surfaces. Furthermore, the regions of flow stagnation and/or flow separation that occur adjacent to the superstructures of these valve designs could promote the deposition of damaged blood elements, leading to thrombus formation on the prosthesis.

The clinical performance of the Medtronic Parallel valve is an example of the effects of these flow patterns on likelihood for thromboembolic complications. This valve showed superior forward flow hemodynamics in an *in vivo* porcine model, suggesting a good clinical performance. However, the Parallel valve performed very poorly in clinical trials; ~20% of patients in these trials developed thrombosis. Patient and material factors were statistically eliminated from the potential reasons for the poor performance. Subsequent *in vitro* analysis of flow through the valve pivot revealed regions of highly disturbed vortical flow within this area during the leakage phase. Thrombi from explant valves were localized within the pivots to these disturbed flow regions.

8.5 DURABILITY OF PROSTHETIC HEART VALVES

The performance of prosthetic valves is in several ways related to structural mechanics. The design configuration affects the load distribution and dynamics of the valve components, which, in conjunction with the material properties, determine durability—notably wear and fatigue life. Valve configuration, in concert with the flow engendered by the geometry, also dictates the extent of low wear (e.g., flow separation) and high shear (e.g., gap leakage) regions. The hinges of bileaflet and tilting-disc valves are particularly vulnerable because their design can produce sites of stagnant flow, which may cause localized thrombosis and restrict occluder motion. As discussed earlier, the rigid circular orifice ring is an unnatural configuration for a heart valve since the elliptically shaped natural valve annulus changes in size and shape during the cardiac cycle.

The choice of valve materials is closely related to structural factors, since the fatigue and wear performance of a valve depends not only on its configuration and loading but also on the material properties as well. Additionally, the issue of biocompatibility is crucial to prosthetic valve design where biocompatibility depends not only upon the material itself but also on its *in vivo* environment. In the design of heart valves, there are engineering design trade-offs—for example, materials that exhibit good biocompatibility may have inferior durability and *vice versa*. For many patients, the implanted prosthetic valve needs to last well over a decade and the need for valve durability may be even greater in the case of young people. Mechanical durability depends on the material properties and the loading cycle with examples of degradation including fatigue cracks, abrasive wear, and biochemical attack on the material.

8.5.1 WEAR

Abrasive wear of valve parts has been, and continues to be, a serious issue in the design of mechanical prosthetic valves. Various parts of these valves come in contact repeatedly for hundreds of millions of cycles over the lifetime of the device. A breakthrough occurred with the introduction of PYC as a valve material because it has relatively good blood compatibility characteristics and wear performance. It has been shown that while wear of PYC upon PYC and PYC upon metals is relatively low, wear of PYC by metals is considerably greater. One example of this is a PYC disc mounted on a metallic orifice/hinge combination. The most durable wear couple is PYC-PYC; therefore, PYC-coated components are very attractive. The first valve to employ a PYC-PYC couple was the St. Jude Medical valve, which has fixed pivots for the leaflets. Tests indicate that it would take 200 years to wear halfway through the PYC coating on a leaflet pivot. By creating designs that allow wear surfaces to be distributed rather than focal (e.g., the Omnicarbon valve, which has a PYC-coated disc that is free to rotate), it is possible to reduce wear even further.

Despite these advances, wear on prosthetic heart valve surfaces can still be problematic, as can be seen by the mechanical failures of the *Edwards-Duromedics* valve. The Edwards-Duromedics valve design was introduced in 1982, but withdrawn from the market after one of the leaflets in a number of these valves fractured and embolized within the vascular system of patients. Scanning electron microscopic examinations of the fractured leaflets revealed regions of pitting on the leaflet and housing surfaces where the leaflet contacts the housing during closure and within the pivot area as well as several regions of concentrated micropores in the carbon surfaces near where the fractures occurred. A subsequent study showed that these micropores existed only in the Edwards-Duromedics design and hypothesized that they were created as a result of the shaping of carbon components with a mandrel, a process that was unique to the Edwards-Duromedics valve. This study linked pitting (indicative of cavitation damage) to the presence of these micropores. Other studies have disputed the connection between micropores and pitting damage. The fact that the cause of leaflet embolization in these valves remains unknown means that wear remains a potential problem in the design of mechanical prostheses.

8.5.2 Fatigue

Metals are prone to fatigue failure. Their polycrystalline nature contains structural characteristics that may produce dislocations under mechanical loading. These dislocations can migrate when subjected to repeated loading cycles and can accumulate at intercrystalline boundaries with the end result being tiny cracks. These tiny cracks are sites of stress concentration in which the fissures may worsen until fracture occurs. The *Haynes 25 Stellite Björk-Shiley* valve, which used a chromium-cobalt alloy, experienced the most severe fatigue problem for a mechanical valve. While previous investigations had suggested that fatigue was not a problem for PYC, recent data contradicts this and suggests that cyclic fatigue-crack growth occurs in graphite/PYC composite materials. This work suggests a fatigue threshold that is as low as 50% of the fracture toughness and views cyclic fatigue as an essential consideration in the design and life prediction of heart valves constructed from PYC. The FDA now requires detailed characterization of PYC materials used in different valve designs (December 1993 FDA heart valve guidelines).

8.5.3 Mineralization

The major cause of both porcine aortic and pericardial bioprosthetic valve failures is calcification, a process that stiffens leaflets and frequently causes cuspal tears. Calcific deposits occur most commonly at the commissures and basal attachments and are most extensive deep in (intrinsic to) the cusps in the spongiosa layer. Ultrastructurally, calcific deposits are associated with cuspal connective tissue cells and collagen. Degenerative cuspal calcific deposits are composed of calcium phosphates that are chemically and structurally related to physiological bone mineral (hydroxyapatite). The flexing bladders in cardiac assist devices, flexing polymeric heart valves, and vascular grafts have also been found to be vulnerable to calcific deposits. In such cases, calcification is usually related to inflammatory cells adjacent to the blood-contacting surface rather than to the implanted material itself.

The mechanisms of calcification and the methods of preventing calcification are an active area of current research. The most common methods of studying calcification involve either valve tissue implanted subcutaneously in 3-week-old weanling rats or valves implanted as mitral replacements in young sheep or calves. Results of both types of studies show that bioprosthetic tissue calcifies in fashion similar to clinical implants, but at a greatly accelerated rate. The subcutaneous implantation mode is a well-accepted, technically convenient, economical, and quantifiable model for investigating mineralization issues. It is also very useful for determining the potential of new anti-mineralization treatments.

Host, implant, and biomechanical factors impact the calcification of tissue valves. Patients who are young or have renal failure are vulnerable to valve mineralization, but immunological factors seem to be unimportant. Pretreatment of valve tissue with an aldehyde cross-linking agent has been found to cause calcification in rat subcutaneous implants; nonpreserved cusps, on the other hand, do not mineralize. Calcification of bioprosthetic valves is greatest at the cuspal commissures and bases where leaflet flexion is the greatest and deformations are maximal. Most data suggest that the basic mechanisms of tissue valve mineralization result from aldehyde pretreatment that changes the tissue microstructure.

In both clinical and experimental bioprosthetic tissue, the earliest mineral deposits have been observed to be localized in transplanted connective tissue cells with the collagen fibers being involved later. Mineralization of the connective tissue cells of bioprosthetic tissue is thought to result from glutaraldehyde-induced cellular "revitalization" and the disruption of cellular calcium regulation. Normal animal cells have a low intracellular-free calcium concentration ($\sim 10^{-7}$ M), while extracellular-free calcium is much higher ($\sim 10^{-3}$ M), yielding a 10,000-fold gradient across the plasma membrane. In healthy cells, cellular calcium is maintained at low concentration by energy-requiring metabolic mechanisms. In addition, organellar and plasma membranes and cell nuclei—the observed sites of early nucleation of bioprosthetic tissue mineralization—contain considerable phosphorus, mainly in the form of phospholipids. In cells modified by aldehyde cross-linking, passive calcium entry occurs unimpeded, but the mechanisms for calcium removal are dysfunctional. This calcium influx reacts with the preexisting phosphorous and contributes to the mineralization.

8.6 CURRENT TRENDS IN VALVE DESIGN

Initially, improvement of hemodynamic performance of bioprosthetic valves was the primary focus of development. The clinical introduction of the bovine pericardial valve solved the hemodynamic problem with such valves exhibiting hemodynamics equal to or better than some mechanical prostheses. Since long-term durability data has now become available; however, clinical durability of bioprosthetic valves is the major impediment to their use. The long-term durability of porcine and bovine bioprostheses can be improved through innovative stent designs that minimize stress concentrations and through improved fixation processing techniques that yield more pliable tissue.

If the aforementioned design challenges are met so that bioprostheses can be produced which are durable and are at the same thromboresistant (and, thus, anticoagulant therapy would *not* be required), there will most likely be another swing back toward increased use of bioprostheses.

The introduction of transcatheter valves gave clinicians the option for a minimally invasive procedure for valve replacement that reduces operative risks, which has been welcomed by patients and clinicians alike. There are plans to extend the transcatheter valves from high-risk patients to normal patients, as an alternative to surgical valves. To enable this, shortcomings of transcatheter valves such as perivalvular leakage and lack of sufficient visual guide for implantation are being addressed.

8.7 CONCLUSIONS

Direct comparison of the "total" performance of artificial heart valves is difficult, if not impossible. The precise definition of criteria used to benchmark valve performance varies from study to study. To study long-term performance, large numbers of patients and lengthy observation periods are required. During these periods, there may be an evolution in valve materials, or design, or in the medical treatment of patients with prosthetic heart valves. The age of the patient at implant and the underlying valvular heart disease(s) are extremely important factors in valve choice and longevity as well. A valve design suited for the aortic position may be inappropriate for the mitral position. Consequently, it is not possible to categorize a particular valve as *the best*. All valves currently in use, mechanical and bioprosthetic, produce relatively large turbulent stresses (that can cause lethal and or sublethal damage to red cells and platelets), and also greater pressure gradients and regurgitant volumes than normal heart valves.

Therefore, there are three promising directions for further advances in heart valves (and, therefore, three challenges for engineers designing new heart valves):

- *Improved thromboresistance* with new and better artificial materials
- *Improved durability* of new tissue valves, through the use of nonstented tissue valves, new anticalcification treatments, and better fixation treatments
- *Improved hemodynamic characteristics*, especially reduction or elimination of low shear stress regions near valve and vessel surfaces and of high turbulent shear stresses along the edges of jets produced by valve outflow and/or leakage of flow

While the current status of artificial valves leaves room for further improvement, the superior prognosis for the patient with a replacement heart valve is dramatic and convincing.

PROBLEMS

8.1 A 27mm bileaflet valve was tested in a pulse duplicator at a mean systolic flow rate of 15Lpm. The corresponding mean pressure drop across the valve was measured to be 5.2mmHg. Assuming a discharge coefficient of 0.61 for the bileaflet valve, compute the effective valve orifice area and the performance index for the valve.

8.2 Describe, qualitatively and quantitatively, the flow fields through the three major types of MHVs: ball and cage; tilting-disc; and bileaflet. Relate the flow fields to distinct design features. Discuss potential design improvements (could be a semester project).

8.3 Tissue mineralization is a major problem with bioprosthetic heart valves. Review the recent literature and discuss advances in treatments to mitigate calcification.

8.4 Describe the fluid mechanic principles of cavitation that may occur in a liquid. How could it occur with a prosthetic heart valve in the human circulation. Quantitatively relate the impact of cavitation to the structural integrity of the formed elements of blood.

8.5 Describe how Equation 8.5 is derived using all of the relevant fluid mechanic assumptions.

REFERENCES

Azadani, A. N., Jaussaud, N., Matthews, P. B., Ge, L., Guy, T. S., Chuter, T. A., and Tseng, E. E. (2009) Energy loss due to paravalvular leak with transcatheter aortic valve implantation. *Ann. Thorac. Surg*. 88(6): 1857–1863.

Bleiziffer, S., Ruge, H., Mazzitelli, D., Schreiber, C., Hutter, A., Laborde, J. C., Bauernschmitt, R., and Lange, R. (2009) Results of percutaneous and transapical transcatheter aortic valve implantation performed by a surgical team. *Eur. J. Cardiothorac. Surg*. 35(4): 615–620; discussion 620–611.

Clavel, M. A., Webb, J. G., Pibarot, P., Altwegg, L., Dumont, E., Thompson, C., De Larochelliere, R., Doyle, D., Masson, J. B., Bergeron, S., Bertrand, O. F., and Rodes-Cabau, J. (2009) Comparison of the hemodynamic performance of percutaneous and surgical bioprostheses for the treatment of severe aortic stenosis. *J. Am. Coll. Cardiol*. 53(20): 1883–1891.

Grube, E., Buellesfeld, L., Mueller, R., Sauren, B., Zickmann, B., Nair, D., Beucher, H., Felderhoff, T., Iversen, S., and Gerckens, U. (2008) Progress and current status of percutaneous aortic valve replacement: Results of three device generations of the CoreValve Revalving system. *Circ. Cardiovasc. Interv*. 1(3): 167–175.

Ionescu, M. I. and Ross, D. N. (1969) Heart valve replacement with autologous fascia lata. *The Lancet* 294(7616): 335–338.

Iung, B., Cachier, A., Baron, G., Messika-Zeitoun, D., Delahaye, F., Tornos, P., Gohlke-Barwolf, C., Boersma, E., Ravaud, P., and Vahanian, A. (2005) Decision-making in elderly patients with severe aortic stenosis: Why are so many denied surgery? *Eur. Heart J*. 26(24): 2714–2720.

Kaiser, B. L. and Beuren, A. J. (1969) Clinical use of a new design stented xenograft heart valve prosthesis. *Surg. Forum*. 20: 137–138.

Kapadia, S. R., Goel, S. S., Svensson, L., Roselli, E., Savage, R. M., Wallace, L., Sola, S., Schoenhagen, P., Shishehbor, M. H., Christofferson, R., Halley, C., Rodriguez, L. L., Stewart, W., Kalahasti, V., and Tuzcu, E. M. (2009) Characterization and outcome of patients with severe symptomatic aortic stenosis referred for percutaneous aortic valve replacement. *J. Thorac. Cardiovasc. Surg*. 137(6): 1430–1435.

Leo, H. L. et al. (2002) *J. Thorac. Cardiovasc. Surg.* 124: 561–574.

Padala, M., Sarin, E., Willis, P., Babaliaros, V., Block, P., Guyton, R., and Thourani, V. (2010) An engineering review of transcatheter aortic valve technologies. *Cardiovasc. Eng. Technol.* 1(1): 77–87.

Senning, A. (1996) Aortic valve replacement with fascia lata. *Acta Chir. Scand. Suppl.* 356B: 17–20.

Travis, B. (2001) The effects of bileaflet valve pivot geometry on turbulence and blood damage potential. PhD thesis, Georgia Institute of Technology, Atlanta, GA, 2001.

Vahanian, A., Alfieri, O., Al-Attar, N., Antunes, M., Bax, J., Cormier, B., Cribier, A., De Jaegere, P., Fournial, G., Kappetein, A. P., Kovac, J., Ludgate, S., Maisano, F., Moat, N., Mohr, F., Nataf, P., Pierard, L., Pomar, J. L., Schofer, J., Tornos, P., Tuzcu, M., van Hout, B., Von Segesser, L. K., and Walther, T. (2008) Transcatheter valve implantation for patients with aortic stenosis: A position statement from the European Association of Cardio-Thoracic Surgery (EACTS) and the European Society of Cardiology (ESC), in collaboration with the European Association of Percutaneous Cardiovascular Interventions (EAPCI). *Eur. Heart J.* 29(11): 1463–1470.

Webb, J. G., Altwegg, L., Boone, R. H., Cheung, A., Ye, J., Lichtenstein, S., Lee, M., Masson, J. B., Thompson, C., Moss, R., Carere, R., Munt, B., Nietlispach, F., and Humphries, K. (2009) Transcatheter aortic valve implantation: Impact on clinical and valve-related outcomes. *Circulation* 119(23): 3009–3016.

Webb, J. G., Pasupati, S., Humphries, K., Thompson, C., Altwegg, L., Moss, R., Sinhal, A., Carere, R. G., Munt, B., Ricci, D., Ye, J., Cheung, A., and Lichtenstein, S. V. (2007) Percutaneous transarterial aortic valve replacement in selected high-risk patients with aortic stenosis. *Circulation* 116(7): 755–763.

Yoganathan, A. P. (1995) Cardiac valve prostheses. In *The Biomedical Engineering Handbook*, Bronzino, J. D., ed., CRC Press, Boca Raton, FL.

Yoganathan, A. P., He, Z., and Casey Jones, S. (2004) Fluid mechanics of heart valves. *Annu. Rev. Biomed. Eng.* 6: 331–362.

9 Vascular Therapeutic Techniques

9.1 VASCULAR GRAFT IMPLANTS

Earlier in Section 3.10, we discussed how atherosclerosis of the major systemic arteries (e.g., coronary, carotid, renal, etc.) is the greatest cause of death in the Western world, leading to conditions such as heart attacks, strokes, and disabilities of the legs. Later, in Section 6.7, we discussed the topic of arterial stenoses and the nature of fluid dynamic changes that are associated with them. From a clinical standpoint, the presence of a stenosis often leads to either reduced blood flow to the corresponding distal organs or to the production of emboli (usually thrombi) which are convected downstream to smaller arterial branches where occlusion occurs. The most critical sites for these events are the coronary (Figure 9.1), carotid, renal, and lower extremity (e.g., iliac, femoral, etc.) arteries.

The primary means of treating these stenosed arteries is to provide an alternative path, or a "bypass," for the blood in order to circumvent the obstruction and reach the dependent end organ. Arterial bypasses can be readily created by implanting a *vascular graft* around the diseased area (Figure 9.2) since arterial stenoses are focal in nature and, thus, leave neighboring segments of the artery relatively unaffected.

In this surgical procedure, the affected vessel is exposed and the bypass graft is placed alongside and sewn to arterial sites well upstream and downstream of the stenosis. The junctions between the artery and the graft are called *anastomoses* and are generally constructed in an *end-to-side* fashion. The primary exception to this is with grafts used for repair of an abdominal aortic aneurysm (AAA) where the anastomoses are placed in an *end-to-end* fashion. Once the graft is in place, blood flow is then reinstituted around the diseased area, often with some residual flow still being carried through the native artery. A variety of surgical procedures are used to perform coronary artery bypass grafting with internal mammary arteries, ranging from the traditional open-chest procedure to newer approaches using either a thoracotomy (*OPCAB*) or only a small incision in the ribcage (*MIDCAB*), both of which avoid the need for simultaneous heart-lung bypass support during the procedure.

9.2 ARTERIOVENOUS FISTULAS

Another clinical purpose for using vascular grafts is to simply provide a direct access to the bloodstream. This is important, for example, when performing hemodialysis on a patient with renal failure or for administering chemotherapy to cancer patients. With this procedure, a bypass is created between an artery and a vein (rather than

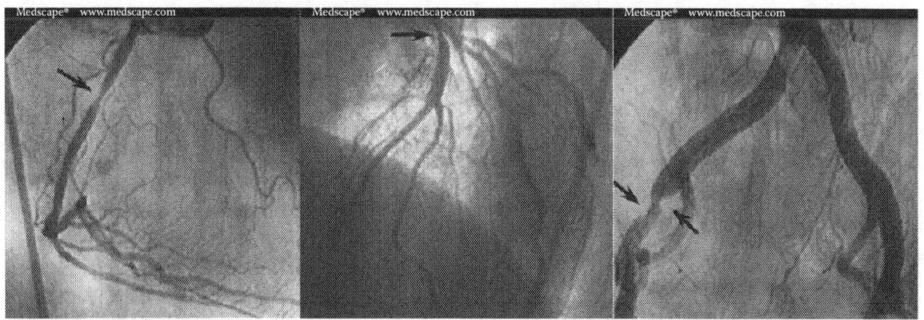

FIGURE 9.1 Angiogram of the left coronary system of a patent with severe coronary artery disease. (From Gotto, A.M., Jr. et al., *Atherosclerosis*, UpJohn, Kalamazoo, MI, 1997. With permission.)

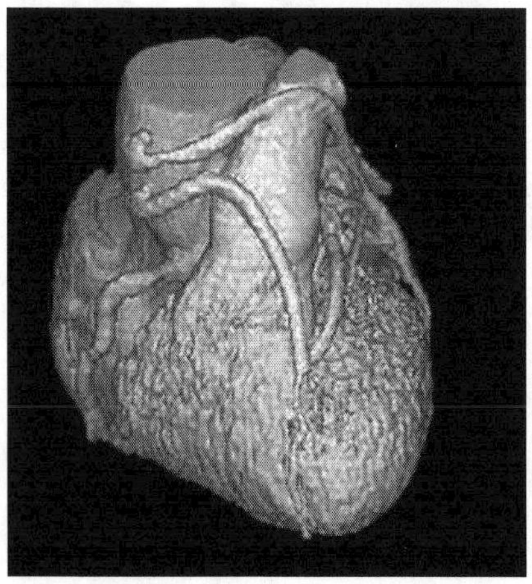

FIGURE 9.2 3D electron beam CT scanner showing bypass grafts. (Courtesy Dr. Alan Boyar, Newport Beach, CA.)

between two points on the same or connected arteries), thus allowing for blood to be withdrawn and then returned to the circulation or for therapeutic agents to be delivered directly into the bloodstream. There are two main types of *arteriovenous fistulas* (AVFs). One is a direct anastomosis between an artery and its adjacent vein in a *side-to-side* fashion (called a native AVF), while the other uses a synthetic graft implant (usually e-PTFE material) which is anastomosed between the artery and vein in an end-to-side fashion (Figure 9.3). The most common locations for native AVFs and synthetic graft fistulas are between the radial artery and vein of the forearm and between the brachial artery and vein of the upper arm, respectively.

Since a fistula directly joins blood at arterial pressures (80–100 mmHg) with blood at venous pressures (10–20 mmHg), fistula flow rates are normally very high (often 10%–20% of total cardiac output depending upon the anatomic site) and the flow often turbulent (Figure 9.4).

This elevated flow rate (often 800–1000 mL/min) is useful in the process of hemodialysis, for example, since a large amount of blood is readily accessible and the

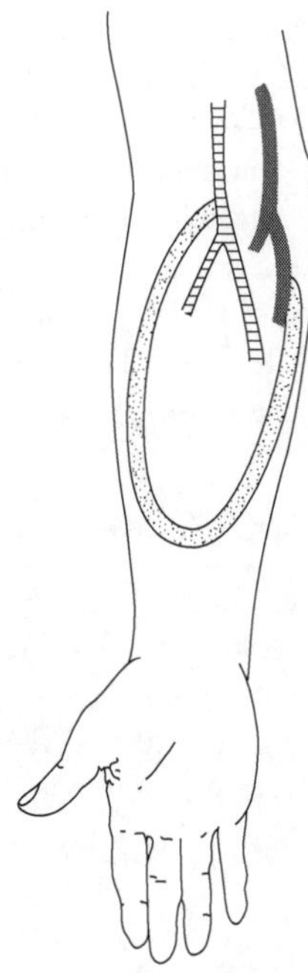

FIGURE 9.3 A brachiobasilic bridge (loop) graft. (From Ernst, C.B. and Stanley, J.C., *Current Therapy in Vascular Surgery*, 2nd edn., B.C. Decker, Philadelphia, PA, 1991. With permission.)

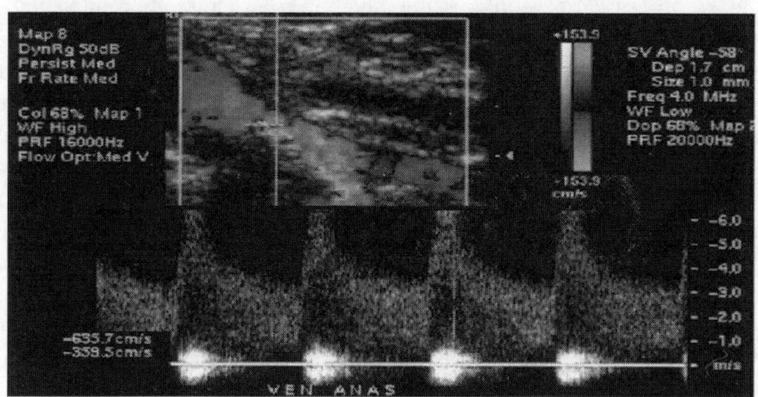

FIGURE 9.4 (Left) Power Doppler image of the distal venous limb of the hemodialysis access graft at the anastomosis with the basilic vein with a normal (4 mm) transverse diameter (crosshairs). This was the narrowest area of the graft. (Right) Power Doppler image at the same level demonstrates normal flow characteristics at spectral analysis, peak systolic velocity of 268 cm/s, and an average flow greater than 1300 mL/min. (From Dumars, M.C. et al., *Radiology*, 222, 103, 2002.)

detoxification process can be accomplished more quickly (~3–4 h). Despite these high flow rates, usually patients do not suffer from major complications other than occasionally experiencing a "steal syndrome" in which enough blood is diverted from distal vessels to cause coolness and numbness of the tissue. These fistulas, however, do have a fairly high failure rate with an average longevity of only 1–2 years. Obviously, this event further increases the patient's overall morbidity. Most failures are immediately due to thrombosis, especially with graft fistulas, which then require surgical revision or replacement of the graft. The thrombosis itself is often secondary to the development of IH at the anastomoses, particularly at the venous anastomosis.

9.3 TYPES OF VASCULAR GRAFT MATERIALS USED

A variety of synthetic and biological materials are used for the construction of bypass grafts. The preferred choice is to use one of the patient's own vessels since this provides the best possible degree of biocompatibility. In practice, either an intrathoracic artery—that is, the internal mammary artery (IMA) or a vein from the leg—that is, the saphenous vein is most commonly harvested for this purpose. The IMA is used exclusively for bypasses of the coronary artery and is nearly ideal because of its similarity in size, availability (i.e., it is not a critically required vessel), and its natural arterial structure. It is limited, however, by the fact that it is short and that only two such vessels (left and right IMAs) exist in the body. The saphenous vein is used for coronary artery bypass procedures but it is also commonly used to construct bypasses of the lower extremity (e.g., femoral/popliteal artery bypasses) as well. The *saphenous vein graft* (SVG) is a good, autologous conduit material with low thrombogenicity but it is also limited in its quantity (especially when multiple bypass grafts and/or procedures are required) and sometimes by its quality in older patients. It also suffers from a process termed "arterialization," in which the vein adapts to the abrupt increase in pressure which it experiences upon implantation in an arterial environment by thickening its walls.

For these reasons, other synthetic materials have also been used as bypass grafts. Chief among these are polyethylene terephthalate (*PET*), or *Dacron*, polytetrafluoroethylene (*PTFE*), or *Teflon*, and polyurethane. Dacron is a strong fabric with long life and is the normal material used in large diameter *AAA* repairs (Figure 9.5).

For smaller caliber grafts, such as those in the leg, PTFE is the main graft material used due to its relatively inert surface properties (Figure 9.6).

A disadvantage of this material, however, is that it is very stiff (Young's modulus, $E > 10^7$ N/m^2). Therefore, a more compliant, expanded version of this material, *e-PTFE*, has been adopted as the current surgical standard. Polyurethane has the advantages of being relatively easy to manufacture and having good mechanical properties although it does not have thromboresistant properties that are comparable with those of PTFE.

An attempt has been made to improve the antithrombogenic properties of synthetic materials and to, thus, exploit their advantage of greater availability by incorporating a natural biological surface on the material. This procedure, known as *endothelial cell seeding*, involves the placing of endothelial cells derived from the same patient onto the surface of the graft (usually e-PTFE material) prior to surgery

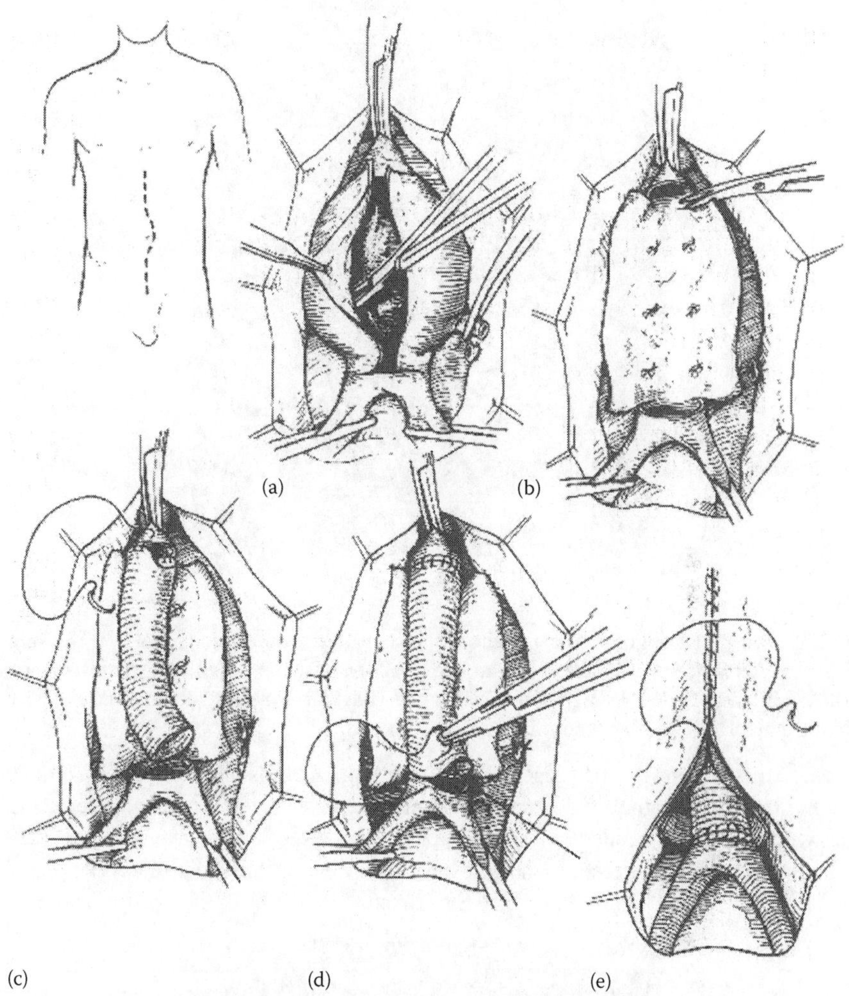

FIGURE 9.5 Technique for resection and replacement of infrarenal aneurysm of abdominal aorta. (a) Method of resection of aneurysm of aorta. Occluding clamps are applied to the aorta immediately above the aneurysm and below the renal arteries and to both common iliac arteries. The inferior mesenteric artery is divided near its origin, and the distal end is ligated. A vertical incision is made through the anterior wall of the aneurysm, and intima and laminated thrombus material are removed. (b) Bleeding lumbar arteries are sutured and ligated. (c) An appropriately sized albumin-coated DeBakey Dacron graft is sutured by end-to-end anastomosis to the proximal opening of the aorta by continuous suture of 000 polypropylene. (d) Distal end of the graft is appropriately tailored to be attached to the distal opening of the aorta just above the bifurcations, and an end-to-end anastomosis is made with 000 polypropylene. (e) Periaortic tissue is closed around the graft by continuous suture of chromic catgut. (From Ernst, C.B. and Stanley, J.C., *Current Therapy in Vascular Surgery*, 2nd edn., B.C. Decker, Philadelphia, PA, 1991. With permission.)

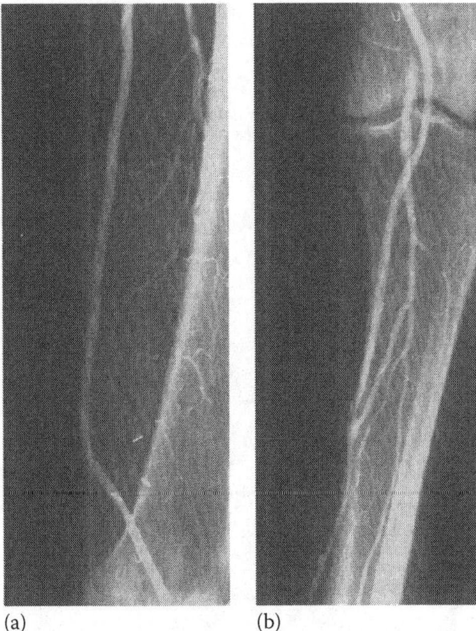

FIGURE 9.6 Arteriogram in a patient with patent femoroposterior tibial e-PTFE graft 10 years after placement of the graft. (a) Proximal graft and (b) distal anastomosis. (From Ernst, C.B. and Stanley, J.C., *Current Therapy in Vascular Surgery*, 2nd edn., B.C. Decker, Philadelphia, PA, 1991. With permission.)

in order that the graft will present a naturally appearing surface to the blood. The technique uses endothelial cells from either a harvested vein or microvascular tissue which are then "seeded" onto the graft surface using either gravitational, adhesive, or electrostatic methods and allowed to replicate until they reach confluence (i.e., full coverage) (Figure 9.7). Once the surface is stabilized, the graft is implanted

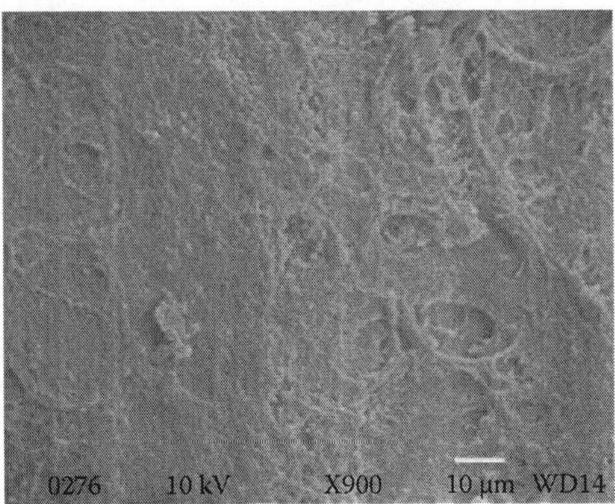

FIGURE 9.7 Scanning electron micrograph illustrating results of the prime electrostatic endothelial cell transplantation onto e-PTFE (GORE-TEX®). (From Bowlin, G.L. et al., *J. Biomater. Appl.*, 16, 157, 2001. With permission.)

and the endothelial cells not only prevent a foreign body response but also may actively reduce the potential for thrombosis and IH by the production of agents, for example, prostaglandins and nitric oxide.

9.4 CLINICAL EXPERIENCE WITH VASCULAR GRAFTS

In most cases, a bypass graft's ability to remain open, called its *patency*, is very good immediately after surgery (>90%) but continually decreases with time (~50% at 5 years) (Figure 9.8).

The reasons for these failures are related to either early (<30 days) thrombus formation or late (>30 days) IH formation. Graft *thrombosis* occurs due to the trauma associated with the implantation surgery and also as part of the body's response to the implantation of a foreign material. It is also more likely to occur in regions of slow or static flow where the tendency for clotting is enhanced. One result of this is that failure rates for grafts extending below the knee, for example, are particularly high due to the low flow rates carried in these smaller caliber (<6 mm ID) vessels. It is for this reason as well that, currently, no grafts made of synthetic materials are used for coronary artery (3–4 mm ID) bypass procedures.

The development of IH is a natural response of the vessel to specific conditions, especially those present at bypass graft anastomoses. As shown in Figure 9.9, IH occurs primarily along the suture line regions between the graft and host artery (known as the anastomotic "heel" and "toe" regions) and also along the "floor" of the host artery directly across from the graft outlet.

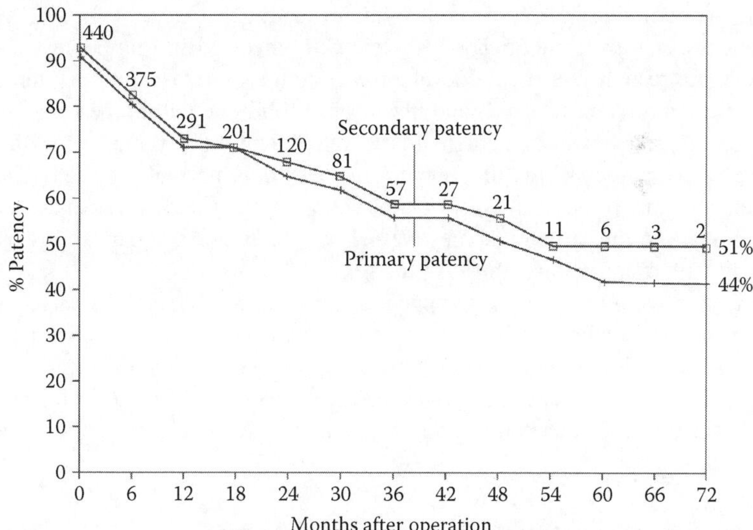

FIGURE 9.8 Cumulative life table patency rates for 440 PTFE femoropopliteal bypasses. The lower line shows primary patency rates, while the upper line shows secondary (achieved after thrombectomy) patency rates. (From Sawyer, P.N., *Modern Vascular Grafts*, McGraw-Hill Book Co., New York, 1987. With permission.)

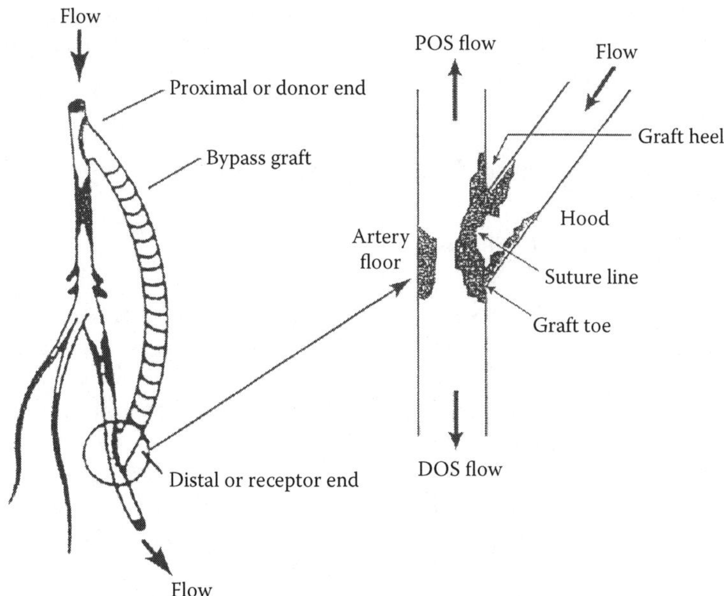

FIGURE 9.9 Sites of intimal hyperplasia formation in a bypass graft distal anastomosis. POS, proximal outflow segment; DOS, distal outflow segment. (From Li, X.-M., *Evaluation of hemodynamic factors at the distal end-to-side anastomosis of a bypass graft with different POS:DOS ratios*, Master's thesis, Department of Biomedical Engineering, The University of Akron, Akron, OH, 1998.)

As its name implies, IH consists of tissue in the intimal layer of the wall which experiences excessive growth. The principle cells involved in this process are the same as those responsible for the development of atherosclerosis (see Section 3.10). Specifically, smooth muscle cells and fibroblasts proliferate within the vessel media and adventitia, respectively, and then migrate into the intimal layer as part of the vessel's healing response. While this process involves only normally present vascular tissue and not other components such as cholesterol, calcium, and necrotic tissue, it can still culminate in the same outcome—vessel occlusion due to a partial obstruction combined with eventual thrombosis of the graft.

The responses of the artery wall appear to coincide with changes in its local biomechanical environment, such as pressure and wall shear stress (see Section 6.5). Since these variables are particularly affected by the geometric configuration of the anastomosis, extensive work has been performed to examine the effect of the choice of graft caliber and the anastomotic angle, in addition to the flow rate, upon eventual patency of the graft.

9.5 BIOMECHANICS AND ANASTOMOTIC IH

While implantation of a bypass graft is usually successful in restoring needed blood flow to distal tissues, it does so by creation of non-anatomic junctions between vessels which, in turn, lead to complex, 3D flow patterns. These flow patterns are mainly confined to

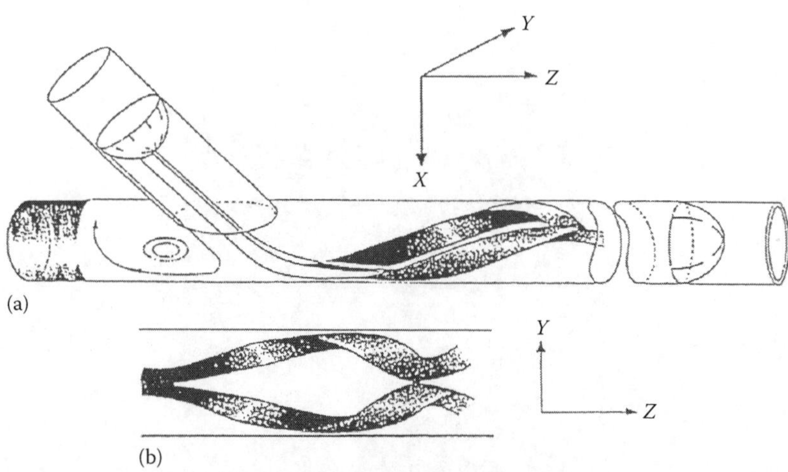

FIGURE 9.10 Three-dimensional sketch of the path line of the high inertia fluid seen under steady flow conditions at $Re = 950$ and 1300, as well as for unsteady flow at around peak flow: (a) side view, showing development of the double helix; (b) top view. (From *J. Vasc. Surg.*, 12, Ojha, M. et al., Steady and pulsatile flow fields in an end-to-side arterial anastomosis model, 747–753, Copyright (1990), with permission from Elsevier.)

either the proximal or distal anastomoses where sharp angles and abrupt changes in vessel diameters are present. Although the flow at these sites is typically laminar in character, complex features such as skewed velocity profiles, separation zones, and reattachment points as well as strong secondary motions (Figure 9.10) are present.

Important consequences of this include the presence of wide variations (i.e., high, low, and reversing) in local wall shear stresses and extended residence times for blood cells and other components to interact with the vessel wall. A compounding factor related to this is the stiffness, or lack of *compliance* (=Δvolume/Δpressure), of the graft material since changes in vessel diameter under pulsatile flow conditions will further alter the local geometry. A mismatch in compliance between the graft and native artery could also lead to significant changes in local fluid and solid wall stresses which might then elicit various tissue responses. We have mentioned earlier, for example, the relatively high stiffness of e-PTFE material that when interposed with more elastic native vessels may produce elevated wall stresses and impedance mismatches. This problem may persist, however, even when using more compliant biological materials, such as veins, since they may also become very stiff when exposed to arterial pressures.

It is not a surprising observation, then, that IH commonly develops at the toe and heel regions as well as along the artery floor of the anastomosis (Figure 9.11).

Since these sites coincide closely with areas of altered biomechanical variables, a number of studies have been performed to look at the effect of geometric and material parameters upon the local fluid dynamics and subsequent vascular responses. Specific variables that have been investigated include (1) material stiffness differences between the two vessels, (2) the angle of the anastomosis, (3) the diameter mismatch between the graft and the host artery, and (4) the flow distribution through

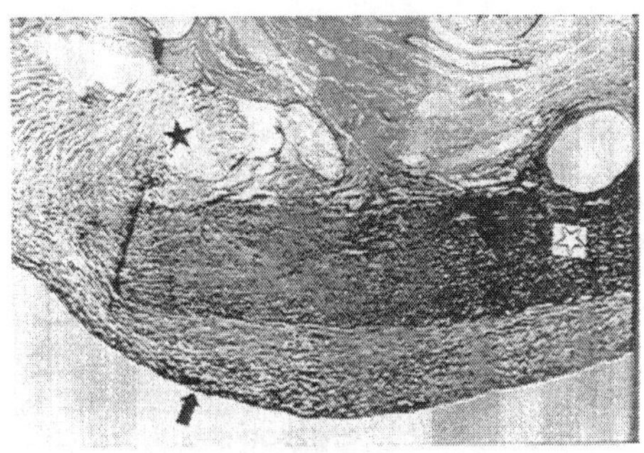

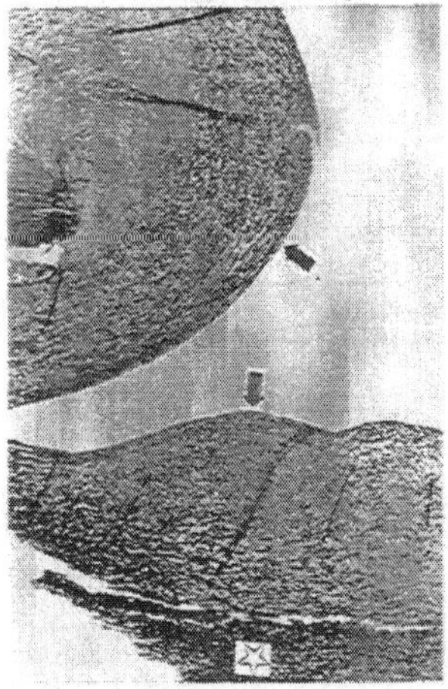

FIGURE 9.11 Longitudinal histological section (7.5×) of a typical distal anastomosis for diameter ratio $DR = 1.5$ showing the development of intimal hyperplasia along (top) the graft toe and (bottom) the graft heel (upper left) and artery floor (bottom). (White star denotes native artery, black star denotes e-PTFE graft, and arrows identify regions of neointimal hyperplasia. Flow is from left to right.) (From Keynton, R.S. et al., *J. Biomech. Eng.*, 123, 464, 2001.)

the artery (i.e., the proximal versus distal outflows), particularly at the distal anastomosis. From these studies, better insights have been gained as to the potential advantages and disadvantages of using various geometric and material configurations.

Specifically, graft-to-artery compliance differences have been shown to correlate with subsequent loss of viability of the graft (Figure 9.12). Thus, a graft, whether biological or synthetic, would be predicted to have higher failure rates as the stiffness of the graft material increases (i.e., graft compliance decreases).

Regarding changes in the graft-to-artery anastomotic angle, results from computational models with anastomoses of 30°, 45°, and 60° showed an increased skewing of the velocity profile and an increased flow separation in the outflow artery segment over that angle range (Figure 9.13).

Computation of the wall shear rates (WSRs) along the vessel wall quantitates these findings in more detail and shows the wide range of forward and reverse shear effects present (Figure 9.14), especially at the larger angle. This suggests that

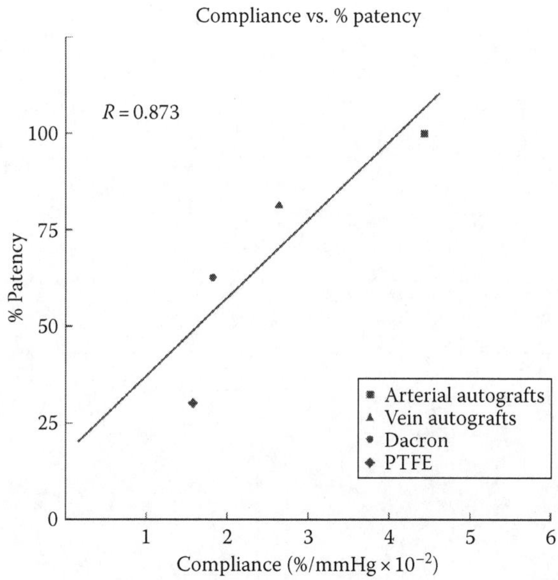

FIGURE 9.12 Linear regression analysis of compliance versus graft patency. (From *Graft Materials in Vascular Surgery*, Dardik, H., Copyright (1978), with permission from Elsevier.)

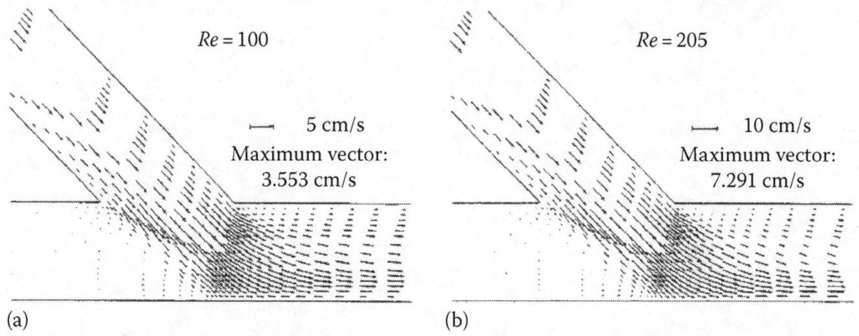

FIGURE 9.13 Velocity vectors in the plane of symmetry for a 45° anastomotic angle at (a) *Re* = 100 and (b) *Re* = 205. (*Note*: Velocity vectors are plotted at mesh nodes and do not lie along tube diameters.) (From Fei, D.Y. et al., *J. Biomech. Eng.*, 116, 331, 1994. With permission from ASME.)

small angles would be preferable—a conclusion that is supported by the fact that grafts anastomosed in an end-to-end fashion generally have higher patency rates than those anastomosed in an end-to-side fashion.

Clearly, these fluid mechanical changes appear to correspond quite closely with earlier observed sites of IH (Figure 9.9) at the heel and toe and along the artery floor of the anastomosis. In the previous figures, it is also evident that graft flow rate (which is proportional to *Re* in these models) plays an important role in determining WSR values with larger regions of the artery being exposed to low WSRs at the lower *Re*. This observation is consistent with clinical findings that, in general,

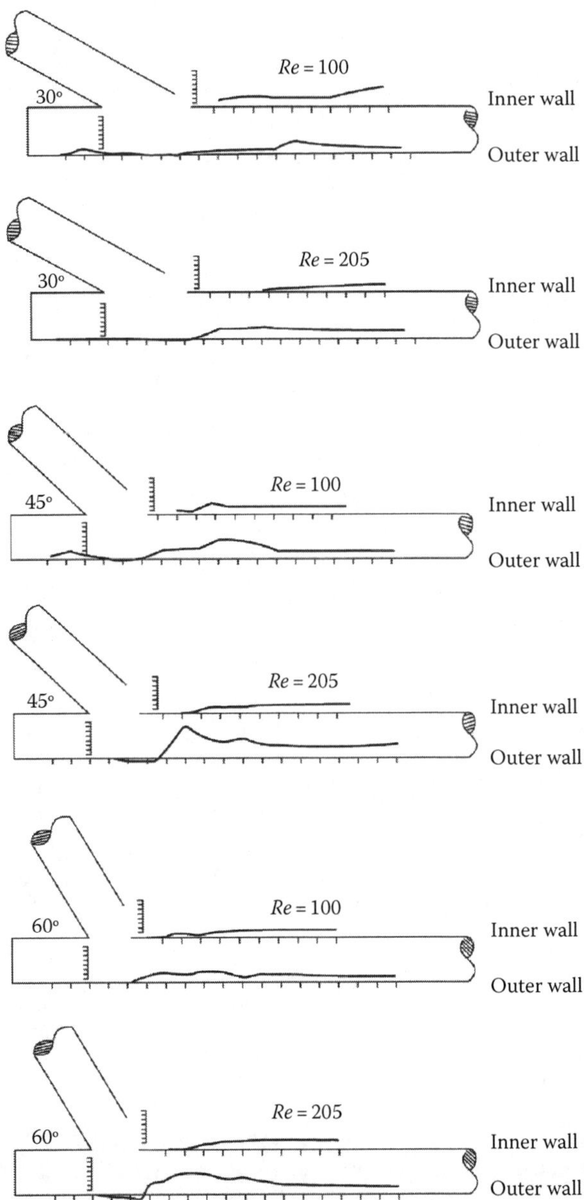

FIGURE 9.14 Normalized axial shear rate in anastomoses of 30°, 45°, and 60° at Re = 100 and 205. (*Note*: Wall shear rates were derived from laser Doppler anemometry velocity measurements.) (From Keynton, R.S. et al., *J. Biomech. Eng.*, 113, 460, 1991. With permission from ASME.)

patency rates of bypass grafts are better under high flow (i.e., larger, more proximal vessels) rather than low flow (i.e., smaller, more distal vessels) conditions.

In many bypass procedures, there is also a discrepancy between the caliber of the graft and the host artery. This occurs because (1) there are limited choices of sizes available with biological grafts, (2) SVGs must be reversed in order to avoid flow obstruction by their intact valves (thus creating a size mismatch at both the proximal and distal anastomoses), and (3) synthetic grafts are normally uniform in diameter while human arteries and veins are tapered. From animal experiments, it was shown that increasing the graft/artery diameter ratio from 1.0 to 1.5 (at the same 30° anastomotic angle) produces a greater magnitude and extent of flow reversal exposure in the anastomotic region (Figure 9.15).

Finally, another factor that is thought to significantly affect the local anastomotic flow patterns is the relative distribution of blood flow to the proximal and distal outflow segments of the artery. This POS:DOS flow ratio depends primarily on the degree of obstruction in the bypassed artery (i.e., whether it is occluded or partially stenosed) and the resistance of the distal bed (i.e., the degree of vasodilatation/vasoconstriction). Presence of proximal arterial outflow tends to reduce flow separation zone at the heel and artery floor but increases that effect at the toe region and, particularly, in the hood region of the graft. It also reduces the wall shear stresses along the entire distal outflow segment of the artery (Figure 9.16).

In clinical practice, it is quite common for many of these factors to occur in combination. For example, a Dacron material might be chosen as a bypass graft for replacement of an AAA and anastomosed distally to the iliac artery in either an end-to-end or end-to-side fashion. Mean wall stresses in the anastomosis are elevated not only due to the compliance mismatch between the artery and graft but also by the choice of anastomotic geometry (Figures 9.17 and 9.18).

While the previous results provide trends that may be useful in surgical treatment, they do not provide a single geometric, hemodynamic, or material factor that is responsible for the development of IH observed in practice. Consequently, many researchers have attempted to identify a possible common intermediate variable that may be directly related to IH development. This parameter might vary in response to changes in the anatomical and physiological conditions investigated earlier and, in turn, produce a predictable effect upon the vessel wall. If such a parameter were identified as having direct influence on the cell/tissue response, it might then be controlled in order to produce the desired clinical outcome (i.e., reduced IH). Several key candidates that have been suggested are mean and oscillatory wall shear and its gradients (spatial and temporal), wall stress, wall strain, and so on. Given our growing knowledge about the vascular wall and its ability to monitor local dynamic conditions and to actively respond to them, data have been obtained which compare the eventual (12 week) development of IH with the level of WSR at the time of implantation (Figure 9.19). These data show a modest inverse relationship ($r = -0.483$) between IH and WSR where IH is greatest at low and reversing WSRs and reaches a near-zero asymptote around $1000\,s^{-1}$—a level comparable with ~2× the normal, mean WSR seen in major arteries. Furthermore, there is a direct correlation ($r = 0.6$) of IH with the OSI, a parameter sensitive to the degree of pulsatility in the flow (see Section 6.4.2).

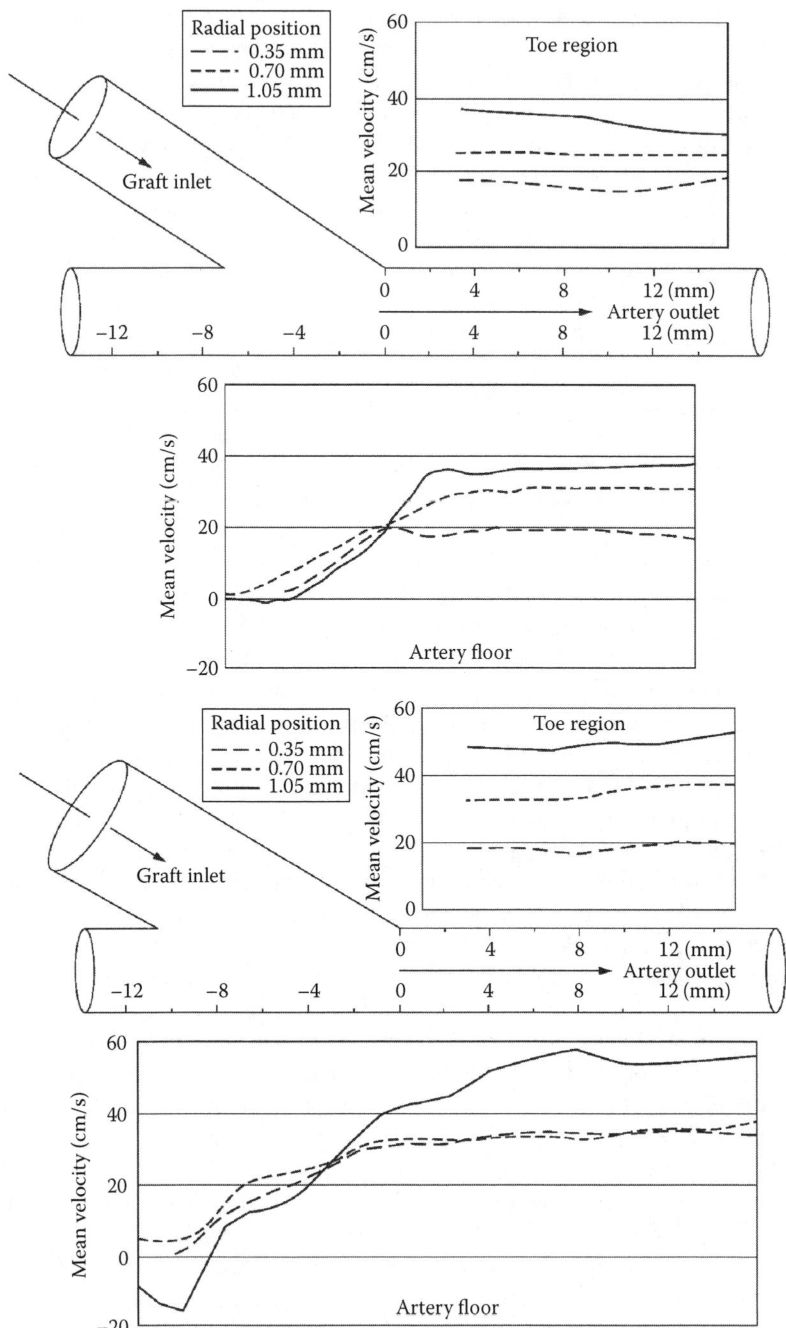

FIGURE 9.15 Typical plots of mean axial velocities at three radial positions along the artery toe and floor regions for diameter ratio $DR = 1.0$ (top) and $DR = 1.5$ (bottom). (*Note*: Velocity measurements made using pulse Doppler ultrasound.) (From Keynton, R.S. et al., *J. Biomech. Eng.*, 121, 82, 1999. With permission from ASME.)

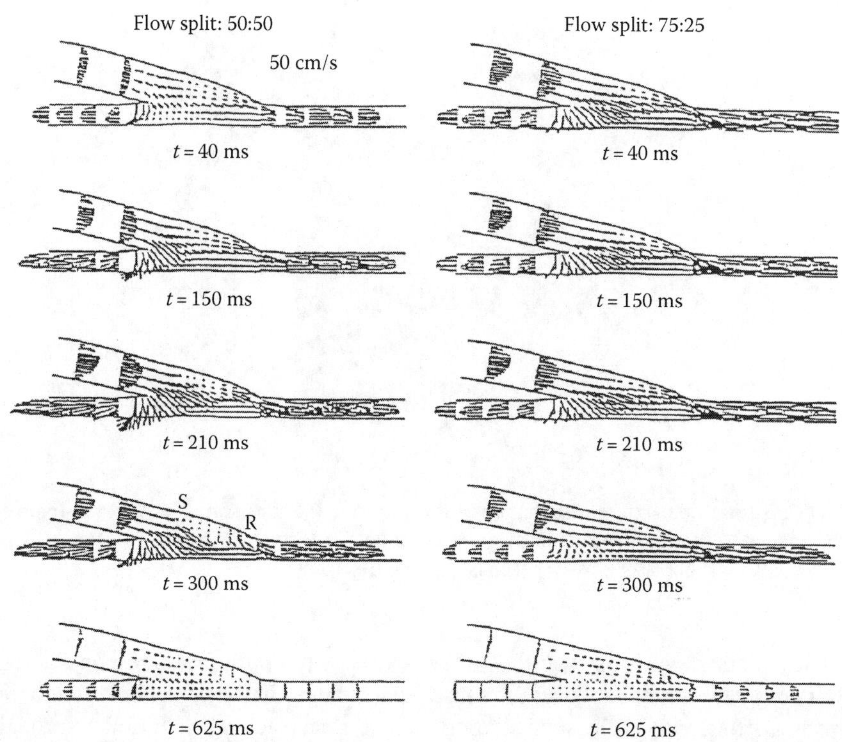

FIGURE 9.16 Vector plots in the ETS anastomosis for flow splits (ratio of distal to proximal arterial outflow) of 50:50 and 75:25 at various times during the flow cycle. Flow separation at S and reattachment at R occur on the graft hood during the systolic deceleration phase (t = 210 and 300 ms) with a flow split of 50:50. (From *J. Vasc. Surg.*, 31, How, T.V. et al., 1011, Copyright (2000), with permission from Elsevier.)

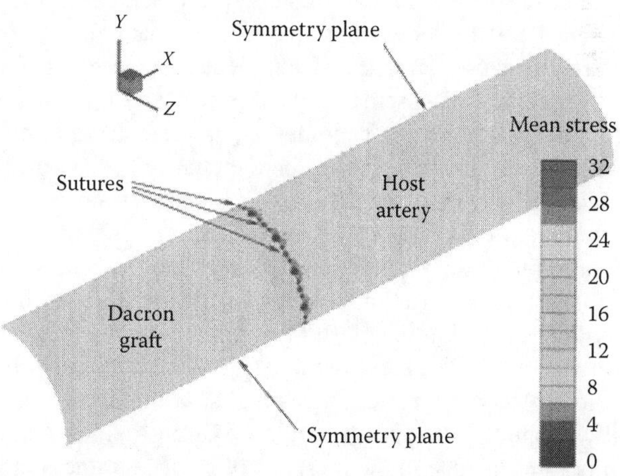

FIGURE 9.17 Mean stress distribution at the end-to-end Dacron graft-artery anastomosis projected onto a three-dimensional image of the geometry. (From *J. Biomech.*, 31, Ballyk, P.D. et al., 232, Copyright (1998), with permission from Elsevier.)

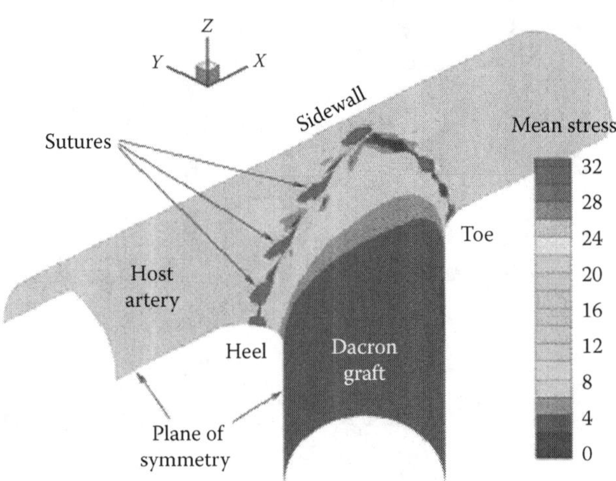

FIGURE 9.18 Mean stress distribution at the end-to-side Dacron graft-artery anastomosis projected onto a three-dimensional image of the geometry. (From *J. Biomech.*, 31, Ballyk, P.D. et al., 232, Copyright (1998), with permission from Elsevier.)

These data suggest that while wall shear is not the *only* factor responsible for IH, it does have an influence on the subsequent changes in the vessel wall following bypass grafting and is at least one important factor that should be controlled through modulation of other physiological (e.g., flow rate) and anatomical (e.g., anastomotic angle, graft caliber) variables.

In practice, it is always desirable to try to "translate" these investigational findings into practical recommendations for use by the surgeon in order to improve the success of an arterial bypass procedure. Certainly, reduction of flow through a vessel has been shown to be a potent stimulant of subsequent changes in the vessel wall. Langille and O'Donnell (1986), for example, have shown that reduction of blood flow in rabbit carotid arteries causes a rapid and significant decrease in the artery diameter and involves regulation of vascular cell migration and mitosis and apoptosis rates, control of matrix synthesis and degradation, and regulation of matrix reorganization. These changes are mediated by the endothelial cells that sense mechanical forces through shear-sensitive ion channels, and the shear strain rate acting on the cell. Thus, it is common to experience better success in bypassing larger arteries with higher flow rates rather than smaller arteries with low flow rates and to attempt to place the distal anastomosis proximal rather than distal to a branch point so that more total flow will be carried in the graft. Furthermore, the use of near-zero graft-to-artery anastomotic angles (i.e., end-to-end) has produced superior clinical results compared with those placed at greater angles and so a low angle, hooded anastomosis is generally created. Although the presence of a proximal outflow segment (POS) from an anastomosis (due to the presence of a partial rather than a complete proximal arterial obstruction) has been shown to dramatically affect the local flow patterns, and especially the wall shear stress, its possible effect on the development of anastomotic IH has not been as clearly confirmed. Thus, the degree of proximal

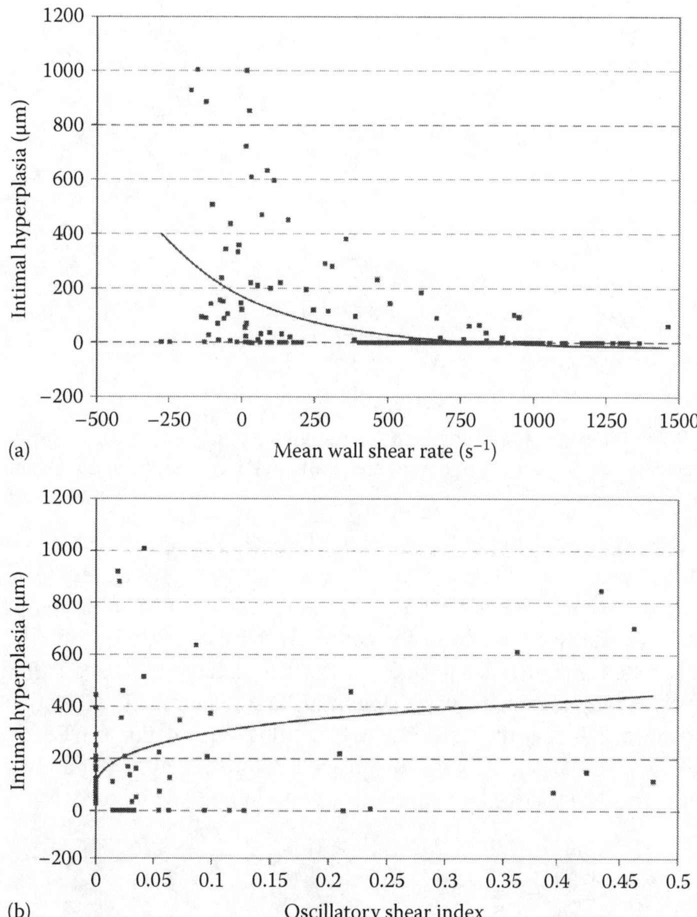

FIGURE 9.19 Nonlinear regression of (a) intimal hyperplasia (IH) versus mean wall shear rate (WSR) ($r = -0.483$) and (b) IH versus oscillatory shear index (OSI) ($r = 0.600$). (From Keynton, R.S. et al., *J. Biomech. Eng.*, 123, 470, 2001. With permission from ASME.)

stenosis (e.g., by tying off the stenosed artery) is not actively controlled in practice as part of a preferred surgical procedure.

Finally, there are inevitable interactions between many of these factors which lead to additional effects upon the vessel response. Clearly, there still remains a need for further research on these questions in order to better understand their importance.

9.6 ANGIOPLASTY, STENT, AND ENDOLUMINAL GRAFT IMPLANTS

More recent methods for treating arterial stenosis include less invasive procedures in which the vessel is not exposed through a direct surgical approach, but rather, is accessed using a catheter delivery system (Figure 9.20).

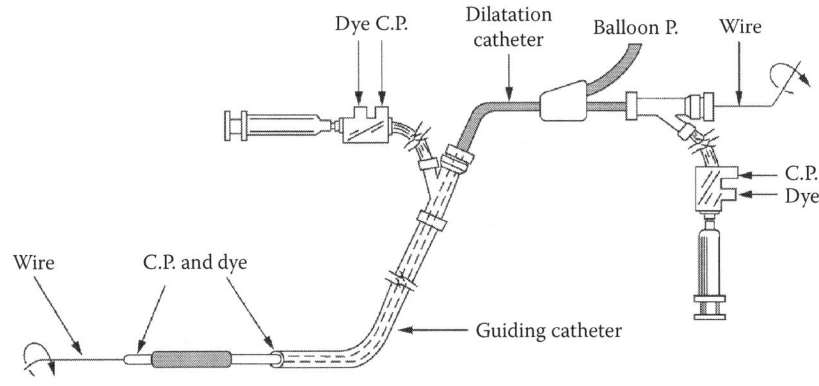

FIGURE 9.20 Schematic of a percutaneous balloon angioplasty device showing guide wire (Wire), catheter, and ports for balloon pressure (Balloon P.), dye injection (Dye), and catheter pressure (C.P.).

With this *percutaneous transluminal angioplasty* (PTA) technique, a balloon device is placed near the tip of a catheter which is then inserted through an artery in an extremity (typically the common femoral artery in the leg). The catheter is then positioned within a stenosis site, such as one of the coronary or carotid arteries, and the balloon inflated at elevated pressures up to 6 atm in order to enlarge the stenotic lumen. The resulting increase in vessel lumen size (Figure 9.21) has a dramatic effect on reducing the pressure drop and, thus, the resistance to blood flow (see Section 1.8, Equation 1.74).

Typically, the initial results with this procedure are very good and far less traumatic than with surgical bypass procedures, with many patients recovering quickly

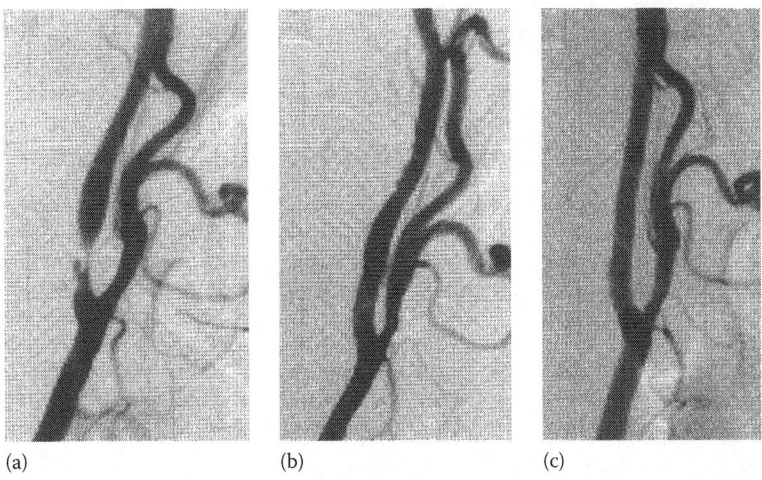

FIGURE 9.21 Digital subtraction angiograms showing excellent immediate and long-term results of percutaneous transluminal angioplasty in a patient with severe ulcerated internal carotid stenosis (a) immediately before angioplasty; (b) immediately after angioplasty; and (c) 1 year after angioplasty. (From *Adv. Vasc. Surg.*, 4, Whittemore, A.D., Copyright (1996), with permission from Elsevier.)

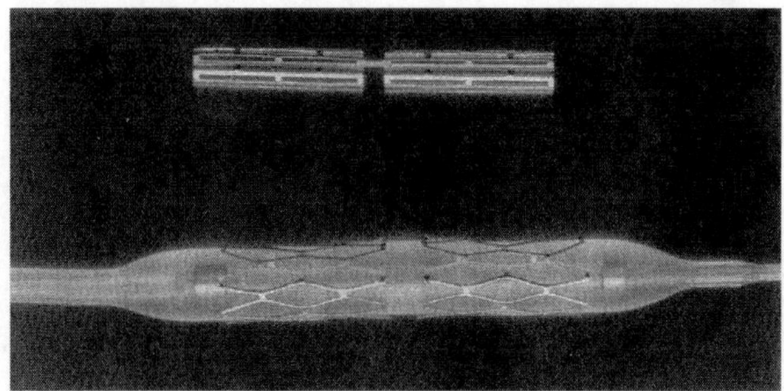

FIGURE 9.22 Balloon-expandable coronary artery stent. (Reprinted from *Biomaterials Science: An Introduction to Materials in Medicine*, Ratner, B.D., Copyright (1996), with permission from Elsevier.)

at lower cost. It has been found, however, that a large number of these patients experience recurrent symptoms similar to those that were originally present only a few months or years after the procedure was performed. When this happens, repeat contrast angiography often shows that the initial atherosclerotic plaque has "reappeared" in the vessel. This is a consequence of the fact that angioplasty does not remove the plaque but only displaces it into the vessel wall that may exhibit a recoil effect due to its elastic nature. Progression of the underlying atherosclerosis is also thought to contribute to this phenomenon of *restenosis*. Therefore, an improvement to this technique has been to combine PTA with placement of a *vascular stent* within the expanded vessel following angioplasty (Figure 9.22).

Vascular stents are made of various metals such as stainless steel and titanium. They are fabricated in tube or wire forms that are then either cut or shaped into a mesh or coil-like pattern. Each stent design is produced in a compact configuration so that it may pass through the stenosis and then be expanded once in position. Thus, the stent is placed over the balloon component of its delivery catheter and then deployed at the site of stenosis following PTA with a separate catheter. Once in place, the stent provides a mechanical scaffold that can help sustain the vessel opening over time (Figure 9.23).

Other variations on this approach involve compressing a coiled wire mesh inside a small plastic sleeve and then deploying it within the stenosis by pulling back the sleeve and allowing the stent to spring open (Figure 9.24).

Another approach is to use a unique metal, *nitinol*, which has "thermal memory" properties. This type of stent is first shaped into a coil at warm temperatures and then straightened into a wire at room temperature (~22°C). Once it is reheated by the body's blood (~37°C) at the site of stenosis, the device then returns to its original coiled shape.

A therapeutic device that evolved subsequent to the use of vascular stents is the *endoluminal stent graft* (Figure 9.25). Endoluminal graft implants are synthetic grafts placed in the circulation to repair a diseased arterial segment but without requiring the use of traditional surgical techniques. The way this is accomplished is to actually deliver the graft to the site using an intra-arterial catheter which then deploys the graft by balloon inflation. The graft is held in place by the inclusion of stents that are positioned at either the proximal only or at both the proximal and

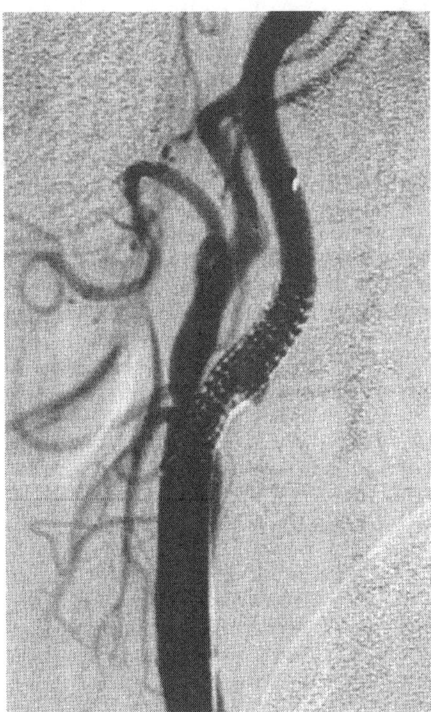

FIGURE 9.23 Digital subtraction angiogram immediately after the percutaneous transluminal insertion of a stent across a carotid stenosis at the bifurcation. (From Brown, M.M., Balloon angioplasty for extracranial carotid diseases, in *Advances in Vascular Surgery*, Vol. 4, Whittemore, A.D., ed., Elsevier, Philadelphia, PA, Copyright 1996, with permission from Elsevier.)

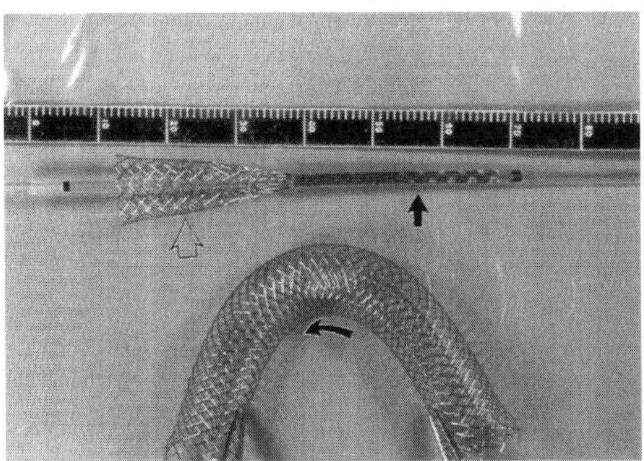

FIGURE 9.24 A photograph of a Wallstent. The tubular, highly permeable braided mesh has considerable longitudinal flexibility and radial strength. (From Marin, M.L. and Veith, F.J., Endovascular stents and stented grafts for the treatment of aneurysms and other arterial lesions, in *Advances in Surgery*, Cameron, J.L., ed., Mosby-Year Book, St. Louis, MO, 1995. With permission.)

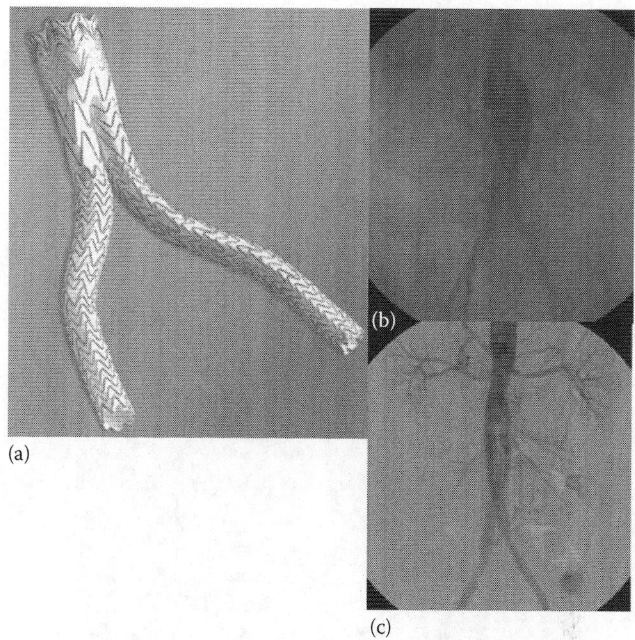

FIGURE 9.25 The AneuRx AAA stent graft system (Medtronic Inc., Santa Rosa, CA). (a) View of AneuRx stent graft, which includes a bifurcated main graft with a left iliac limb. Additional iliac and aortic extender cuffs are available. This polyester graft is supported by a nitinol exoskeleton. (b) A planning anteroposterior aortogram taken before stent graft placement in a 78 year old man with a 6 cm infrarenal AAA. The aortic neck was determined to be 25–26 mm in diameter and 1.5 cm long. (c) This aortogram was taken after AneuRX stent graft placement. The main body of the stent graft was 28 mm in diameter and 13.5 cm long. Bilateral iliac extenders (16 mm diameter) were inserted. (Reprinted with permission of Anderson Publishing Ltd. from Kinney, T.B. et al., *Appl. Radiol.*, 34(3), 9, 2005. © Anderson Publishing Ltd.)

distal ends of the endoluminal graft and that are also deployed by balloon inflation. The primary application for this device is that of AAA repair in patients who are at high risk of mortality during open abdominal surgery. The graft material is usually a Dacron fabric and the stents are usually stainless steel or nitinol strands in a crossed or zigzag configuration. The device is collapsed over the delivery catheter and covered by a smooth plastic sheath until it is in position for deployment. The catheter used for this procedure is a heavier design than that used for intra-arterial stent delivery since it carries a larger object and passes only through the larger arteries of the upper leg and abdomen. In constructing an endoluminal graft for AAAs which also extend down into the iliac arteries from the aorta (and, thus, require distal anastomoses to each iliac artery), additional modular components are available (Figure 9.26).

Endoluminal grafts have proven to be relatively effective devices, especially in patients who would not have successfully tolerated surgery. However, there are several technical difficulties associated with this procedure which include the need to pass

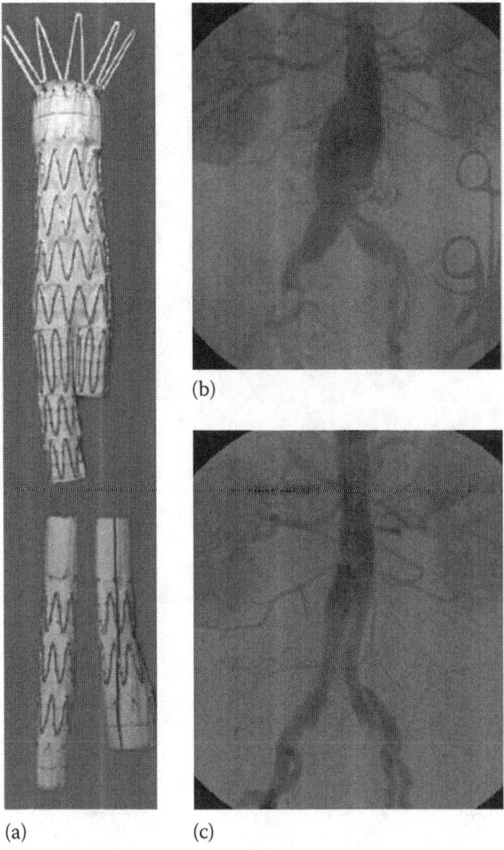

FIGURE 9.26 Zenith endovascular graft (Cook, Inc., Bloomington, IN). (a) A disassembled Zenith stent graft. This graft has an uncovered z-stent with barbs at the superior end for suprarenal fixation. The graft is made of polyester material attached to a frame of stainless steel stents. The two lower components are the iliac legs. Additional modular components are available to extend both the main aortic body and the iliac limbs. An occluder and a converter are available to convert a bifurcated graft into an aorto-uni-iliac graft. (b) Planning angiogram before placement of the Zenith stent graft in a 70 year old man with a 5.4 cm infrarenal AAA. The neck of the AAA measures 21 mm in diameter and is 1.5 cm long. The aneurysm extends into both common iliac arteries. Because of a history of stable angina, an endograft was inserted. (c) An angiogram taken after zenith stent graft placement shows exclusion of the AAA. A 30 mm main body and bilateral iliac legs (24 mm left and 20 mm right) were inserted, and the aneurysm was successfully excluded. (Reprinted with permission of Anderson Publishing Ltd. from Kinney, T.B. et al., *Appl. Radiol.*, 34(3), 9, 2005. © Anderson Publishing Ltd.)

this large object through a potentially diseased femoral or iliac artery and the need to achieve proper placement of the graft such that it does not interfere with flow to the renal arteries. The primary long-term complication experienced with this device has been the development of *perivascular leaks*. These occur because of an incomplete seal between the graft and the artery, resulting in blood at relatively high pressure entering the gap between the two vessels. This buildup of blood pressure could eventually cause a rupture of the aorta very similar to that of an untreated aneurysm.

Finally, another type of stenting procedure (*intracranial stenting and coiling*) has been developed to treat otherwise *inoperable* intracranial aneurysms that, while not being common, can be the cause of stroke in up to 5% of cases. The procedure involves insertion of a stent into the dilated (preferably, fusiform) mid-cerebral artery and then using that as a scaffold to create a distinct "neck" and a channel through the aneurysm. Once in place, microcatheters are used to insert detachable coils through the stent mesh which effectively act as initiators of thrombosis. When the region between the stent and vessel wall clots, the risk of further expansion and rupture is reduced while still allowing for continued flow through the vessel.

9.7 BIOMECHANICS OF STENT IMPLANTS

The addition of stents to the catheter-based treatment of arterial stenoses has brought a dramatic improvement in patency rates of these procedures and has become the method of choice for treating many patients. Since these procedures are still relatively new, however, there is some uncertainty over their long-term effectiveness. The main concern involves the possible responses of the artery wall to the altered fluid and solid dynamic environment caused by the presence of a small, but exposed, metallic intraluminal device that is in place for an extended period of time. Part of this response is the production of additional support tissue in the form of smooth muscle cells and fibroblasts which, in turn, produce elastin and collagen fibers as well as extracellular matrix. In some vessels, this response is controlled and limited in scope, but in others, the process can continue until excess tissue begins to intrude on the vessel lumen (Figure 9.27).

One implication of the presence of stents in the flow stream is the disruption of blood flow patterns, especially along the inner surface of the lumen. Since the stent struts are thin (~0.05–0.15 mm), this effect is relatively small and does not produce gross alterations in the main flow stream. However, these flow "obstacles" may produce unusually low and reversed shear stresses on the local level, especially within vortices generated just in front of and just behind the strut (Figure 9.28) which could contribute to the development of IH (see Section 6.5).

Another effect is that stents possess a much higher stiffness than the surrounding arterial tissue. This produces a sharp reduction in vessel compliance in the stented region and also produces impedance mismatches at the stent/artery interfaces. In addition, stents are typically deployed at very high pressures (≥6 atm) and are often overexpanded in order to seat them in place. This causes the tissue surrounding the stent to be in a permanent state of elevated wall stress which may elicit a healing or remodeling response.

One proposed design is to taper the stent stiffness along its length in such a way as to reduce it from maximum at its center to minimum at its ends (Figure 9.29).

This compliance matching stent leads to a more gradual transition of material properties and produces a more uniform distribution of circumferential stress in the artery than earlier designs (Figure 9.30).

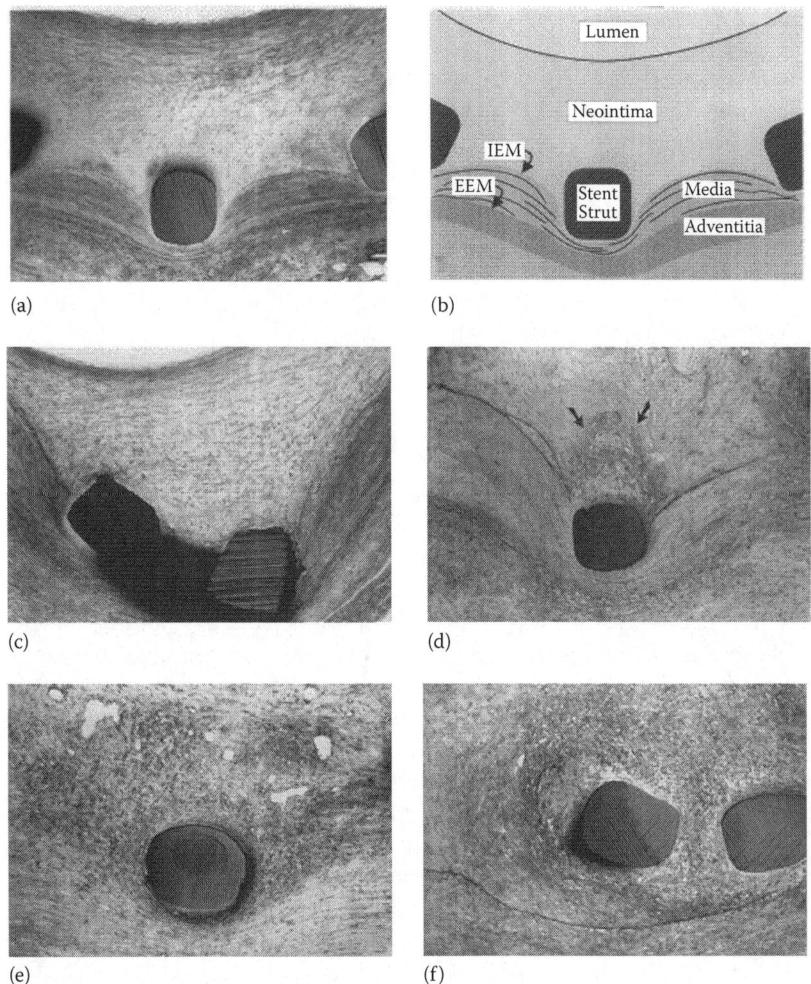

(a) (b) (c) (d) (e) (f)

FIGURE 9.27 Histological examples of the neointimal response to inflammation or injury, or both, and representative types of inflammatory cells. (a) Inflammatory score = 0: There is normal neointima over the strut, with normal complement of smooth muscle with no histiocytes or lymphocytes around. No mural injury or neovascularization of the strut is present. (b) A schematic representation of the histological sections to signify the position of the stent struts in relation to the arterial wall structures. EEM, external elastic membrane; IEM, internal elastic membrane. (c) Inflammatory score = 1: There is a light, widespread lymphohistiocytic infiltrate adjacent to the lumen surface of two adjoining struts. Compression of the media is present without mural injury. (d) Inflammatory score = 2: The moderate, localized cellular aggregate of mononucleated and multinucleated histiocytes along with dispersed lymphocytes adjacent to the lumen surface of the strut (*arrows*). (e) Inflammatory score = 3: There is dense, circumferential inflammatory cell infiltration of the strut, with neovascularization and loss of the internal elastic membrane. (f) Inflammatory score = 3: Each of the two struts is surrounded by the mixed lymphohistiocytic cell infiltrates, with the paler staining histiocytes immediately adjacent to the struts. The internal elastic membrane is intact, and no significant mural injury caused by the strut is noted.

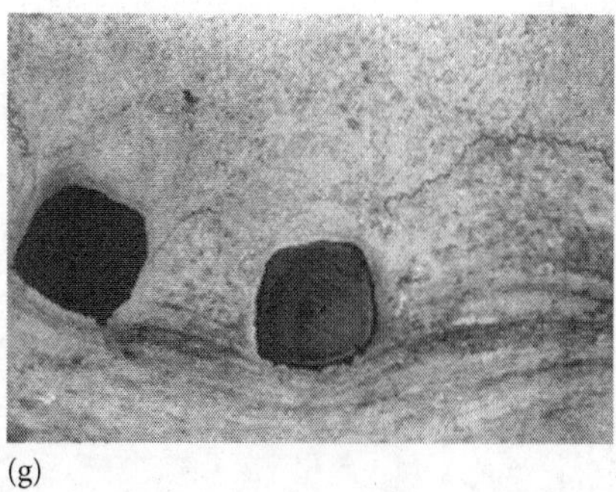

FIGURE 9.27 (continued) (g) There is perforation of the internal elastic membrane and tunica media of the artery, with only grade 1 inflammatory reaction around the strut. (a), (c)–(g), 160×, reduced by 50%. (From Kornowski, R. et al., *J. Am. Coll. Cardiol.*, 31, 224, 1998.)

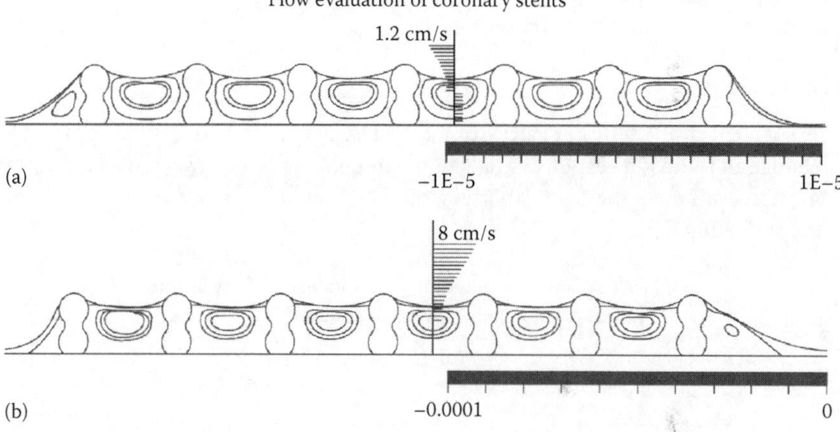

FIGURE 9.28 Streamlines (m^2/s) (for L/D = 3.53, resting conditions, 4 mm vessel) at (a) midsystole and (b) peak diastolic forward flow. (From Berry, J.L. et al., *Ann. Biomed. Eng.*, 28, 386, 2000. With permission.)

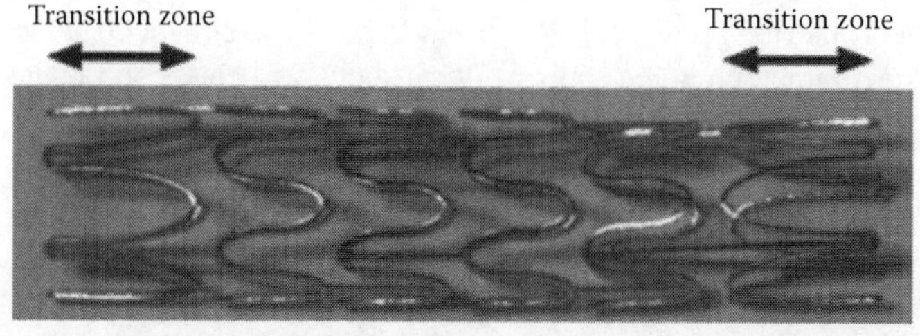

FIGURE 9.29 Illustration of the CMS. The ends of the stent are gradually more flexible toward the ends, providing a smooth transition in compliance when deployed in an artery. (From Moore, J.E., Jr. and Berry, J.L., *Ann. Biomed. Eng.*, 30, 498, 2002. With permission.)

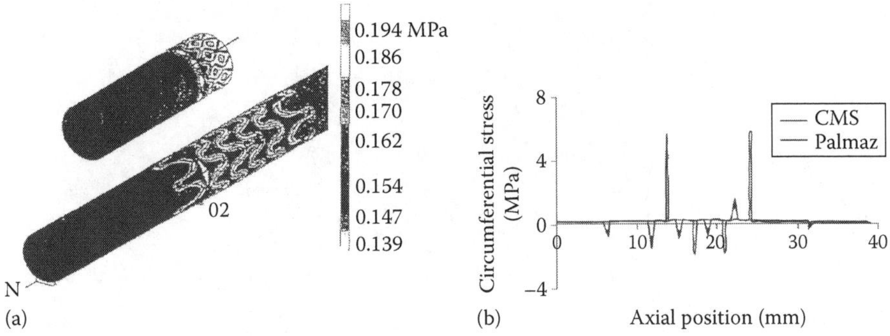

FIGURE 9.30 Color-encoded maximum principal stress in an artery into which the Palmaz stent (a) or the CMS (b) has been deployed. (From Moore, J.E., Jr. and Berry, J.L., *Ann. Biomed. Eng.*, 30, 498, 2002. With permission.)

Further investigations are currently being made of other design modifications and also of applying coatings to the stent which are capable of releasing various drugs (*drug-eluting*) that can inhibit IH formation.

PROBLEMS

9.1 A segment of the femoral artery of a dog is replaced with an arterial graft. The change in radius in response to a change in pulse pressure was measured in the graft as well as in the femoral artery on the other side ("contralateral") to yield the following data:

	Pulse Pressure (mmHg)	Internal Radius (mm)	Change in Radius (%)	Wall Thickness (mm)
Artery	50	4.0	15	1.0
Graft	50	5.0	10	1.0

For each of these vessels, compute the compliance and the incremental elastic modulus at the mean pressure.

9.2 A catheter-tip balloon is designed to expand diseased regions of arteries that have a normal (nondiseased) internal diameter of 6 mm. The balloon has a wall thickness of 0.1 mm and becomes fully distended at 6 mm. It can withstand up to 6 atm of internal pressure. If the artery can only tolerate a 20% increase over its normal diameter before rupturing, what should the elastic modulus of the balloon material be to provide full dilatation at maximum pressure?

Is this a *maximum* or *minimum* value?

REFERENCES

Ballyk, P. D. et al. (1998) Compliance mismatch may promote graft-artery intimal hyperplasia by altering suture-line stresses. *J. Biomech.* 232: 229–237.

Berry, J. L. et al. (2000) Experimental and computational flow evaluation of coronary stents. *Ann. Biomed. Eng.* 28: 386.

Bowlin, G. L. et al. (2001) The persistence of electrostatically seeded endothelial cells lining a small diameter expanded polytetrafluoroethylene vascular graft. *J. Biomater. Appl.* 16: 157.

Brown, M. M. (1996) Balloon angioplasty for extracranial carotid diseases. In *Advances in Vascular Surgery*, Vol. 4, Whittemore, A. D., ed., Elsevier, Philadelphia, PA.

Cameron, J. L., ed. (1995) *Advances in Surgery*, Mosby-Year Book, St. Louis, MO.

Dardik, H. (1978) *Graft Materials in Vascular Surgery.*

Dumars, M. C. et al. (2002) *Radiology*, 222: 103.

Ernst, C. B. and Stanley, J. C. (1991) *Current Therapy in Vascular Surgery*, 2nd edn., B.C. Decker, Philadelphia, PA.

Fei, D. Y. et al. (1994) *J. Biomech. Eng.* 116: 331.

Gotto A.M. Jr. et al. (1997) *Atherosclerosis*, UPJohn, Kalamazoo, MI.

How, T. V. et al. (2000) Interposition vein cuff anastomosis alters wall shear stress distribution in the recipient artery. *J. Vasc. Surg.* 31: 1008–1017.

Keynton, R. S. et al. (1991) The effect of angle and flow rate upon hemodynamics in distal vascular graft anastomoses: An in vitro model study. *J. Biomech. Eng.* 113: 460.

Keynton, R. S. et al. (1999) The effect of graft caliber upon wall shear within in vivo distal vascular anastomoses. *J. Biomech. Eng.* 121: 82.

Keynton, R. S. et al. (2001) Intimal hyperplasia and wall shear in arterial bypass graft distal anastomoses: An in vivo model study. *J. Biomech. Eng.* 123: 464.

Kinney, T. B. et al. (2005) Stent grafts for abdominal and thoracic aortic disease. *Appl. Radiol.* 34(3): 9.

Kornowski, R. et al. (1998) In-stent restenosis: Contributions of inflammatory responses and arterial injury to neointimal hyperplasia. *J. Am. Coll. Cardiol.* 31: 224.

Langille, B. L. and O'Donnell, F. (1986) Reductions in arterial diameter produced by chronic decreases in blood flow are endothelium-dependent. *Science* 231: 405–407.

Li, X.-M. (1998) Evaluation of hemodynamic factors at the distal end-to-side anastomosis of a bypass graft with different POS:DOS ratios, Master's thesis, Department of Biomedical Engineering, The University of Akron, Akron, OH, p. 6.

Moore J. E. Jr. and Berry, J. L. (2002) *Ann. Biomed. Eng.* 30: 498.

Ojha, M. et al. (1990) Steady and pulsatile flow fields in an end-to-side arterial anastomosis model. *J. Vasc. Surg.* 12: 747–753.

O'Rourke, M. F. (1982) Vascular impedance in studies of arterial and cardiac function. *Physiol. Rev.* 62: 570–623.

Ratner, B. D. et al. (1996) *Biomaterials Science: An Introduction to Materials in Medicine.*

Sawyer, P. N. (1987) *Modern Vascular Grafts*, McGraw-Hill Book Co., New York.

10 Fluid Dynamic Measurement Techniques

10.1 INTRODUCTION

We have now used models for steady (Chapter 5) and unsteady (Chapter 6) flow through rigid or elastic tubes to understand the flow dynamics in the blood vessels. Analysis of the governing equations resulted in expressions for pressure pulse, flow rate, and velocity profiles. To verify the accuracy of our models, data on these variables must be obtained from *in vitro*, or, preferably from *in vivo* measurements. Moreover, measurements of pressure, flow rate, and resistance within specific segments of the circulatory system are also important diagnostically to the physician. Measurement of detailed velocity profiles and other flow parameters will also be helpful in understanding the factors involved in the initiation of disease processes such as thrombus formation and atherosclerosis (see Chapter 6).

10.2 BLOOD PRESSURE MEASUREMENT

Earlier, we discussed the pressure pulse in the arteries and the systolic and diastolic pressures. These values are again an important measurement for the physician to have for diagnostic purposes. Indirect method of pressure measurement can be performed with the familiar pressure cuff method. In this method using a sphygmomanometer (*sphygmos* means pulse), a pneumatic cuff encircling the upper arm is inflated to a pressure larger than the blood pressure. Thus, the brachial artery in the arm collapses and occludes the flow of blood through the artery. As the cuff pressure is slowly released and when the cuff pressure decreases to a value slightly lower than the peak systolic blood pressure, the blood squirts through the collapsed segment of the artery. The flow through the segment is turbulent and generates sound referred to as the "Korotkoff" sound which can be detected by a stethoscope placed over the brachial artery. The pressure at the initiation of this sound is the systolic pressure. As the cuff pressure is further decreased, the Korotkoff sound ceases to exist at a point when there is no constriction of the artery and hence flow is no more turbulent. The pressure corresponding to the cessation of the sound is the diastolic pressure. Replacing the stethoscope with a microphone to detect the sound, this pressure measurement technique can be automated. This technique is noninvasive and pressure can be measured with minimal discomfort to the patient. However, the error in measurement in this technique can be as high as 10 mmHg.

For more accurate determination of blood pressure, direct methods require gaining access to the blood vessel through catheterization. Usually, a fluid-filled catheter is introduced into an artery and is connected to a pressure transducer where the fluid comes in contact with the transducing element. The pressure transducers described earlier work on the principle that the resistance of that element changes in proportion to the pressure applied on the element. This resistance change is converted into an electrical output signal. For a bridge containing four active elements, the output voltage can be shown to be

$$e_0 = E\frac{\Delta R}{R}$$

Commercial transducers will have a transducer sensitivity factor provided and the sensitivity factor F is given as volts output per volt of excitation per unit of the physical quantity measured. Thus, the output voltage e_0 will be given by

$$e_0 = FEQ \tag{10.1}$$

where

E is the excitation voltage

Q is the quantity being transduced, such as pressure

Thus, the measurement of any physical quantity depends upon the accuracy of the sensitivity factor, the accuracy of the excitation voltage, and the accuracy of the measurement of the output voltage. Many transducers also have a calibration resistor incorporated in the circuit.

The fluid-filled catheter system is commonly used in the clinical setting for continuous monitoring of the patient's blood pressure. However, the catheter-tipped transducer that avoids the fluid-filled flexible tubing has a higher frequency response and, hence, is preferred particularly in a research setting when an accurate reproduction of the pressure pulse is of importance. The fluid-filled catheter is filled with heparinized saline to prevent clotting of the blood in the catheter and periodic flushing of the catheter is necessary to prevent blood coagulation. Also, care must be taken to prevent trapped air bubbles in the catheter since the air bubbles will distort the pressure pulse due to damping. Figure 10.1 shows a comparison of pressure signals obtained with a fluid-filled catheter with and without air bubbles with that obtained from a catheter-tipped transducer. When the fluid-filled catheter is introduced in a large diameter blood vessel, due to the flailing motion of the catheter, low frequency oscillations are superposed on the pressure signal as shown in Figure 10.2.

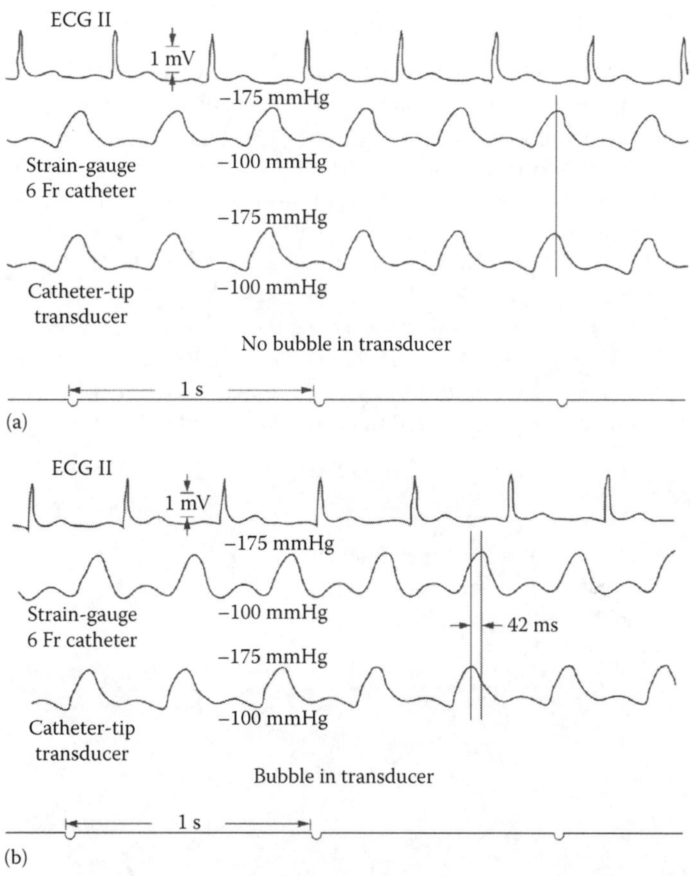

FIGURE 10.1 Comparison of pressure signals recorded with fluid-filled catheter transducer and catheter-tipped transducer. Note the similarity of the signals between the two transducers in the absence of air bubble in the catheter. Changes in pulse shape and a time delay are observed with the presence of the air bubble with the fluid-filled catheter. (a) No bubble in transducer. (b) Bubble in transducer. (Geddes, L.A.: *Cardiovascular Devices and Applications*. 1984. Copyright Wiley-VCH Verlag GmbH & Co. KGaA. With permission.)

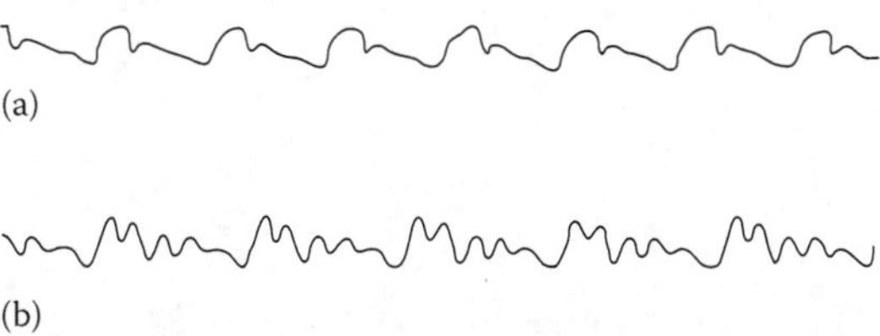

FIGURE 10.2 Distorted pressure signals in a fluid-filled catheter due to catheter whip: (a) good quality pressure recording and (b) the distorted signal due to catheter whip. (Geddes, L.A.: *Cardiovascular Devices and Applications*. 1984. Copyright Wiley-VCH Verlag GmbH & Co. KGaA. With permission.)

10.3 BLOOD FLOW MEASUREMENT

Ultimately, the delivery of essential nutrients and oxygen to tissues and the removal of waste products is the overriding purpose of the circulation. Therefore, measurement of the volume rate of flow of blood through the heart and vessels is very important in assessing the function of the system. The *electromagnetic flow meter* (EMF) is a device currently used for such measurements. It operates by determining the mean velocity of flow through a blood vessel of known cross-sectional area and then derives the flow rate through the vessel as the product of these two values. The theory on which this measurement technique is based is Faraday's law. According to this law, when a conductive fluid such as blood flows between the lines of force of a magnetic field, an electromagnetic force is generated in the fluid which is perpendicular to the direction of the magnetic field as well as the direction of motion of the fluid (Figure 10.3). The voltage generated between the electrodes, E_f (volts), is given by the relationship

$$E_f = B\ell V$$

where

B is the flux density of the magnetic field (Wb/m^2)
ℓ is the spacing between electrodes (m)
V is the mean flow velocity (m/s)

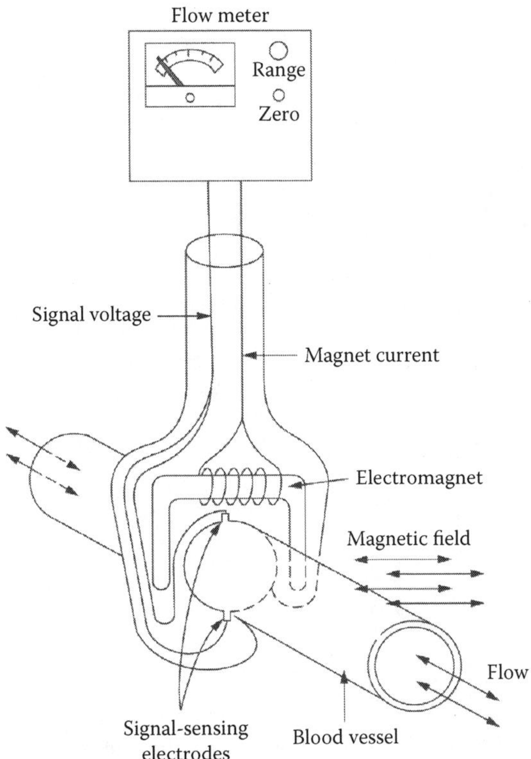

FIGURE 10.3 Schematic of an electromagnetic flow probe used for blood flow measurement.

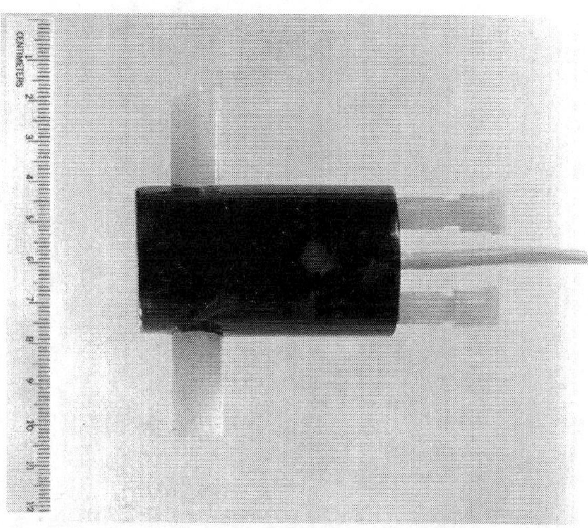

FIGURE 10.4 Typical electromagnetic flow probes: extracorporeal. (Courtesy of Carolina Medical Electronics Inc., King, NC.)

Relating the flow rate through the vessel, Q (m^3/s) and area of cross section A (m^2) with the mean velocity by

$$Q = VA$$

The flow rate can be computed from the relationship

$$Q = \frac{A}{B\ell} E_f \tag{10.2}$$

The ratio $A/B\ell$ is a constant specified for a given flow meter system.

The electromagnetic flow probe, which is attached to the blood vessel, consists of an electromagnet that generates the magnetic force and two electrodes to detect the flow signal. These are encapsulated in probes of varying sizes to adapt to the various vessels in the circulation. The extracorporeal probe shown in Figure 10.4 is inserted by cannulation of the blood vessel for acute *in situ* measurements or is used for flow measurements in extracorporeal circulation. The intracorporeal probes have an opening slot so that it can be fit snugly around the vessel as shown in Figure 10.5.

The relationship derived in Equation 10.2 assumes a dc magnetic field that would produce a dc flow signal. However, problems from electrode offset potentials, amplifier drift, and so on make it difficult to delineate the actual flow signal and ac excitation is used in the common flow meters. The flow meters use either a square wave excitation or sine wave excitation. In ac excitation, the time variation of the magnetic flux, dB/dt, must be included in Equation 10.2. In the commercial systems, measurements are obtained when the time varying component is zero. In the sine wave excitation, the dB/dt component is effectively zero only for a relatively shorter time and the voltage-sensing circuits must be gated for a short time. On the other hand, with square wave excitation, the time varying component is effectively zero except during the short periods in which the signals are switched. The signal-to-noise ratio is

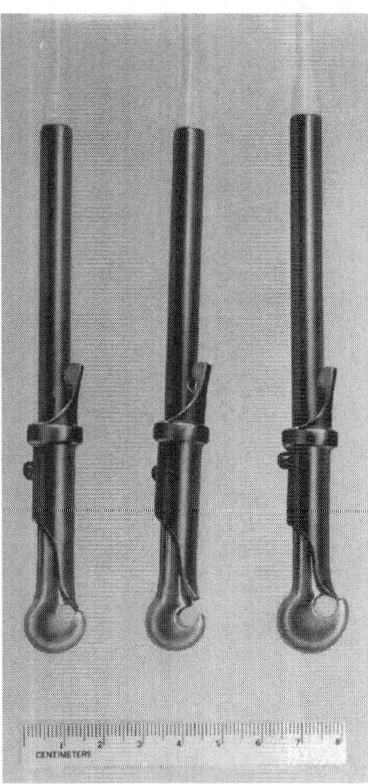

FIGURE 10.5 Typical electromagnetic flow probes: intracorporeal. (Courtesy of Carolina Medical Electronics Inc., King, NC.)

proportional to the peak-to-peak value of excitation and for the same signal-to-noise ratio, the square wave excitation requires twice as much power as the sine wave excitation. Hence, the meters for the square wave devices are larger and must operate at higher temperatures. A typical flow rate signal from an *in vitro* pulse duplicator distal to a heart valve is shown in Figure 10.6 in which measurements were made with a Carolina square wave EMF and an *in vivo* metric extracorporeal flow probe. The time-averaged flow rate (cardiac output) and other information such as the amount of back flow can be determined from such curves.

Even though the EMF is an ideal device for *in vitro* testing, there are several drawbacks in using it for *in vivo* measurements. One is that this is an invasive technique so that the vessel must be exposed and that the flow probe fitted around the vessel. Second, if left in the body for some time, problems of contact of the electrodes with the arterial wall, such as protein or thrombus coating, and subsequent deterioration of the signals may occur. Moreover, this device actually measures the *mean flow velocity*, and, thus, the area of the probe lumen must be accurately known to determine the flow rate. The EMF theory also assumes that the fluid has a flat velocity profile at the mean velocity magnitude. Since in blood vessels the lumen is not an ideal circular cross section and the flow is asymmetric, some errors will occur in measuring the flow rate using this technique.

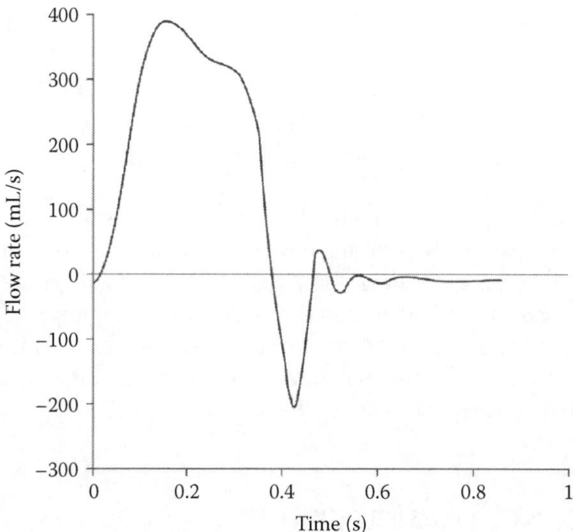

FIGURE 10.6 A typical flow rate signal distal to a heart valve from an electromagnetic flow meter in a pulse duplicator.

A more recent flow measuring device is the *transit time flow meter*. This instrument is based on the fact that sound waves travel through a fluid at slightly greater or lower velocities depending upon whether the flow is forward or reverse, respectively. The transit time flow meter, then, utilizes ultrasonic energy in the kilohertz range (as opposed to ultrasound imaging and Doppler devices which operate in the megahertz range) which is transmitted through a vessel along the axis of the flow in alternate directions (Figure 10.7). The device then detects small differences (order of nanoseconds) in transit times between the two signals, t_f and t_r, as

$$t_f = \frac{\ell}{(c+u)}$$

$$t_r = \frac{\ell}{(c-u)}$$

where $\ell = 2d/(\sin\theta)$.

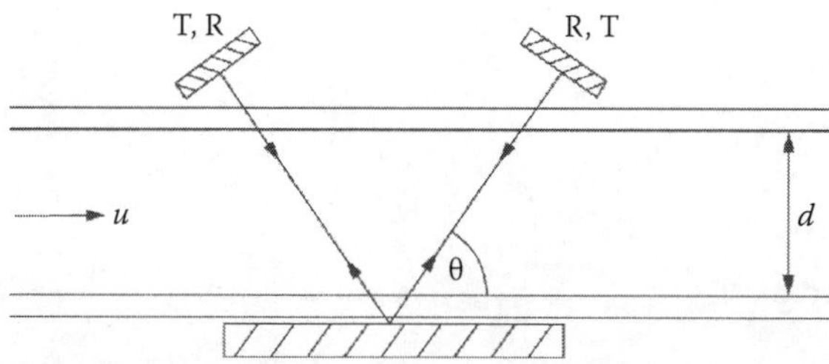

FIGURE 10.7 Transit time flow probe with two ultrasonic crystals alternately transmitting and receiving signals passing through a fluid and reflecting off of a backplate.

It then computes the flow velocity, u, from

$$u = \frac{c^2 \Delta t}{(2d \cos\theta)}$$

where $\Delta t = t_r - t_f$.

The volume flow rate is determined by multiplying this velocity by the known vessel cross-sectional area. While this device is also invasive (i.e., the probe must be placed around the vessel), it does not depend on any special features of the vessel (e.g., electrical conductivity) other than the presence of reflectors in the form of red blood cells. Since the flow rate is proportional to the transit time of the sound signals, it is a very linear and easily calibrated device that is very stable (i.e., not susceptible to other electrical signals) and that can be left in place for long-term (i.e., days to weeks) experiments.

10.4 IMPEDANCE MEASUREMENT

In developing the steady flow models for blood flow, we discussed the *resistance* to blood circulation as being given by the relationship

$$R = \frac{\Delta p}{Q}$$

When measuring the resistance across the systemic circulation, the mean pressures at the aorta and at the vena cava were used along with the mean flow rate (cardiac output). Using a familiar electrical analogy, the resistance in dc circuits is given by $R = E/I$ where E is the voltage and I is the current in a branch of the circuit. In ac circuits, the corresponding measure is the electrical *impedance*. Thus, impedance to flow in the circulation under unsteady flow can be defined similar to resistance under steady flow conditions. Three different impedance relationships are defined by Milnor (1989) as

Longitudinal impedance:

$$Z_L = \frac{-dp/dz}{Q} \tag{10.3}$$

Input impedance:

$$Z_z = \frac{p}{Q} \tag{10.4}$$

Transverse impedance:

$$Z_w = \frac{p}{-dQ/dz} \tag{10.5}$$

Longitudinal impedance is the ratio of the pressure gradient to the flow and, hence, is directly analogous to the vascular resistance defined in steady flow. The longitudinal impedance depends only on the local properties of the vessel across which the pressure gradient is measured. Input impedance, on the other hand, is the ratio of the pressure and flow at a *particular site* in the vasculature and is dependent on the local properties as well as those in the segments distal to it. The input impedance at the end of the vessel is called the *terminal impedance*, Z_t. If the distal bed were just a continuation of the vessel in which measurements are made (i.e., without any change in characteristics), then this value is termed the *characteristic impedance*, Z_0.

From the theoretical models developed for pulsatile blood flow in elastic tubes by Womersley and others, the impedances can be computed from the relationships given earlier. The impedances will be complex quantities which depend upon the Womersley parameter as well as the elastic properties of the tube. Thus, the complex impedance can be resolved into real and imaginary quantities where the real part is the resistive component and the imaginary component is the reactive component of the impedance. The computed results can also be presented as the modulus and phase lag. Several models have been used to theoretically calculate the input or characteristic as well as the longitudinal impedance (Milnor, 1989).

To determine the input impedance experimentally, the pressure as well as the flow is measured simultaneously at the selected point in the circulation. The pressure can be measured with high-fidelity pressure transducers discussed earlier and the flow can be measured by an EMF or by ultrasound methods. The frequency response of the flow and pressure transducers must be determined and the distortion of modulus and phase must be taken into account in computing the impedance (O'Rourke, 1982). The signals are then subjected to a frequency analysis and the input impedance at any frequency component is the ratio of the pressure and the flow at that frequency. Thus, at a frequency, n, the input impedance will be given by

$$|Z_z|_n = \frac{|P|_n}{|Q|_n} \tag{10.6a}$$

and

$$\theta_n = \phi_n - \xi_n \tag{10.6b}$$

where

ϕ_n is the phase angle of the pressure
ξ_n is the phase angle of the flow

Frequency analysis, or decomposition, is usually performed by *Fourier analysis* where the phase and amplitude of each frequency component is obtained. A basic assumption of this technique is that the system is linear so that there is no interaction between signals of different frequencies. A limitation of the characteristic impedance is that it cannot be directly measured *in vivo*. However, in larger arteries, the input impedance is essentially independent of the frequency except for a drop in the

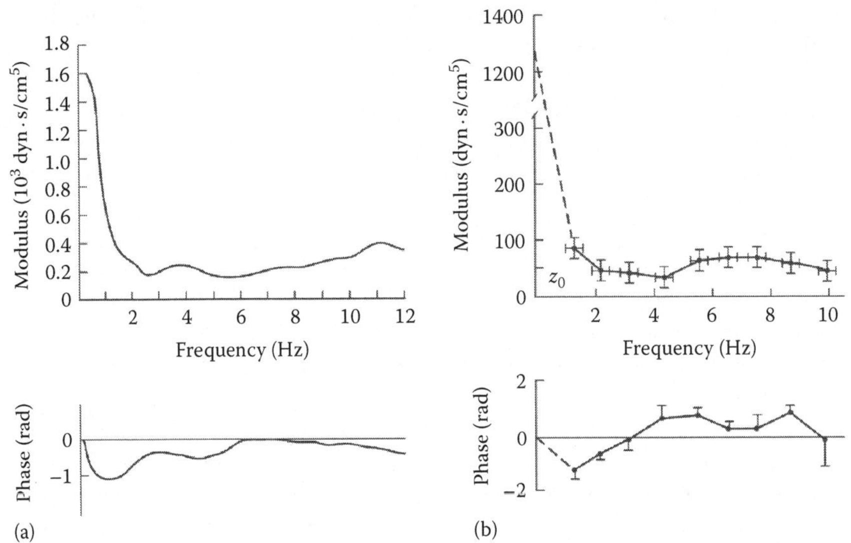

FIGURE 10.8 Input impedance in the aorta of (a) dog and (b) human. (Redrawn from Milnor, W.R., *Hemodynamics*, 2nd edn., Williams & Wilkins, Baltimore, MD, 1989.)

impedance at low frequencies. Thus, the characteristic impedance, Z_0, is computed by averaging the modulus of the input impedance across the frequency spectrum, neglecting the low frequencies where the steep drop in impedance occurs.

The input impedance in the ascending aorta for a dog and a human is given in Figure 10.8 where it is seen to fall steeply from 0 to 2 Hz and then fluctuate with frequency thereafter. Such an input impedance spectrum usually shows a minimum of the impedance modulus between 2 and 8 Hz. The phase angle of the input impedance is usually zero at the first minimum of the modulus. Oscillations in the modulus of the impedance depend upon reflections of the waves in the peripheral arteries as they encounter discontinuities (i.e., branches, end organs, etc.), and vasoconstriction will increase the reflections and, hence, increase the oscillations in the impedance. The ratio of Z_z/Z_0 and also the ratio of

$$\frac{Z_z(\max) - Z_z(\min)}{Z_0}$$

are useful measures of the oscillations in the impedance. In this ratio, the first maximum and first minimum of the modulus are used. Under normal resting conditions, this ratio is about 0.6–0.85 in man and dogs.

The input impedance in the main pulmonary circulation is shown in Figure 10.9. As can be observed, the shape of the profile is similar to that for the aorta even though the magnitude is smaller. The first minimum of the modulus occurs between 2 and 4 Hz and the next maximum occurs at 6–8 Hz. The characteristic impedance in pulmonary circulation is obtained by averaging the impedance modulus at higher frequencies and it is about 190 dyn · s/cm^5 in dogs and about 23 dyn · s/cm^5 in man.

As mentioned earlier, the impedance will change due to alterations in the vascular tone as well as changes in the elastic properties of the distal vessels.

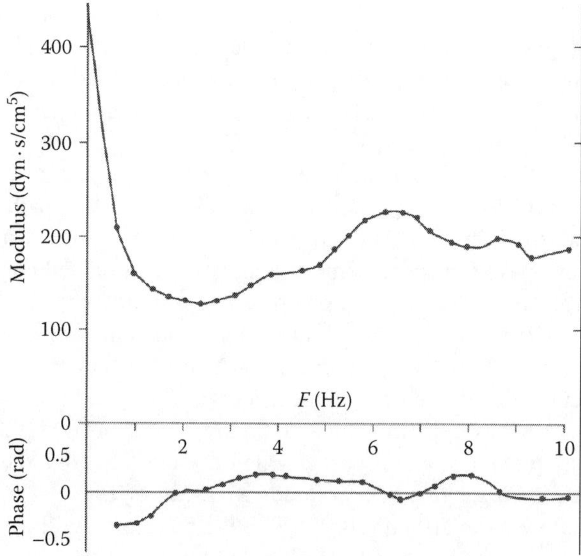

FIGURE 10.9 Input impedance in the main pulmonary circulation of a dog. (Redrawn from Milnor, W.R., *Hemodynamics*, 2nd edn., Williams & Wilkins, Baltimore, MD, 1989.)

Thus, measurements of vascular impedance can be used for diagnostic purposes to determine changes in the vasculature in the distal vessels. For example, pulmonary vascular hypertension increases the vascular impedance to as much as three times the normal value and, as a consequence, the minimum of the modulus is displaced from 3 Hz to about 8 Hz. Systemic vascular hypertension is also known to increase the input impedance from normal values in a similar way. Further discussion on the impedance characteristics with arterial disease can be found in Milnor (1989).

10.5 FLOW VISUALIZATION

A useful technique for obtaining visual information about the flow characteristics in various cardiovascular anatomies and devices is *flow visualization*. Flow visualization, which is widely used in the automotive and aircraft industries, is performed by inserting a visible marker into the flow stream and then making a photographic record of the markers movement. With this technique, it is possible to obtain a general overview of the flow field, to identify fine details of flow structures such as jets, separation zones, secondary motions, and so on, and to provide an indication of the stability of the flow (i.e., laminar versus turbulent). This information can be obtained relatively simply and cheaply and serves as a good starting point for designing subsequent experiments for obtaining more quantitative data.

The key assumption of a flow visualization technique is that the marker accurately follows the actual flow movement. To do so, there must be a balance of the inertial, viscous, buoyant, and gravitational forces acting on the marker and it must not disturb the flow. The best way to satisfy these requirements is to use small, neutral density particles. Advantages of flow visualization over other techniques are its simplicity and ability to provide full-field (i.e., 2D) information at any instant of time. Disadvantages are its requirement for optically transparent fluids and materials and, traditionally, its nonquantitative nature although newer advances with *particle image velocimetry* (PIV) now make it possible to derive *quantitative* information from flow visualization data as well.

Most flow visualization techniques provide information in the form of either *path lines* or *streak lines*. Path lines represent the actual trajectory or path followed by a single particle in the flow field while streak lines show the present positions of all particles that have passed through some common point. A related concept is that of "*streamlines*" that are curves superimposed on the flow field that are tangent to the velocity vectors of particles at a particular position and at a specific instant in time. In some cases, *time lines* may also be obtained which show the movement of a region of flow that occurs between successive time intervals.

Depending upon the application and the nature of data desired, there are a variety of flow visualization methods used which are classified by the type of flow marker employed. For example, a colored dye is an effective way of obtaining streak lines in a flow system (Figure 10.10). This method can be performed with virtually any visible dye (e.g., ink, food coloring, fluorescein, etc.) that dissolves in the fluid medium (usually an aqueous solution). The dye can then be injected at a specific location, generally using a fine needle, and then its path tracked using photographs or video recordings. One disadvantage of dye flow visualization is the eventual buildup of the dye in the fluid which then clouds the visual field. Another disadvantage is that it is not useful for either pulsatile or turbulent conditions. Solid particles (e.g., aluminum flakes or microspheres) are often used to obtain path lines, especially if either the light source or the camera shutter is strobed (Figure 10.11).

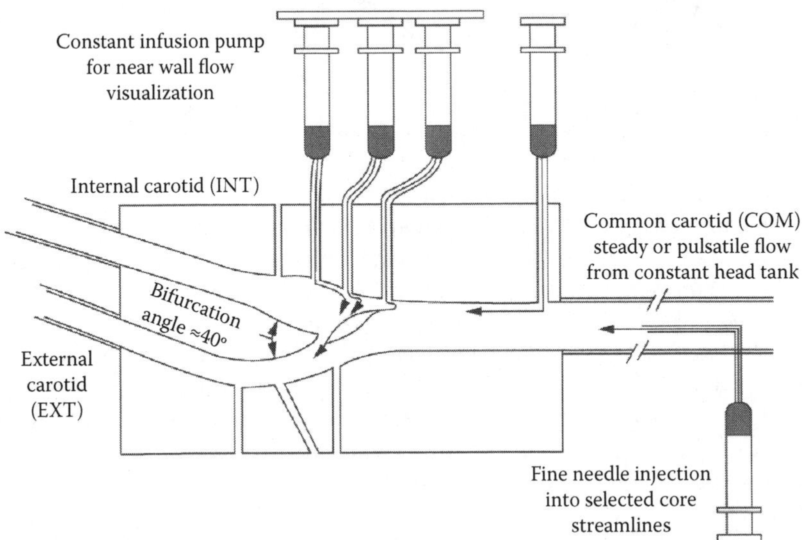

FIGURE 10.10 Schematic of the experimental setup for flow visualization using colored dye. (From LoGerfo et al., *J. Vasc. Surg.*, 2, 263, 1985.)

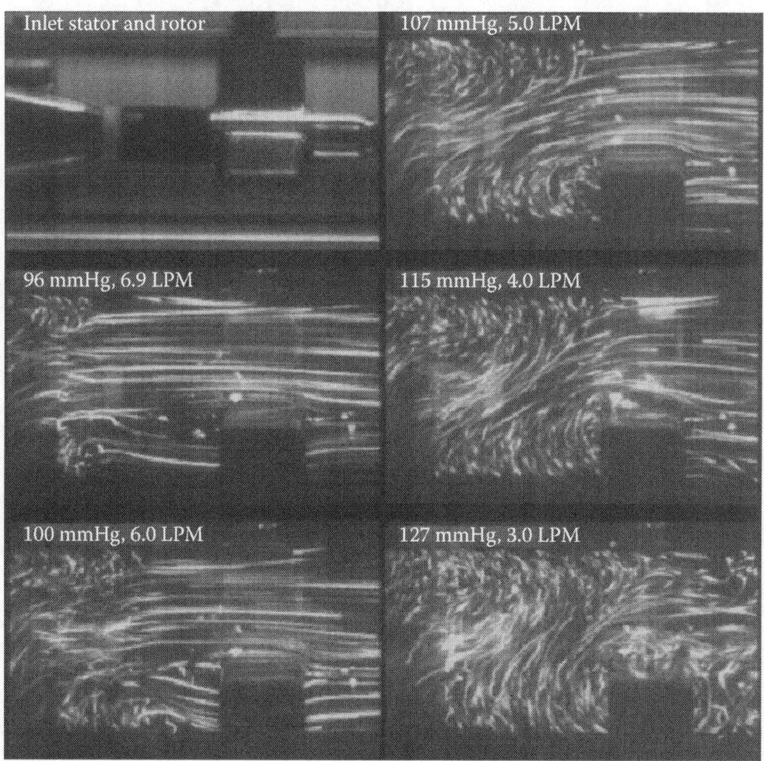

FIGURE 10.11 Flow visualization study of HeartMate II; area of inlet stator and rotor are seen with various pressure–flow conditions. Note variation in flow pattern. The microvortices predicted by CFD were not apparent (LPM 5 L/min). (From Griffith B.P. et al., *Ann. Thorac. Surg.*, 71, S116, 2001. With permission.)

The particles must be chosen so that they are good reflectors of light, have densities similar to that of the fluid medium, and are small in comparison with the finest flow structure being imaged.

A technique sometimes used in an aqueous fluid medium is called *hydrogen bubble* flow visualization. This technique actually generates flow markers within the fluid by the process of electrolysis, thereby creating H_2 and O_2 molecules at a cathode and an anode, respectively. Advantages of this method are that no external markers need to be added to the fluid and there is no buildup of them, for example, with dye. Disadvantages of the technique are that electrodes must be introduced into the fluid that must be an electrical conductor and the density of the gas particles generated is much less than that of the fluid medium. Despite these drawbacks, however, this technique may be adequate for cases where high flow velocities exist and the transit time of the gas bubbles through the imaging field is brief. (Note: Hydrogen bubble flow visualization was the technique used in earlier images of symmetric, carotid stenosis model.)

A fairly ingenious flow visualization approach is the use of a transparent compound that is mixed into the fluid medium and that can then be selectively converted to a colored state upon activation by laser light illumination (Figure 10.12).

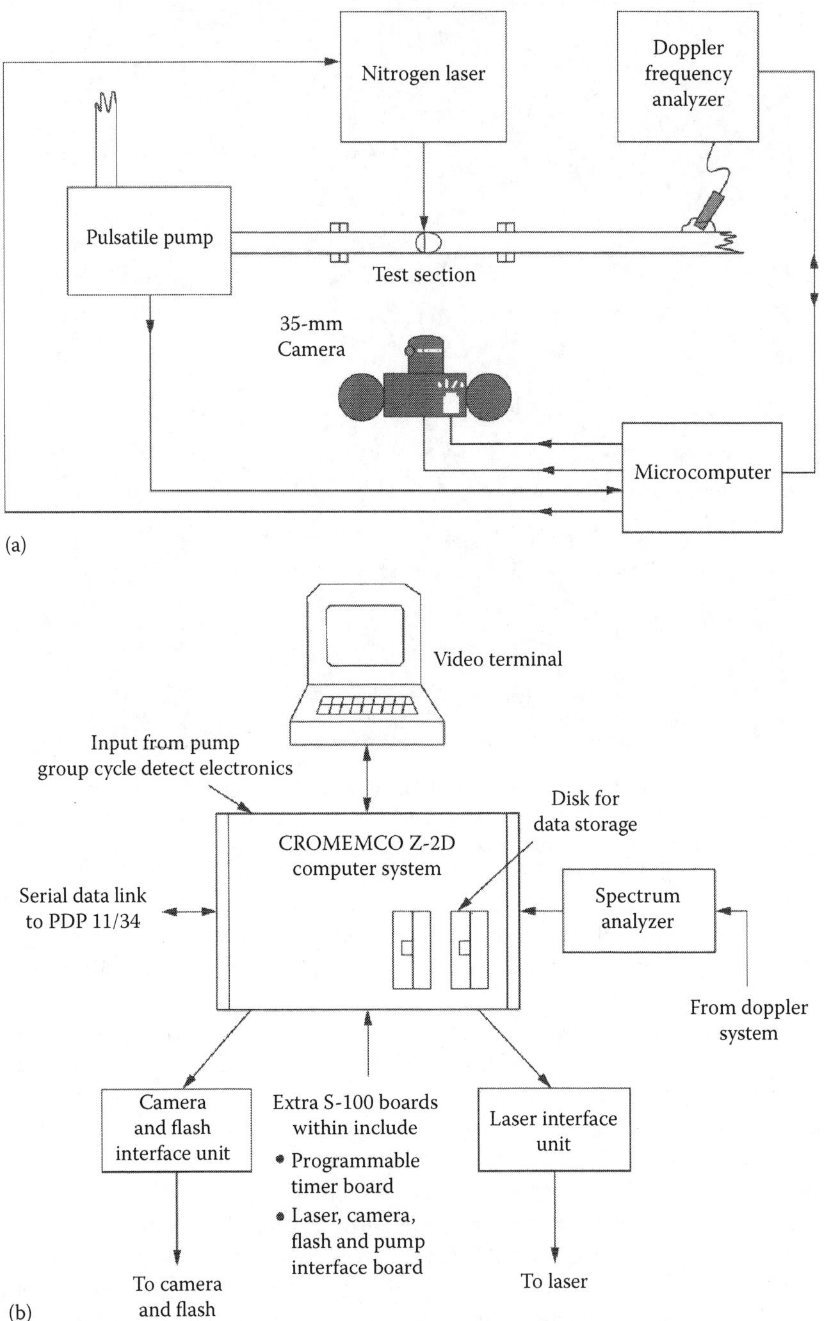

FIGURE 10.12 Schematic of the experimental setup for flow visualization using photochromic dye technique. (a) Overall system and (b) computerized control and data handling system. (From *Ann. Biomed. Eng.*, 14, Poots, K. et al., 203–218, Copyright (1986), with permission from Elsevier.)

This *photochromic dye* technique utilizes the chemical TNSB that has the property of becoming opaque when exposed to the ultraviolet light emitted from a nitrogen laser. Images of the movement of regions of the flow rendered visible by the laser beam activation can then be recorded by standard photographic methods. Advantages of this technique are that the laser beam can be positioned at any site in the flow field, the chemical reaction is completely reversible with a half-time of only a few seconds (i.e., there is no accumulation of dye), and the dye is clearly seen and recorded. The major disadvantage of this technique is that TNSB is not water soluble and must instead be dissolved in a hydrocarbon-based fluid such as kerosene, a flammable and toxic substance.

Since each of aforementioned techniques is an optical technique, it is critical to provide a transparent, distortion-free system for making recordings. A common approach is to place the test model within a flat-surfaced *view box* filled with a fluid having a refractive index similar to that of the model construction material. In this way, light penetrating through the viewing area will follow a straight path and not be diffracted by irregular or curved surfaces.

10.6 ULTRASOUND DOPPLER VELOCIMETRY

While several of the previous techniques are invaluable for providing important qualitative and quantitative information about flow conditions within *in vitro* models, there are some cases where they cannot be used due to their optical nature and their requirement for transparent models and fluids. Examples of this would be testing of an actual prototype device that is opaque or translucent, the use of blood as a test fluid, or testing in an *in vivo* animal model. An approach that can be used to make velocity measurements in these cases is *ultrasound Doppler velocimetry*. Here, the term "ultrasound" denotes frequencies that are much higher than those of audible sound (i.e., >20,000 Hz).

Ultrasound Doppler velocimetry is based on a phenomenon first described by Christian Doppler in 1842. It was his observation that the apparent tone of a sound changes if the source and the listener were moving relative to each other. He demonstrated this with a musician riding on a train car that passed a second musician standing along the tracks. As the car approached and then departed, the second musician recorded the perceived tone, or note, of the sound. The result was an apparent increase in tone as the car approached and a decrease in tone on departure. This "Doppler shift" effect can be described mathematically to show that the change in frequency is proportional to the relative speed between source and observer.

Specifically, if a source emits a sound at a frequency, f_s, and a *receiver* is moving at a velocity, V_r, relative to the source (Figure 10.13), then the number of wave peaks received per unit time would equal the number of peaks transmitted from the source plus the extra number of peaks intercepted due to the advancing position of the receiver, or

$$N_r = N_s + \Delta N \tag{10.7}$$

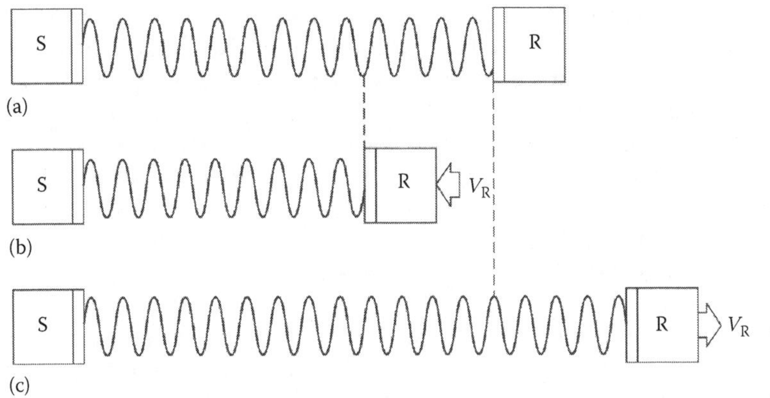

FIGURE 10.13 Doppler effect caused by a moving receiver. (From Atkinson, P. and Woodcock, J., *Doppler Ultrasound and Its Use in Clinical Measurement*, Academic Press, London, U.K., 1982.)

Since the number of wave peaks in a given time interval, Δt, would be equal to the corresponding frequency times Δt and the additional peaks would be the distance traveled divided by the wavelength, λ,

$$f_r(\Delta t) = f_s(\Delta t) + \frac{V_r(\Delta t)}{\lambda_s} \tag{10.8}$$

Therefore,

$$f_r = f_s + \frac{V_r}{\lambda_s} \tag{10.9}$$

Rewriting the wavelength, λ_s, in terms of its frequency, f_s, and the speed of sound in the medium, c (=1540 m/s for water and 1560 m/s for blood)

$$\lambda_s = \frac{c}{f_s} \tag{10.10}$$

we can now solve for the frequency difference, f_d,

$$f_d = f_r - f_s = \frac{V_r}{\lambda_s} = \left(\frac{V_r}{c}\right) f_s \tag{10.11}$$

The same analysis can be carried out for the case of a moving *source*, yielding

$$f_d = \left(\frac{V}{c}\right) f_s \tag{10.12}$$

Both of these equations show that the amount of frequency shift caused by the motion between the source and receiver is directly proportional to the relative velocity between them.

In practice, most fluid velocity measurements are made using a sound wave that is transmitted to an object and then echoed back to the source where it is received. Examples of this would be a particle reflector in the fluid medium (*in vitro*) or a red blood cell in the blood (*in vivo*). In this configuration, the frequency shift, Δf, becomes

$$\Delta f = \frac{2Vf_s}{c} \tag{10.13}$$

Finally, ultrasound Doppler transducers are usually not placed directly in the flow stream in order to either avoid disturbing the flow (*in vitro*) or become invasive to the body (*in vivo*). Thus, they are generally positioned *outside* the vessel and directed at an angle, θ, to the flow axis. In this case, the velocity detected represents only a *component* of its axial magnitude and, thus, a modified Doppler shift equation is used:

$$\Delta f = \frac{2Vf_s}{c} \cos\theta \tag{10.14}$$

To obtain the axial flow velocity, the Doppler shift equation is simply rewritten in terms of V:

$$V = \frac{\Delta f}{f_s} \frac{c}{2\cos\theta} \tag{10.15}$$

or

$$\frac{V}{c} = \frac{\Delta f}{f_s 2\cos\theta} \tag{10.16}$$

In this last expression, we can see the direct proportionality between the ratio of reflector velocity to sound wave speed and the ratio of frequency shift to source frequency. Also note in Equation 10.14 that a forward velocity will produce an upshifted frequency while a reverse velocity will produce a downshifted frequency—thus, the device has *directional* capability.

In order to obtain the flow velocity from the Doppler shift waveform, the received signal must be processed for its frequency content and, in particular, for the frequency shift information. This outcome is accomplished in three steps. The first step, called *phase quadrature demodulation* (Figure 10.14), extracts the frequency

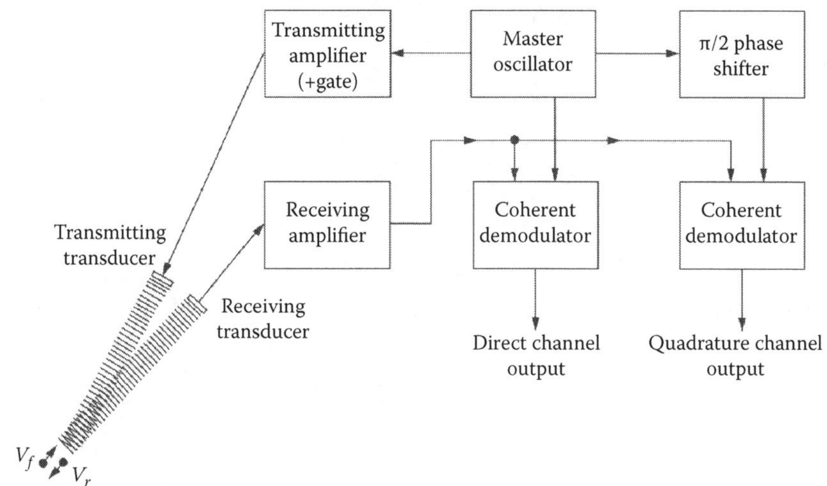

FIGURE 10.14 Phase quadrature demodulation. (From Atkinson, P. and Woodcock, J., *Doppler Ultrasound and Its Use in Clinical Measurement*, Academic Press, London, U.K., 1982.)

shift of the received signal from the frequency of the transmitted signal by mixing the two together. This process produces a combination of signals at both summed and differenced frequencies. Those that are summed are all in the range of f_s while those that are differenced are in the range of Δf. By running all signals through a low-pass filter (e.g., one with a cutoff frequency $\geq 2\Delta f$), only those signals with Doppler-shifted frequencies will remain. The second step, called *phase domain demodulation* (Figure 10.15b), separates out those signals that were upshifted in frequency

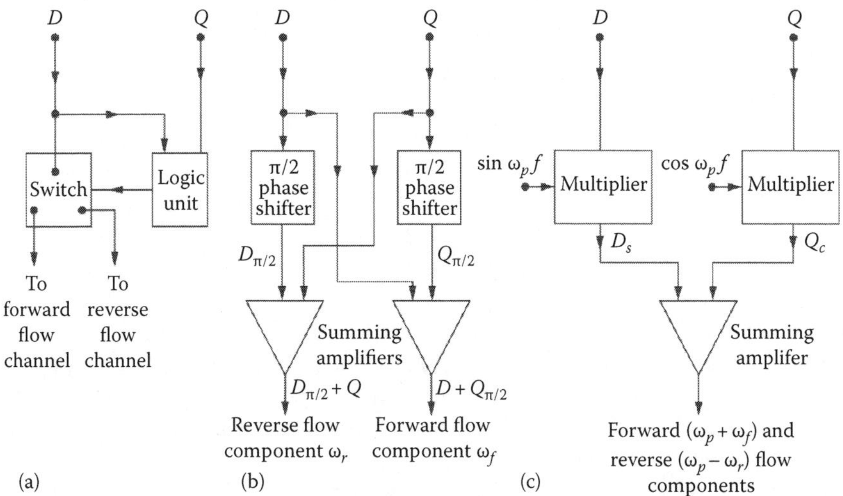

FIGURE 10.15 Directional processing in (a) the time domain, (b) the phase domain, and (c) the frequency domain. (From Atkinson, P. and Woodcock, J., *Doppler Ultrasound and Its Use in Clinical Measurement*, Academic Press, London, U.K., 1982.)

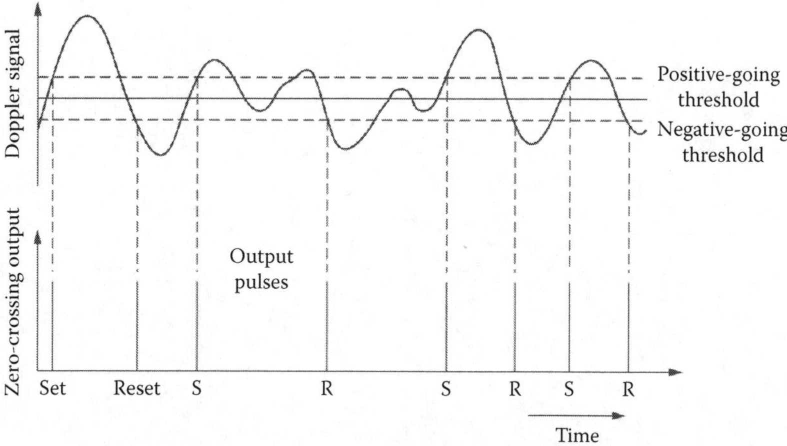

FIGURE 10.16 SET-RESET zero-crossing counter. (From Atkinson, P. and Woodcock, J., *Doppler Ultrasound and Its Use in Clinical Measurement*, Academic Press, London, U.K., 1982.)

(i.e., forward velocity) from those that were downshifted in frequency (i.e., reverse velocity). The final step involves actually quantifying the frequencies of those analog signals. This can be done using one of two common signal processing methods—either zero-crossing detection (ZCD) or Fourier transformation.

ZCD or *zero-crossing counting* (ZCC) simply counts the number of times an oscillatory signal crosses the zero baseline (Figure 10.16). Thus, a signal with high frequency has a larger count than a signal with low frequency over a fixed period of time. This is a simple and inexpensive approach that can be built into any ultrasound Doppler device. However, it does not give a true mean frequency as its output is actually proportional to the RMS value of the signal. An alternate approach to the *ZCD/ZCC* is to perform a *fast Fourier transformation* (FFT) on the signal (Figure 10.17). This process converts the signal from a *time domain* to a *frequency*

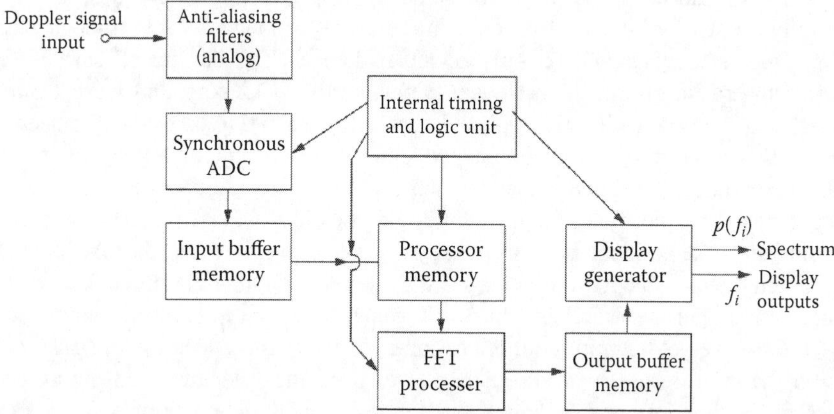

FIGURE 10.17 The FFT analyzer. (From Atkinson, P. and Woodcock, J., *Doppler Ultrasound and Its Use in Clinical Measurement*, Academic Press, London, U.K., 1982.)

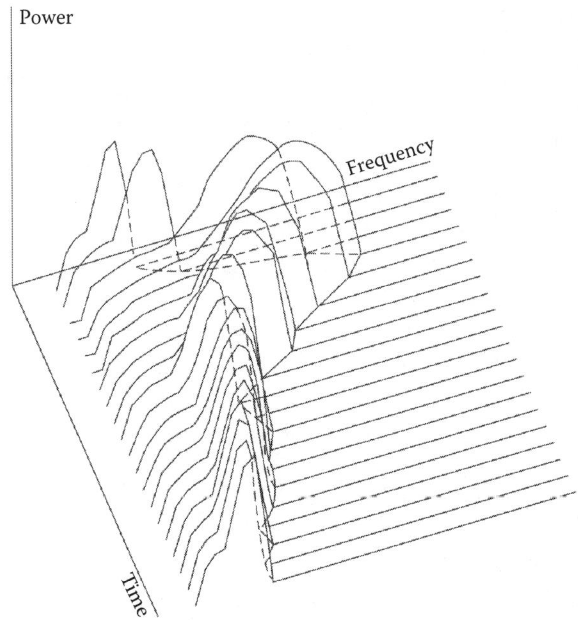

FIGURE 10.18 3D plot of time-variable spectrum. (From Hatle, L. and Angelson, B., *Doppler Ultrasound in Cardiology: Physical Principles and Clinical Applications*, Lea & Febiger, Philadelphia, PA, 1985.)

domain representation in terms of its *harmonics*. By doing this, the relative magnitude of each harmonic is determined and a resultant spectrum of frequencies can be obtained (Figure 10.18). The result is that the frequency shift (α particle velocity) and the power of the signal (α number of particle reflectors present) can be obtained over time.

While all ultrasound Doppler velocimeters are based on the same fundamental principles and utilize virtually the same signal processing techniques, they are typically constructed in two different configurations or modes: (1) continuous wave (CW) Doppler devices and (2) pulse Doppler devices. *CW* devices (Figure 10.19) operate by transmitting a high-frequency (generally >1 MHz) sound wave from a crystal and then collecting the returned echo from a moving object with a second crystal. Since the crystals operate independently, each one either continuously transmits or continuously receives signals which are then compared with determining the instantaneous frequency shifts and, thus, velocities of the target objects. Since the transmit and receive sound beams virtually overlap with each other, the CW Doppler is characterized by having a relatively large *sample volume*—that is, region within which motion can be detected. Thus, it is generally easy to obtain a clear recording from the vessel but with no information as to the specific location of that signal within the entire cross section. Furthermore, since the velocities from many particles are being detected simultaneously, the resultant signal contains a wide range or *spectrum* of shifted frequencies. Thus, in practice, the signal is usually averaged or processed by simply identifying the maximum velocity for use.

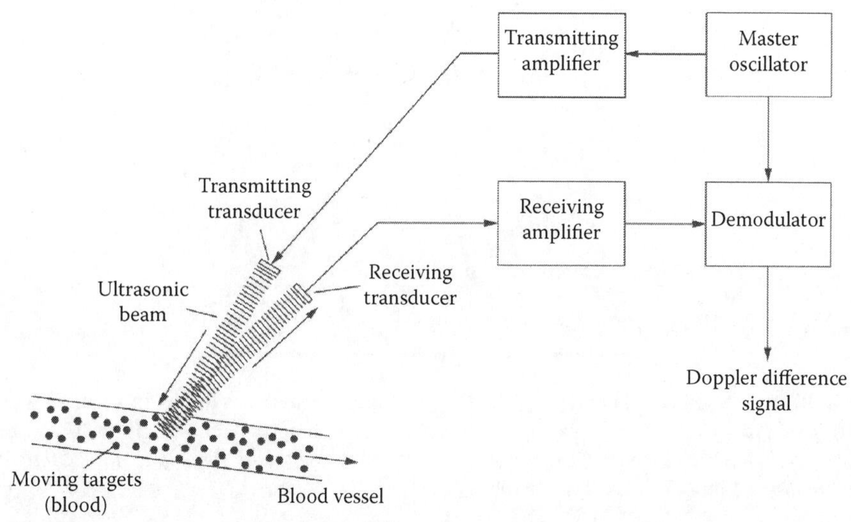

FIGURE 10.19 The continuous wave flow meter. (From Atkinson, P. and Woodcock, J., *Doppler Ultrasound and Its Use in Clinical Measurement*, Academic Press, London, U.K., 1982.)

These recordings have proven valuable, especially for clinical diagnostic purposes, because of the ability of ultrasound to readily penetrate soft tissues. We have mentioned earlier (Section 5.3), how important pressure measurements may be indirectly obtained through the use of blood flow velocity measurements. In valvular stenosis, for example, an obstruction to blood flow is provided by a valve that does not open to its full extent. Such an obstruction results in an elevated pressure gradient across the valve, thereby placing additional pumping requirements on the heart which can result in hypertrophy. Since the systemic pressure is essentially independent of valvular disorders, the elevated pressure is reflected mainly in the proximal chamber (such as the left ventricle in aortic stenosis) and can lead to regurgitation in associated valves (such as the mitral valve). Therefore, it is the pressure gradient across the valve which best characterizes the severity of the lesion. Traditionally, this gradient was measured invasively by catheterization techniques. However, since conservation of energy requirements state that the pressure drop (or loss of potential energy) is accompanied by an increase in velocity (or kinetic energy), elevated velocities can be used to calculate decreased pressures. The physiological impact of the stenosis is most accurately assessed by the maximum pressure drop or the maximum velocity. Since this maximum velocity may occur at the level of the leaflets or distal to them—if a significant *vena contracta* exists—a technique with which maximum velocity could be obtained regardless of its location along the entire path of blood would be the most effective in obtaining this clinically relevant quantity.

CW Doppler fits such specifications perfectly. Due to the continuous emission/reception of signals, the locations of the velocity measurements cannot be defined due to lack of spatial resolution. Therefore, for a given CW spectrum, velocities present within the entire range of the ultrasound beam are displayed. Consequently, by reading the peak signal displayed at a given temporal location on the spectrum,

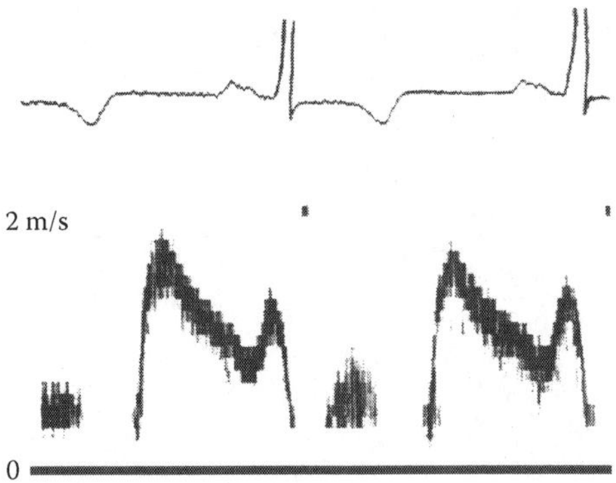

FIGURE 10.20 Spectral analysis of the Doppler signal from the mitral jet in a patient with mitral stenosis. Continuous wave spectrum of patient with aortic stenosis. (From Hatle, L. and Angelson, B., *Doppler Ultrasound in Cardiology: Physical Principles and Clinical Applications*, Lea & Febiger, Philadelphia, PA, 1985.)

one automatically obtains the *maximum velocity*, regardless of where it occurs along the ultrasound beam. Clinically, then, if the CW beam is passed down the ascending aorta and through the barrel of the stenotic aortic valve, for example, the maximum systolic velocity is immediately obtained and can be converted to the maximum pressure gradient by the use of Equation 1.54. Figure 10.20 shows a CW Doppler spectrum of a patient with aortic stenosis and a peak aortic ejection velocity of 2 m/s. The velocity can then be converted into a pressure gradient of 16 mmHg via the simplified Bernoulli equation to provide an estimate of the severity of the stenosis. Traditionally, such a pressure gradient would have been measured painstakingly by catheterization.

Techniques developed to replace catheterization in the assessment of stenosis using CW Doppler have been quite successful over the past decade. The only limitation to such a modality is the lack of range resolution which is actually an advantage for the assessment of valvular stenosis, and because of the continuous nature of ultrasound emission in this modality, there is no maximum velocity limit.

The *pulse Doppler* (Figure 10.21), on the other hand, uses only a single crystal, which transmits a signal for a brief time (i.e., a "burst") and then pauses to listen for returning echos from previous transmissions. In this way, the device can not only acquire the frequency shift (i.e., velocity) information but it can also determine the location of the moving reflector by recording the time required for the sound waves to travel out and back from the reflector. This capability is known as *range resolution* and is very useful when it is important to be able to detect velocities at specific locations. The resolution of the measurement along the beam axis is dependent upon the length of the signal burst sent out (Figure 10.22). Typically, the number of cycles transmitted in a pulse Doppler burst, n, is of the order of 4–6 so that there is sufficient information in the echo for Doppler shift frequencies to be detected. Thus, the sample volume length along the beam axis and the device resolution is $n\lambda$. Consequently, high spatial revolution is achieved by using a high-frequency system. Situations where this feature is useful would be in obtaining a

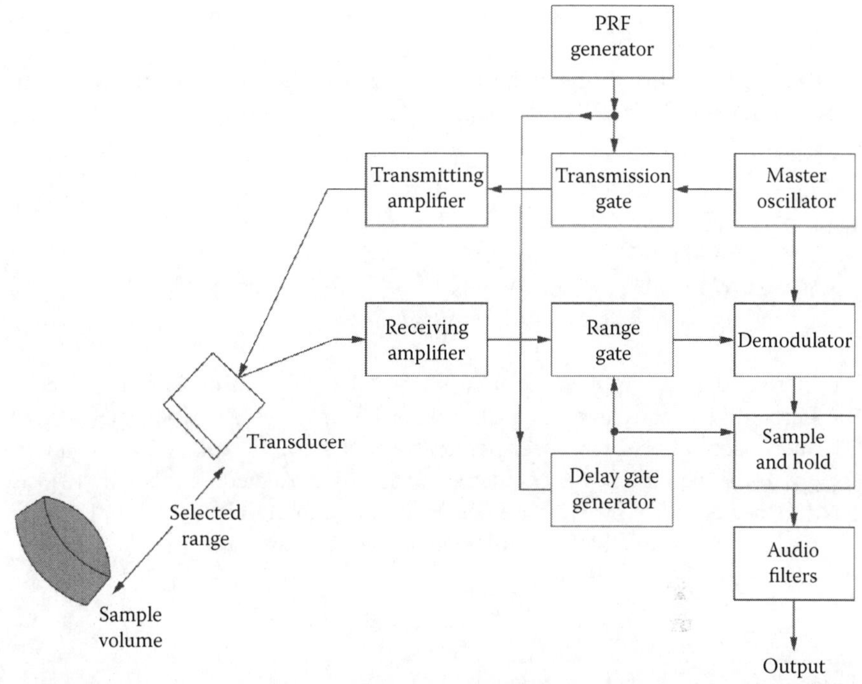

FIGURE 10.21 Pulse Doppler layout. (From Atkinson, P. and Woodcock, J., *Doppler Ultrasound and Its Use in Clinical Measurement*, Academic Press, London, U.K., 1982.)

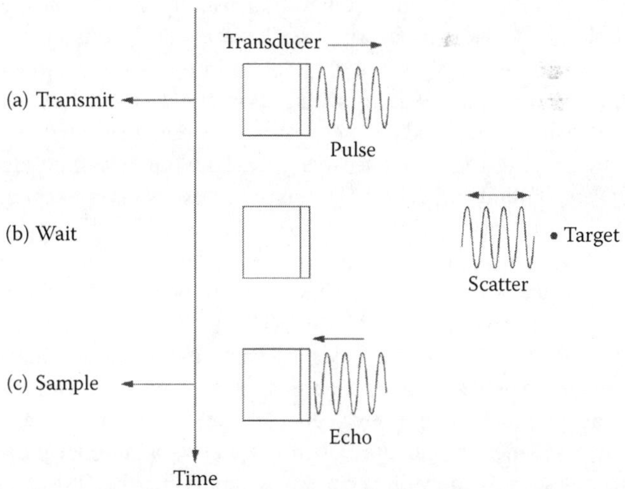

FIGURE 10.22 Pulse Doppler basic principles. (a) Transmit, (b) wait, (c) sample. (From Atkinson, P. and Woodcock, J., *Doppler Ultrasound and Its Use in Clinical Measurement*, Academic Press, London, U.K., 1982.)

velocity profile across an artery or in determining the maximum blood velocity through a stenosed heart valve.

As mentioned earlier, the relationship used to convert Doppler velocities to stenotic pressure gradients is generally the *simplified Bernoulli equation*:

$$p_1 - p_2 = 4V_2^2 \tag{1.65}$$

where

p_1 and p_2 are in mmHg
V_2 is the CW maximal velocity in m/s
The constant term, 4, has units of (mmHg/(m/s)^2)

To derive such a simplified equation, three deletions were made from the complete Bernoulli (energy balance) equation 1.62. The first two, the absence of acceleration and viscous effects, have been demonstrated to be valid omissions both *in vitro* and *in vivo* for the obstructive geometries generally presented in valvular stenosis. The third, neglecting of proximal velocities, is not always clinically valid. If such an assumption is *not* made, the Bernoulli equation appears as

$$p_1 - p_2 = \frac{1}{2}\rho\left(V_2^2 - V_1^2\right) \tag{1.63}$$

where

V_2 is the maximal distal velocity
V_1 is the proximal velocity

The distance between points 1 and 2 is the distance over which the pressure drop occurs.

Since the distal velocity V_2 in a stenotic jet usually significantly exceeds any proximal velocity (and this is especially true for the values squared), the proximal velocity is neglected to enable ease of application in the form of Equation 8.1 with CW Doppler. However, in some cases such as combined valvular insufficiency and stenosis for the same valve, blood cell velocities are already elevated beyond normal at a location proximal to the stenotic valve. These situations can be identified with 2D echocardiography and in such cases, measurement of the proximal velocity is necessary using pulse Doppler techniques to correct, in effect, Equation 1.55.

Another useful *in vivo* application of pulse Doppler velocimetry is in determining the *velocity profile* across a vessel. This can be important in evaluating complex flow patterns such as exist in the aortic arch (Figure 10.23), branches, and bifurcations and in key arteries such as the coronaries and carotids (see Section 6.6). It is also helpful in pathological situations such as arterial stenoses and aneurysms where the flow patterns are greatly altered by sudden changes in geometry. Once a velocity profile is obtained (either in real time or in the mean), additional parameters may be derived from it such as the wall shear stress (including the OSI and shear stress gradients) and also local residence times.

While range resolution is a valuable feature, the act of pulsing the transmitted signal imposes certain limitations on the operation of the system. First, the maximum

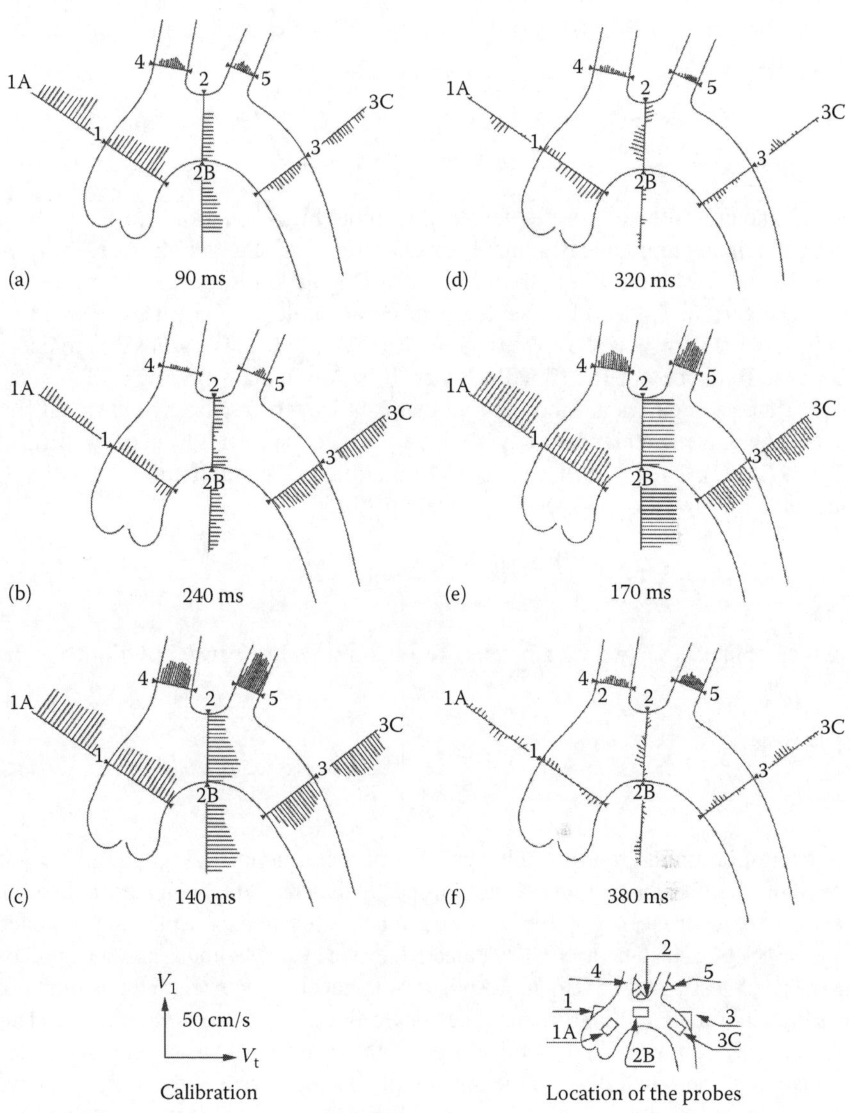

FIGURE 10.23 Velocity profiles in the aorta of a dog using ultrasound Doppler velocity measurement technique: (a) 90 ms, (b) 240 ms, (c) 140 ms, (d) 320 ms, (e) 170 ms, and (f) 380 ms after the opening of the valve. 1A, 2B, and 3C represent profiles in perpendicular planes corresponding to the profiles shown in the plane of the figure. (Redrawn from Farthing, S. and Peronneau, P., *Cardiovasc. Res.*, 13(11), 607, 1979. With permission.)

range of the device is directly restricted by the time period between pulses since the distance traveled to the target is the product $c \cdot \Delta t$. The period between successive transmissions is determined by the instrument's pulse repetition frequency, *PRF*, and can be expressed as 1/PRF (s/cycle). Thus, a pulse Doppler device's maximum range, Z_{max}, becomes

$$Z_{max} = \frac{c(\Delta t)}{2} = \frac{c}{2(PRF)} \tag{10.17}$$

Second, the pulsed nature of the device also limits the amount of information that can be obtained from a measurement since a returning echo is only received once every 1/*PRF* s. Therefore, the frequency of a Doppler-shifted signal, Δf_{max}, must be within certain values in order for it to be accurately determined. Exceeding this limit, also known as the *Nyquist sampling limit*, will cause "*aliasing*" to occur where the frequency of the signal appears to be lower than it really is. Since the Nyquist theory requires a sampling rate that is at least *twice* that of the signal frequency, the pulse Doppler can only accurately collect data with frequency shifts of $\Delta f_{max} < (PRF/2)$. This, in turn, imposes a limitation on the maximum velocity, V_{max}, obtainable through the Doppler shift equation 10.15:

$$V_{max} < \frac{(PRF/2)c}{2(f_s)} \quad \text{for } \theta = 0^\circ \tag{10.18}$$

If we combine these two parameters, we obtain a *range* × *velocity* limit for the device, or

$$Z_{max}(V_{max}) < \left[\frac{c}{2(PRF)}\right]\left[\frac{(PRF)c}{4(f_s)}\right] < \frac{c^2}{8(f_s)} \tag{10.19}$$

It is interesting to observe that although each of these parameters (Z_{max} and V_{max}) is limited by the PRF, their *product* is not. Instead, it depends simply on the wave speed, c, and the source frequency, f_s. Hence, for a given flow location, or depth, only a limited range of velocities can be accurately detected, or vice versa, without producing aliasing (i.e., underestimates of velocity). And, the *only* recourse to extending this limit (for the same fluid medium) is to change the source frequency, f_s, to a *lower* value. This can be done, but it turns out that this impacts other features of the system such as the attenuation of the sound through the medium ($\propto f_s$) and the size of the sample volume [$\propto(1/f_s)$]. As an example, a pulse Doppler velocimeter that transmits a 1 MHz signal through a water-based medium (c = 1540 m/s) will have a "range × velocity" limit of 0.30 m²/s while one operating at 10 MHz would have a product limit of 0.03 m²/s. The implication of this is that at a distance of 10 cm from the transducer, the 1 MHz device could measure velocities up to about 30 cm/s without aliasing while the signal from the 10 MHz device would alias at velocities above 3 cm/s.

In light of these considerations, a decision must be made in practice regarding the trade-off between these two factors. Increasing pulse repetition frequency allows higher velocity measurements, but increases the chance of range ambiguity.

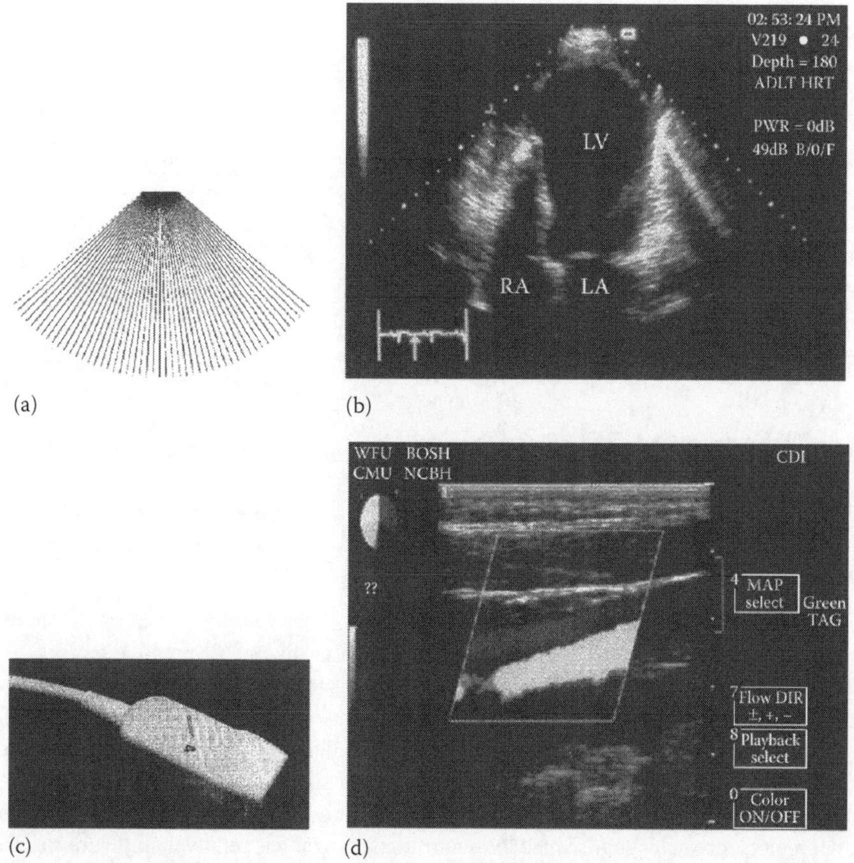

FIGURE 10.24 Linear array transducer. (a) A vector array sends pulses out in different directions from different starting points across the flat surface of the array. (b) A cardiac scan produced by a vector array. (c) A vector array. (d) A phased linear array producing a parallelogram-shaped color Doppler display. (From Kremkau, F.W., *Diagnostic Ultrasound Principles and Instruments*, 6th edn., W.B. Saunders Co., Philadelphia, PA, 2002.)

Decreasing pulse repetition frequency results in the opposite, so the nature of the clinical situation at hand must be examined constantly when making this decision. In general, the normal upper limit of pulsed wave Doppler measurements is around 2 m/s. Using high PRF, velocities of around 4–5 m/s can be obtained.

Newer ultrasound Doppler techniques have greatly expanded the capabilities of a single crystal device by incorporating a large number of crystals into a single array (either linear or annular) which allows detection of velocities at many points in a 2D field of view (Figure 10.24). The resultant device combines velocity detection (Doppler) with an imaging capability (called *brightness* or *B-mode*), thus forming an ultrasound *duplex* system (Figure 10.25) that can provide flow information at known anatomical locations. In order to display all these data, the device displays point velocities in a color-coded presentation where velocity amplitudes vary as intensities and flow directions are typically displayed as reds (toward the transducer) or blues (away from the

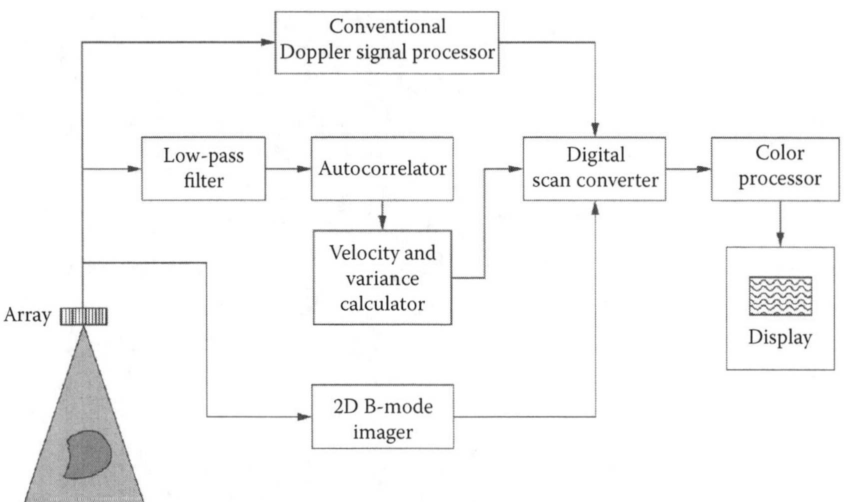

FIGURE 10.25 Schematic of a color Doppler imaging system. (From Shung, K.K., *Principles of Medical Imaging*, Academic Press, Inc., San Diego, CA, 1992.)

transducer). The resultant ultrasound *color Doppler flow mapping* (CDFM) systems are now widely used clinically in many cardiovascular diagnostic applications.

One of the main advances of the CDFM systems is that their transducers have many crystals (from 64 to 128 or 256) arranged along the face of the transducer. Furthermore, by gating the signal, many sample volumes (typically 64) can be arranged along a single line extending perpendicular to the face of the transducer. This line may then be swept laterally or rotationally back and forth at a frequency of 7–30 frames/s to form either a block or sector scan. Since the scanning frequency is relatively high compared with characteristic cardiac cycle frequencies that are on the order of 1 Hz, temporally varying blood flow velocities are displayed throughout the 2D sector in what essentially appears as real time. These velocities are then color-coded (in *RGB* format), usually with red for flow toward the transducer (i.e., upshifted Doppler frequencies) and blue for flow away from the transducer (i.e., downshifted Doppler frequencies) in order to compress all this information into a single display. Within a certain pixel location, increasing image intensity corresponds to a higher velocity in that beam direction. Therefore, a cardiac CDFM image consists of moving white or gray anatomical structures (i.e., B-mode images) on a black background, with superimposed color-coded blood flow (i.e., pulse Doppler)—all imaged in quasi-real time. It should be noted that in addition to these very sophisticated signal processing and display techniques, the CDFM device still offers the capability of single point pulse Doppler measurements by simply tracking the reflected echo from one selected crystal and then gating it to a specific axial location. Using this feature, it is then possible to better interrogate a point of particular interest (e.g., within a cardiac septal defect or stenosed valve, at or downstream of a stenosis, etc.) and obtain accurate, pulsatile waveforms.

In its present state, however, the full, 2D CDFM display provides only semiquantitative velocity information. This occurs because the system utilizes a faster autocorrelation technique in place of direct spectral analysis due to the greatly increased amount of data processing requirements of CDFM compared with conventional Doppler. Also, pulse repetition frequencies are set very low to avoid range ambiguity and to obtain greater depth penetration (Equation 10.16) and, thus, Nyquist velocity limits also become very low. With these low Nyquist velocities, aliasing frequently occurs with physiological flows, especially in high-velocity situations such as mitral regurgitation or aortic stenosis. The concept of aliasing in color flow results, in a "wrap-around" of color to a value, corresponds to flow in the opposite direction. In these cases, multiple aliasing effects have restricted color image quantification to a simple measurement of the color boundary location since quantitative distinction of velocities within the jet is virtually impossible for high-velocity flows.

Another important function of Doppler ultrasound is the clinical determination of severity of heart valve regurgitation. Severe heart valve regurgitation can be fatal if untreated, since it can lead to extreme remodeling of the ventricle and heart failure. It has been observed that the timing of the required surgical treatment can affect the outcome of the treatment. Accurate quantification of valvular regurgitation is important since it can determine the timing of surgery. The gold standard method for quantifying valvular regurgitation flow is the 2D proximal isovelocity surface area (PISA) method, and is recommended by American Society of Echocardiography as the standard tool for such evaluations.

The principle of the PISA technique is based on the fact that a fluid that enters a regurgitant orifice must accelerate to reach a peak velocity at the throat of the orifice. If the orifice is circular, this acceleration region should be axisymmetric about the center of the orifice (Figure 10.26). Thus, upstream of the regurgitant orifice, a series of hemispherical isovelocity contours can be defined within the flow field. For a control volume that does not change in size, the same amount of fluid that enters the volume must exit it as well (see Section 1.4.1). If the control volume is constructed to coincide with a hemispherical contour and the regurgitant orifice, the regurgitation volume (RV) can be expressed as

$$RV = 2\pi r^2 v_{ups} t \tag{10.20}$$

where

v_{ups} is the temporal average of the velocity at a radial distance r upstream of the regurgitant orifice during forward flow

t represents the time during which regurgitation takes place during a single beat

The expression $2\pi r^2$ in this equation represents the surface area of the hemispherical shell surrounding the control volume

The most serious limitation of the PISA technique is its assumption that isovelocity contours around regurgitant orifices are hemispherical in shape. This assumption has been reported to function quite well for estimating regurgitant volume in patients with functional mitral regurgitation from natural valves. However, it is likely invalid for patients with mechanical prostheses. Such valves have several asymmetric regurgitant orifices, some of which are partially surrounded by solid boundaries.

With the advent of 3D echocardiography, researchers have tried to extend the 2D PISA methodology to its 3D version to reduce the errors caused by ultrasound probe

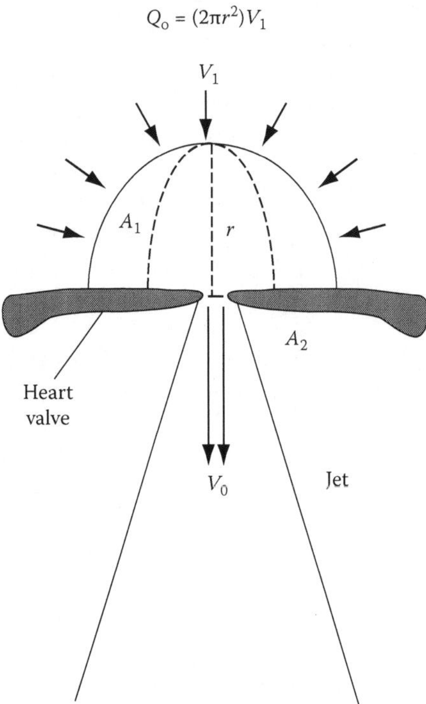

FIGURE 10.26 Illustration of the PISA methodology. In the upstream zone, velocity converges onto the regurgitation hole, resulting in isovelocity surfaces that are approximately hemispherical in shape. The surface area of these hemispherical isovelocity surfaces can be used to quantify the regurgitation flow.

misalignment which are common in the 2D version. Such errors can be reduced by not having to assume a perfectly hemispherical shape for the proximal isovelocity surface. However, Doppler ultrasound can only be used to measure one-component velocities—that is, the component toward/away from the ultrasound probe. Currently proposed 3D PISA methods cannot yet correct for the missing velocity components in order for the measurements to be accurate.

10.7 LASER DOPPLER VELOCIMETRY

Laser Doppler velocimetry (LDV) (also referred to as *laser Doppler anemometry* [LDA]) is a technique used to measure fluid velocity accurately by detecting the Doppler frequency shift of laser light that has been scattered by small particles moving within the fluid. The LDV provides precise velocity data within a small volume element, and by using a traverse system to move the laser probe volume point-by-point, it is possible to perform an area investigation. The technique is *noninvasive* since only light is used as the measuring tool. Furthermore, it can reach difficult measurement locations without disturbing the flow. LDV offers a wide flexibility and is used in many applications such as transonic and supersonic flows, boundary layers, and flames.

Over the past three decades, LDV systems have been used extensively for *in vitro* biofluid mechanics studies. These studies have been performed under both steady and pulsatile flow conditions to measure 1D, 2D, and 3D flow fields. From these data, it is possible to compute parameters such as velocity fields, turbulent normal stresses, and laminar and turbulent shear stresses. Examples of such studies include (1) measurements in the immediate vicinity of prosthetic heart valves, (2) flow fields in arterial bifurcation geometries, (3) flow fields downstream arterial stenoses, and (4) flow fields in vascular bypass geometries.

10.7.1 General Features

A typical LDV system uses a plasma tube, such as an argon-ion gas laser, to produce the laser beam. This intense laser beam is directed toward a fiber-optic drive unit through a *Bragg cell* that splits the incoming laser into two parallel beams of equal power, but of different frequencies. The Bragg cell adds a frequency shift to one beam of each focal pair, that is, one beam (called the zero-order beam) retains the frequency of the incident beam while the other beam (called the first-order beam) is typically shifted by 40 MHz in frequency. The two beams are then manipulated by dispersion prisms that separate them into individual colors (i.e., wavelength)—for example, green (514.5 nm), blue (488 nm), and violet (476.4 nm) in the case of the argon-ion laser. This process creates two beams for each color, for a total of six beams. Each color pair forms a plane of measurement and the optical arrangement is such that the three color pairs are perpendicular to one another.

Fiber-optic transceiver probes are coupled to the fiber drive, allowing the crossing of the individual color beam pairs to produce an ellipsoidal probe volume. Thus, a two-component measurement entails the crossing of four laser beams while a three-component measurement entails the crossing of six laser beams. Since a single transceiver is required for two-component measurement, a three-component investigation requires the use of two transceivers placed at right angle to each other (Figure 10.27). The *backscattering mode* is commonly used in a

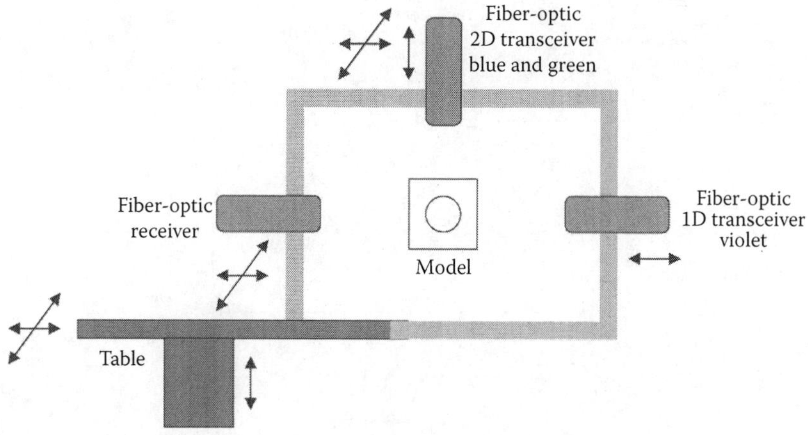

FIGURE 10.27 Transceiver and receiver orientation around flow model.

two-component study where a single optic fiber probe can act as both a transmitter as well as a receiver. An additional receiver is usually required in the *forward* and *side scattering modes* for three-component investigation. The spatial resolution of this technique is determined by the beam width and the angle of the beam intersection.

10.7.2 Probe Volume Specifications

Figure 10.28 shows the intersection of two arbitrary color beams which creates a probe volume with the shape of an ellipsoid. Since the beams are coherent sources, the probe volume is a stable interference pattern characterized by alternating light and dark fringes. In this figure, l_m represents the length dimension of the probe volume, d_m is the diameter dimension, d_f is the fringe spacing, α is the half-angle of the beam intersection, d is the prefocal beam spacing, and f is the beam focal length.

10.7.2.1 Calculation of Probe Volume Dimensions

In the case where the beam pairs intersect in air, α can be calculated from d and f using the following equation:

$$\tan\alpha = \frac{d/2}{f} \quad (10.21)$$

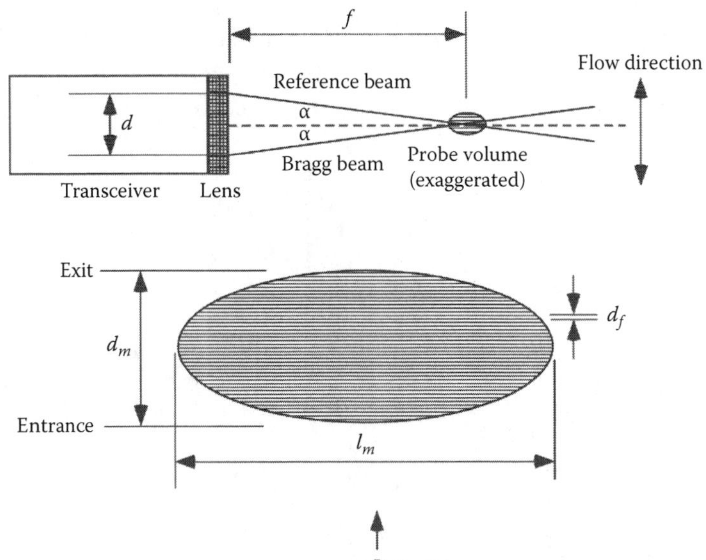

FIGURE 10.28 Probe volume formed by intersection of laser beam pair.

The dimensions of the ellipsoidal probe volume, d_m and l_m, formed by a pair of intersecting beams are given by

$$d_m = \frac{4\lambda f}{\pi D_e E} \tag{10.22}$$

$$l_m = \frac{d_m}{\tan\alpha} \tag{10.23}$$

where

λ is the wavelength of the beam in air
f is the focal length of the transceiver lens
D_e is the original beam diameter
E is the beam expansion ratio

10.7.2.2 Fringe Patterns

Since the beams are coherent sources, the probe volume is a stable interference pattern characterized by alternating light and dark fringes (Figure 10.28). When a particle passes through the probe volume formed by the intersection of all beam pairs, it scatters the light from within the probe volume, generating a signal called a Doppler burst. The time required for a particle to traverse the probe volume, called its gate time, is recorded for each valid particle. In order to measure multiple velocity components of a given particle, the probe volumes formed by each beam pair are aligned so that they intersect at the same spatial location.

Within the destructive fringes (dark fringes) of the probe volume, the light intensity is zero. Within the constructive fringes (bright fringes) of the probe volume, however, the light intensity varies in a Gaussian fashion from the probe volume entrance to the exit. Thus, the signal amplitude modulates as the particle alternately intersects dark and bright fringes. Consequently, when a particle crosses a dark fringe, the intensity is zero, and when it crosses a light fringe, the intensity is high. The output voltage then peaks when the particle crosses the central light fringe of the probe volume where the intensity is the highest. The crossing of the particle through the alternate light and dark fringes gives a characteristic "on-off intensity" Doppler burst as illustrated in Figure 10.29. The variation in light intensity causes a low-intensity background pedestal to be superimposed on the burst. This pedestal is removed during signal processing.

The frequency relationship between a forward scattered light wave and the incident light wave is given by the following vector equation:

$$f_s = f_i + \frac{1}{\lambda}\bar{V}\cdot(j_s - j_i) \tag{10.24}$$

where

f_i is the frequency of incident light
f_s is the frequency of scattered light
j_i is the unit vector in incident direction
j_s is the unit vector in scattering direction
$\bar{V}$ is the velocity vector
λ is the wavelength of incident light

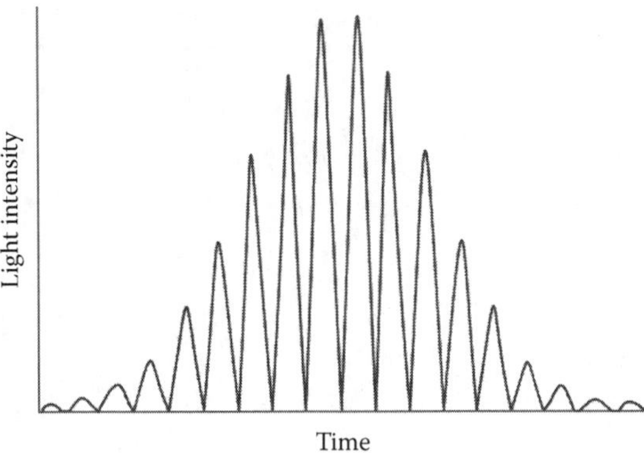

FIGURE 10.29 Schematic of raw Doppler burst.

The Doppler frequency f_d is given by

$$f_d = f_s - f_i \tag{10.25}$$

Therefore,

$$f_d = \frac{1}{\lambda}\overline{V}\cdot(j_s - j_i)$$

The distance between the fringes is fixed by the wavelength of the laser beam and the beam angle between the intersecting beams. The light scattered by the particle passing through the probe volume is modulated with a frequency that is related to the velocity of the particle by the equation:

$$V = f_d\frac{\lambda}{2\sin\alpha} \tag{10.26}$$

where V is the component of local velocity which is normal to the bisector of the beam intersecting angle. Alternately,

$$V = f_d d_f \tag{10.27}$$

and

$$d_f = \frac{\lambda}{2\sin\alpha} \tag{10.28}$$

It can be seen from Equation 10.27 that the Doppler frequency is directly proportional to the velocity. The constant of proportionality is a direct function of the wavelength of the laser and of the optical arrangement of the experiment.

10.7.3 Photodetectors

Particles moving through the measuring volume scatter light of varying intensity. However, the light signals are usually too weak to be analyzed, and, thus, *photomultipliers* (PM) are needed to amplify and convert the input to a voltage output for analysis. A photomultiplier tube consists of a photocathode, a multiplier chain, and an anode. When photons from the scattered laser beam of a passing particle hit a PM tube, they are converted into electrons by means of the photoelectric effect. These electron emissions are amplified and accelerated by a string of successive electron absorbers called dynodes to produce enhanced secondary emission. Finally, the anode at the end of the tube is used to collect the resulting voltage that is large enough to be picked up and analyzed. Some laser systems make use of photodiodes for the signal amplification; however, the main advantage of using photomultiplier tubes over photodiodes is the high gain and low noise levels, which allow the system to operate with a light signal of low intensity. The light signal picked up by the photodetectors contains the Doppler signal as well as the frequency shift from the Bragg cell.

10.7.4 Signal Processing

The optical frequency shift introduced by the Bragg cell causes the fringe pattern in the probe volume to move up on the frequency axis, thereby displacing the zero velocity away from the zero frequency. This frequency shift is necessary in order to discriminate between negative and positive velocities, which might otherwise produce the same detected frequency shift (since frequency cannot be negative). It is also necessary because the Doppler frequency (f_d) of the particle is very small compared with the frequency of the laser beams. For example, the frequency of visible light is on the order of 10^{15} Hz, while the Doppler frequencies can be on the order of 10^6 Hz. Thus, the frequency shift permits the resolution required to process the positive and negative velocity fluctuations that typically occurs in each of the measured directions.

The raw Doppler signal and a superimposed pedestal are created whenever a particle crosses the probe volume. The resultant signal thus consists of (1) the true Doppler frequency of the particle, (2) the 40 MHz Bragg shift, and (3) the frequency of the pedestal. The signal is passed through a preamplifier and through real-time signal analyzers (RSA). In the RSA, a high-pass filter is applied to the signal to remove the low-intensity pedestal. The signal is then down-mixed, a process that removes the 40 MHz shift and leaves the Doppler frequency f_d. After down-mixing, the signal is passed through a low-pass filter, which eliminates high-frequency noise. The down-mixed, filtered Doppler signal appears as illustrated in Figure 10.30.

10.7.5 Phase Window Averaging of LDV Data in Pulsatile Flow

The first step in processing LDV measurements made in simulated cardiac pulsatile flow is to divide the heart cycle into discreet intervals, called phase windows

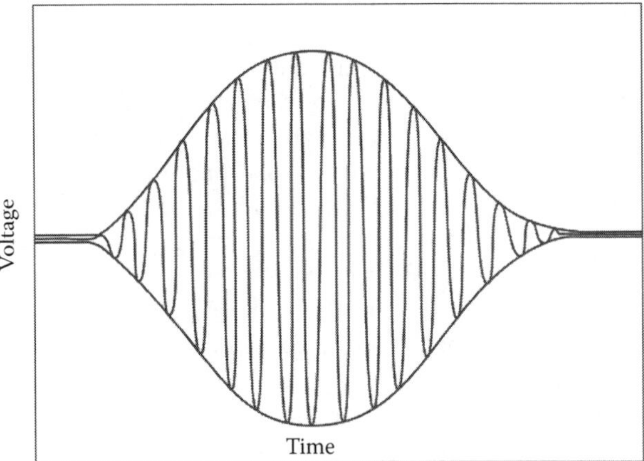

FIGURE 10.30 Down-mixed filtered Doppler signal.

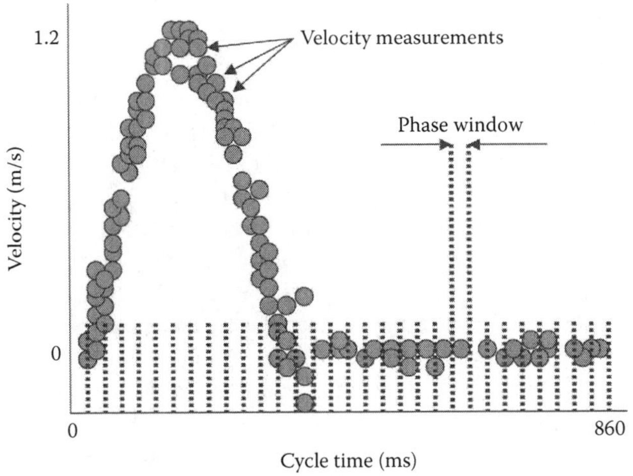

FIGURE 10.31 Phase window averaging.

(Figure 10.31). Within these phase windows, the flow is assumed to be steady, allowing the use of ensemble averaging to describe the statistics of the flow. In choosing the size of the phase windows, there is a trade-off between temporal resolution and statistical accuracy. The choice of a relatively small phase window allows a fine definition of the temporal characteristics of the flow and increases the strength of the steady flow assumption. However, a relatively small phase window also contains a relatively small number of discreet velocity samples for ensemble averaging and limits statistical accuracy. Conversely, choosing a large phase window limits the temporal definition of the flow and decreases the strength of the steady flow assumption but increases statistical accuracy of the velocity measurements.

In typical measurements, velocities are usually phase-averaged within 10–30 ms time windows. The averaging procedure is summarized as follows. The mean and standard deviation of the measurements are calculated as

$$Mean = \frac{\sum_{i=1}^{a}\sum_{j=1}^{n} u_{ij}G_{ij}}{\sum_{i=1}^{a}\sum_{j=1}^{n} G_{ij}} \tag{10.29}$$

$$SD = \sqrt{\frac{\sum_{i=1}^{a}\sum_{j=1}^{n} (u_{ij} - mean)^2 G_{ij}}{\sum_{i=1}^{a}\sum_{j=1}^{n} G_{ij}}} \tag{10.30}$$

where

a represents the total number of cycles during which measurements from a specific location are collected

n represents the number of measurements at that location with a specific combination of cycle number and phase window

G_{ij} is the gate time associated with instantaneous velocity, u_{ij}

10.8 MRI AND VELOCITY MAPPING TECHNIQUES

MRI is a widely used clinical imaging modality that provides high-quality images with detailed anatomical information. Unlike x-ray or echocardiography, MRI uses various properties of tissues submersed in a magnetic field, rather than attenuation or reflection characteristics, to generate a signal. Thus, by making changes to the magnetic field excitation sequence applied to the tissue, the signal characteristics can be manipulated to yield a wide array of information for a given subject. One example is the direct measurement of velocity, such as from blood flow, from the phase shift of the signal.

The main component of an MRI system is the *superconducting magnet*, which produces the strong, static magnetic field. However, it is the systematic perturbation of this static magnetic field with *radiofrequency* (rf) *pulses* about the region of interest that actually produces a usable signal to reconstruct an image. For this, a combination of smaller coils is used to either transmit the perturbations (*gradients*) or receive the signal.

The principles of MRI have been extensively published and, therefore in this chapter, only the main points will be discussed briefly. Consider a nucleus with an odd number of particles (sum of protons and neutrons). Due to its charge and spin, a magnetic field is inherently present. If the nucleus is placed inside a static magnetic field, the vector of the magnetic moment will tend to align parallel (the low-energy state) or antiparallel (the high-energy state) to the vector of the magnetic moment of the applied static magnetic field. However, rather than static alignment, the combination of the external magnetic field and the angular momentum will force the nucleus to a composite motion called precession (Figure 10.32). The frequency of precession,

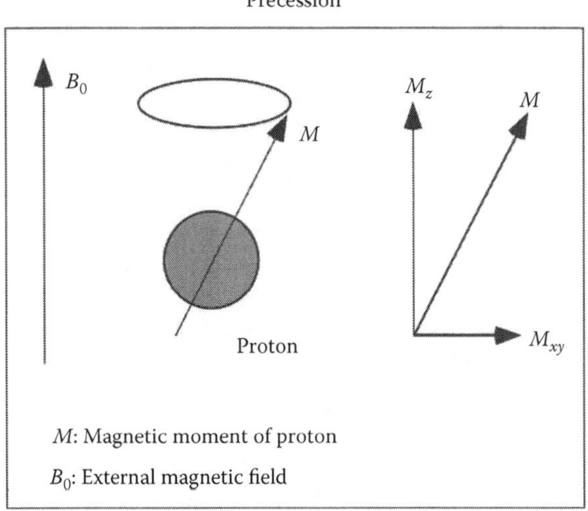

FIGURE 10.32 The combination of the angular momentum and external magnetic field results in a complex motion called precession.

called the *Larmor frequency*, depends on the strength of the magnetic field and on the type of material according to the following equation:

$$\Phi = \gamma B_0 \tag{10.31}$$

where

- Φ is the angular frequency of the precession or Larmor frequency
- γ is the material-specific gyromagnetic ratio ($T^{-1} \cdot s^{-1}$)
- B_0 is the strength of the static magnetic field (T)

Since hydrogen with a single proton in its nucleus is most commonly used as the target atom in clinical MRI, the term "nucleus" will be replaced hereafter by the term "proton."

Of the two possible orientations for the proton's magnetic moment vector, the parallel orientation prevails slightly over the antiparallel. It is this net magnetic moment of the whole mass of protons directed parallel to the magnetic moment of the static magnetic field that is actually responsible for detecting a signal at the end of the acquisition procedure.

An advantage of MRI compared with other imaging techniques is that any region in the body at any orientation can be imaged without limitations related to acoustic windows or to the depth of the region of interest (e.g., in contrast to ultrasound). The sequence of events that manipulate the magnetic field in such a way as to allow for this freedom and flexibility can be broken down into four primary steps. These are (1) slice selection or *excitation*, (2) encoding in the phase and frequency directions or *spatial encoding*, (3) *signal readout*, and (4) *image reconstruction*. The remainder of this section will focus on the details of the first two of these steps, which constitute the bulk of MR sequence design.

10.8.1 Slice Excitation

The first step during the MRI examination is to select and energetically excite the region to be imaged. Since protons within a magnetic field B_0 precess with the Larmor frequency, Φ, they can be energetically excited to move between the parallel and the antiparallel energy states by another field with a frequency equal to f. This excitation is achieved by the application of another magnetic field B_1 that acts very rapidly as a pulse with a frequency in the radio wave band, called "RF pulse." Before the RF pulse is applied, the sum of the vectors of the magnetic moments of all protons in a sample volume is the net magnetization vector M aligned with the static magnetic field along the bore of the scanner. This direction is conventionally referred as the "z-direction." By applying the RF pulse, protons are forced to move between the lower- and higher-energy states. Since the number of protons with a magnetic momentum vector parallel to B_0 is larger than that with antiparallel orientation, the result is a net transition from the lower-energy state to the higher-energy state or an excitation. Therefore, M is "tipped" (i.e., rotated) from the z-axis toward the x-y plane (Figure 10.33). The angle that M is tipped with respect to the z-axis is called "flip angle."

To ensure that a specific thin slice in the body will be excited, the precession frequency of the protons to be imaged can be varied by proper application of magnetic field gradients. These gradients create a spatial variation in the strength of the static magnetic field, $B_0 \pm \Delta B(r)$, where r is the direction of slice selection. Therefore, the Larmor frequency varies depending on the position along the slice selection direction. Upon application of the RF pulse, only those protons within a slice having a Larmor frequency equal to that of the RF pulse will be excited. Therefore, axial resolution is achieved since these are the only protons that will contribute to the resulting image.

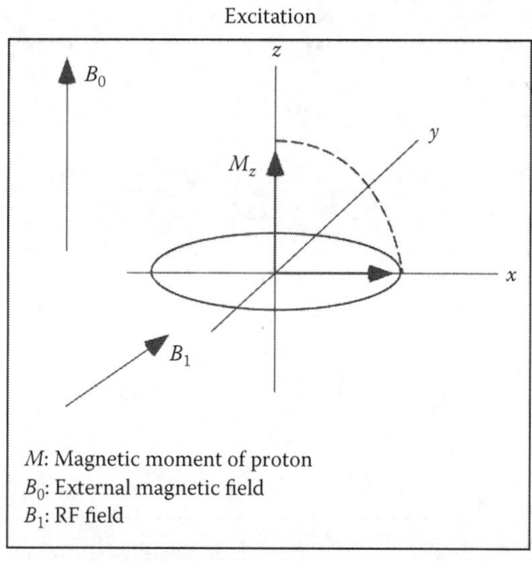

FIGURE 10.33 Proton excitation: By applying an RF pulse, B_1, the magnetization vector is tipped from the z-axis toward the x-y plane.

10.8.2 Spatial Encoding

At the end of the application of the RF pulse, all protons within a thin slice are excited such that the magnetic moment, M, is tipped from the z-direction toward the x-y plane. After the excitation, the protons relax by releasing the excessive energy in the form of a detectable signal through a process called "free induction decay" (FID), as shown schematically in Figure 10.34. If signal readout were the only event to follow slice excitation, the protons would relax by emitting the excessive energy in the form of a signal with a single frequency, since all protons under the same magnetic field resonate with the same Larmor frequency. The reconstructed image would contain no information about structures, function, or flow. Therefore, it is necessary to encode the position of each proton or, in practice, a small group of protons within a volume element (*voxel*) in order to ensure a strong signal. The slice can then be divided into voxels, each of which will correspond to a different resonant frequency; thus, it will be spatially encoded. To achieve such an encoding, the signal information in each voxel must be unique. This is accomplished by applying proper magnetic field gradients in the two planar directions of the slice. One of those directions is used for *phase encoding* and the other for *frequency encoding.*

During the phase-encoding step, the magnetic field gradient is applied solely to differentiate the precession frequency in each row of voxels for a short period of time. At the end of this step, all rows return to the original precessing frequency but now include a small differentiation with respect to the phase of this precession from row to row. After phase encoding, another magnetic field gradient is applied in the frequency-encoding direction. This creates a change in the precession frequency along each row. Since each row already had an identity in space through the

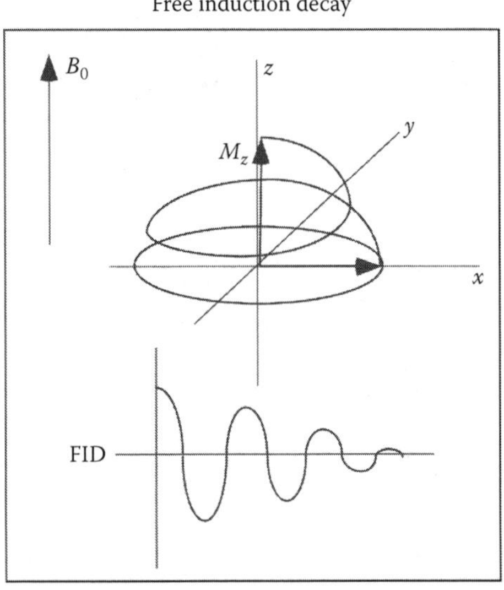

FIGURE 10.34 Free induction decay: After termination of the RF pulse, the excited protons emit their excessive energy while returning to their original condition. The magnetization vector returns to the z-direction alignment. It is during this period that the image data are actually acquired.

differentiation in the phase of precession, the second encoding causes an identification of each separate voxel with a unique frequency and phase. This is also the stage when the signal is read by the receiving coil. This signal fills the frequency *k*-space and through 2D Fourier transform the final image is reconstructed.

10.8.3 Imaging Procedure and Pulse Sequences

To obtain an initial idea about the location of the region of interest, a series of "scout" or "localizer" images is acquired. This is usually a multislice acquisition procedure. In the scout images, it is possible to isolate and observe an organ or a vessel and plan the main acquisitions in the region of specific interest. Depending on the type of information needed, imaging can be performed using a variety of pulse and gradient sequences. Here, we will consider two pulse sequences that may be used: *spin echo* and *gradient echo.*

10.8.3.1 Spin Echo

In this imaging modality, a 90° RF pulse is used to tip the net magnetization vector M by 90°, moving it completely into the X-Y plane (Figure 10.35). Then, FID

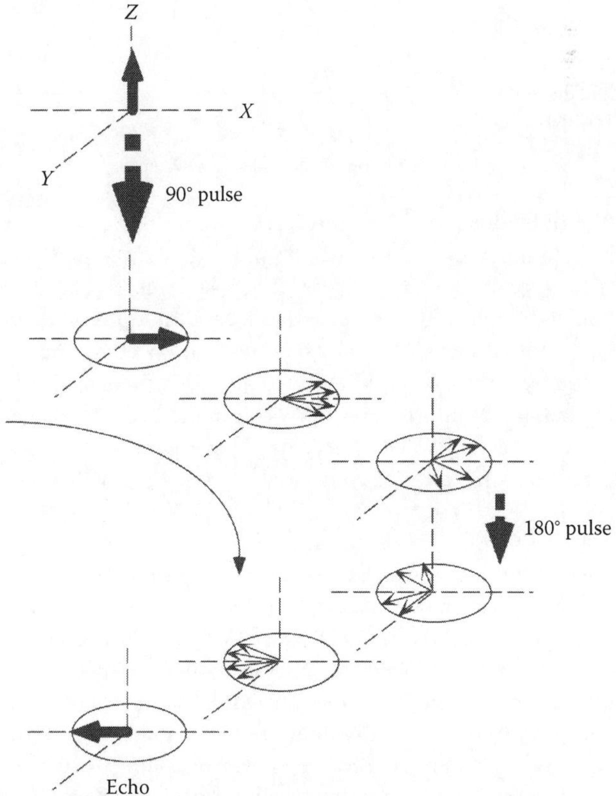

FIGURE 10.35 Spin-echo sequence: Initially, the magnetization vector (bold upward arrow) is tipped 90°. Then, spins start to de-phase until another 180° pulse re-phases them and an echo is generated.

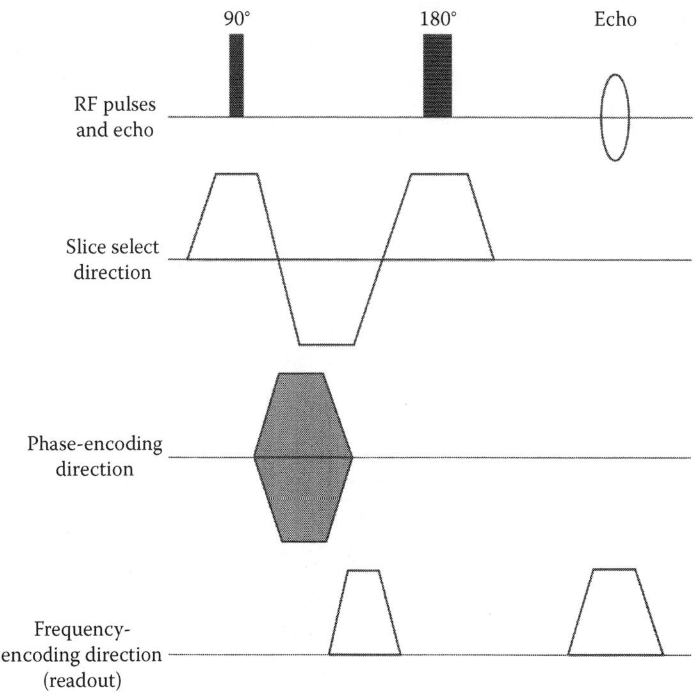

FIGURE 10.36 Diagram of a typical spin-echo pulse sequence.

occurs while the individual spins begin to precess out-of-phase or de-phase due to local magnetic field inhomogeneity. Since de-phasing reduces the amplitude of the received signal, re-phasing of the spins is desirable. This can be achieved by the application of an additional 180° RF pulse that forces the spins to re-phase, producing an echo. The emitted signal is read when this echo occurs. The components of the spin-echo sequence are shown in Figure 10.36. It is widely used clinically, especially to obtain anatomical information anywhere in the body. In the heart, it is used mainly to observe vessel walls that appear bright compared with blood that appear dark (also referred to as *MR angiography*).

10.8.3.2 Gradient Echo

This is the most commonly used pulse sequence for cardiovascular imaging, especially to obtain flow information, either qualitatively or quantitatively. In gradient echo, the RF pulse tips the magnetization vector M to an angle >90°. This provides a faster acquisition procedure, since less time is required for relaxation, which is important for cine cardiac imaging. After excitation, the relaxation process and the de-phasing of the individual spins begin. Application of an additional magnetic field gradient in the frequency-encoding direction causes the de-phasing to accelerate. Then, another gradient of opposite polarity re-phases the spins and an echo is formed and read. The great advantage of the gradient-echo pulse sequence is its speed compared with spin echo, since the flip angle is usually much less than 90°. A cine acquisition throughout a specific time period

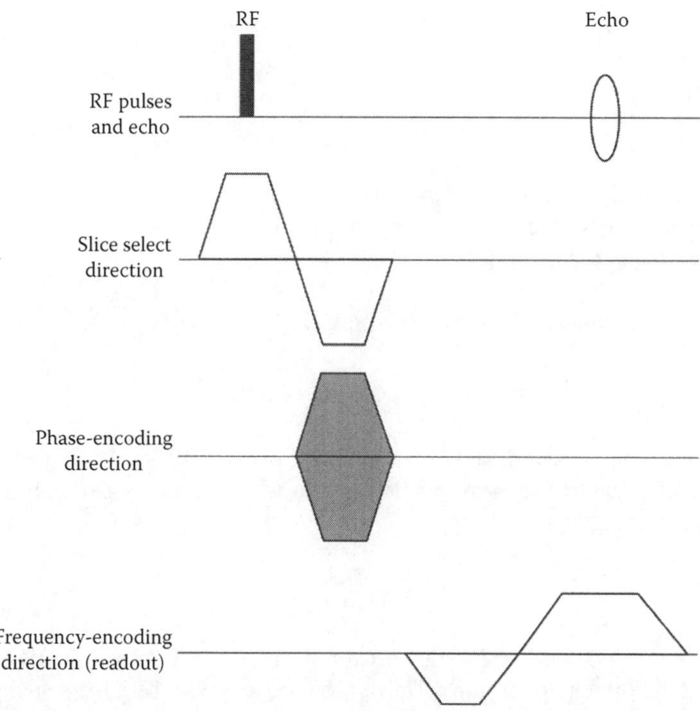

FIGURE 10.37 Diagram of a typical gradient-echo pulse sequence.

can be thus achieved. This is very important when imaging structures which are in motion such as the heart or arteries. The components of the gradient-echo sequence are shown in Figure 10.37.

10.8.4 Phase Contrast MRI

The result from the conventional imaging acquisition and display process is the reconstruction of an image where contrast is based on variations of the magnitude or intensity of the received signal. MRI can also be used to directly measure the velocity of moving protons based on the following principle. When a proton moves along a magnetic field gradient, it acquires a phase shift in its precession proportional to the strength and duration of the magnetic field gradient. This shift is expressed by the following equation:

$$\Phi = \int \gamma G(t)[r(t)]dt \tag{10.32}$$

where

- Φ is the phase of the signal
- γ is the gyromagnetic ratio
- $G(t)$ is the vector of the magnetic field gradient (T/m)
- $r(t)$ is the position vector of the protons (m)

For the case of motion in only a single direction where acceleration and higher-order motion terms are neglected, the position vector is

$$r(t) = Z_0 + u \cdot t \tag{10.33}$$

where

Z_0 is the initial position of the proton (m)
u is the velocity of the proton in the z-direction (m/s)
t is the time of the motion (s)

Combining Equations 10.32 and 10.33 results in

$$\Phi = \int \gamma G_z(t) Z_0 dt + \int \gamma G_z(t) u \cdot t dt \tag{10.34}$$

By applying a bipolar gradient $G_z(t)$, as shown in Figure 10.38, the first term on the right side of Equation 10.34 becomes zero. In addition, if the particle velocity is assumed constant, then

$$\Phi = \gamma u \int G_z(t) t dt \tag{10.35}$$

As seen from Equation 10.35, a linear relationship exists between the phase of the signal and the velocity of protons. Thus, if the phase is obtained, the velocity can be determined by

$$u = \frac{\Phi}{\left[\gamma \int G_z(t) t dt\right]} \tag{10.36}$$

The velocity can be measured in all three Cartesian coordinates in space. By using the bipolar velocity-encoding gradient, in which the total area under the lobes is

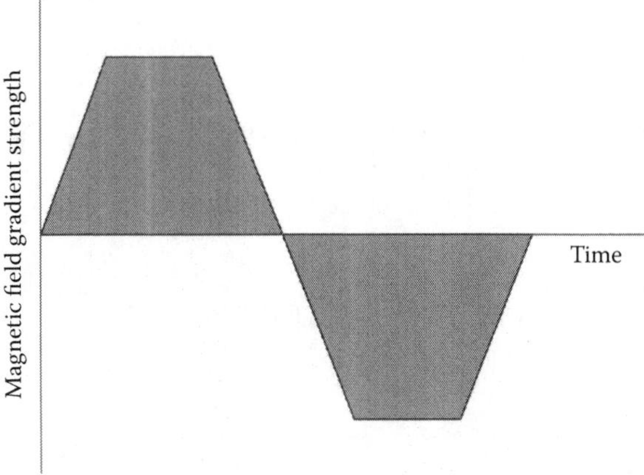

FIGURE 10.38 A schematic of a bipolar gradient, $G_z(t)$: The total area of the two lobes is zero, resulting in a linear relationship between signal phase and proton velocity.

zero, stationary protons will not have any resulting phase, whereas moving protons will. This linear relationship between signal phase and proton velocity is the principle of phase velocity mapping or phase contrast (PC) MRI.

10.8.5 Clinical Applications of PC MRI

This section will highlight a few of the many clinical applications that utilize the strengths of MRI with regard to direct velocity measurement at arbitrary depths and orientations within the body.

10.8.5.1 Flow in the Aorta

The characteristics of flow through the aorta are relevant in many clinical settings, including

- As a surrogate measure of ventricular function and health (by measuring the cardiac output)
- As an indication of aortic valve function in cases of stenosis or other disease
- To understand the hemodynamic implications and risk factors for vascular diseases, such as atherosclerosis, aneurysms, or congenital coarctation

The most basic measurement of aortic flow can be performed using a 2D plane to measure the through-plane velocity in the ascending aorta, just above the aortic valve (Figure 10.39). Using these data, the cardiac output can be derived (by integrating the measured velocity over the vessel cross section), and asymmetries in the velocity profile can be appreciated.

Recent improvements in MRI hardware and sequence design have also allowed for the development of four-dimensional (4D; 3D + time) imaging of velocity gated to the cardiac cycle. As a result, it is now possible to image flow through the entire aorta as a single volume. Figure 10.40 shows an example of such data, visualized using particle streak lines color-coded by local velocity magnitude. Given the complex, 3D nature of aortic flow fields, such techniques allow for the robust visualization of the entire domain of interest with minimal time postprocessing data.

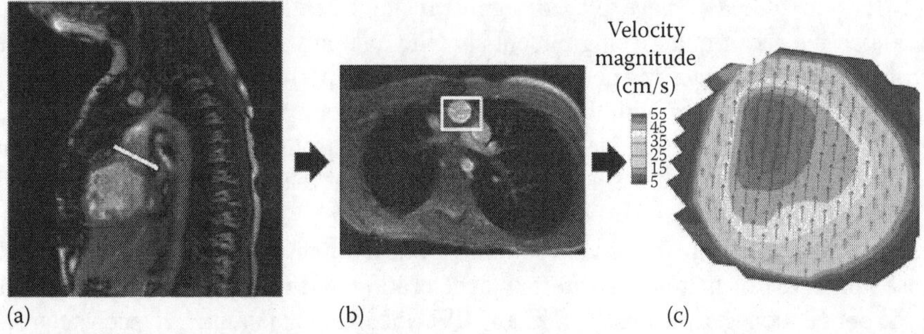

FIGURE 10.39 Sample placement of a 2D phase velocity plane through the ascending aorta as viewed through a sagittal magnitude image (a) and an axial (b) phase velocity image. The (c) panel shows the subsequent velocity contours and vectors derived from this slice from early systole. A slight skew toward the anterior wall is evident.

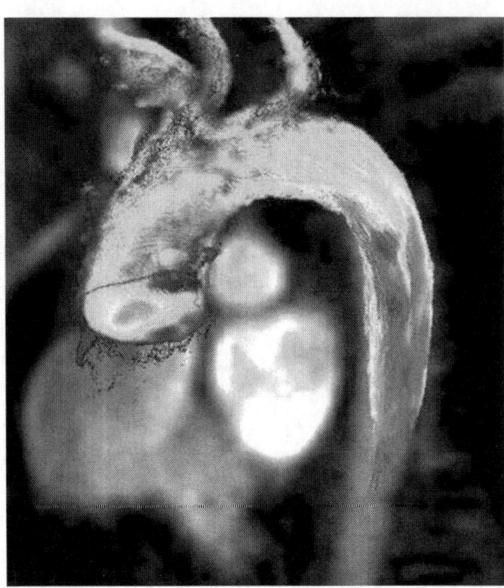

FIGURE 10.40 "Candy-cane" view of 3D velocity streak lines through the aorta during late systole, derived from a 4D velocity acquisition.

10.8.5.2 Single Ventricle Congenital Heart Defects

Single ventricle defects are the most severe form of congenital heart disease and are often surgically corrected by connecting the superior and inferior venae cavae (SVC and IVC, respectively) to the pulmonary arteries to bypass the right side of the heart. An MRI-derived patient-specific reconstruction of such a connection (called the total cavopulmonary connection, TCPC), in relation to the aorta, is shown in Figure 10.41. Having only a single pressure source to power both the systemic and pulmonary circulations places a tremendous burden on the single ventricle, and significant research has been done in an effort to hemodynamically optimize the TCPC.

MRI and PC MRI have played significant and central roles in these efforts, both as a means of quantifying patient-specific anatomy as well as measuring the through-plane flow rates in each vessel to facilitate experimental and computational studies. Furthermore, as with the aorta, the phase velocity plane (or volume) can be repositioned to better visualize the hemodynamics through the connection. As an example, Figure 10.42 shows a coronal perspective of the TCPC (highlighted with border on the left), the corresponding 3D anatomy (top right), and the 3D velocity vectors extracted from that slice (bottom right). Despite the localized presence of noise in the vector field, the local flow acceleration and recirculation at the center of the connection (i.e., where the IVC and SVC meet) are apparent. Yet, such acquisitions are not able to fully capture the whole picture.

Again, technological advancements have progressed to allow for full 4D visualization of *in vivo* TCPC flows. Actual volumetric imaging, as in Figure 10.40, is quickly becoming a clinical standard; however, complex interpolation schemes have

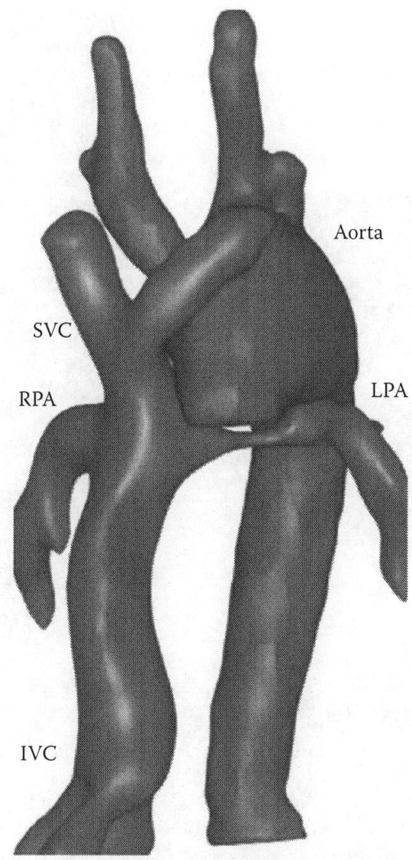

FIGURE 10.41 Patient-specific reconstruction of the total cavopulmonary connection (TCPC—left) relative to the aorta (right), both derived from axial MRI. The TCPC is made up of the connection of the IVC and SVC to the left and right pulmonary arteries (LPA and RPA, respectively).

also been effectively used for such purposes. For example, Figure 10.43 shows two examples of *in vivo* flow fields in patient TCPCs reconstructed from a novel divergence-free interpolation scheme using a stack of coronal 3D phase velocity images. The additional information gained from this 3D approach, compared with the 2D approach shown in Figure 10.42, is clearly evident. The complex interactions can be seen between the superior and inferior flows in the case on the left, and the large vortex in the center of the flow on the right. For the purposes of future connection design or revision, such detail is useful for understanding the inherent coupling between the anatomy of the surgical connection and the resulting hemodynamics.

10.8.5.3 Intraventricular Flows

Understanding the hemodynamics of flow within the ventricles, and, particularly the left ventricle, allows scientists and clinicians to better understand and diagnose pathology states. While echocardiography is traditionally used for many imaging

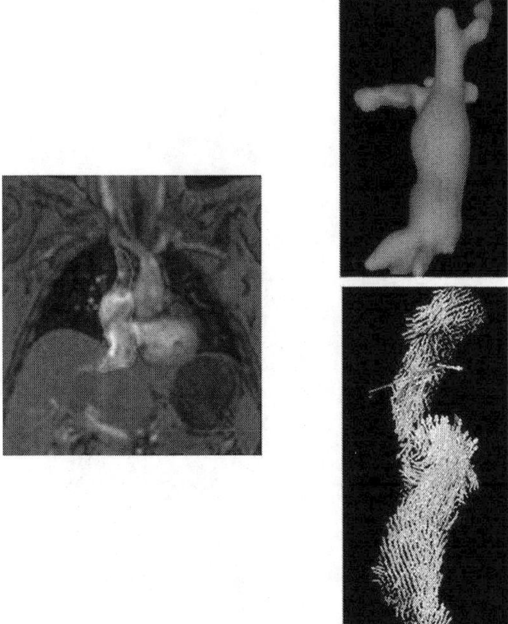

FIGURE 10.42 Coronal view of the TCPC (highlighted with border on left) and the associated anatomical reconstruction (top right) and 3D velocity vector field (bottom right).

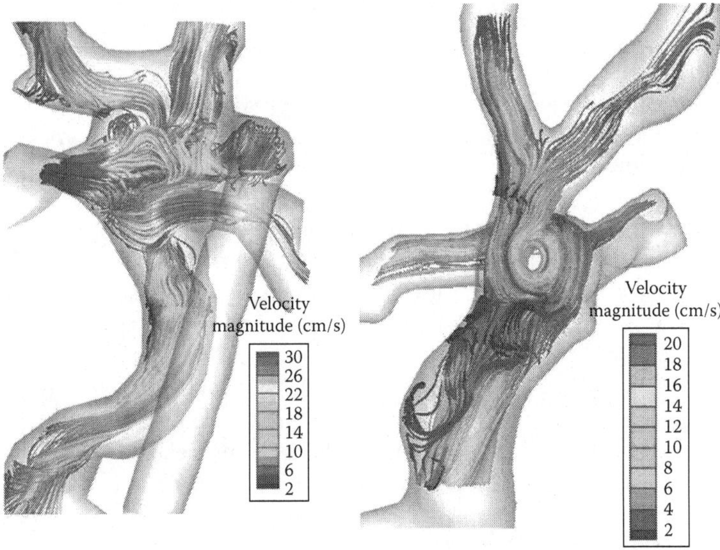

FIGURE 10.43 3D *in vivo* velocity stream traces for two TCPCs. These volumes were interpolated from a coronal stack of 3D phase velocity acquisitions using a novel divergence-free scheme. The depth of information contained in 3D visualization is evident.

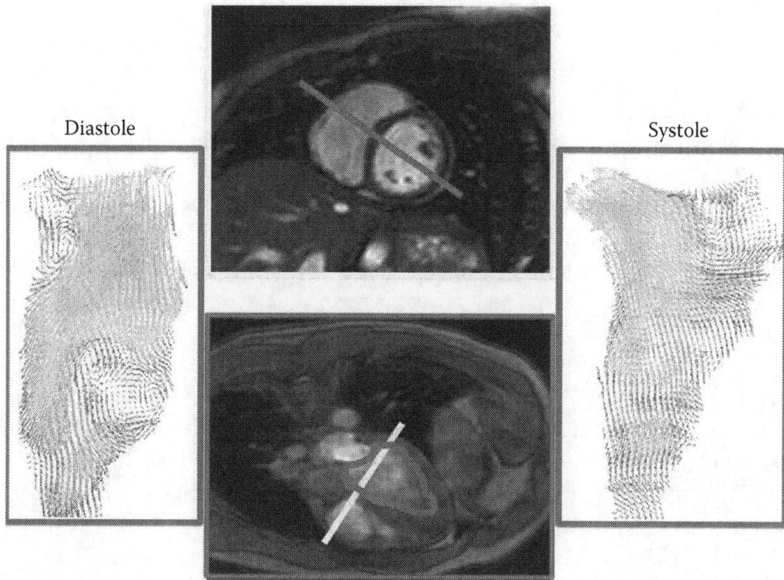

FIGURE 10.44 The center images display various orientations (short axis on top, long axis on the bottom) for viewing the left ventricle. The superposed lines are included to guide the reader in resolving the relations of the planes to each other. The images on either side show the velocity vectors in the long-axis orientation during diastolic (left) and systolic (right) phases of heart contraction.

applications related to the ventricle (see Section 10.6), MRI can also provide a great deal of quantitative information while not being limited by "windows," and easily capturing the entire ventricular volume. Figure 10.44 shows an excellent representation of these features by demonstrating the ability to select from multiple viewing planes to obtain the desired orientation of interest within the ventricle (such as the long-axis cut through the left ventricular outflow tract and mitral valve) and visualize the velocity vectors resolved with the cardiac cycle. Flow disturbances due to localized infarction, transvalvular abnormalities, diastolic dysfunction, or mechanical dysynchrony could all be evaluated in such a fashion. In fact, the advancement of these imaging capabilities is quickly opening up new avenues for research by allowing clinicians and engineers to measure and quantify more physiological characteristics than ever before, thus improving diagnostic and treatment abilities.

PROBLEMS

10.1 For a typical electromagnetic flow probe, the following values are specified: $B = 0.02\,\text{Wb/m}^2$ and ℓ 0.01 m. If the probe has a cross-sectional area of $0.05 \times 10^{-3}\,\text{m}^2$, compute the output voltage for 0.1 L per minute of flow.

10.2 Blood flow is being measured in an 8 mm diameter artery using a transit time flow meter. If the ultrasound beam angle is 45° and the speed of sound in blood is 1560 m/s, what is the resolution of the velocity measurement if the transit time clock is sensitive to intervals of 1×10^{-10} s?

10.3 The sensitivity factor of a typical catheter-tipped pressure transducer is 4 μ V/V/mmHg. If you desire the output voltage to be 40 μV per mmHg of pressure, compute the required excitation voltage to the transducer bridge.

10.4 What percent error occurs in measured velocity compared with the true velocity in a given ultrasound Doppler system when the error in the Doppler angle is 20° versus the true Doppler angle of 0°?

10.5 What are the advantages of measuring blood velocity using an ultrasound Doppler technique as opposed to volume flow measuring techniques?

10.6 What are the Doppler shift conversion factors (in Hz/m/s) for the following cases?

a. $F = 8\,\text{MHz}, \theta = 45°$

b. $F = 8\,\text{MHz}, \theta = 60°$

c. $F = 8\,\text{MHz}, \theta = 72°$

10.7 How would the (range × velocity) limit of a pulse Doppler change if the ultrasound beam were *not* perpendicular to the target but rather at an angle of θ?

10.8 a. What is the *maximum* transmitting frequency, F_0, that should be used to detect aortic velocity if

CO = 5 L/min
HR = 72 bpm
Systole = Diastole/2
Aortic diameter = 2 cm

b. What is the PRF? Is this a *maximum* or a *minimum*?

10.9 Consider phase velocity mapping using a bipolar gradient as shown in Figure 10.38. If the velocity changes due to flow acceleration in systole as

$$u(t) = U_0 + at$$

How will this acceleration affect the

a. Estimate of velocity compared with a constant velocity of U_0?

b. Average velocity during the gradient sequence?

REFERENCES

Atkinson, P. and Woodcock, J. (1982) *Doppler Ultrasound and Its Use in Clinical Measurement*, Academic Press, London, U.K.

Farthing, S. and Peronneau, P. (1979) Flow in the thoracic aorta. *Cardiovasc. Res.* 13(11): 607–620.

Geddes, L. A. (1984) *Cardiovascular Devices and Applications*, Wiley-VCH Verlag GmbH & Co. KGaA, New York.

Griffith, B. P. et al. (2001) *Ann. Thorac. Surg.* 71: S116.

Hatle, L. and Angelson, B. (1985) *Doppler Ultrasound in Cardiology: Physical Principles and Clinical Applications*, Lea & Febiger, Philadelphia, PA.

Kremkau, F. W. (2002) *Diagnostic Ultrasound Principles and Instruments*, 6th edn., W.B. Saunders Co., Philadelphia, PA.

LoGerfo, F. W. et al. (1985) *J. Vasc. Surg.* 2: 263.

Milnor, W. R. (1989) *Hemodynamics*, 2nd edn., Williams & Wilkins, Baltimore, MD.

Poots, K. et al. (1986) *Ann. Biomed. Eng.* 14: 203–218.

Shung, K. K. (1992) *Principles of Medical Imaging*, Academic Press, Inc., San Diego, CA.

11 Computational Fluid Dynamic Analysis of the Human Circulation

11.1 INTRODUCTION

As is evident from the material covered in the earlier chapters, the etiology and the progression of arterial and valvular diseases and the problems associated with cardiovascular implants have generally been linked to the local blood flow mechanics in the vicinity of the region of interest. Hence physicians, basic scientists, and engineers have been interested in characterizing the flow of blood in various regions of interest in the human circulation. One method is to measure the velocity profiles directly in the arterial segments in the human or animal model. Measurements in humans require exposure of the vessels and the introduction of probes for velocity or pressure measurement which is often impractical and involves ethical considerations as well. More recently, noninvasive measurements of velocity profiles have been possible, but data obtained from such measurements also have practical limitations to obtain detailed flow characteristics within the region of interest. Measurements in animal models are also expensive with limited data acquisition due to practical limitations. Additionally, the use of animal models in research and development needs full justification as well. Nonetheless, the data obtained from *in vivo* human subjects or animal models have provided a wealth of information in increasing our knowledge about the physiological blood flow dynamics in various organs of interest and also the alterations in flow with the onset of pathology.

An alternative method to this is to employ benchtop experimental studies where flow analysis in the organ of interest is obtained employing sophisticated velocity measurement techniques. Earlier experiments were restricted to models of regular geometry such as long rigid pipes representing arterial segments in which detailed velocity measurements were obtained both under steady and pulsatile flow conditions. Such studies were followed by advances in obtaining morphologically realistic models for the organs of interest such as the human aorta or the left ventricle in which the detailed flow dynamic measurements were obtained. Numerous studies have also been reported with the use of flexible models that simulate compliant organs. These benchtop experimental studies have complemented *in vivo* studies in providing more detailed results on the complex flow dynamics in the human circulation. Even with sophisticated experimental techniques, there are practical limitations to obtaining detailed measurements in restricted regions such as in the vicinity of the leaflets of the heart valves or in the small diameter vessels such as the coronary arteries. Moreover, sophisticated velocity measurement techniques such as LDV or PIV require optical access and, hence, in most cases are restricted to rigid, transparent models of the arterial segment or the heart chamber. Furthermore, the sophisticated measurement devices require substantial investment that makes these *in vitro* experimental studies relatively expensive.

In the last several decades, engineers, scientists, and mathematicians have been interested in analytical or numerical solutions for the fluid mechanics in the human circulation in order to determine the flow characteristics in detail to relate the fluid mechanics to the etiology of diseased states. Such detailed fluid mechanical analyses also become powerful tools in the design and evaluation of cardiovascular implants as well as in the development of tissue-engineered organ substitutes. The detailed analysis of fluid mechanics in the human circulation requires solving the conservation of mass (continuity equation) and the Navier–Stokes (conservation of momentum) equations. Since the Navier–Stokes equations are highly nonlinear partial differential equations, closed form solutions are available only for a handful of cases with restrictive assumptions (see Section 1.5.3). Typical examples include the Bernoulli equation applied for 1D flow of inviscid fluid and the Poiseuille relationship for 1D steady laminar flow in a tube which have found limited applications in our attempts to describe the flow characteristics in the human circulation (see Chapters 1 and 5). Even the closed form solution obtained for unsteady 1D flow of viscous fluid in a rigid tube (see Section 6.3.1.2) invoked several assumptions that are clearly violated in the flow within the human circulation. Nevertheless, the results from the Womersley solution have also found applications in our understanding of the physiology and pathophysiology in the human circulation. These solutions, however, are limited to regular geometrical flow regimes, which do not describe the complex flow dynamics anticipated in various segments of the human arterial circulation.

An alternative for this dilemma is to resort to pursuing *approximate* solutions employing numerical analysis techniques where such solutions fall under the category of CFD. With the advancement of CFD solution algorithm development and also with the advent of high performance computers, the development of computational simulations for the understanding of the physiology and pathophysiology in the human circulation has experienced rapid advancement. Once a basic simulation is set up and *validated with appropriate experimental data*, the simulation can be extrapolated to various applications with relatively little cost and effort, and hence, it is not surprising that computational simulations are increasingly sought out by the researchers. In this chapter, we will present the basic ideas behind the CFD techniques, discuss the various requirements for obtaining reasonable and realistic solutions for application to the human circulation, and review some of the applications of these techniques that are available in the literature. We will also discuss the possible future directions in order to improve our understanding of the physiology of the normal circulation, fluid dynamic factors in the etiology of circulatory diseases, and in the design and evaluation of cardiovascular implants. Further details on (1) the various imaging modalities employed to acquire images, (2) methods for segmentation and reconstruction of morphologically realistic geometry of the organ of interest, (3) computational details for simulation of blood, biological soft tissue, fluid-structure interaction (FSI) analysis, and the dynamics of the blood elements, and (4) several examples of application of simulations to address cardiovascular diseases are included in Chandran et al. (2011) for interested readers.

11.2 COMPUTATIONAL FLUID DYNAMIC ANALYSIS TECHNIQUES

11.2.1 Governing Equations

A fluid whose shear stress is linearly proportional to the velocity gradient in the direction perpendicular to the plane of shear is considered *Newtonian*. The behavior of such a fluid was described earlier by Equation 1.1. Blood is a fluid that does *not* obey the relation of Equation 1.1 and is thus called *non-Newtonian* because its viscosity changes with the applied shear forces. Consequently, non-Newtonian fluid behavior is extremely complex, and the assumption of a Newtonian fluid is commonly made in order to predict flow dynamics using numerical simulation tools. Another simplification commonly used is to consider the fluid as being incompressible. In this case, the fluid density ρ is assumed to be constant throughout the flow field and over time. Despite the fact that in reality all fluids are compressible to some extent, this idealization holds in most cases.

Again, the equations that govern the motion of Newtonian fluids are called the Navier–Stokes equations given by Equations 1.43a through 1.43c. These equations are derived from the conservation laws of mass, momentum, and energy. The governing equations for an incompressible isothermal flow can be expressed in Cartesian coordinates (from Table 1.1 with the gravitational force terms neglected in the momentum equations) as follows

Continuity equation

$$\frac{\partial u}{\partial x}+\frac{\partial v}{\partial y}+\frac{\partial w}{\partial z}=0 \tag{11.1}$$

Momentum equations

$$\begin{aligned}
\rho\left[\frac{\partial u}{\partial t}+u\frac{\partial u}{\partial x}+v\frac{\partial u}{\partial y}+w\frac{\partial u}{\partial z}\right]&=-\frac{\partial p}{\partial x}+\mu\left[\frac{\partial^2 u}{\partial x^2}+\frac{\partial^2 u}{\partial y^2}+\frac{\partial^2 u}{\partial z^2}\right]\\
\rho\left[\frac{\partial v}{\partial t}+u\frac{\partial v}{\partial x}+v\frac{\partial v}{\partial y}+w\frac{\partial v}{\partial z}\right]&=-\frac{\partial p}{\partial y}+\mu\left[\frac{\partial^2 v}{\partial x^2}+\frac{\partial^2 v}{\partial y^2}+\frac{\partial^2 v}{\partial z^2}\right]\\
\rho\left[\frac{\partial w}{\partial t}+u\frac{\partial w}{\partial x}+v\frac{\partial w}{\partial y}+w\frac{\partial w}{\partial z}\right]&=-\frac{\partial p}{\partial z}+\mu\left[\frac{\partial^2 w}{\partial x^2}+\frac{\partial^2 w}{\partial y^2}+\frac{\partial^2 w}{\partial z^2}\right]
\end{aligned} \tag{11.2}$$

Since the fluid density is assumed constant, the continuity and momentum equations constitute a closed system of equations, that is, there are four equations for the four unknowns—three velocity components and pressure.

To simplify programming and algorithm implementation, the Navier–Stokes equations are commonly written in vector form. To do so, all governing equations are regrouped into a single equation for a vector containing all flow variables (i.e., density, velocity components, pressure, etc.). For instance, the incompressible Newtonian Navier–Stokes equations in vector form are given by

$$\Gamma\frac{\partial Q}{\partial t}+\frac{\partial E}{\partial x}+\frac{\partial F}{\partial y}+\frac{\partial G}{\partial z}-\frac{\partial E_{\upsilon}}{\partial x}-\frac{\partial F_{\upsilon}}{\partial y}-\frac{\partial G_{\upsilon}}{\partial z}=0 \tag{11.3}$$

where

- Γ is a diagonal matrix
- Q is the vector containing the flow variables
- E, F, and G are the convective flux vectors
- E_{υ}, F_{υ}, and G_{υ} are the viscous flux vectors

These terms are specifically defined as

$$\Gamma=\text{diag}(0,1,1,1) \tag{11.4}$$

$$Q=\begin{bmatrix}P\\u\\v\\w\end{bmatrix} \quad\text{and}\quad E=\begin{bmatrix}u\\u^2+\dfrac{P}{\rho}\\uv\\uw\end{bmatrix}$$

$$F=\begin{bmatrix}v\\uv\\v^2+\dfrac{P}{\rho}\\vw\end{bmatrix} \quad\text{and}\quad G=\begin{bmatrix}w\\uw\\vw\\w^2+\dfrac{P}{\rho}\end{bmatrix} \tag{11.5}$$

$$E_{\upsilon}=\begin{bmatrix}0\\\dfrac{\partial u}{\partial x}\\\dfrac{\partial v}{\partial x}\\\dfrac{\partial w}{\partial x}\end{bmatrix},\quad F_{\upsilon}=\begin{bmatrix}0\\\dfrac{\partial u}{\partial y}\\\dfrac{\partial v}{\partial y}\\\dfrac{\partial w}{\partial y}\end{bmatrix},\quad\text{and}\quad G_{\upsilon}=\begin{bmatrix}0\\\dfrac{\partial u}{\partial z}\\\dfrac{\partial v}{\partial z}\\\dfrac{\partial w}{\partial z}\end{bmatrix} \tag{11.6}$$

11.2.2 Grid Generation

Most flow fields in the cardiovascular system involve flows though complex geometries (i.e., blood flow in the heart, flows through heart valves, flow in arteries, etc.). To compute such flows, the geometries have to be described in detail and computational grids have to be generated. This constitutes the first step toward computing the flows and is generally referred to as the *grid generation problem.* This step consists of choosing an appropriate coordinate system that facilitates the description of the geometry under consideration.

For instance, to simulate flow through a straight, circular blood vessel, one choice to generate a grid would be to use a Cartesian coordinate system (Figure 11.1a). However, it is evident that the use of such a system will not guarantee the presence of grid nodes located near the surface of the blood vessel. This will make the enforcement of the physical boundary conditions challenging. For this rather simple problem, a more suitable coordinate system is the cylindrical polar system shown in Figure 11.1b. The coordinate system consists of two coordinate lines: (1) radial lines of constant θ and (2) and circumferential lines of constant r (Figure 11.1b). As shown in the figure, a coordinate line coincides with the body surface. Hence, the boundary conditions can be easily applied to all nodes located along that line. Such a coordinate system is called a *body-fitted coordinate system.*

For complex body shapes, the choice of a body-fitted coordinate system is not always straightforward. For instance, consider the aortic arch geometry depicted in Figure 11.2. The body-fitted coordinates do not resemble any commonly used coordinate systems (i.e., cylindrical, spherical, etc.). Such a system can be described by a *generalized non-orthogonal coordinate system.* With this coordinate system, body-fitted grids can be generated for any geometrical body.

With the use of body-fitted coordinates, flows around and through arbitrarily complex geometries can be treated as easily as flows in simple geometries. This is done by transforming the complex physical domain, defined by the generalized coordinates, into a simple *computational domain.* This computational domain, also called the transformed domain, is essentially an equally spaced Cartesian grid—it is a rectangular domain for 2D problems or a parallelepiped for 3D problems. The transformation from the physical flow domain to the computational domain

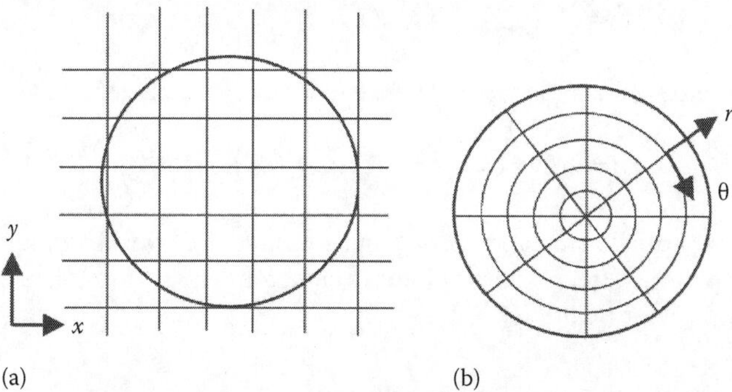

FIGURE 11.1 Grid generation for flow through a model of a straight blood vessel using: (a) Cartesian coordinates and (b) polar coordinates.

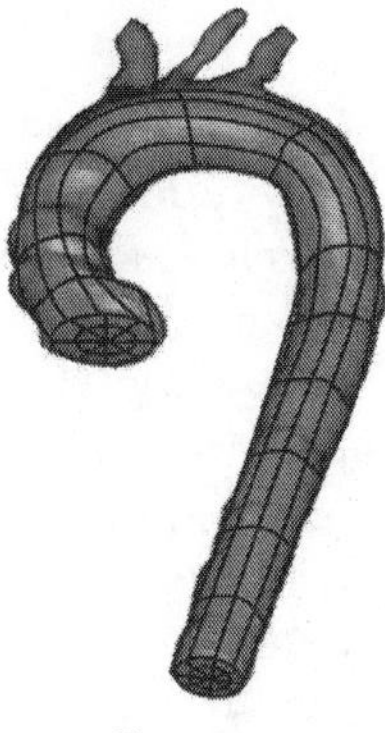

FIGURE 11.2 Generalized coordinate grid for an aortic arch model.

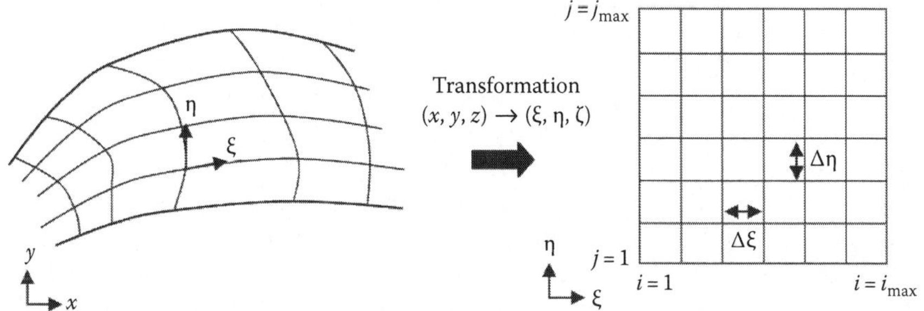

FIGURE 11.3 Transformation from the physical flow domain to the computational domain shown for a 2D coordinate transformation.

is depicted in Figure 11.3. In a 2D case, the physical domain is described using Cartesian coordinates (x, y) and the computational domain using generalized coordinates (ξ, η). The transformation, in general, for the 3D case $(\xi, \eta, \zeta) \rightarrow (x, y, z)$ can be described as

$$\xi = \xi(x, y, z), \quad \eta = \eta(x, y, z), \quad \varsigma = \varsigma(x, y, z) \tag{11.7}$$

and the inverse transformation $(x, y, z) \rightarrow (\xi, \eta, \zeta)$ can also be defined as

$$x = x(\xi, \eta, \varsigma), \quad y = y(\xi, \eta, \varsigma), \quad z = z(\xi, \eta, \varsigma) \tag{11.8}$$

Using these coordinate transformations and formulas for transforming the various differential operators, the 2D Navier–Stokes equations can be formulated in generalized curvilinear coordinates as

$$\frac{1}{J}\Gamma\frac{\partial Q}{\partial t} + \frac{\partial \bar{E}}{\partial \xi} + \frac{\partial \bar{F}}{\partial \eta} - \frac{\partial \overline{E_\upsilon}}{\partial \xi} - \frac{\partial \overline{F_\upsilon}}{\partial \eta} = 0 \tag{11.9}$$

where J is the Jacobean of the geometric transformation defined as

$$J = \det\begin{bmatrix} \xi_x \eta_x \\ \xi_y \eta_y \end{bmatrix} = \xi_x \eta_y - \xi_y \eta_x \tag{11.10}$$

$$\bar{E} = \frac{1}{J}(\xi_x E + \xi_y F), \quad \bar{F} = \frac{1}{J}(\eta_x E + \eta_y F) \tag{11.11}$$

$$\overline{E_\upsilon} = \frac{1}{J}(\xi_x E_\upsilon + \xi_y F_\upsilon), \quad \overline{F_\upsilon} = \frac{1}{J}(\eta_x E_\upsilon + \eta_y F_\upsilon) \tag{11.12}$$

and E, F, E_υ, and F_υ are defined as previously in Equations 11.5 and 11.6. Furthermore, the so-called shape derivatives due to the coordinate transformation appear in the equations in the general form $\xi^i_{x_j} = \partial\xi^i/\partial x_j$ with x_j the jth direction coordinate in the physical domain and ξ^i the ith direction coordinate in the computational domain.

As seen from Equations 11.9 through 11.12, the use of a generalized curvilinear coordinate system simplifies the shape of the computational domain at the expense of complicating the governing equations.

11.2.3 Discretization Techniques

As mentioned in the previous section, the first step in simulating flows is to transform the continuous physical flow domain into a discretized computational domain consisting of a finite number of points, called *nodes*. In the computational domain, a continuous function can then be represented by a set of discrete values at each node and every continuous derivative of such a function can be approximated by algebraic expressions involving only values of the function at the nodes. The second step toward simulating flows is to reduce the continuous governing equations to a system of algebraic equations which represents discrete approximations of the original equations at nodes of the computational domain. This step relies on *spatial discretization techniques*. A successful spatial discretization scheme should (1) have good spatial resolution, (2) ensure accuracy and stability of the numerical algorithm, and (3) be simple to implement. The accuracy of these discretization techniques depend on two main criteria: (1) the size of the grid spacing (which defines how well the discretized domain approximates the continuous domain) and (2) the order of accuracy of the discretization formulas used to approximate the function derivatives (which corresponds to the rate at which discretization-related errors approach zero as the grid spacing tends to zero). Several discretization methods have been developed for computational fluid dynamic simulations including the *finite difference*, *finite volume*, and *finite element* methods. We will illustrate the discretization technique employing the *finite difference* method later.

The general concept of the finite difference method is simple and based on the calculus definition of the derivative. Consider the first-order derivative of the function $u = u(x)$. By definition, this derivative is

$$\frac{\partial u}{\partial x} = \lim_{\Delta x \to 0} \frac{u(x+\Delta x) - u(x)}{\Delta x} \tag{11.13}$$

Assuming Δx to be small but finite, the derivative can be approximated by

$$\frac{\partial u}{\partial x} \approx \frac{u(x+\Delta x)-u(x)}{\Delta x} \tag{11.14}$$

and the accuracy of this approximation can be estimated by expanding the function $u(x)$ in a Taylor series as follows:

$$u(x+\Delta x) = u(x) + \Delta x \frac{\partial u}{\partial x} + \frac{\Delta x^2}{2}\frac{\partial^2 u}{\partial x^2} + \frac{\Delta x^3}{6}\frac{\partial^3 u}{\partial x^3} + \frac{\Delta x^4}{24}\frac{\partial^4 u}{\partial x^4} + \cdots \tag{11.15}$$

Substituting Equation 11.15 into Equation 11.14, the first-order derivative can be expressed as

$$\frac{u(x+\Delta x)-u(x)}{\Delta x} = \frac{\partial u}{\partial x} + T \quad \text{with} \quad T = \frac{\Delta x}{2}\frac{\partial^2 u}{\partial x^2} + \frac{\Delta x^2}{6}\frac{\partial^3 u}{\partial x^3} + \frac{\Delta x^3}{24}\frac{\partial^4 u}{\partial x^4} + \cdots \tag{11.16}$$

where T is the *truncation error* of the approximation.

The leading term of the truncation error, T, indicates the *order of accuracy* of the expression. In the present case, the discrete approximation equation is first-order accurate in space. Using the notation ϑ for the order of accuracy, the discretization scheme can be written as

$$\frac{u(x+\Delta x)-u(x)}{\Delta x} = \frac{\partial u}{\partial x} + \vartheta(\Delta x) \tag{11.17}$$

It is important to note that as the grid spacing approaches zero all the terms in the truncation error series approach zero.

Using Taylor series expansions or polynomial fitting, one can derive discrete approximations of any order of accuracy for continuous derivatives. As an example, several discretization schemes for the first-order derivative of the function $u(x)$ using the notation given in Figure 11.4 are listed in Table 11.1.

The finite difference method discretization is relatively simple to implement. Nonetheless, one of the main disadvantages of this method is that the computational grid has to be sufficiently smooth in order to maintain a high order of accuracy on nonuniform meshes. Alternative discretization techniques using finite volume or finite element techniques are also being employed in the CFD simulations.

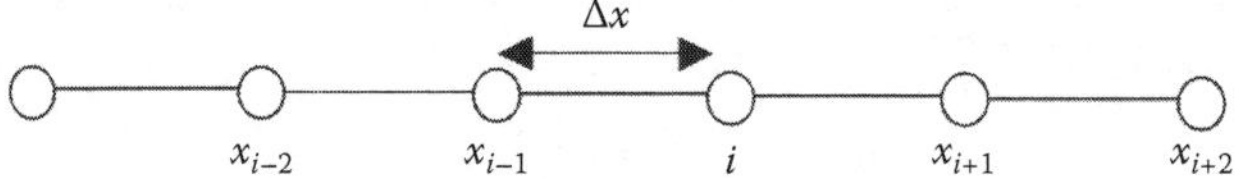

FIGURE 11.4 Discretized domain.

TABLE 11.1
Examples of Discretization Schemes for a First-Order Derivative

Schemes		Formulas
Central second-order accurate formula		$\frac{\partial u}{\partial x} = \frac{u_{i+1} - u_{i-1}}{2\Delta x} + \vartheta(\Delta x^2)$
First-order accurate one-sided formula	Forward	$\frac{\partial u}{\partial x} = \frac{u_{i+1} - u_i}{\Delta x} + \vartheta(\Delta x)$
	Backward	$\frac{\partial u}{\partial x} = \frac{u_i - u_{i-1}}{\Delta x} + \vartheta(\Delta x)$
Second-order one-sided formula	Forward	$\frac{\partial u}{\partial x} = \frac{-3u_i + 4u_{i+1} - u_{i+2}}{2\Delta x} + \vartheta(\Delta x^2)$
	Backward	$\frac{\partial u}{\partial x} = \frac{3u_i - 4u_{i-1} + u_{i-2}}{2\Delta x} + \vartheta(\Delta x^2)$

11.2.4 Temporal Integration

The governing equations of fluid motion contain both spatial and temporal derivatives and similar finite difference schemes are commonly used to discretize the temporal derivatives. The system of governing equations is integrated in time using suitable time-stepping techniques. Several of these time marching techniques have been developed and they can be classified into two main categories: (1) *explicit* and (2) *implicit* methods. The general concept of these two categories can be explained using, for instance, the 1D linear advection-diffusion equation that governs the propagation of waves subjected to dissipation:

$$\frac{\partial u}{\partial t} + c\frac{\partial u}{\partial x} - \upsilon\frac{\partial^2 u}{\partial x^2} = 0 \qquad (11.18)$$

where

c represents the wave speed
υ is the kinematic viscosity

This equation can be discretized in space using finite difference schemes such as

$$\frac{\partial u_i}{\partial t} + c\frac{u_{i+1} - u_{i-1}}{2\Delta x} - \upsilon\frac{u_{i+1} - 2u_i + u_{i-1}}{\Delta x^2} = 0 \qquad (11.19)$$

Using a first-order backward differencing scheme, the equation can also be discretized in time:

$$\frac{u_i^{n+1} - u_i^n}{\Delta t} + c\frac{u_{i+1}^n - u_{i-1}^n}{2\Delta x} - \upsilon\frac{u_{i+1}^n - 2u_i^n + u_{i-1}^n}{\Delta x^2} = 0 \qquad (11.20)$$

where

n denotes the time level
Δt is the time increment

Equation 11.20 can be rewritten as

$$u_i^{n+1} = u_i^n - \Delta t\left(\frac{u_i^{n+1} - u_i^n}{\Delta t} + c\frac{u_{i+1}^n - u_{i-1}^n}{2\Delta x} - \upsilon\frac{u_{i+1}^n - 2u_i^n + u_{i-1}^n}{\Delta x^2}\right) \tag{11.21}$$

It can be seen that if the solution is known at the time level n, the solution at the time level $(n + 1)$ can be simply evaluated using Equation 11.21. Such a method is called *explicit time marching scheme.* However, if one wants to evaluate the spatial derivative at the time level $(n + 1)$, then Equation 11.20 becomes

$$\frac{u_i^{n+1} - u_i^n}{\Delta t} + c\frac{u_{i+1}^{n+1} - u_{i-1}^{n+1}}{2\Delta x} - \upsilon\frac{u_{i+1}^{n+1} - 2u_i^{n+1} + u_{i-1}^{n+1}}{\Delta x^2} = 0 \tag{11.22}$$

It is clear that the solution for u_i^{n+1} cannot be calculated without knowing the solutions of the surrounding nodes (in this case, u_{i+1}^{n+1} and u_{i-1}^{n+1}). This particular time integration scheme, therefore, requires the solution of a coupled set of equations. Such schemes are called *implicit time marching schemes* and several algorithms have been proposed to solve the coupled set of equations. The choice between the explicit and implicit scheme requires considerations of stability of the solution as well as the solver employed. The algorithm for explicit time marching is relatively simple whereas the implicit scheme requires relatively complex matrix solvers. Once discretization schemes have been selected and all terms of the Navier–Stokes equations have been discretized, the system of governing equations can be solved to numerically obtain the flow fields in the geometry of interest.

The earlier description of the various steps involved in the setting up of a computational fluid dynamic simulation is intended to provide an overview of the efforts involved in developing algorithms for such simulations. The field of computational fluid dynamics is vast and relatively mature with numerous commercial codes available for users to perform increasingly sophisticated simulations for biological flows. Numerous textbooks and monographs are available in the literature on the techniques employed in computational fluid dynamics (e.g., Anderson, 1995). Interested students may consult such publications or enroll in courses on computational fluid dynamics in order to pursue a career in biological flow simulation applications.

11.2.5 Poiseuille Flow Simulation, Validation, and Mesh Independence

We will consider an example of setting up a simulation for steady laminar flow in a circular cylindrical pipe in order to describe the various steps in setting up the simulation, validating the results, and demonstrating that a sufficient density mesh is chosen for the problem in order to yield reasonably accurate results. Use of this particular example enables us to compare the results of our simulation with theoretical results for Poiseuille flow derived in Section 1.5.3.2.

The 2D geometry of the cylindrical pipe in the diametrical plane with a diameter of 0.5 cm and an axial length of 4.0 cm is shown in Figure 11.5. The simulation is started with a coarse mesh with five evenly spaced nodes along the radial direction

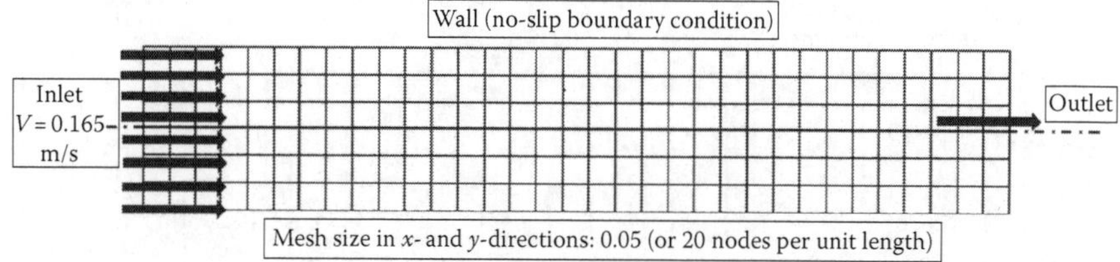

FIGURE 11.5 The simulated geometry with boundary conditions for Poiseuille flow simulation.

and 80 nodes along the axial direction. The no-slip boundary condition ($u|_{r=a} = 0$) is specified for the nodes on the wall surfaces of the pipe. A uniform inlet velocity of 0.165 m/s is specified with the pressure at the outlet boundary set to be zero. The density and viscosity coefficient for blood as a Newtonian fluid were specified as 1060 kg/m^3 and 0.0035 Pa s, respectively, as representative of the properties of whole blood. The computed Reynolds number for the flow (based on the inlet diameter and velocity) is 500 and hence laminar flow simulation is employed with a convergence limit specified as $1 \times e^{-5}$ in the computational software (ANSYS {FLUENT} version 12.1.4—Canonsburg, PA) employed for the simulation. For the coarse mesh (5 × 80) employed in this initial simulation, the solution converged after 35 iterations. In order to show the effect of grid size on the results, the simulation was repeated with three additional mesh densities: fine (10 × 160), finer (20 × 320), and finest (40 × 640). The number of iterations needed for convergence dramatically increased with the finer mesh densities as shown in Figure 11.6. Note the particularly large increase in the number of iterations between the finer and the finest mesh densities. As the mesh becomes finer, the computational time and memory requirements will dramatically increase especially if the flow regime for the simulation is complex requiring millions of nodes like in the simulations typically performed in biological fluid dynamic analyses.

The velocity profiles at various cross sections from the simulations employing the finer mesh are shown in Figure 11.7. As can be observed, the velocity profiles

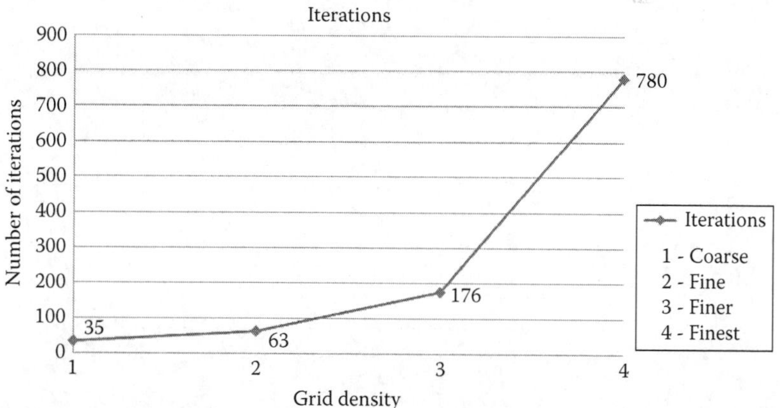

FIGURE 11.6 The number of iterations required for convergence of solution as a function of mesh density.

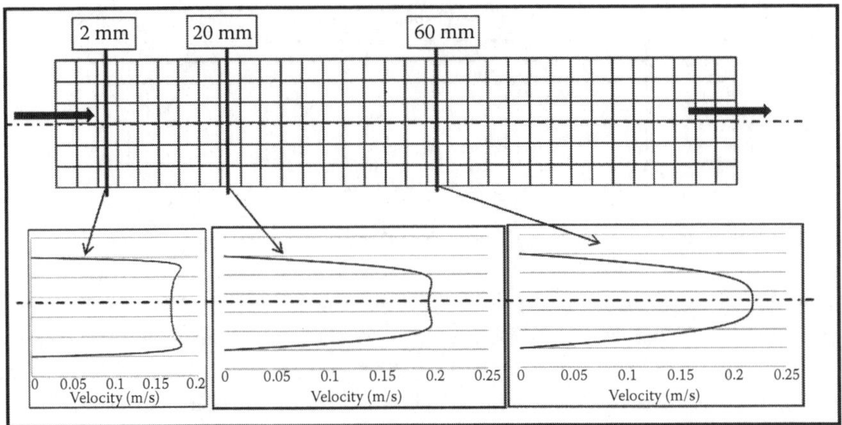

FIGURE 11.7 Velocity profiles at various locations along the axis in the tube.

develop from the uniform entry conditions into a fully developed parabolic velocity profile further into the pipe. A judicious choice of mesh density is needed for such simulations in order to obtain results with reasonable accuracy and an optimal use of computational time and memory. In this simulation, the computational results can be compared with the results from closed form solution. For example, we showed that the wall shear stress (WSS) for the Poiseuille flow can be expressed as

$$\tau_w = \frac{4\mu Q}{\pi R^3} \qquad (1.80)$$

Substituting the magnitudes for the viscosity coefficient, volume flow rate, and the radius of the tube employed in this simulation, the theoretical value for the WSS is computed as 0.0559 Pa. The computational results for the WSS (from the results at the wall in a cross section closer to the outlet where the flow is fully developed) as a function of mesh density are plotted in Figure 11.8. The computed WSS between the

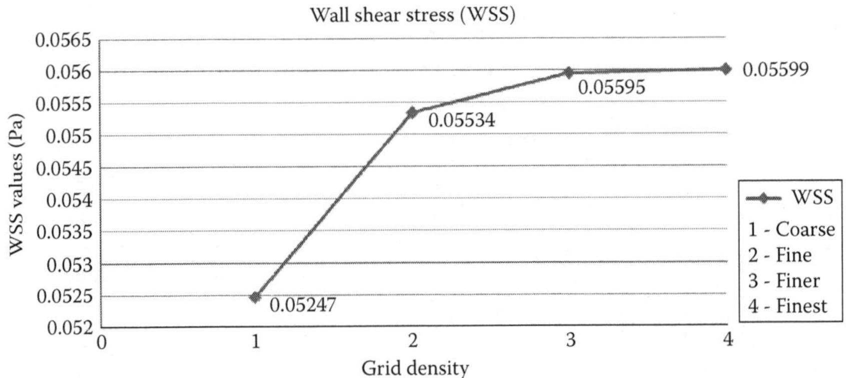

FIGURE 11.8 Computed wall shear stress in the fully developed flow region as a function of grid density. The results can be compared with the results from the closed form solution magnitude of 0.0559 Pa.

simulations with finer and finest mesh is very close and in agreement with the theoretical value. Hence, the computations with the finer mesh are acceptable and the increase in computational time and memory required for the use of the finest mesh is clearly not justified. It should also be noted that when dealing with large number of mesh points, in order to minimize the storage and computational time requirements, any symmetric planes in the flow regime can be identified and taken advantage of. In this particular simulation, the center line of the geometry is also symmetric line and hence same results can be obtained by performing the computations in either the top or bottom half of the geometry and specifying the boundary condition $\partial u/\partial y = 0$ at the line of symmetry. The mirror image of the resulting velocity profile can be plotted on the other half of the geometry and the results should be the same.

In most of the biological simulations, such closed form results are not available for validation. Then the usual practice is to compare prespecified results (e.g., maximum shear stress in a certain region of interest) between two different mesh densities and if the percentage change in results is relatively small (e.g., <5%), further simulations are performed with the lesser density mesh. This process is generally known as the demonstration of mesh independence in the simulations. In addition, since the results from complex simulations cannot be compared with closed form solutions, additional validation of the results of such simulations cannot be overemphasized. In order to gain confidence on the validity of the simulations before the results can be extrapolated and important conclusions are drawn from the same, the results should be critically compared with *in vivo* or *in vitro* experimental data for similar applications or with computational simulations already published in comparable simulation domains.

11.3 MODELING CONSIDERATIONS FOR BIOFLUID MECHANICAL SIMULATIONS

In order to describe the nature of fluid flow in the various organs in the human circulation, the simulation must be as realistic as possible. Requirements for realistic simulations include (1) morphologically realistic time-dependent 3D geometry of the region of the interest, (2) appropriate discretization of the region for accurate computations, (3) appropriate boundary conditions specification, (4) rheological property specifications for the human blood and biological soft tissue (in cases where the interaction between blood and the soft tissue such as the arterial wall is included for modeling considerations), and (5) interpretation and presentation of results. Depending up on the specific questions to be answered from the results of the simulation, some assumptions are also usually made in order to simplify the problem at hand and the assumptions invoked in the simulations also need thorough consideration. In this section, we will discuss several of the issues that are normally encountered in the simulation of fluid mechanics in the human circulation.

11.3.1 Geometry of the Region of Interest

With the interest spurred by several publications on the potential relationship between WSS and the atherosclerotic lesion formation in the late 1960s onward

(Fry, 1968; Caro et al., 1971), researchers concentrated on describing the flow field (such as the velocity profiles and WSS distribution) in specified sites such as regions of curvature and bifurcation in the arterial system. As described in Section 3.10, atherosclerotic lesions in the human arterial system are found in specific sites such as in the aortic arch, coronary vessels, carotid arterial bifurcation, ileofemoral arterial bifurcation, and the renal arterial branching sites. Hence, modeling and experimental measurements of fluid dynamics are of interest at these sites in order to determine a possible relationship between fluid-induced stresses and etiology of atheroma. In the 1970s, due to the limitation in the computational power and lack of commercially available CFD codes, most studies were restricted to simplified geometries. For example, flow development in the human aortic arch (a site of significant curvature in the vessel) was modeled as a mildly curved tube of circular cross section with a vessel radius-to-radius of curvature ratio of about 0.1 (Chandran et al., 1974) compared with the actual magnitude of about 0.42 (Yearwood and Chandran, 1980). Examples of simplified 2D and 3D models can be found in other works as well. For example, Perktold and Hilbert (1986) employed a 2D model of the carotid artery bifurcation with the dimensions averaged from human carotid artery bifurcation angiographic images (Ku and Giddens, 1983). These modeling studies paralleled experimental studies with simplified geometries of curved or bifurcating vessels using flow visualization and/or velocity measurements to describe the local fluid dynamics. With increase in computational power and memory, 3D models were introduced and the solution for pulsatile flows was included in the simulations. Examples include analysis of fluid dynamics in the carotid arterial bifurcation (Perktold and Rappitsch, 1995), coronary arteries (Chandran et al., 2006), and ileofemoral bifurcations (Taylor et al., 1998).

In the latter half of the twentieth century, several new imaging modalities were introduced for diagnosis of problems in the human circulation which include 2D/3D ultrasound (echocardiography, trans-esophageal echocardiography (TEE), and intravascular ultrasound), multidetector computed tomography (MDCT), and MRI. Several of these imaging modalities are noninvasive or minimally invasive (i.e., require the introduction of contrast agent for image enhancement) and afford information about the anatomy of the organs of interest. Advances in image storage, segmentation, and reconstruction of morphologically realistic geometries have also resulted in the availability of the geometric information necessary for more realistic simulations. Details of the physics of the imaging modalities and examples of acquired images are included in Thedens (2011), and the various techniques employed for processing of the images and segmentation are included in Wahle et al. (2011). An example of the geometry of the mitral valve reconstructed from TEE imaging is shown in Figure 11.9 with the leaflets in the open position. The chordae tendineae attached to the free edges of the leaflets on one end and to the tip of the papillary muscles at the other end are also represented in the figure. The geometrical data is usually imported into the preprocessors of the commercial software employed for the solution and the computational mesh is generated. Additional examples of arterial segment reconstructions from imaged data are also included in the following sections.

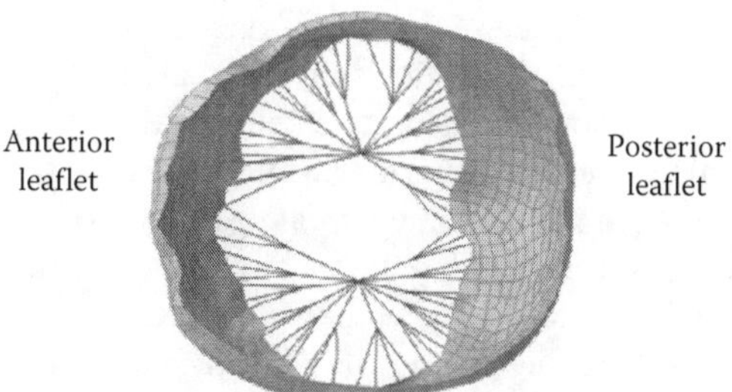

FIGURE 11.9 Typical geometrical reconstructions of a mitral valve obtained from transesophageal ultrasound images. (Courtesy of Dr. Hynggun Kim, Department of Internal Medicine, University of Texas Health Science Center at Houston, TX.)

11.3.2 Simulation of Blood Rheology

In Section 1.2.2, we discussed the constitutive relationship and presented the shear stress versus rate of shear relationship for a Newtonian fluid and for non-Newtonian fluids (power law, Bingham plastic, and Casson fluids). In Section 4.1.3, we reviewed the studies pertaining to the rheological behavior of plasma and whole human blood and concluded that, in general, whole human blood follows the Casson fluid constitutive relationship. However, we also showed that for rates of shear larger than 50–100 s^{-1}, the apparent viscosity for blood asymptotically reaches a constant magnitude around 3.5 cP. In modeling blood flow in arterial vessels such as the coronary, carotid, and femoral arteries or in flow past implants such as heart valves, vascular grafts, and stents in these arteries, it is generally accepted that the rates of shear encountered during most of the cardiac cycle will be higher than 50–100 s^{-1}. Hence, employing a Newtonian fluid for *in vitro* experiments or the use of a fluid specification with a constant viscosity coefficient representing the whole human blood (3.0–4.0 cP) in computational simulations is a commonly accepted practice (Ramaswamy et al., 2004, 2006; Krishnan et al., 2006; Fu et al., 2010). Since the hemodynamic theories discussed in Section 6.4 have suggested a strong relationship between WSS and atherogenesis, our interests lie in the determination of the shear stress magnitudes as well as spatial and temporal variation of the same that endothelial cells are being subjected to in the arterial sites of interest. Similarly, in relating the fluid dynamics with intimal hyperplasia formation with stent implants or in the analysis of thrombus deposition in prosthetic heart valves, once again the flow fields near the implant structures are of importance since wall shear is relatively low. Hence, a number of other studies have questioned the validity of employing a Newtonian fluid description for such simulations and have incorporated a non-Newtonian constitutive relationship in the simulations. In Section 4.1.4, we have employed the constitutive relationships for the power law, Bingham plastic, and Casson fluid and have analyzed the changes in the WSS magnitude with each of the models in a fully developed steady flow of a straight rigid tube of circular cross section. The results shown in Table 4.3 showed a maximum difference of about 12% in WSS magnitude between the Newtonian and non-Newtonian fluids in this simple geometry. However, when creating biological flow simulations, other considerations such as complex unsteady flows through 3D geometries need to be taken into account. Hence, it is not surprising to see a range of publications suggesting that the non-Newtonian effect is important while others suggest that these effects are secondary. As shown in the plot of apparent viscosity as a function of shear rate in Figure 4.8, blood is a shear-thinning fluid approaching a constant viscosity coefficient, μ_∞ at larger shear rates. Typical examples of the nonlinear constitutive relationship employed in comparing the results of flow simulation through a cerebral aneurysm can be found in Fisher and Rossman (2009). The relationships employed in that study were

1. A generalized power law incorporating a local shear rate, a consistency index λ, and n given by

$$\mu = \lambda \left|\dot{\gamma}\right|^{n-1} \tag{11.23}$$

The parameters λ and n depend on the limiting Newtonian viscosity coefficient and constants a–d given by

$$\lambda = \mu_\infty + \Delta\mu \exp\left[-\left(1+\left(\frac{|\dot{\gamma}|}{a}\right)\right)\exp\left(\frac{-b}{|\dot{\gamma}|}\right)\right] \tag{11.24a}$$

$$n = n_\infty + \Delta n \exp\left[-\left(1+\left(\frac{|\dot{\gamma}|}{c}\right)\right)\exp\left(\frac{-d}{|\dot{\gamma}|}\right)\right] \tag{11.24b}$$

The constants were specified from Johnston et al. (2004, 2006) as

$$\mu_\infty = 0.0035 \text{ Pa s}; \quad \Delta\mu = 0.025 \text{ Pa s}; \quad a = 50;$$

$$b = 3; \quad c = 50; \quad d = 4; \quad n_\infty = 1; \quad \text{and} \quad \Delta n = 0.45$$

The Casson model employed in this study is given by the relationship

$$\mu = \frac{\mu_\infty^2}{\dot{\gamma}} + \frac{2\mu_\infty N_\infty}{\sqrt{\dot{\gamma}}} + N_\infty^2 \tag{11.25}$$

In this relationship, the model parameters depend on the plasma viscosity μ_p and hematocrit

$$N_\infty = \sqrt{\mu_p(1 - Hct)^{-0.25}}$$

and

$$\mu_\infty = \sqrt{(0.625\ Hct)^3}$$

Typical values employed in this study were (Johnston et al., 2004, 2006)

$$\mu_p = 0.00145 \text{ Pa s}; \quad Hct = 0.4$$

2. The Carreau-Yasuda model (Bird et al., 1987) is given by the relationship

$$\mu = \mu_\infty + (\mu_0 + \mu_\infty)[1 + (\lambda\dot{\gamma})^a]^{(n-1)/a} \tag{11.26}$$

Two sets of parameter values for the previous equation were specified from previous publications (Cho and Kensey, 1991; Chen and Lu, 2004). For example, the parameter values from Cho and Kensey (1991) were μ_∞ = 0.00345 Pa s; μ_0 = 0.056 Pa s; λ = 1.902 s; a = 1.25; and n = 0.22. Generally, values for such parameters are obtained by curve fitting of experimental data. Figure 11.10 shows the resulting streamlines within a saccular aneurysm with the various rheological models for the blood employed in the simulation. Subtle changes in the flow patterns near the wall of the aneurysm can be observed with the various rheological models. After a detailed comparison of the flow dynamic analysis in various aneurysm models, the authors concluded that the non-Newtonian behavior of blood was found to have a more significant effect within aneurysms than in the parent vessel, and that the effect was more important during the diastolic phase of the cardiac cycle rather than during the systolic phase. The authors also concluded that the aneurysm geometry is more important in the assessment of hemodynamic stresses rather than the non-Newtonian behavior in the simulation. Numerous other studies have been reported in the literature on the importance of employing a non-Newtonian relationship for blood. For example, Gijsen et al. (1999) compared the effect of shear-thinning behavior of blood on the flow through a carotid artery bifurcation model and pointed out the importance of including this effect on the flow through large arteries. These studies suggest that alterations in the velocity profiles and WSS can be predicted with changes in the constitutive law specified for the behavior of blood in analyzing flow through arterial segments. In studies where there are significant changes in the morphology of the regions under investigation such as in flow past stenoses, aneurysms, and implant devices, the effect of fluid dynamic alterations due to geometrical changes may become dominant compared with that of the blood flow behavior. Most of the commercial CFD software includes the commonly employed nonlinear rheological models and the use of incorporating the additional complexity will depend on the applications of the results of such simulations.

11.3.3 Inlet, Outlet, and Solid Interface Boundary Conditions

Specification of appropriate and realistic boundary conditions is very important in order to obtain physiologically realistic simulations. Even though desirable, data on *in vivo* inlet velocity profiles in an arterial segment such as the ascending aorta or the carotid artery are not generally available. Hence, the alternative inlet boundary conditions include the inlet pressure or velocity profile based on the known flow rate

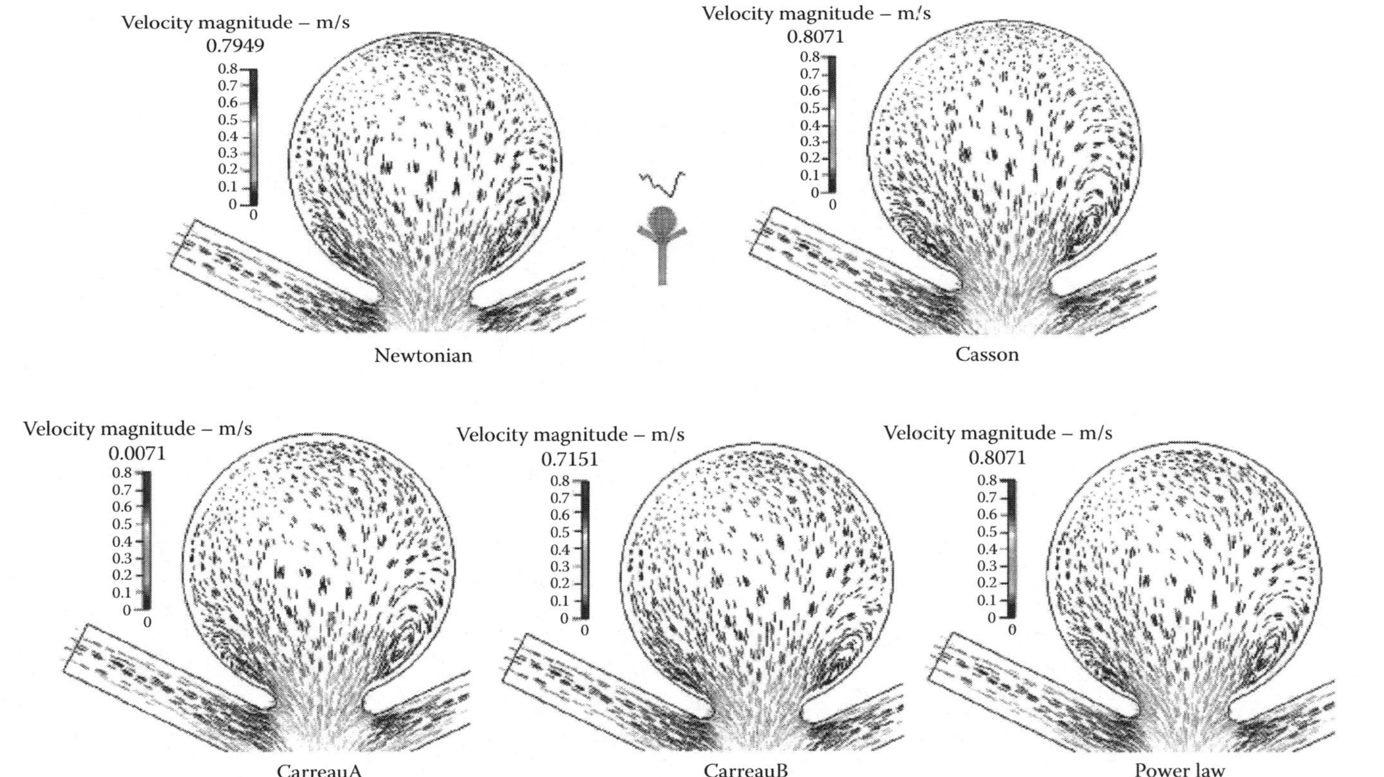

FIGURE 11.10 Comparison of flow dynamics in a cerebral saccular aneurysm geometry with various rheological models for blood employed in the simulation. (Reprinted from Fisher, C. and Rossman, J.N., *Biomech. Eng.*, 131, 091004.1–9, 2009. With permission from ASME Publications.)

through the segment. In the case of arterial simulations, it is a common practice to specify a uniform velocity or a fully developed parabolic velocity profile at the inlet cross section based on the flow rate. In a study on the analysis of flow development past a stenosis in the femoral artery of an animal model, Liu et al. (2004) employed an inlet velocity profile that was derived from discrete Doppler velocity measurements at several points in the inlet cross section. In order to overcome the entrance effects from the uncertainties in the specified inlet velocity profile, they extended the geometry on the upstream side by seven diameters. It is also important to point out that, in most of the studies, the inflow boundary condition only specifies the axial velocity profile and ignores any secondary flow velocity components. For example, in the analysis of flow in the renal arterial branches or in the iliac bifurcation, studies (Frazin et al., 1990; Kilner et al., 1993) have shown that the flow in the descending aorta is helical with a significant secondary flow component. Shipkowitz et al. (2000) have reported that the flow development in the renal arteries and in the iliac bifurcations is significantly altered when the inlet velocity profile includes the secondary velocity components as well. Generally, pressure is specified as the outflow boundary condition and the outflow segment is also extended by several diameters in order to avoid any influence of the downstream boundary condition on the flow development in the segment of interest. When the simulation segment includes branch vessels (such as in the study of the carotid artery bifurcation), either pressure boundary conditions are specified at the outlet of each of the branches or, alternatively, the flow rate split among the branches (Taylor et al., 1998) is specified. In the case of analysis in segments with multiple branches such as in the pulmonary vasculature, the outlet boundary conditions in each of the branch vessels are specified as impedances computed from the structured trees of the distal vessels (Clipp and Steele, 2009). Ideally, realistic simulations will result from specifications of inlet velocity (or pressure) and outlet resistance (or impedance) derived from *in vivo* data when available.

The treatment of the boundary between the fluid and solid is also challenging in biological flow simulations due to the fact that the 3D geometry of the cardiovascular system is usually complex and the boundaries representing the biological soft tissue such as the wall of the arteries are flexible and deform over a cardiac cycle. In the case of steady flow simulations for arterial segments, it is reasonable to assume that the blood vessels are rigid and to apply the no-slip boundary conditions. However, if unsteady flow is being simulated, the blood vessels distend with pulse pressure and the radius increases by an order of 10% during a cardiac cycle. Once again, numerous unsteady simulations have been performed by neglecting the distensibility of the vessel. In analyzing the flow past native human or prosthetic heart valves, relatively large and complex motion of the leaflets can be anticipated in the valve opening and closing phases of the cardiac cycle and cannot be ignored. Several studies have attempted to solve a quasi-steady problem in valvular flow dynamics in which the leaflets are fixed at a time in the cardiac cycle (e.g., in the fully open position) and the steady flow analysis performed with the appropriate blood flow rate across the orifice prescribed as the inflow boundary condition. The flexible boundary of biological soft tissue can be handled in the simulations either as a moving boundary problem or by employing a comprehensive FSI analysis. These methods will be briefly discussed in Section 11.3.6.

11.3.4 Steady and Unsteady Flow Analysis

In performing simulations for any given segment of the cardiovascular system, it is a common practice to initially simulate the steady-state fluid dynamics. The time-averaged or peak forward flow rate is used for the inlet velocity flow boundary condition and the flow development in the segment is analyzed in detail and the results presented on velocity profiles at various cross sections of interest, as well as WSS distribution. Regions of flow separation, relative stasis, and reattachment are of interest especially in flow dynamics distal to the throat of a stenosis. In the flow past heart valves, the flow distal to the leaflets with the leaflets fixed in the fully open position is analyzed in order to study the details of vortex shedding distal to the tip of the leaflets and bulk fluid shear stresses downstream. Steady flow analysis serves a useful purpose in understanding the time-averaged fluid dynamics in the region of interest and identifying specific regions being subjected to WSS extremes and its spatial variations and also regions of flow separation and vortex formation where blood particles may be trapped. In regions where the Womersley parameter, α, is less than or close to unity, the flow can be considered as quasi-steady as well. The steady flow analysis will generally be followed with a pulsatile flow analysis. The time-varying WSS and flow separation regions will be analyzed and correlated with the pathology being studied. The time-varying flow rate will be the basis for the inlet velocity boundary condition and, in addition to the WSS maximum and minimum, its temporal and spatial variations will be of interest in the analysis.

Typical path line plots for a steady flow 2D computational simulation of flow past stenosis geometry are shown in Figure 11.11. A uniform inlet velocity of 0.165 m/s

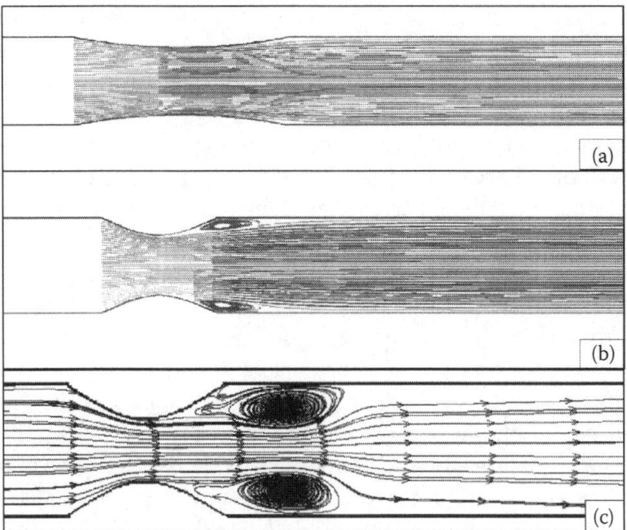

FIGURE 11.11 Plots of path lines in flow past stenoses: (a) 40% occlusion with respect to the area of cross section at the inlet, (b) 60%, and (c) 80%. Note the region of flow separation and recirculation with 60% occlusion and the growth in the recirculation region with increased area of occlusion.

and a Reynolds number of 500 based on the inlet diameter were employed for this simulation. The figure includes the flow behavior with (a) 40%, (b) 60%, and (c) 80% occlusion by area compared with that at the inlet. As can be observed, with the 40% occlusion, no flow separation is evident distal to the stenosis at this flow rate whereas flow separation and recirculation region are clearly visible in the 60% and 80% occlusion cases with the recirculation region becoming larger and the flow reattachment point moving away from the throat of the occlusion with increasing degree of occlusion. Such simulations can be used effectively to model plaque growth in atherosclerosis once the initial lesion forms in an arterial segment, to assess the flow past the stenosis and use the same to characterize the degree of occlusion, and to identify plaques with potential to rupture (see discussions on simulations for arterial stenoses in the following).

Steady flow simulation past arterial aneurysm is shown in Figure 11.12. The inlet velocity for this simulation was also 0.165 m/s with the resulting Reynolds number of 500. As can be seen from the figure, with a bulge in the arterial segment with the radius at the bulge 25% larger than at the inlet, no recirculation region is observed in the aneurysmal region at the flow rate employed in the simulation. However, with corresponding increase in the bulge at 50%, 75%, and 100% radius at the bulge

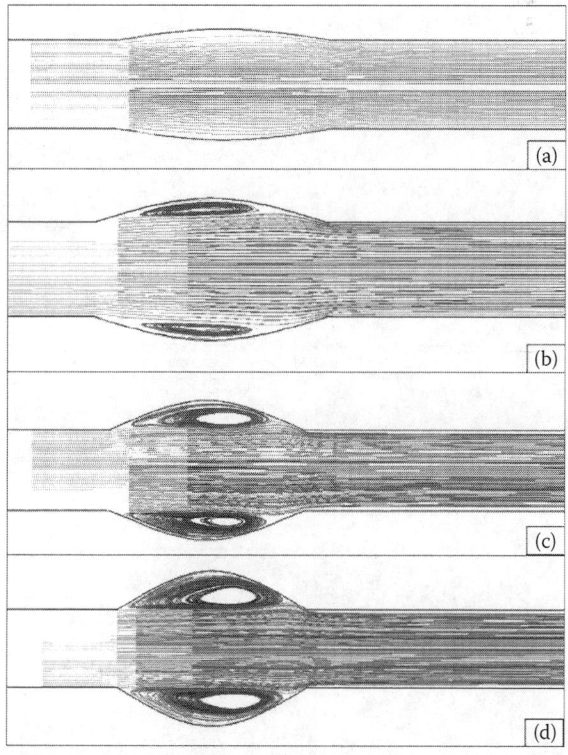

FIGURE 11.12 Path line plots on steady flow simulation past aneurysms with varying degree of radial expansion in the aneurysmal region: (a) 25% increase in diameter at the middle of the aneursym; (b) 50%; (c) 75%; and (d) 100%.

compared with the inlet radius, recirculation region is observed within the enlarged region of the arterial segment. Simulations involving abdominal and cerebral aneurysm geometries have been reported in the literature where the details of the flow dynamics within the bulge is studied in detail in order to relate the effect of pressure and shear stress distribution with intraluminal thrombus deposition in this region as well as to analyze the effect of flow-induced stresses on the potential for the aneurysm to rupture.

Steady flow simulation examples described earlier give us an idea on the nature of flow development past stenosis or aneurysm in the artery and to identify regions of interest such as the flow separation region observed distal to the stenosis for more detailed analysis. However, flow in the human circulation is pulsatile as described in Chapter 6 and hence unsteady simulation is necessary to understand the realistic flow dynamics in such regions. Results of a steady flow simulation past a 60% arterial stenosis is compared with that with an oscillatory flow in Figure 11.13. For the unsteady flow analysis, a uniform inlet velocity profile that is varying sinusoidally in time (Figure 11.13A) is employed. The oscillatory flow simulation is used as a simple example of unsteady flow analysis and as described in Chapter 6, a true pulsatile flow will have a steady average flow component superposed with several harmonics of the oscillatory flow. In the case of unsteady flow simulation, in addition to a

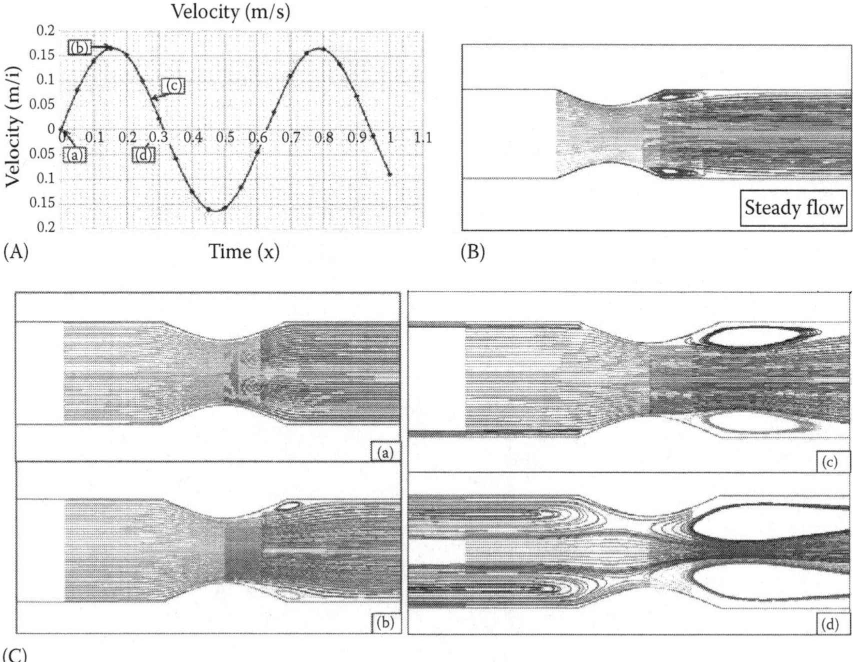

FIGURE 11.13 Comparison of steady flow dynamics past a 60% stenosis with the simulation with oscillatory flow: (A) plot of inlet velocity profile as a function of time; (B) steady flow simulation results; and (C) unsteady flow at times indicated in the inlet velocity plot in panel (A).

judicious choice of the mesh density, the appropriate choice of the time increment, Δt, is also important. In CFD analysis, the Courant-Friedrichs-Lewy (CFL) number defined as

$$C = \frac{u\Delta t}{\Delta x} \leq 1$$

where u is the velocity employed to determine the appropriate time step for a given mesh density. This criterion (Courant et al., 1967) is a necessary but not sufficient condition for convergence and stability in the solution. If a particle is traveling across a grid with size Δx, the aforementioned condition states that the time step Δt chosen must be less than the time taken for the particle to travel across the grid. Thus, as the grid size becomes smaller, smaller time steps need to be employed in the simulation resulting in corresponding increase in computational time and cost.

The results for steady flow with a uniform inlet velocity of 0.165 m/s is shown in Figure 11.13B. The path lines for the unsteady flow analysis at times (*a*), (*b*), (*c*), and (*d*) as indicated in the velocity-time plot at the top of the figure are plotted directly in the following for comparison with the steady flow results. As can be observed, while the steady flow simulation shows a constant flow separation region distal to the stenosis, the unsteady flow simulation depicts the time-varying nature of the flow separation distal to the stenosis. As the flow accelerates past the stenosis, the recirculation region grows and the reattachment point varies with respect to time when an unsteady simulation is employed. Modeling of the time-varying flow dynamics distal to the stenosis is important in increasing our understanding of the nature of plaque growth and potential for plaques to rupture.

11.3.5 2D and 3D Modeling

In the past, with limited computer memory and processing power and lack of adequate CFD code availability, simulations were essentially restricted to 2D or axisymmetric geometries. With advancement in imaging and 3D reconstruction of cardiovascular segments, high-speed computational capabilities, and the availability of sophisticated CFD codes, 3D simulations are becoming more common. Yet, 2D models have their own usefulness. For a beginner in the area of computational simulations, it will be advisable to start with 2D (or axisymmetric) models and become familiar with all aspects of the simulation requirements including the mesh generation, boundary condition specification, running the flow solver, and then interpreting, plotting, and validating the results. In addition, when the flow simulations involve extremely complex geometry, 2D simulations will once again prove useful in identifying regions of interest where the local fluid dynamics provide particularly interesting results for further detailed analysis with the 3D geometry.

11.3.6 FSI Analysis

In order to study the effect of the wall motion on the fluid mechanics within the segment of interest, a moving boundary specification is included if the boundary displacement and velocity magnitudes can be obtained from *in vivo* measurements. In biological flows, the usual moving boundary technique employed is the arbitrary Lagrangian-Eulerian (ALE) approach. In this boundary-conforming method, the computational mesh deforms with the moving boundary. The ALE method has been employed in numerous arterial flow problems (e.g., Taylor et al., 1998) and generally works very well in simulations with relatively uncomplicated geometry and moderate boundary deformation. Application of the ALE method for mechanical valve flow dynamics (Cheng et al., 2004) involves interpolation of mesh between time steps and smoothing of the interpolated mesh (Sotiropoulos et al., 2010). Another class of moving boundary analysis is the nonboundary-conforming methods such as the immersed boundary method. In this method, the fluid computational domain is discretized with a single, fixed grid system (e.g., a fixed Cartesian mesh). The structural domain is discretized with a separate mesh whose nodes comprise a set of Lagrangian points used to track its motion within the fluid domain. The effect of moving boundary on the fluid is accounted for by adding body forces to the governing equations of motion. Various immersed boundary methods applied for biological flows include the diffused interface method (Peskin, 1982), fictitious domain method (de Hart et al., 2003), and the sharp interface method (Borazjani et al., 2008; Vigmostad et al., 2010). Hybrid approaches with a combination of body-fitted and immersed boundary methods have also been reported (Ge and Sotiropoulos, 2007).

A more rigorous approach would be to perform a FSI analysis. In biological flows, FSI analysis requires the specification of the usually nonlinear anisotropic material property of the biological soft tissue such as the arterial wall segment or the tissue valve leaflet. In a partitioned FSI approach, the fluid and solid domains are separated and the interactions between the two domains accounted for at the fluid-solid interface with appropriate boundary conditions. In a loosely coupled approach explicit in time, the domain solutions are obtained sequentially with the boundary conditions for the analysis at a current time step obtained from the solutions from the previous time step. In a strongly coupled approach implicit in time, the boundary conditions are obtained by carrying out a number of sub-iterations at each physical time step and updating the boundary conditions with each sub-iteration. Details of the computational techniques for the moving boundary and FSI problems in the circulatory system and the common problems encountered in the application of FSI analysis for biological flows are included in Sotiropoulos et al. (2010), Vigmostad et al. (2010), and Vigmostad and Udaykumar (2011).

11.4 FLUID DYNAMIC SIMULATIONS IN THE HUMAN CIRCULATION

In Section 3.10, we noted that the atherosclerotic lesions in the human arterial system occur in specific sites such as the coronary arteries, carotid bifurcation, aortic arch, renal arterial branch sites, and in the ileofemoral bifurcation. The common geometrical features in these arterial segments include curvature and bifurcation or branching of the arteries. The fluid dynamics at these sites can be anticipated to be complex with regional and temporal variations in pressure and WSS, as well as in the stresses within the material of the arterial wall structure. In Section 6.4, we reviewed several

TABLE 11.2
Typical Diameter and Inlet Velocity Magnitudes in the Various Arterial Segments of Interest

Arterial Segment	Inlet Diameter (cm)	Uniform Inlet Velocity (cm/s) Peak	Uniform Inlet Velocity (cm/s) Time-Averaged	*Re* Peak	*Re* Time-Averaged	α	τ_p (dyn/cm²) Peak	τ_p (dyn/cm²) Time-Averaged
Ascending aorta[a]	3.00	43.2	10.5	3920	956	22.7	4.03	0.98
Carotid[b]	0.63	75.4	19.3	1439	368	4.76	33.5	8.58
LAD coronary[c]	0.36	9.04	5.01	99	55	2.72	7.03	3.90
Aortoiliac bifurcation[d]	2.20	75.9	16.7	5057	1113	16.6	9.67	2.13

$Re(=\rho VD/\mu)$: Reynolds number based on the inlet diameter and uniform inflow velocity; $\alpha(=R\sqrt{\omega\rho/\mu})$: Womersley parameter; and the computed Poiseuille WSS ($\tau_p = 4\mu Q/\pi R^3$).

[a] Yearwood and Chandran (1980, 1982).
[b] Milner et al. (1998).
[c] Perktold et al. (1998).
[d] Shipkowitz et al. (2000).

hemodynamic theories for atherogenesis relating local WSS and its temporal and spatial gradients with atherogenesis. In that chapter, we also discussed the basic nature of flow development in curved and branching/bifurcating geometries such as regions of high, low, and oscillating WSS and regions of flow stagnation. Hence, it is not surprising that numerous experimental as well as computational studies have been reported on the fluid dynamics in these segments in an attempt to determine a specific relationship between WSS and atherosclerosis. Table 11.2 includes typical magnitudes of the diameter at the entrance and inflow velocity magnitudes employed in the aorta, carotid, and coronary arteries, and descending aortoiliac bifurcation reported in the literature. It should be noted that the magnitudes reported are based on a single study and a range of values have been employed in various publications for the same arterial location. The values chosen in this table is merely to calculate typical Reynolds numbers and Womersley parameters as shown, and these magnitudes are representative of the values to be anticipated in these segments. The Reynolds number and the Womersley parameter in the table are computed based on viscosity coefficient of 0.035 P, density of 1.06 g/cc, and a heart rate of 72 beats/min. The table also provides the computed values of the Poiseuille WSS ($\tau_p = 4\mu Q/\pi R^3$) by assuming a fully developed flow through the arterial segment in order to provide an order of magnitude for the anticipated WSS in these arterial segments. These representative magnitudes may be helpful to students in developing and working on simulations.

In Sections 6.6 and 6.7, we also reviewed typical experimental studies on flow development in arterial segments of interest. A brief description of important anatomical features and representative computational simulations of these including the aortic arch, carotid, and aortoiliac bifurcation, and the coronary arteries are given in the following. Additional simulation studies in these segments of interest can be found in leading journal publications as well as in research monographs.

11.4.1 Human Aorta

The human aorta is the main artery through which blood from the left ventricle flows into the systemic circulation. Distal to the aortic valve, the ascending aorta has three sinuses corresponding to the three aortic valve leaflets and the coronary arteries originate from two of the sinuses. Distal to the sinuses, the aorta has a complex geometry with a major curvature at the aortic arch. Secondary and tertiary curvatures are present as the aorta arches around the esophagus and the left atrium and three major branches arise at the aortic arch feeding blood to the upper extremities. A typical computer-enhanced MR image of the aorta and the reconstructed model are shown in Figure 11.14 (Canstein et al., 2008) and the complex geometry with the major branches at the arch can be appreciated from this figure. The inner curvature of the aortic arch is a common site for the predilection of atherosclerotic lesions (Caro et al., 1971), and, hence, the fluid mechanics in this artery have been extensively studied in order to establish a relationship between WSS and lesion formation (Shahcheraghi et al., 2002). Due to the curved arch segment, secondary flows develop in the aorta as explained in Section 6.6.1, resulting in a helical flow in the ascending aorta. Canstein et al. (2008) have reported on a comparison between *in vivo* velocity profiles measured from magnetic resonance velocity mapping and CFD results in the thoracic aorta in order to assess the accuracy of the simulations. Jin et al. (2003) have also reported on the simulations of helical flow development

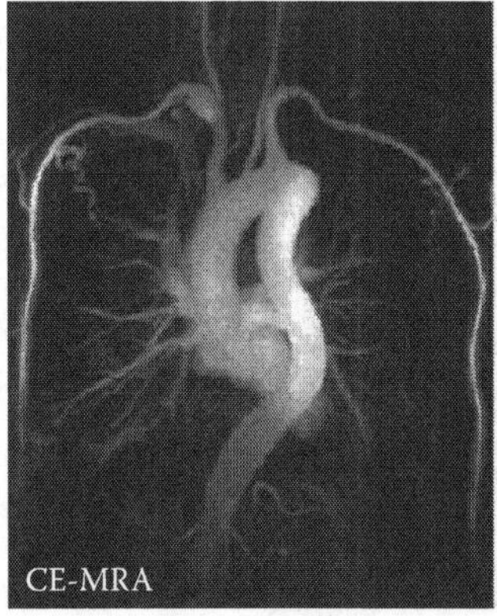

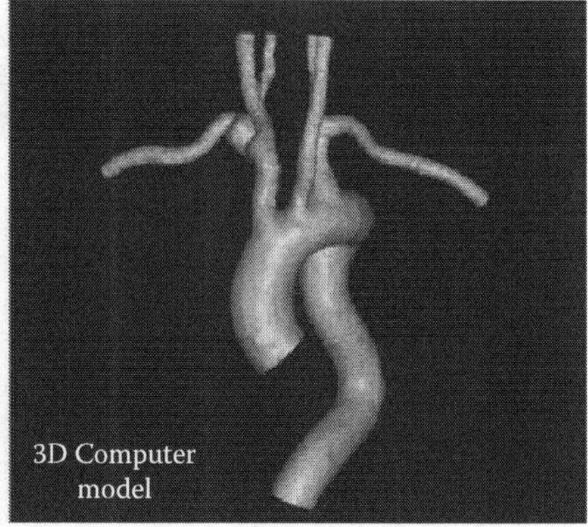

FIGURE 11.14 A computer-enhanced MR image and a segmented and reconstructed model of the human aortic arch with major branch vessels at the aortic arch. (Canstein, C. et al.: 3D MR flow analysis in realistic rapid-prototyping model systems of the thoracic aorta: Comparison with in vivo data and computational fluid dynamics in identical vessel geometries. *Magn. Reson. Med.* 2008. 59. 535–546. Copyright Wiley-VCH Verlag GmbH & Co. KGaA. Reprinted with permission.)

in the ascending aorta. It has also been demonstrated that such helical flow persists even in the descending thoracic aorta (Frazin et al., 1990). It should be pointed out that for the demonstration of complex 3D helical flow in the region of interest, a detailed unsteady 3D simulation is required and such complexities cannot be delineated with 2D models. Experimental and computational studies have shown that relatively low WSS values are found along the inner wall of curvature of the aortic arch. Moreover, during the diastolic phase, flow reversal along the inner wall has also been demonstrated and hence this region is also subjected to oscillating WSS during a cardiac cycle (Chandran, 1993). Due to the large size of the aortic vessel, presence of atherosclerosis in these segments may not result in clinical symptoms in patients since the relative obstruction would be small. Furthermore, it can be anticipated that patients with lesions in the aorta may also be prone to have such lesions in the coronary and carotid arterial segments where the presence of the lesions may be more critical. Even so, the detailed studies on the fluid mechanics in the aortic arch with complex curved geometry with branches may be of advantage in establishing a definitive relationship between the WSS distribution and atherogenesis. Furthermore, detailed computational studies in the aorta can also be very useful in understanding the relationship between the flow-induced stresses and other pathologies in the aorta such as aneurysms (Bogren et al., 1995).

11.4.2 Carotid Arterial Bifurcation

The common carotid arteries bifurcate into internal and external carotid arteries in the neck region providing blood supply to the brain and the facial and skull regions, respectively. The carotid sinus is located at the site of bifurcation for the internal carotid artery, and this bifurcation site is a common site for atherosclerotic plaque formation. Both the fluid mechanics at this bifurcation site, including those within the arterial bulge at the carotid sinus as well as anatomical variations of the bifurcation, have been implicated in the plaque formation (Schulz and Rothwell, 2001). A typical geometry of the carotid artery bifurcation reconstructed from MR images is shown in Figure 11.15 where the carotid sinus bulge is clearly visible at the internal carotid arterial bifurcation site. Geometric reconstructions obtained from MR imaging have been employed in numerous simulations (Milner et al., 1998; Steinman et al., 2002). A typical path line plot during the peak forward flow phase of a pulsatile flow cycle in the bifurcation is shown in Figure 11.16. Results from such simulations indicate a correspondence between vessel wall thickening and low and oscillating WSS in the carotid bulb region (Steinman et al., 2002).

11.4.3 Aortoiliac Bifurcation

Distal to the renal arterial branching sites, the descending aorta bifurcates into the iliac arteries and, subsequently, into the femoral arteries. Atherosclerotic plaques are commonly observed in this region resulting in peripheral arterial disease that endangers the lower limbs. Hence, it is not surprising that the fluid mechanics in this region have been studied in detail as well (Long et al., 2000; Shipkowitz et al., 2000). Typical computed WSS contours in the iliac bifurcation during the acceleration,

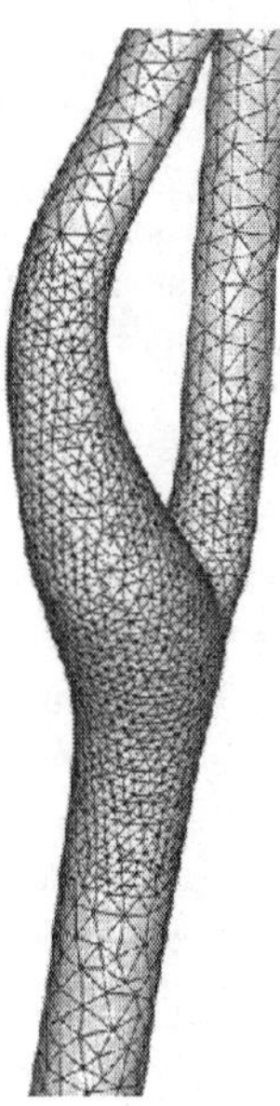

FIGURE 11.15 A typical reconstructed geometry obtained from MR images with FE mesh for CFD analysis of the carotid artery bifurcation. (Reprinted from *J. Vasc. Surg.*, 27, Milner, J.S. et al., Hemodynamics of human carotid artery bifurcations: Computational studies with models reconstructed from magnetic resonance imaging of normal subjects, 143–156, Copyright (1998), with permission from Elsevier.)

deceleration, and reversed flow phases in a geometry reconstructed from MR images are shown in Figure 11.17 (Long et al., 2000). Relatively higher WSS in the flow divider region and distinct differences in the WSS magnitudes in the two branches can be noted from these results.

A study by Shipkowitz et al. (2000) in a simulated geometry of the renal arterial branches together with the iliac bifurcation in the descending aorta also highlighted the importance of the appropriate inlet flow boundary conditions for realistic flow simulations. Frazin et al. (1990) have demonstrated that the helical flow in the aorta persists even in the descending aortic segments. The study by Shipkowitz et al. (2000) compared computations employing a uniform entry flow at the inlet and an inlet boundary condition including secondary flow components. Important differences in the WSS distribution in the flow divider and the outer wall regions were observed between the two boundary condition specifications.

11.4.4 Coronary Arteries

As discussed in Section 3.5, the left and right coronary arteries arise out of the aortic sinuses and are embedded on the epicardial surface of the left and right ventricles, respectively. The main coronary arteries bifurcate into various branches in covering the ventricular surfaces. The curved and branching sites of the coronary vessels are also sites for atherosclerotic plaques and coronary artery disease. Plaques at

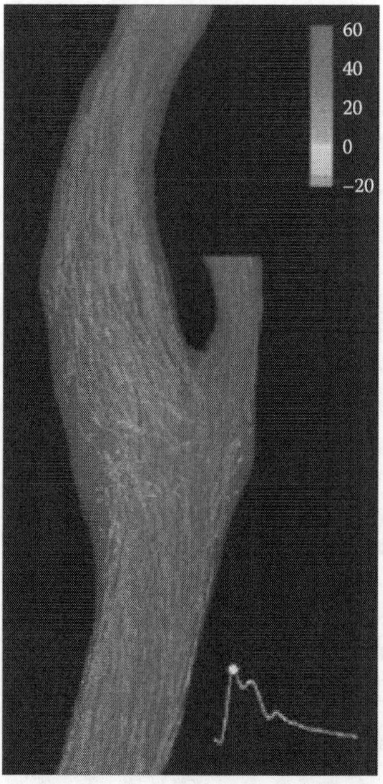

FIGURE 11.16 CFD path line visualization in the carotid bifurcation during the peak forward flow phase. (Steinman, D.A. et al.: Reconstruction of carotid bifurcation hemodynamics and wall thickness using computational fluid dynamics and MRI. *Magn. Reson. Med.* 2002. 47. 149–159. Copyright Wiley-VCH Verlag GmbH & Co. KGaA. Reprinted with permission.)

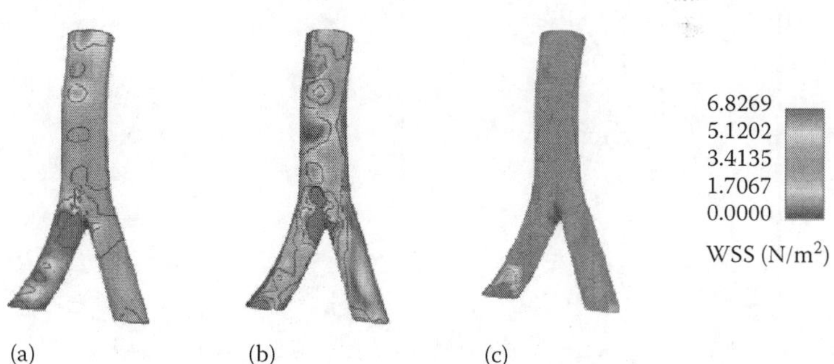

FIGURE 11.17 Computed WSS distribution in the iliac bifurcation segment during (a) acceleration phase; (b) deceleration phase; and (c) the flow reversal phase of a cardiac cycle with the geometry of the segment reconstructed from MR images. (Long, Q. et al.: Numerical study of blood flow in an anatomically realistic aorto–iliac bifurcation generated from MRI data. *Magn. Reson. Med.* 2000. 43. 565–576. Copyright Wiley-VCH Verlag GmbH & Co. KGaA. Reprinted with permission.)

advanced stages occlude the vessels, preventing blood supply to the cardiac muscles and are still the leading cause of death in western countries. Hence, it is not surprising that the fluid mechanics in the coronary arteries and the relationship between the WSS and plaque development have been the subject of numerous investigations. However, since the coronary arteries are embedded on the cardiac muscles and move during the contraction and relaxation of the heart, these arteries are subject to translational and rotational motion during the cardiac cycle and also alter in length and shape. Pao et al. (1992), Ding and Friedman (2000), and Ramaswamy et al. (2004, 2006) have reported on the quantitative measurement of the arterial motion during a cardiac cycle. A plot of the typical motion of the centerline of the left anterior descending coronary artery during a cardiac cycle is shown in Figure 11.18. The data for this analysis were obtained by the fusion of biplane angiographic and intravascular images from a patient with coronary artery disease (Ramaswamy et al., 2004). Even though simulations have been reported in the coronary arteries with the motion of the artery during a cardiac cycle neglected (Qiu and Tarbell, 2000), several recent studies have investigated the effect of incorporating the arterial motion in experimental studies (Moore et al., 1994; Schilt et al., 1996) and in computational simulations (Santamarina et al., 1998; Zeng et al., 2003; Ramaswamy et al., 2004, 2006). Several of these studies indicate significant alterations in the flow development in the coronary arterial segment when the arterial motion was included in the

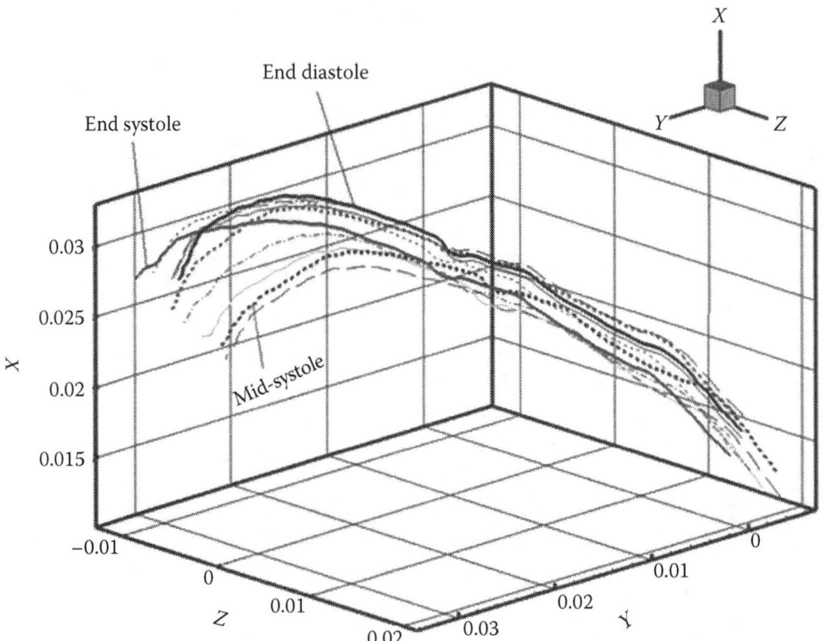

FIGURE 11.18 Measured arterial motion of a segment of the left anterior descending coronary artery during a cardiac cycle. (Reprinted with kind permission from Springer Science+Business Media: *Ann. Biomed. Eng.*, Fluid dynamic analysis in a human left anterior descending coronary artery with arterial motion, 32, 2004, 1628–1641, Ramaswamy, S.D. et al.)

analysis (Santamarina et al., 1998; Ramaswamy et al., 2004, 2006) whereas other studies claim that the effect of arterial motion on the flow development is not important (Zeng et al., 2003).

Several important points can be drawn from the simulations relating fluid mechanical stresses and the initiation and development of atherosclerosis. Both experimental and computational studies performed to date indicate a stronger correlation between low and oscillating WSS and atherosclerotic plaque development. However, the range of computed low or high WSS varies widely based on the arterial segment studied, local geometric variations, and the specified boundary conditions. In other words, one cannot come to a general conclusion that atherosclerotic plaque development will occur if the time-averaged WSS is below a specific magnitude or specific demarcation of magnitudes of other indices such as the OSI for atherogenesis. Morphologically realistic models of the segments are increasingly being employed in the simulations, and the arterial wall compliance is also being incorporated in models incorporating FSI analysis. It should also be pointed out that in these arterial segments with complex geometries, the stresses within the arterial wall will also be a function of local geometry and the effect of these stresses on the arterial wall components may also play a crucial role in the plaque development. The simulations described earlier only consider the effect of mechanical stresses on the endothelial cells. The process of plaque formation and progression is also dependent on the local mass transport of low-density lipoproteins, monocytes, and other biochemical and mass transport processes. All these factors must be considered for our complete understanding of this complicated disease process.

11.4.5 Arterial Aneurysms (AAA and Cerebral)

In Section 6.7, we discussed aneurysm formation in the arterial system due to the weakened arterial wall. Aneurysms are more often found in the abdominal aorta (AAA), thoracic aorta, or in the cerebral region. Rupture of aneurysms in the aorta often results in mortality and morbidity and, hence, physicians are interested in the identification of aneurysms that have an increased potential to rupture. In the cerebral region, the rupture of an aneurysm will lead to stroke and, once again, physicians are interested in identifying aneurysms that can potentially rupture for effective management of the disease. For the AAA, a number of studies employing stress analysis of the complex geometry of the vessel wall at the site of the aneurysm have suggested that regions of abnormal stress concentrations may be a more important consideration rather than the size of the aneurysm for rupture potential (Raghavan and Vorp, 2011). In addition to the structural analysis of the wall of the aneurysm, fluid mechanical stresses on the walls of the aneurysm have also been extensively studied with CFD analysis. The hydrostatic pressure and the WSS distribution may play an important role in the growth of the aneurysm leading to rupture in both AAA and cerebral aneurysms. Papaharilaou et al. (2007) and Scotti and Finol (2007) compared the stresses on the wall of patient-specific AAA geometry computed with solid structural analysis alone and by including the effect of the nonuniform fluid-induced stress loads on the walls. Their results suggest that the maximum stresses on the aneurysm wall are underestimated by as much

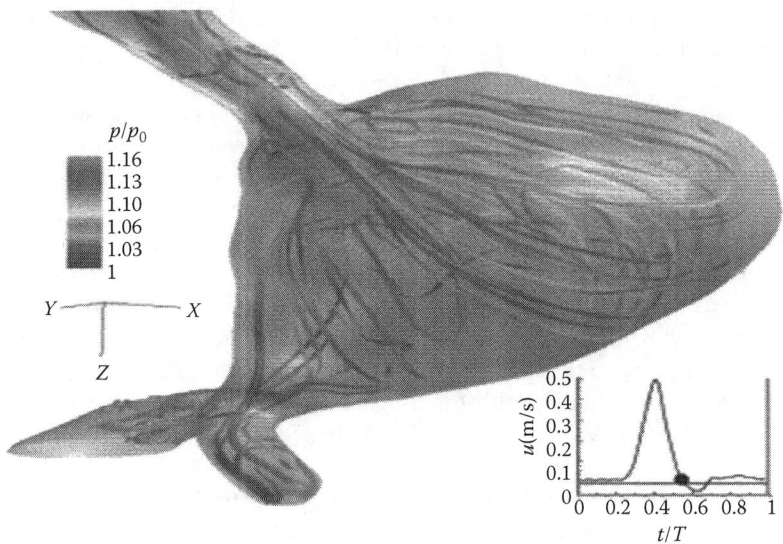

FIGURE 11.19 Stream ribbons of computed flow field in a patient-specific AAA geometry during the deceleration phase of systolic phase. (Reprinted from *J. Biomech.*, 40, Papaharilaou, Y. et al., A decoupled fluid structure approach for estimating wall stress in abdominal aortic aneurysms, 367–377, Copyright (2007), with permission from Elsevier.)

as 25% if the fluid forces are not included. In the case of saccular aneurysms in the cerebral region, the WSS in the aneurysm cavity is suspected of being a major factor in the cavity growth and potential for rupture and, hence, detailed studies on the flow development within the cavity have been the subject of a number of reports (Shojima et al., 2004; Fisher and Rossman, 2009; Torii et al., 2009). Figure 11.19 is an example of the computed flow field in the cavity of an aneurysm during end systolic deceleration flow.

11.4.6 Arterial Stenoses

CFD simulations in arterial sites of interest described previously were aimed toward a specific relationship between fluid-induced stresses and the formation of atherosclerotic lesions. Once a lesion is initiated, growth toward advanced stages of arterial stenosis may take several years. The lesions at advanced stages generally include a calcified cap containing fibrous and lipidous material within the plaque. Unfortunately, clinical symptoms are manifested only at the advanced stages of the disease, either with significant occlusion of the artery preventing adequate blood supply to the distal tissue fields or sudden rupture of the plaque with acute thrombosis completely occluding the arterial site resulting in heart failure in the case of coronary arterial disease or stroke in the case of carotid arterial plaques. In Section 6.7, we also reviewed the fluid dynamics past a stenosis which included accelerated flow at the throat of the occlusion, flow separation, and development of turbulent flow in the distal flow field and spatially varying WSS exist on the surface of the stenosis (Long et al., 2001), particularly when the

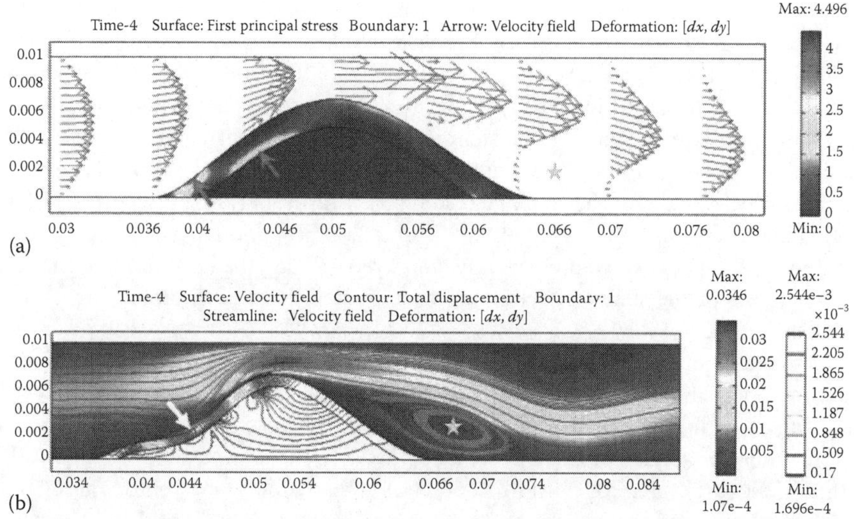

FIGURE 11.20 Computational simulation of pulsatile flow past a stenosed carotid artery occlusion: (a) 70% stenosis—the velocity vectors in the arterial lumen and maximum principal stress distribution within the plaque; arrows indicate regions of stress concentration and (b) 80% stenosis—streamline plots in the lumen and strain contours in the plaque. The arrow indicates the site for maximum plaque deformation and the star indicates the large recirculation zone. (Reprinted from Li, Z.-Y. et al., *Stroke*, 37, 1195, 2006. With permission from Wolters Kluwer Health.)

arterial occlusion covers >50% of the cross-sectional area. Detailed fluid dynamic analysis of flow past stenoses has been of interest in potential identification of flow characteristics that can be used to detect plaque growth during early stages (Cebral et al., 2002), in modeling the fluid dynamical effects on plaque growth (Bluestein et al., 1997), and, particularly, in identifying vulnerable plaques that can potentially rupture (Stroud et al., 2000; Tang et al., 2003; Li et al., 2006; Kock et al., 2008) resulting in acute clinical symptoms. Figure 11.20 shows a plaque stability analysis in flow through a carotid arterial segment with a 70% and 80% stenosis. In addition to showing the velocity vectors and streamlines for flow through the arterial lumen, the plot also includes the computed principal stress and strain distributions within the plaque.

11.4.7 Interventional Treatment and Surgical Planning

There are two forms of treatment for patients with advanced stages of coronary artery occlusion. In the first treatment method, the blood flow to the cardiac muscles is restored by anastomosing a vascular graft from the aorta to the coronary artery distal to the occlusion. As described in Section 9.3, either saphenous vein or internal mammary artery grafts are employed in this bypass surgery. Unfortunately, subsequent loss of patency with vascular grafts is still a major problem. A number of simulations in these bypass grafts have been reported in the literature relating the fluid mechanical factors with eventual intimal hyperplasia formation in the distal anastamosis (Kute and Vorp, 2001). A treatment alternative to bypass grafting is a balloon angioplasty procedure (PTCA) in which a balloon inserted through a catheter to the site of the occlusion is inflated to compress the plaque and re-open the occlusion. Subsequently, a metallic stent is implanted as a scaffold to keep the arterial segment in the open position, reducing the possibility of restenosis. However, a significant percentage of the implanted stents also result in intimal hyperplasia formation and occlusion of the stent at the distal end. CFD simulations of arterial flow with stent implants are also increasingly employed to study the local fluid mechanics at the surface of the stents in detail and have related them to thrombus deposition (LaDisa et al., 2004).

Computational simulations are being suggested as objective assessment tools for planning optimal surgical treatment and it is anticipated that such simulations will find increasing in number of applications in the foreseeable future. One example is the treatment of single ventricle heart defect (SVHD) that is present in 2 per 1000 births (Zclicourt ct al., 2011). In this condition, there is only one ventricular chamber in the heart and, hence, the oxygenated and deoxygenated blood mixes in the single ventricle. Surgical intervention is necessary for the survival of the patient and total cavopulmonary connection is the currently accepted treatment procedure. This surgery is done in three stages as described in detail in Zelicourt et al. (2011). Acquisition of patient-specific imaging, reconstruction of the geometry for image-based simulations, and suggestion of an optimal geometry to surgeons based on the simulations is the process that is currently being used to improve the outcome from such surgical procedures. Numerous other applications are being investigated and it can be anticipated that patient-specific simulations will play a more significant role in surgical planning in the foreseeable future.

11.4.8 Simulation of Valvular Dynamics

The anatomy and the functional characteristics of the native human valves have been described in Chapter 7. The diseases of the human heart valves such as valvular stenosis and regurgitation are commonly treated with surgical repair or with prosthetic valve replacement. The valvular diseases are more often found in the aortic and mitral positions as the valves are subjected to high-pressure conditions compared with that of the valves in the right heart. In addition, congenitally malformed bicuspid valves are also found in the aortic position. The commonly available mechanical and biological tissue valve prostheses that are implanted as replacement of diseased valves along with the complications of thrombus deposition with mechanical valves and loss of durability with bioprostheses were discussed in Chapter 8. Current advancements in catheter-based valve replacements were also discussed in that chapter. The mechanical stresses that the leaflets are subjected to during a cardiac cycle and regions of abnormal stresses have been linked to leaflet calcification and failure. Valvular regurgitation has also been related to structural alterations such as the enlargement of the valve root. Hence, it is not surprising that researchers have been interested in detailed simulations of valve dynamics in order to (1) understand the mechanical factors that induce valvular diseases, (2) make objective decisions on valvular repair techniques, and (3) identify design improvements toward minimizing the problems with prosthetic implants. A complete understanding of the dynamics of the valvular function will also be valuable in the development of tissue-engineered valve replacements.

Dynamic simulations of native heart valves and biological prostheses involve 3D simulation of the complex deformation of the aortic and mitral valve apparatus (including the leaflets, the valve root, chordae, etc.), particularly during the opening and closing phases. A recent review of the current status of the simulations of heart valve dynamics can be found in Chandran (2010). With the tissue leaflet heart valves (both native valves and biological prostheses), the primary interest in the dynamic analysis is on the stresses that the leaflets are being subjected to during a cardiac cycle. One of the common methods for such simulations is to perform a dynamic finite element structural analysis employing appropriate pressure loads on the leaflet surfaces as described in Chandran (2010). In such an analysis, a uniform pressure load is applied on the appropriate leaflet surface and, as such, the analysis ignores the local fluid dynamic effects such as nonuniform pressure distribution and the shear forces exerted by the surrounding fluid on the leaflet surfaces. For a more realistic simulation of the valve dynamics, and also to assess the flow dynamics distal to the valves in the case of diseased or malformed valves, a complete FSI analysis is necessary. FSI analysis for tissue valves is challenging due to the complex deformation of the leaflets and significant changes in the geometry throughout the cardiac cycle. Numerical issues are also present in the fluid flow analysis due to the large deformation of relatively thin and extremely flexible leaflets (Vigmostad et al., 2010). The FSI analysis of tissue valves reported in the literature to date have been restricted to leaflets either with material properties much stiffer than those of biological tissue or with nonphysiological flow Reynolds numbers. Further details of the FSI computational techniques employed for tissue leaflet valve dynamics and the common problems encountered are included in Sotiropoulos et al. (2011) and Vigmostad and Udaykumar (2011). A typical example of a 2D FSI analysis for an aortic valve leaflet with realistic physiological material property specifications during the opening phase of the valve dynamics is described in Vigmostad et al. (2010) as shown in Figure 11.21. The challenges present with a complete 3D simulation of tissue heart valve dynamics is currently being addressed by several research groups and further advances can be anticipated in the near future.

In the case of mechanical valve simulations, the structural components of the valve like the disks and the housing are made entirely of pyrolytic carbon with the housing made of steel alloys in some tilting disc valves. These structures can be considered as rigid and thus, stresses within the disc material are not of interest. However, tendency for thrombus deposition and need for long-term anticoagulant therapy with the mechanical valves are suspected to be due to platelet activation and aggregation due to large shear stresses that these cells are subjected to in the blood flow past the valves. Hence, a number of studies have reported on the detailed fluid mechanics past mechanical valves during the forward and closing flow phases of the cardiac cycle. FSI analysis with mechanical valve dynamics is comparatively simpler because the disc motion can be predicted by

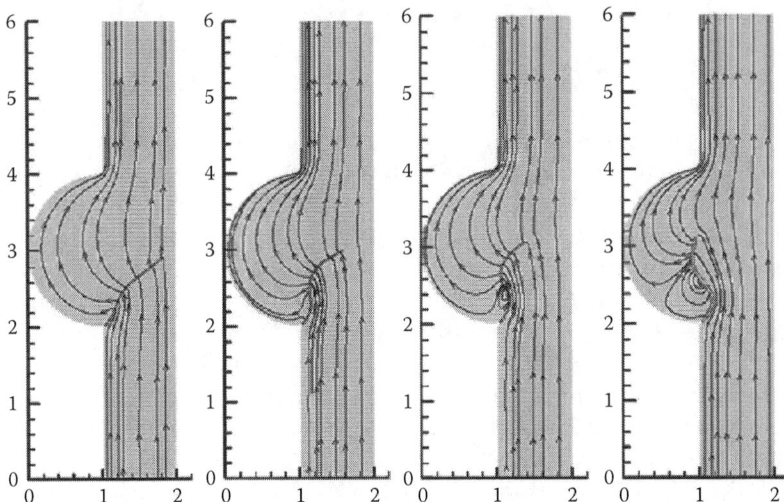

FIGURE 11.21 FSI analysis of a preserved pericardial tissue valve leaflet with experimentally determined material properties. The plots show the leaflet position and flow streamlines during four time points during the opening phase of the valve dynamics. (Vigmostad, S.C. et al.: Fluid–structure interaction methods in biological flows with special emphasis to heart valve dynamics. *Int. J. Numer. Methods Biomed. Eng.* 2010. 26. 435–470. Copyright Wiley-VCH Verlag GmbH & Co. KGaA. Reprinted with permission.)

the governing equation for rotational motion rather than detailed finite element dynamic analysis. However, the geometry of the hinge region in bileaflet valves is where the detailed analysis of the interaction between the rotating disks and the valve housing presents a challenge in the simulations. In addition, the flow analysis requires transitional turbulence modeling, particularly during the deceleration phase. The flow through the hinge region for the bileaflet valves and the clearance region between the disc edge and the valve housing at the instant of valve closure requires dense meshing for highly resolved and accurate results. A number of studies have been reported on the forward flow dynamics past the mechanical valves in the aortic position in order to compute the turbulent and viscous shear stresses downstream from the valves in the ascending aorta and then relating the stress magnitudes to possible platelet activation. Another school of thought is that the fluid mechanics through the narrow hinge and clearance regions at the instant of closure results in flows with abnormally high shear stresses very close to the valve structures which correlate with thrombus deposition on the valve structures. The details of the simulations in mechanical valves to date have also been reviewed by Chandran et al. (2011) and Sotiropoulos et al. (2011). Typical 3D simulation results of flow past a bileaflet valve during the forward flow phase and 2D simulation results of flow through the clearance region of a bileaflet valve at the instant of valve closure are included in Figure 11.22a and b, respectively.

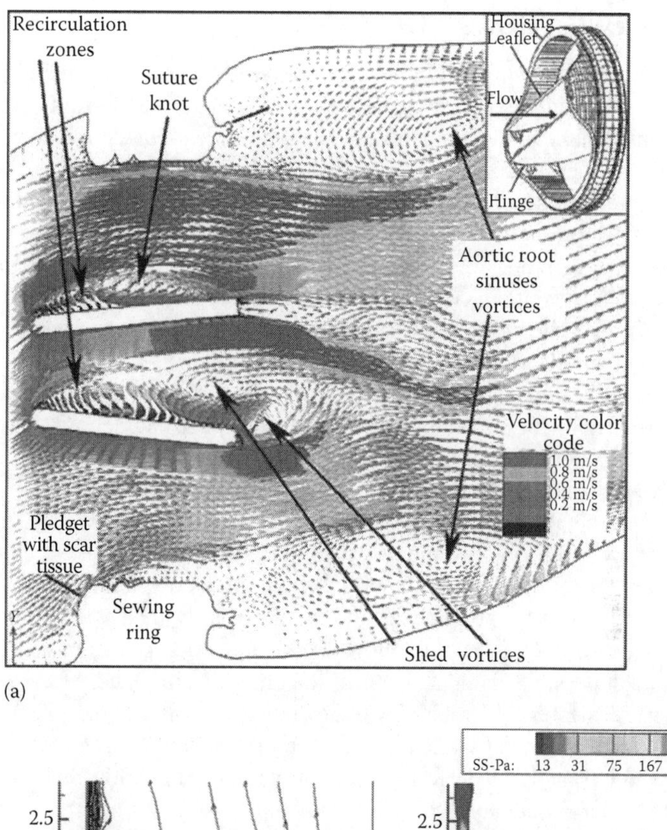

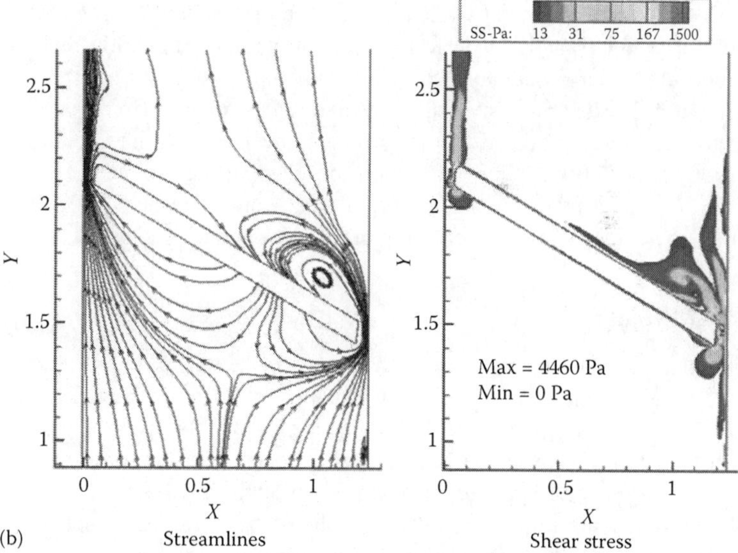

FIGURE 11.22 (a) Computed flow field through a bileaflet mechanical valve during the deceleration period of the forward flow phase and (b) streamline and viscous shear stress distribution plots for flow through the clearance region (right) and the central gap between the leaflets (left) of a bileaflet valve at the instant of closure. (Reprinted with kind permission from Springer Science+Business Media: *Ann. Biomed. Eng.*, Towards non-thrombogenic performance of blood recirculating devices, 38, 2010, 1236–1256, Bluestein, D. et al.)

11.5 FUTURE DIRECTIONS: MULTISCALE MODELING

The physiological processes in the human circulation are a complex interaction of mass, momentum, and energy transport as well as chemical reactions. These processes occur at multiple levels of temporal and spatial scales. For example, an arterial disease such as atherosclerosis can take years to develop and grow to advanced stages when symptoms related to the pathology appears. However, the local transport of low-density lipoproteins across the endothelial cells occurs in nanoseconds. Similarly, in the flow of blood in arteries where the diameter of the vessel can be considered to be relatively large compared with the predominantly red blood cells that have a dimension in the order of several microns, blood can be considered to be a continuum for the dynamic analysis. However, when considering the flow of blood in arterioles and capillaries where the vessel diameter is of the order of the dimensions of cells, the dynamics of the individual cells or the complex interaction of a group of cells must be considered. Similarly, in the determination of fluid dynamics past mechanical valve prostheses, at the organ level where the valve dimensions are of the order of centimeter, the blood can be considered as a continuum. However, when the details of blood flow and formed elements of blood in the hinge region of a bileaflet valve are to be analyzed, the continuum assumption breaks down and the complex interaction of red blood cells and platelets and the flow of plasma should be considered in detail. In the discretization of the flow regime at the organ level in such applications, the smallest possible element size is of the order of 1 mm and the dimension of the smallest mesh size will be relatively large compared with the individual cells. Even with the increasing computational and memory capabilities of modern day computers, it is not feasible to perform direct numerical simulation ranging from the organ level to micro- and nanoscales. Efforts are now being concentrated on the development of detailed analysis at the multiple scales ranging from macro-, meso- and micro- to nanoscales and strategies are being developed to integrate the results from various scales both in time and dimension. Such efforts on the development of multiscale analysis are an important area of advancement in our understanding of the normal physiology as well as etiology of diseases and pathophysiology.

11.6 SUMMARY

Computational simulations have emerged to play an increasingly important role in our understanding of normal physiology, pathophysiology, surgical and interventional treatment planning, and the development of implants in the human circulation. In this chapter, we have introduced the basic concepts of the computational fluid dynamic techniques and application of the simulations in the human circulation. We have discussed the requirements of morphologically realistic geometry of the segment of interest, blood and soft tissue rheology, boundary conditions, and validation of the results before extrapolating these for clinical applications. We have also touched upon the potential future areas of development in the simulations involving multiscale models. Students interested in pursuing applications in CFD simulations can gain valuable experience by initially working on 2D simulations in simplified geometries and some typical assignments are given in the following.

11.7 CFD SIMULATION ASSIGNMENTS

These exercises are based on the ability of the student to build meshes for simple geometries using the preprocessors of the CFD program available at your institution. Run the CFD analysis, and use software such as Tech Plot to plot and interpret the results.

1. Axisymmetric rigid pipe computational model with symmetry assumption. Assume 0.3 cm radius and 90 cm in length with uniform entry flow with a velocity of 20 cm/s. Assume a viscosity coefficient representative of (a) water—0.01 Pa and (b) whole blood—0.035 Pa.

   Determine the entry length before the flow becomes fully developed and compare the same with the entry length computed using the empirical equation for entry length presented in Chapter 1. Express your results as percentage error in comparison with the results from the equation. Double the mesh density in your model, repeat the analysis, and determine the reduction in error with increasing mesh density in your computations.

   You will notice that, in general, in the computational studies presented in the literature, there will be a paragraph on mesh independence study. Repeat the analysis with two or three different mesh densities (varying from coarse to very fine) and decide on an appropriate mesh density based on considerations on accuracy of results and the cost and time associated with computations.
2. Modify the axisymmetric model described earlier by choosing the appropriate dimensions reported in the literature representing a relatively straight segment without any branches of (a) an aorta, (b) left coronary artery, (c) a common carotid artery, and (d) descending thoracic aorta. Choose values for the flow rate into the segment reported in the literature and specify appropriate magnitude for uniform entry flow for a steady flow simulation. Plot the cross-sectional velocity profiles at various intervals moving toward the outflow cross section. Compute and plot the WSS as a function of axial distance in the artery. Compare your results with WSS magnitudes published in the literature.
3. Repeat the previous exercise employing a Poiseuille flow parabolic velocity profile at the inlet with appropriate maximum velocity at the center with the same flow rates employed in the previous exercise. Plot the velocity profiles and the WSS distribution as done earlier and discuss any significant alterations in results between the two input velocity conditions.
4. Construct 2D models of symmetric arterial stenosis with the cross-sectional area occlusion ranging from 20% to 80%. Assuming a time-averaged flow rate through the stenosis, compute the flow dynamics and plot the results as a function of area of occlusion for (a) the peak WSS in the vicinity of the plaque; (b) the reattachment point distal to the occlusion; and (c) maximum velocity at the throat of the stenosis. Repeat the exercise with asymmetric stenosis models and compare the results between symmetric and asymmetric stenosis geometries on the flow parameters (a)–(c).

5. Repeat the previous exercise for simulated aneurysms with the maximum diameter of the aneurysm ranging from 1.5 to 3.0 times the diameter at the inlet of the model.
6. Construct a 2D model representing the aortoiliac bifurcation with representative dimensions of the parent and daughter vessels and typical bifurcation angle reported in the literature. Employing typical flow rates at the inlet, study the fluid dynamics at the bifurcation site for uniform and parabolic inlet velocity profiles. Plot the velocity profiles in the daughter vessels and also the shear stress distribution on the flow divider and outer walls of the daughter vessels.
7. Perform the previous exercises with oscillatory flow inflow conditions and compare the results with those for corresponding steady flow analysis.
8. Perform the previous exercises with physiological pulsatile flow inflow conditions and compare the results with those for corresponding steady flow analysis.

REFERENCES

Anderson, J. D., Jr. (1995) *Computational Fluid Dynamics: The Basics with Applications*, McGraw-Hill, New York.

Bird, R. B., Armstrong, R. C., and Hassager, O. (1987) *Dynamics of Polymer Liquids*, Vol. 1, 2nd edn., Wiley, New York.

Bluestein, D., Chandran, K. B., and Manning, K. B. (2010) Towards non-thrombogenic performance of blood recirculating devices. *Ann. Biomed. Eng*. 38: 1236–1256.

Bluestein, D., Niu, L., Schoephoerster, R. T., and Dewanjee, M. K. (1997) Fluid mechanics of arterial stenosis: Relationship to the development of mural thrombosis. *Ann. Biomed. Eng*. 25: 344–356.

Bogren, H. G., Mohiaddin, R. H., Yang, G. Z., Kilner, P. J., and Firmin, D. N. (1995) Magnetic resonance velocity vector mapping of blood flow in the thoracic aortic aneurysms and grafts. *J. Thorac. Cardiovasc. Surg*. 110: 704–714.

Borazjani, I., Ge, L., and Sotiropoulos, F. (2008) Curvilinear immersed boundary method for simulating fluid-structure interaction with complex 3D rigid bodies. *J. Comput. Phys*. 227: 7587–7620.

Canstein, C., Cachot, P., Faust, A., Stalder, A. F., Bock, J., Frydrychowicz, A., Kuffer, J., Hennig, J., and Markl, M. (2008) 3D MR flow analysis in realistic rapid-prototyping model systems of the thoracic aorta: Comparison with in vivo data and computational fluid dynamics in identical vessel geometries. *Magn. Reson. Med*. 59: 535–546.

Caro, C. G., Fitz-Gerald, J. M., and Schroter, R. C. (1971) Atheroma and arterial wall shear. Observation, correlation, and proposal of a shear-dependent mass transport for mechanism for atherogenesis. *Proc. R. Soc. Lond. B* 177: 109–159.

Cebral, J. R., Yim, P. J., Lohner, R., Soto, O., and Choyke, P. L. (2002) Blood flow modeling in carotid arteries with computational fluid dynamics and MR imaging. *Acad. Radiol*. 9: 1286–1299.

Chandran, K. B. (1993) Flow dynamics in the human aorta. *J. Biomech. Eng*. 115: 611–616.

Chandran, K. B. (2010) Role of computational simulations in the heart valve dynamics and design of vascular prostheses. *Cardiovasc. Eng. Technol*. 1: 18–38.

Chandran, K. B., Swanson, W. M., Ghista, D. H., and Vayo, H. W. (1974) Oscillatory flow of viscous fluid in thin-walled curved elastic tubes. *Ann. Biomed. Eng*. 2: 392–412.

Chandran, K. B., Udaykumar, H. S., and Reinhardt, J. M., eds. (2011) *Image-Based Computational Modeling of the Human Circulatory and Pulmonary Systems: Methods and Applications*, Springer, New York.

Chandran, K. B., Wahle, A., Vigmostad, S., Olszewski, M. E., Rossen, J. D., and Sonka, M. (2006) Coronary arteries: Imaging, reconstruction, and fluid dynamic analysis. *Crit. Rev. Biomed. Eng.* 34: 23–103.

Chen, J. and Lu, X.-Y. (2004) Numerical investigation of the non-Newtonian blood flow in a bifurcation model with a non-planar branch. *J. Biomech.*, 37: 1899–1911.

Cheng, R., Lai, Y. G., and Chandran, K. B. (2004) Three-dimensional fluid-structure interaction simulation of bileaflet mechanical heart valve flow dynamics. *Ann. Biomed. Eng.* 32: 1471–1483.

Cho, Y. I. and Kensey, K. R. (1991) Effects of non-Newtonian viscosity of blood on flows in a diseased arterial vessel. Part 1: Steady flows. *Biorheology* 28: 241–262.

Clipp, R. B. and Steele, B. N. (2009) Impedance boundary conditions for the pulmonary vasculature including the effects of geometry, compliance, and respiration. *IEEE Trans. Biomed. Eng.* 56: 862–870.

Courant, R., Friedrichs, K., and Lewy, H. (1967) On the partial difference equations of mathematical physics. *IBM J.* 11: 215–234.

Ding, Z. and Friedman, M. H. (2000) Dynamics of human coronary arterial motion and its potential role in atherogenesis. *J. Biomech. Eng.* 122: 488–492.

Fisher, C. and Rossmann, J. N. (2009) Effect of non-Newtonian behavior on hemodynamics of cerebral aneurysms. *J. Biomech. Eng.* 131: 091004.1–9.

Frazin, L. J., Lanza, G., Vonesh, M., Khasho, F., Spitzzeri, C., McGee, S., Mehlman, D., Chandran, K. B., Talano, J., and McPherson, D. D. (1990) Functional chiral asymmetry in the descending thoracic aorta. *Circulation* 82: 1985–1994.

Fry, D. L. (1968) Acute vascular endothelial changes associated with increased blood velocity gradients. *Circ. Res.* 22: 165–197.

Fu, W., Gu, Z., Meng, X., and Chu, B. (2010) Numerical simulation of hemodynamics in stented internal carotid aneurysm based on patient-specific model. *J. Biomech.* 43: 1337–1344.

Ge, L. and Sotiropoulos, F. (2007) A numerical method for solving the 3D unsteady incompressible Navier-Stokes equations in curvilinear domains with complex immersed boundaries. *J. Comput. Phys.* 225: 1782–1809.

Gijsen, F. J. H., van de Vosse, F. N., and Janssen, J. D. (1999) The influence of non-Newtonian properties of blood on the flow in large arteries: Steady flow in a carotid bifurcation. *J. Biomech.* 32: 601–608.

de Hart, J., Baaijens, F. P., Peters, G. W., and Schreurs, P. J. (2003) A computational fluid-structure interaction analysis of a fiber-reinforced stentless aortic valve. *J. Biomech.* 36: 103–112.

Jin, S., Oshinski, J., and Giddens, D. P. (2003) Effect of wall motion and compliance on flow patterns in the ascending aorta. *J. Biomech. Eng.* 125: 347–354.

Johnston, B. M., Johnston, P. R., Corney, S., and Kilpatrick, D. (2004) Non-Newtonian blood flow in human coronary arteries: Steady state simulations. *J. Biomech.* 37: 709–720.

Johnston, P. R., Johnston, B. M., Corney, S., and Kilpatrick, D. (2006) Non-Newtonian blood flow in human right coronary arteries: Transient simulations. *J. Biomech.* 39: 1116–1128.

Kilner, P. J., Yang, G. Z., Mohiaddin R. H., Firmin, D. N., and Longmore, D. B. (1993) Helical and retrograde secondary flow patterns in the aortic arch studied by three-directional resonance velocity mapping. *Circulation* 88: 2235–2247.

Kock, S. A., Nygaard, J. V., Eldrup, N., Frund, E-T., Klaerke, A., Paaske, W. P., Falk, E., and Kim, W. Y. (2008) Mechanical stresses in carotid plaques using MRI-based fluid–structure interaction models. *J. Biomech.* 41: 1651–1658.

Krishnan, S., Udaykumar, H. S., Marshall, J. S., and Chandran, K. B. (2006) Dynamic analysis of platelet activation during mechanical valve operation. *Ann. Biomed. Eng.* 34: 1519–1534.

Ku, D. N. and Giddens, D. P. (1983) Pulsatile flow in a model carotid artery bifurcation. *Arteriosclerosis* 3: 31–39.

Kute, S. M. and Vorp, D. A. (2001) The effect of proximal artery flow on the hemodynamics at the distal anastomosis of a vascular bypass graft: Computational study. *J. Biomech. Eng*. 123: 277–283.

LaDisa, J. F., Jr., Olson, L. E., Guler, I., Hettrick, D. A., Audi, S. H., Kersten, J. R., Warltier, D. C., and Pagel, P. S. (2004) Stent design properties and deployment ratio influences indexes of wall shear stress: A three-dimensional computational fluid dynamics investigation within a normal artery. *J. Appl. Physiol*. 97: 424–430.

Li, Z.-Y., Howarth, S. P. S., Tang, T., and Gillard, J. H. (2006) How critical is fibrous cap thickness to carotid plaque stability?: A flow-plaque interaction model. *Stroke* 37: 1195–1199.

Liu, Y., Hamilton, A., Nagaraj, A., Yan, L. L., Liu, K., Lai, Y., McPherson, D. D., and Chandran, K. B. (2004) Alterations in fluid mechanics in porcine femoral arteries with atheroma development. *Ann. Biomed. Eng*. 32: 544–554.

Long, Q., Xu, X. Y., and Griffith, T. M. (2000) Numerical study of blood flow in an anatomically realistic aorto–iliac bifurcation generated from MRI data. *Magn. Reson. Med*. 43: 565–576.

Long, Q., Xu, X. Y., Ramnarine, K. V., and Hoskins, P. (2001) Numerical investigation of physiologically realistic pulsatile flow through arterial stenosis. *J. Biomech*. 34: 1229–1242.

Milner, J. S., Moore, J. A., Rutt, B. K., and Steinman, D. A. (1998) Hemodynamics of human carotid artery bifurcations: Computational studies with models reconstructed from magnetic resonance imaging of normal subjects. *J. Vasc. Surg*. 27: 143–156.

Moore Jr., J. E., Guggenheim, N., Delfino, A., Doroit, P.-A., Dorsaz, P.-A., Rutishauser, W., and Meister, J.-J. (1994) Preliminary analysis of the effects of blood vessel movement on blood flow patterns in the coronary arteries. *J. Biomech. Eng*. 116: 302–306.

Pao, Y. C., Lu, J. T., and Ritman, E. (1992) Bending and twisting of an in vivo coronary artery at a bifurcation. *J. Biomech*. 25: 287–295.

Papaharilaou, Y., Ekaterinaris, J. A., Manousaki, E., and Katsamouris, A. N. (2007) A decoupled fluid structure approach for estimating wall stress in abdominal aortic aneurysms. *J. Biomech*. 40: 367–377.

Perktold, K. and Hilbert, D. (1986) Numerical simulation of pulsatile flow in a carotid artery bifurcation. *J. Biomed. Eng*. 8: 193–199.

Perktold, K. and Rappitsch, G. (1995) Computer simulation of local blood flow and vessel mechanics in a compliant carotid artery bifurcation model. *J. Biomech*. 28: 845–856.

Perktold, K., Hofer, M., Rappitsch, G., Loew, M., Kuban, B. D., and Friedman, M. H. (1998) Validated computation of physiologic flow in a realistic coronary artery branch. *J. Biomech*. 31: 217–228.

Peskin, C. S. (1982) The fluid-dynamics of heart-valves—Experimental, theoretical, and computational methods. *Annu. Rev. Fluid Mech*. 14: 235–259.

Qiu, Y. and Tarbell, J. M. (2000) Numerical simulation of pulsatile flow in a compliant curved tube model of a coronary artery. *J. Biomech. Eng*. 122: 77–85.

Raghavan, M. L. and Vorp, D. A. (2011) Biomechanical modeling of aneurysms. In *Image-based Computational Modeling of the Human Circulatory and Pulmonary Systems*, Chandran, K. B., Udaykumar, H. S., and Reinhardt, J. M., eds., Springer, New York, Chapter 8, pp. 313–341.

Ramaswamy, S. D., Vigmostad, S. C., Wahle, A., Lai, Y.-G., Olszewski, M. E., Braddy, K. C., Brennan, T. M. H., Rossen, J. D., Sonka, M., and Chandran, K. B. (2004) Fluid dynamic analysis in a human left anterior descending coronary artery with arterial motion. *Ann. Biomed. Eng*. 32: 1628–1641.

Ramaswamy, S. D., Vigmostad, S. C., Wahle, A., Lai, Y.-G., Olszewski, M. E., Braddy, K. C., Brennan, T. M. H., Rossen, J. D., Sonka, M., and Chandran, K. B. (2006) Comparison of left anterior descending coronary artery hemodynamics before and after angioplasty. *ASME J. Biomech. Eng*. 128: 40–48.

Santamarina, A., Weydahl, E., Siegel, J. M., and Moore, J. E. (1998) Computational analysis of flow in a curved tube model of the coronary arteries. *Ann. Biomed. Eng.* 26: 944–954.

Schilt, S., Moore Jr., J. E., Delfino, A., and Meister, J.-J. (1996) The effect of time-varying curvature on velocity profiles in a model of the coronary arteries. *J. Biomech.* 29: 469–474.

Schulz, U. G. R. and Rothwell, P. M. (2001) Major variation in carotid bifurcation anatomy: A possible risk factor for plaque development. *Stroke* 32: 2522–2529.

Scotti, C. M. and Finol, E. A. (2007) Compliant biomechanics of abdominal aortic aneurysms: A fluid–structure interaction study. *Comput. Struct.* 85: 1097–1113.

Shahcheraghi, N., Dwyer, H. A., Cheer, A. Y., Barakat, A. I., and Rutanganira, T. (2002) Unsteady and three-dimensional simulation of blood flow in the human aortic arch. *J. Biomech. Eng.* 124: 378–387.

Shipkowitz, T., Rodgers, V. G. J., Frazin, L. J., and Chandran, K. B. (2000) Numerical study on the effect of secondary flow in the human aorta on local shear stresses in the abdominal aorta. *J. Biomech.* 33: 717–728.

Shojima, M., Oshima, M., Takagi, K., Torii, R., Hayakawa, M., Katada, K., Morita, A., and Kirino, T. (2004) Magnitude and role of wall shear stress on cerebral aneurysm: Computational fluid dynamic study of 20 middle cerebral artery aneurysms. *Stroke* 35: 2500–2505.

Sotiropoulos, F., Aidun, C., Borazjani, I., and MacMeccan, R. (2010) Computational techniques for biological fluids. In *Image-based Computational Modeling of the Human Circulatory and Pulmonary Systems*, Chandran, K. B., Udaykumar, H. S., and Reinhardt, J. M., eds., Springer, New York, Chapter 3, pp. 105–155.

Sotiropoulos, F., Aidun, C., Borazjani, I., and MacMeccan, R. (2011) Computational techniques for biological flows: From blood-vessel hemodynamics to blood cells. In *Image-Based Computational Simulations: Applications in the Cardiovascular and Pulmonary Systems*, Chandran, K. B., Udaykumar, H. S., and Reinhardt, J. M., eds., Chapter 4, Springer, New York.

Steinman, D. A., Thomas, J. B., Ladak, H. M., Milner, J. S., Rutt, B. K., and Spence, J. D. (2002) Reconstruction of carotid bifurcation hemodynamics and wall thickness using computational fluid dynamics and MRI. *Magn. Reson. Med.* 47: 149–159.

Stroud, J. S., Berger, S. A., and Saloner, D. (2000) Influence of stenosis morphology on flow through severely stenotic vessels: Implications for plaque rupture. *J. Biomech.* 33: 443–455.

Tang, D., Yang, C., Kobayashi, S., Zheng, J., and Vito, R. P. (2003) Effect of stenosis asymmetry on blood flow and artery compression: A three-dimensional fluid–structure interaction model. *Ann. Biomed. Eng.* 31: 1182–1193.

Taylor, C. A., Hughes, T. J. R., and Zarins, C. K. (1998) Finite element modeling of three-dimensional pulsatile flow in the abdominal aorta: Relevance to atherosclerosis. *Ann. Biomed. Eng.* 26: 975–987.

Thedens, D. (2011) Image acquisition for cardiovascular and pulmonary applications. In *Image-Based Computational Modeling of the Human Circulatory and Pulmonary Systems: Methods and Applications*, Chandran K. B., Udaykumar, H. S., and Reinhardt, J. M., eds., Chapter 1, Springer, New York.

Torii, R., Oshima, M., Kobayashi, T., Takagi, K., and Tezduyar, T. F. (2009) Fluid–structure interaction modeling of blood flow and cerebral aneurysm: Significance of artery and aneurysm shapes. *Comp. Methods Appl. Mech. Eng.* 198: 3613–3621.

Vigmostad, S. C. and Udaykumar, H. S. (2011) Algorithms for fluid–structure interaction. In *Image-Based Computational Simulations: Applications in the Cardiovascular and Pulmonary Systems*, Chandran, K. B., Udaykumar, H. S., and Reinhardt, J. M., eds., Chapter 6, Springer, New York.

Vigmostad, S. C., Udaykumar, H. S., Lu, J., and Chandran, K. B. (2010) Fluid structure interaction methods in biological flows with special emphasis on heart valve dynamics. *Int. J. Numer. Methods Biomed. Eng.* 26: 435–470.

Wahle, A., Zhang, H., Zhao, F., Lee, K., Downe, R. W., Olzewski, M. E., Ukil, S., Tshirren, J., Shikata, H., and Sonka, M. (2011) 3D and 4D cardio-pulmonary image analysis. In *Image-Based Computational Modeling of the Human Circulatory and Pulmonary Systems: Methods and Applications*, Chandran K. B., Udaykumar, H. S., and Reinhardt, J. M., eds., Chapter 2, Springer, New York.

Yearwood, T. L. and Chandran, K. B. (1980) Experimental investigation of steady flow through a model of the human aortic arch. *J. Biomech.* 13: 1075–1088.

Yearwood, T. L. and Chandran, K. B. (1982) Pulsatile flow experiments in a model of the human aortic arch. *J. Biomech.* 15: 683–704.

Zeng, D., Ding, Z., Friedman, M. H., and Ethier, C. R. (2003) Effects of cardiac motion on right coronary artery hemodynamics. *Ann. Biomed. Eng.* 31: 420–429.

de Zelicourt, D. A., Steele, B. N., and Yoganathan, A. P. (2011) Advances in computational simulations for interventional treatments and surgical planning. In *Image-Based Computational Modeling of the Human Circulatory and Pulmonary Systems: Methods and Applications*, Chandran K. B., Udaykumar, H. S., and Reinhardt, J. M., eds., Chapter 9, Springer, New York.

Index

C

D

K

L

M

R

S

T

V

W

Y

Z

Solid mechanics equations:

$$\varepsilon = \frac{\ell - \ell_0}{\ell_0}$$

Strain and stresses for Hookean material:

$$\sigma = E\varepsilon; \quad \tau = G\gamma$$

Poisson's ratio:

$$\nu = -\frac{\varepsilon_{lateral}}{\varepsilon_{axial}}$$

True strain:

$$\varepsilon_t = \ln(1+\varepsilon)$$

Thin-walled elastic tube:

$$\varepsilon_\theta = \frac{\Delta R}{R}; \quad \sigma_\theta = \frac{pR}{t}$$

Thick-walled elastic tube:

$$E = \left\{ \frac{p_1 R_1^2 (1+\nu)(1-2\nu)}{\left(R_2^2 - R_1^2\right)} \frac{r}{u} \right\} + \left\{ \frac{p_1 R_1^2 R_2^2 (1+\nu)}{\left(R_2^2 - R_1^2\right) r^2} \frac{r}{u} \right\}$$

Arterial flow relationships:

Casson's equation for whole blood:

$$\sqrt{\frac{\tau}{\mu_{plasma}}} = 1.53\sqrt{\dot{\gamma}} + 2.0$$

Elastic modulus for arterial wall:

Thin-walled elastic material model:

$$E_\theta = \frac{pR^2}{t\Delta R}$$

Thick-walled elastic material model (Bergel):

$$E_{inc} = \frac{2(1-\nu^2)R_1^2 R_2}{\left(R_2^2 - R_1^2\right)} \frac{\Delta p}{\Delta R_2}$$

Vascular resistance:

$$R = \frac{\Delta p}{Q}$$

Vascular impedance (longitudinal):

$$\left|Z_z\right|_n = \frac{\left|p\right|_n}{\left|Q\right|_n}$$

Arterial wall compliance:

$$C = \frac{\Delta \vee / \vee}{\Delta p}$$

Gorlin equation for effective valve orifice area:

$$A = \frac{Q_{mean}}{C_d} \sqrt{\frac{\rho}{\Delta p}}$$

Pressure wave velocity (Moens–Kortweg relationship):

$$C_0 = \sqrt{\frac{hE}{2R\rho}}$$

Womersley relationship for blood flow:

$$V_z = \frac{AR^2}{i\mu\alpha^2}\left[1 - \frac{J_0(\alpha r' i^{3/2})}{J_0(\alpha i^{3/2})}\right] e^{i\omega t}$$

$$Q = \frac{A\pi R^4 e^{i\omega t}}{i\mu\rho}\left[1 - \frac{2J_1(\alpha i^{3/2})}{i^{3/2}\alpha J_0(\alpha i^{3/2})}\right]$$